Guide to health informatics

Second edition

Enrico Coiera
Professor and Foundation Chair of Medical Informatics,
University of New South Wales, Sydney, Australia

Hodder Arnold
A MEMBER OF THE HODDER HEADLINE GROUP

First published in Great Britain in 2003 by
Hodder Arnold, a member of the Hodder Headline Group,
338 Euston Road, London NW1 3BH

http://www.hoddereducation.com

Distributed in the United States of America by
Oxford University Press Inc.,
198 Madison Avenue, New York, NY10016
Oxford is a registered trademark of Oxford University Press

British Library Cataloguing in Publication Data
A catalogue record for this book is available from the British Library

Library of Congress Cataloging-in-Publication Data
A catalog record for this book is available from the Library of Congress

ISBN-10: 0 340 76425 2
ISBN-13: 978 0 340 76425 1

4 5 6 7 8 9 10

Commissioning Editor: Georgina Bentliff
Development Editor: Heather Smith
Project Editor: Zelah Pengilley
Production Controller: Lindsay Smith
Cover Design: Amina Dudhia

Typeset in 10/13pt Minion by Charon Tec Pvt. Ltd, Chennai, India
Printed and bound in India by Replika Press Pvt. Ltd

Contents

Note xiii
Preface xiv
Preface to the first edition xvi
Acknowledgements xviii
Publishers' acknowledgements xx
Introduction to health informatics xxi

PART 1 BASIC CONCEPTS IN INFORMATICS

1 Models 3

1.1 Models are abstractions of the real world 4
1.2 Models can be used as templates 7
1.3 The way we model the world influences the way we affect the world 9
Conclusions 10
Discussion points 11

2 Information 12

2.1 Information is inferred from data and knowledge 12
2.2 Models are built from symbols 13
2.3 Inferences are drawn when data are interpreted according to a model 14
2.4 Assumptions in a model define the limits to knowledge 16
2.5 Computational models permit the automation of data interpretation 18
Conclusions 20
Discussion points 20

3 Information systems 22

3.1 A system is a set of interacting components 22
3.2 A system has an internal structure that transforms inputs into outputs for a specific purpose 23

3.3 Information systems contain data and models 29
Conclusions 31
Discussion points 31

PART 2 INFORMATICS SKILLS

4 Communicating 35

4.1 The structure of a message determines how it will be understood 36
4.2 The message that is sent may not be the message that is received 37
4.3 Grice's conversational maxims provide a set of rules for conducting message exchanges 41
Conclusions 42
Discussion points 42

5 Structuring 44

5.1 Messages are structured to achieve a specific task using available resources to suit the needs of the receiver 44
5.2 The patient record can have many different structures 49
Conclusions 53
Discussion points 53

6 Questioning 55

6.1 Clinicians have many gaps and inconsistencies in their clinical knowledge 56
6.2 Well-formed questions seek answers that will have a direct impact on clinical care 59
6.3 Questions to computer knowledge sources are structured according to the rules of logic 60
6.4 Well-formed questions are both accurate and specific 62
Conclusions 65
Discussion points 65

7 Searching 66

7.1 Successful searching for knowledge requires well-structured questions to be asked of well-informed agents 66
7.2 Search strategies are optimized to minimize cost and maximize benefit 67
7.3 The set of all possible options forms a search space 68
7.4 Search strategies are designed to find the answer in the fewest possible steps 69
7.5 The answer is evaluated to see if it is well formed, specific, accurate and reliable 77
Conclusions 79
Discussion points 79

8 Making decisions 81

8.1 Problem-solving is reasoning from the facts to create alternatives, and then choosing one alternative 81
8.2 Hypotheses are generated by making inferences from the given data 83
8.3 Decision trees can be used to determine the most likely outcome when there are several alternatives 88
8.4 Heuristic reasoning guides most clinical decisions but is prone to biases and limited by cognitive resources 89
8.5 An individual's preferences for one outcome over another can be represented mathematically as a utility 93
Conclusions 96
Discussion points 97

PART 3 INFORMATION SYSTEMS IN HEALTHCARE

9 Information management systems 101

9.1 Information systems are designed to manage activities 101
9.2 There are three distinct information management loops 103
9.3 Formal and informal information systems 105
Discussion points 109

10 The electronic medical record 111

10.1 The EMR is not a simple replacement of the paper record 112
10.2 The paper-based medical record 113
10.3 The EMR 117
Conclusions 122
Discussion points 123

11 Designing and evaluating information systems 124

11.1 Design and evaluation are linked processes 125
11.2 The formative assessment cycle defines clinical needs 128
11.3 Summative evaluations attempt to determine the measurable impact of a system once it is in routine use 129
11.4 Interaction design focuses on the way people interact with technology 130
11.5 Designing for change 134
11.6 Designing the information management cycle 136
Discussion points 139

PART 4 PROTOCOL-BASED SYSTEMS

12 Protocols and evidence-based healthcare 143

12.1 Protocols 145
12.2 The structure of protocols 148
12.3 Care pathways 150
12.4 The protocol life cycle 151
12.5 Departures from a protocol help drive protocol refinement 152
12.6 The application of protocols 153
Discussion points 154

13 Computer-based protocol systems in healthcare 156

13.1 Passive protocol systems 156
13.2 Active protocol systems 158
13.3 Protocol representations and languages 164
Conclusions 169
Discussion points 169

14 Disseminating and applying protocols 171

14.1 The uptake of clinical guidelines will remain low as long as the costs perceived by clinicians outweigh the benefits 172
14.2 The clinical impact of a guideline is determined both by its efficacy as well as its adoption rate 173
14.3 Strategies for improving the uptake of evidence into practice may alter either actual or perceived costs and benefits 174
14.4 Socio-technical barriers limit the use of evidence in clinical settings 178
Discussion points 178

15 Designing protocols 180

15.1 Protocol construction and maintenance 180
15.2 The design of protocols 183
15.3 Protocol design principles 185
Discussion points 187

PART 5 LANGUAGE, CODING AND CLASSIFICATION

16 Terms, codes and classification 191

16.1 Language establishes a common ground 191
16.2 Common terms are needed to permit assessment of clinical activities 192

16.3 Terms, codes, groups and hierarchies 193
16.4 Compositional terminologies create complicated concepts from simple terms 196
16.5 Using coding systems 197
Discussion points 200

17 Healthcare terminologies and classification systems 201

17.1 The International Classification of Diseases 202
17.2 Diagnosis related groups 205
17.3 Read codes 206
17.4 SNOMED 208
17.5 SNOMED Clinical Terms 210
17.6 The Unified Medical Language System (UMLS) 213
17.7 Comparing coding systems is not easy 215
Discussion points 216

18 The trouble with coding 217

18.1 Universal terminological systems are impossible to build 218
18.2 Building and maintaining terminologies is similar to software engineering 222
18.3 Compositional terminologies may be easier to maintain over time despite higher initial building costs 223
18.4 The way forward 226
Discussion points 228

PART 6 COMMUNICATION SYSTEMS IN HEALTHCARE

19 Communication system basics 231

19.1 The communication space accounts for the bulk of information transactions in healthcare 232
19.2 A communication system includes people, messages, mediating technologies and organizational structures 233
19.3 Shared time or space defines the basic contexts of communication system use 236
19.4 Communication services 239
Conclusions 242
Discussion points 242

20 Communication technology 244

20.1 Machine communication is governed by a set of layered protocols 244
20.2 Communication channels can be dedicated or shared 246

20.3 Wireline communication systems 249
20.4 Wireless communication systems 252
20.5 HL7 defines standards for the electronic exchange of clinical messages 255
20.6 Computer and communication systems are merging 258
Discussion points 259

21 Clinical communication and telemedicine 261

21.1 Telemedicine supports clinical care with communication technologies 261
21.2 The evidence for the effectiveness of telemedicine remains weak 262
21.3 Communication needs in healthcare vary widely 267
21.4 Communication and home healthcare 268
21.5 Communication and primary care 270
21.6 Communication and hospitals 273
21.7 Researching clinical communication 276
Discussion points 281

PART 7 THE INTERNET

22 The Internet and World Wide Web 285

22.1 The Internet has evolved through four stages 286
22.2 The Internet as a technological phenomenon 287
22.3 The Internet as a social phenomenon 288
22.4 The Internet as a commercial phenomenon 289
22.5 The Internet as an enterprise phenomenon 290
22.6 Communication on the Internet 291
22.7 The World Wide Web 294
22.8 Security on the Internet 299
22.9 Future Web advances 300
Discussion points 302

23 Web health services 303

23.1 The Web can support rapid publication and distribution of clinical information resources 304
23.2 The electronic patient record can be built using Web technologies 306
23.3 The dissemination of peer-reviewed scientific knowledge is enhanced through use of the Web 308
23.4 Online systems can support continuing education and decision-making 309
23.5 Patients may access healthcare information on the Web 311
23.6 Notification systems offer a rapid way of communicating with the clinical community 314
23.7 The Internet has given rise to new types of healthcare service 315
Discussion points 317

24 Information economics and the Internet 319

24.1 Information has a value 320
24.2 Consuming information on the Web is associated with search costs 324
Conclusions 327
Discussion points 327

PART 8 DECISION SUPPORT SYSTEMS

25 Clinical decision support systems 331

25.1 AI can support both the creation and the use of clinical knowledge 332
25.2 Reasoning with clinical knowledge 333
25.3 Machine learning systems can create new clinical knowledge 337
25.4 Clinical decision support systems have repeatedly demonstrated their worth when evaluated 338
Conclusions 343
Discussion points 343

26 Intelligent systems 345

26.1 Before reasoning about the world, knowledge must be captured and represented 346
26.2 Rule-based expert systems 348
26.3 Belief networks 349
26.4 Neural networks 350
26.5 Model-based systems 352
26.6 The choice of reasoning and representation methods should be based on the needs of the task 352
26.7 Intelligent decision support systems have their limits 353
Discussion points 354

27 Intelligent monitoring and control 355

27.1 Automated interpretation and control systems can assist in situations with high cognitive loads or varying expertise 355
27.2 Intelligent systems require access to additional data in the EMR before they can perform many complex functions 357
27.3 There are different levels of signal interpretation, each of which requires increasing amounts of clinical knowledge 358
27.4 Intelligent monitoring systems use a variety of methods for interpretation 364
27.5 Use of intelligent monitors can produce new types of error because of automation bias in the user 364
Conclusions 365
Discussion points 366

28 Biosurveillance 367

28.1 Event reporting = detection + recognition + communication 368
28.2 Infectious disease surveillance systems play a key role in bioagent detection 370
28.3 Clinical education alone is unlikely to enhance event detection and recognition 372
28.4 Online evidence retrieval and CDSS can help support education and decision-making 373
28.5 The Web will need to be used in combination with other communication technologies to support biosurveillance 374
Conclusions 377
Discussion points 378

29 Bioinformatics 379

29.1 Genome science is rich in sequence data but poor in functional knowledge 380
29.2 Genome data can allow patient treatments to be highly tailored to the individual 383
29.3 Bioinformatics can answer many questions about the role of genes in human disease, but is limited by our ability to model biological processes 385
29.4 Bioinformatics is made possible by the development of new measurement and analysis technologies 386
Conclusions 395
Discussion points 395

Glossary 397

References 408

Index 433

Note

Preface

As with the first edition, the present edition of this book has been written for healthcare professionals who wish to understand the principles and applications of information and communication systems in healthcare. The text is presented in a way that should make it accessible to anyone, independent of their knowledge of technology. It should be suitable as a textbook for undergraduate and postgraduate training in the clinical aspects of informatics, and as an introductory textbook for those undertaking a postgraduate career in informatics.

It is said that books are never finished, but that they are just abandoned. The first edition was certainly never finished. Informatics is still exploring its shape as a principled science, and at some point it is more important to come to a view of what that shape is, rather than to await perfection. Unlike novelists, however, authors of textbooks are given the rare privilege of retelling their story in new editions, and changing their mind about what needs to be emphasized or how the story should unfold.

In this second edition I have kept the essential backbone of the informatics story the same. We start with foundational chapters that try to explain simply the abstract concepts that are core to informatics and subsequent chapters are built upon those foundations. Every chapter has been updated and many have been almost completely rewritten to reflect the emergence of new ideas and results. Each chapter now ends with a new element – questions intended to test the reader's understanding of the chapter or stimulate discussion of the material. Not all the answers to the questions are easy or obvious, and some are specifically designed to challenge.

A new set of chapters on clinical informatics skills forms Part 2 of this book and represents the major new element in this edition. I remain deeply conscious that practising clinicians need to translate knowledge into action, and in Part 2 I have attempted to identify those clinical activities that are essentially informatic – communicating, structuring information, asking questions, searching for answers, and making decisions. Informatics is as much about doing as it is about the tools we use in the doing, and I hope these new chapters will, once and for all, establish to clinicians why the study of health informatics is the foundation of all other clinical activities. New specialist chapters on biosurveillance and bioinformatics appear at the end of the book, representing areas where there has been a significant surge in research and development activity since the book was first written in 1996.

The change from 'medical' to 'health' informatics in the title does not represent a major change in emphasis of the text, but rather should make clearer to readers that the text is designed to be used by *all* healthcare professionals, including nurses and allied health professionals, and not just medical practitioners. When I use the term 'clinician' in this book I am referring to any healthcare practitioner directly involved in patient care. I have kept the term electronic medical record (EMR) in the text more as a historical convenience than anything else, and the discussion of record-keeping and its principles is intended to be applied across all the health professions.

Finally, it may have seemed a foolhardy mission for a single author to attempt to write a comprehensive text on health informatics in 1997. I can assure you that in 2003 the task was significantly greater, and the sense of foolhardiness ever more present as I struggled to decide what material should come into a core introductory text, what to exclude, and tried to faithfully extract the major results form an ever-expanding literature. When it came to the bioinformatics chapter, which covers what has now become a discipline in its own right, I elected to call in the expert assistance of Zac Kohane rather than carry on unaided. I am indebted to Zac for providing me the material, drawn from his own excellent bioinformatics text, which is now assembled as Chapter 29.

My one guiding hope during this task was that as a single author I could still write with a single voice and keep the story coherent and simple. Most other informatics texts have multiple authors and usually suffer because of it. I hope that the clarity of this text makes up for any limitations in its comprehensiveness. As before, I hope that readers who find elements of the book they disagree with, or would like to see improved, take the time to let me know. I may one day contemplate a third edition!

EC
ewc@pobox.com
http://www.coiera.com
Sydney, Australia
March, 2003

Preface to the first edition

This book has been written for healthcare professionals who wish to understand the principles and applications of information and communication systems within healthcare. It is presented, I hope, in a way that will make it accessible to anyone, independent of their knowledge of technology. It should thus also be suitable as a component of undergraduate and postgraduate training.

It has not always been easy to explain to those outside the field what medical informatics is all about. Its terminology and concepts, and perhaps more than anything its focus on technology, have made it hard to bridge the gap to the concerns of those working day to day in clinical practice.

However, computing technology is now commonplace in healthcare, and the 'communications revolution' is transforming our daily lives through the likes of the Internet and mobile telephony. So now the technology gap does not seem so great. As importantly, clinicians are starting to understand that some of their biggest problems may only yield to the concerted application of information and communication technologies. Evidence-based clinical practice, for example, can only truly be possible within a clinical community that is set up to attack the mounds of clinical evidence, and then share the distillate through a richly woven communications web.

Yet, amidst all this change, it is often unclear what is fundamental and what is just the fleeting detail of ever-changing technology. Thus the very pace of change is both ally and enemy. It is one of the biggest barriers to informatics concepts and skills becoming a natural part of every healthcare worker's knowledge.

It is with this perspective that I have written this book. It is not so much about the details of the different information or communication technologies. Rapid technological change is a given, and it is impossible to track it all in a single text. More importantly, the finer details of different technologies are probably not relevant or even of interest to most healthcare workers. They want to drive the car, not know what goes on under the hood.

The book is also intended as an introductory text for those who wish to undertake a postgraduate career in informatics. For these readers, I have tried to include more advanced material where possible, along with a strong emphasis on basic principles throughout. Given the introductory nature of this book, I have intentionally avoided some more advanced or specialized areas that might properly be considered a part of informatics, such as formal decision analysis. The text also assumes that informatics students will be taught other more technological modules in parallel. Thus, this book intentionally does not explore subjects like statistics, the principles of programming computers, the basics of computer or communications hardware, computer networking, security or database design. There are many excellent texts available in these fields, and an informatics professional will need a solid grounding in these areas. A single text like the present one cannot, and should not, attempt to provide that. Nevertheless, I have included some introductory material on communications technologies and computer networks because this area is so rapidly changing that it may be difficult to obtain an appropriate text.

Finally, I have tried, however imperfectly, to do justice to history. It is a constant source of amazement to me when I read a mid-nineteenth century text like Oesterlen's *Medical Logic* to find a mind with a richer understanding of the nuances of informatics than many of us have today. It is easy to always look to those close to us in time, but we are richer if we can steal the wider view. It is harsh when it reminds us how little has changed, or how little further we have understood. It whispers encouragement too, because things do change and we do move forward. What would someone like Oesterlen have made of the World Wide Web, or of an expert system?

As enthusiastic as I am with the current shape of the book, I am very conscious that it will fall short of the mark in many places. It is my hope that readers will take the time to let me know where I have succeeded, and where I need to improve the text. I would like to see the book evolve over the next few years, to meet the changing needs of healthcare professionals, just as it needs to evolve because of the pace of technological change.

Bath, UK
March, 1997

Acknowledgements

I have been greatly helped, supported and influenced by many people as I wrote this book.

Michael Power and Jeremy Wyatt provided generous and insightful comments that improved the early foundational chapters, and John Fox's comments on the protocol chapters were much appreciated. This book is much better for the detailed comments of Rose Spencer, Pam Logan, and Vitali Sintchenko. Rosemary Roberts reviewed Chapter 17, and very kindly provided the examples in Table 17.7. Rob Loneragan always reminds me to try and think the way that clinicians do, and that hoofbeats occasionally do mean zebras are approaching.

Since the appearance of the first edition of this text I have left the United Kingdom and returned to work in my homeland, Australia. It has been my great good fortune to meet many generous individuals who have all, in their own way, helped me re-establish my career or worked hard with me to set up the Centre for Health Informatics (CHI) at the University of New South Wales in Sydney. The large team now assembled at CHI is conducting what I think is some of the most exciting health informatics research anywhere on the globe, and I'm very proud to be associated with it.

In particular, I'd like to thank the following people. Bruce Dowton, Dean of the UNSW Medical Faculty, championed the creation of CHI and the first Chair in Medical Informatics in Australia, and without his faith and vision, I doubt we would have started or prevailed. Max Thorpe, with friendship, kindness and wisdom, worked behind the scenes to make all the connections that were needed, and provided counsel and support in the early difficult days. I have also had the great support of many other leading Australian health informaticians and academics including the ever-wise Michael Kidd, Branko Cesnik, Branko Celler, Paul Glasziou, Evelyn Hovenga and the late Chris Silagy who is greatly missed. I am heavily indebted to Dianne Ayers, without whose support the resources for many of our early projects would not have been forthcoming, and our continued existence is a tribute to her early foresight and courage. It is a small, but welcoming, supportive and stimulating informatics world down-under and many colleagues quickly become friends, including Joan Edgecumbe, Jenny Hardy, and Terry Hannan.

I must thank the CHI team who provided the backdrop and continued motivation that supported me as I wrote. I would like to thank Steve Tipper, who joined the centre when we only owned a paperclip and who managed the business meticulously and passionately as we grew rapidly; Branko Celler and Nigel Lovell, who worked hard with me to establish the multidisciplinary heart of CHI, and Johanna Westbrook for her simply outstanding professionalism, support and good humour. The whole CHI team that I work with are there because they are committed to the cause and talented, and I thank you all (alphabetically!): George Alvarez, Keri Bell, Luis Chuquipiondo, Nerida Creswick, Hugh Garsden, Sophie Gosling, Annie Lau, Pamela Logan, Farah Magrabi, Merryn Mathie, Ken Nguyen, Alexander Polyanovskyi, Vitali Sintchenko, Rosemary Spencer, Victor Vickland, Mailis Wakeham, Martin Walther, and Tatjana Zrimec.

The ever-patient team at Hodder needs my thanks as they watched one deadline slip after another, but still believed in this project. I'd specifically like to thank Heather Smith and Georgina Bentliff for being both delightful to work with, and patient and calm in adversity.

My biggest North American fans are my in-laws Bob and Aline Palese, and I'm sure that the local community is in for another battering as they try and sell the second edition to every living soul that they meet. God bless you. Bill Caldicot, you are a wise and great man, and your friendship has been inspiring and nurturing.

As it was with the first edition, writing a book is a long and lonely marathon, and if I have finished, it is only because I have been sustained by the love of my parents and family, and most of all, my wife Blair. It is to you that I dedicate this book.

Publishers' acknowledgements

Material in the introduction, and in Chapters 14 and 23 has been adapted from *BMJ* 1995; **310**: 1381–1387, 1996; **311**: 2–4, and 1998; **317**: 1469–1470, with kind permission from the BMJ Publishing Group. Material from my paper in the *Medical Journal of Australia* 2001; **174**: 467–470 contributed to Chapter 14, and appears with kind permission. Material from my papers in *Journal of the American Medical Informatics Association* 2000; **7**: 215–221, 2000; **7**: 277–286, and 1996; **3**: 363–366, and the *Proceedings of the American Medical Informatics Association Autumn Symposium* (1996), 17–21, has been adapted within Chapters 20, 21 and 24, and appears with permission.

Some material in Chapter 25 was based on work prepared for the report *Electronic Decision Support Activities in Different Healthcare Settings in Australia*, for the Health Online programme of the Australian Federal Department of Health and Ageing, authored by Vitali Sintchenko, Johanna Westbrook, Steven Tipper, Merryn Mathie and Coiera.

Chapter 28 is based on a work supported by AHRQ contract no. 29-00-0020: Bioterrorism: Automated decision support and clinical data collection. Chapter 29 is based on material drawn from Kohane, Kho and Butte's *Microarrays for an Integrative Genomics*, published by MIT Press, Boston.

Figure 4.1 is taken from *BMJ* 1999; **318**: 1527–1531 and appears with permission. Figure 13.1 is taken from a paper by Fox *et al.* in *Proceedings of Medical Informatics Europe* (1996), pp. 516–520 and appears with kind permission of the copyright holder, John Fox. Figure 23.1 appears courtesy of the New South Wales Department of Health. Figures 26.1, 26.2, 26.3, 26.5 and some material in Chapter 26 appear with permission of W.B. Saunders Company Ltd, London. They are adapted from my chapter on automated signal interpretation, in P. Hutton, C. Prys-Roberts (eds.) *Monitoring in Anaesthesia and Intensive Care*, Baillière Tindall Ltd, London (1994).

Introduction to health informatics – the systems science of healthcare

> Of what value, it may be urged, will be all the theorizing and speculation through which it would profess to guide us, when we come to practise at the bedside? Who has not heard so-called practical men say that medicine is a purely empirical science; that everything depends upon facts and correct experience; or, perhaps, that the power to cure is the main point? All arguments and theories, they say, do not enable the physician to treat his patients more correctly; in an art like medicine they rather do harm, or, at best, no positive good. It is there we are in need of experience – facts, and above all, remedies and their correct employment: all the rest is evil. *Oesterlen, Medical Logic (1855), p. 8.*

If physiology literally means 'the logic of life', and pathology is 'the logic of disease', then health informatics is the logic of healthcare. It is the rational study of the way we think about patients, and the way that treatments are defined, selected and evolved. It is the study of how clinical knowledge is created, shaped, shared and applied. Ultimately, it is the study of how we organize ourselves to create and run healthcare organizations. With such a pivotal role, it is likely that in the next century, the study of informatics will become as fundamental to the practice of medicine as anatomy has been to the last.

Health informatics is thus as much about computers as cardiology is about stethoscopes. Rather than drugs, X-ray machines or surgical instruments, the tools of informatics are more likely to be clinical guidelines, formal health languages, information systems or communication systems like the Internet. These tools, however, are only a means to an end, which is the delivery of the best possible healthcare.

Although the term 'health informatics' only came into use around 1973 (Protti, 1995), it is a study that is as old as healthcare itself. It was born the day that a clinician first wrote down some impressions about a patient's illness, and used these to learn how to treat their next patient. Informatics has grown considerably as a clinical discipline in recent years, fuelled in part, no doubt, by the advances in computer technology. What has fundamentally changed is our ability to describe and manipulate health knowledge at a highly abstract level, as has our ability to build up rich communication systems to support the process of healthcare.

We can formally say that health informatics is the study of information and communication systems in healthcare. Health informatics is particularly focused on:

- understanding the fundamental nature of these information and communication systems, and describing the principles which shape them
- developing interventions which can improve upon existing information and communication systems
- developing methods and principles which allow such interventions to be designed
- evaluating the impact of these interventions on the way individuals or organizations work, or on the outcome of the work.

Specific subspecialties of health informatics include **clinical informatics**, which focuses on the use of information in support of patient care and **bioinformatics**, which focuses on the use of genomic and other biological information.

The rise of health informatics

Perhaps the greatest change in clinical thinking over the last two centuries has been the ascendancy of the scientific method. Since its acceptance, it has become the lens through which we see the world, and governs everything from the way we view disease, through to the way we battle it.

It is now hard to imagine just how controversial the introduction of theory and experimental method into medicine once was. Then, it was strongly opposed by the views of the empiricists, who believed that observation, rather than theoretical conjecture, was the only basis for the rational practice of medicine.

With this perspective, it is almost uncanny to hear again the old empiricists' argument that 'healthcare is an art', and not a place for unnecessary speculation or formalization. This time, the empiricists are fighting against those who wish to develop formal theoretical methods to regulate the communal practice of healthcare. Words like quality and safety, clinical audit, outcome measures, healthcare rationing and evidence-based practice now define the new intellectual battleground.

While the advance of science pushes clinical knowledge down to a fine-grained molecular and genetic level, it is events at the other end of the scale that are forcing us to change. Firstly, the enterprise of healthcare has become so large that it now consumes more national resources than any country is willing to bear. Despite sometimes heroic efforts to control this growth in consumption, the healthcare budget continues to expand. There is thus a social and economic imperative to control healthcare and minimize its drain on social resources.

The structure of clinical practice is also coming under pressure from within. The scientific method, long the backbone of medicine, is now in some ways under threat. The reason for this is not that experimental science is unable to answer our questions about the nature of disease and its treatment. Rather, it is almost too good at its job. As clinical research ploughs ahead in laboratories and clinics across the world, like some great information machine, health practitioners are being swamped by its results. So much research is now published each week that it can literally take decades for the results of clinical trials to translate into changes in clinical practice.

So, healthcare workers find themselves practising with ever restricting resources and unable, even if they had the time, to keep abreast of the knowledge of best practice hidden in the literature. As a consequence, the scientific basis of clinical practice trails far behind that of clinical research.

Two hundred years ago, enlightened physicians understood that empiricism needed to be replaced by a more formal and testable way of characterizing disease and its treatment. The tool they used then was the scientific method. Today we are in an analogous situation. Now the demand is that we replace the organizational processes and structures that force the arbitrary selection amongst treatments with ones that can be formalized, tested and applied rationally.

Modern healthcare has moved away from seeing disease in isolation, to understanding that illness occurs at a complex system level. Infection is not simply the result of the invasion of a pathogenic organism, but the complex interaction of an individual's immune system, nutritional status, environmental and genetic endowments. By seeing things at a system level, we come ever closer to understanding what it really means to be diseased, and how that state can be reversed.

We now need to make the same conceptual leap and begin to see the great systems of knowledge that enmesh the delivery of healthcare. These systems produce our knowledge, tools, languages and methods. Thus, a new treatment is never created and tested in intellectual isolation. It gains significance as part of a greater system of knowledge, since it occurs in the context of previous treatments and insights, as well as the context of a society's resources and needs. Further, the work does not finish when we scientifically prove a treatment works. We must try to communicate this new knowledge and help others to understand, apply and adapt it.

These then are the challenges for healthcare. Can we put together rational structures for the way clinical evidence is pooled, communicated and applied to routine care? Can we develop organizational processes and structures that minimize the resources we use and maximize the benefits delivered? And finally, what tools and methods need to be developed to help achieve these aims in a manner that is practicable, testable and in keeping with the fundamental goal of healthcare – the relief from disease? The role of health informatics is to develop a systems science for healthcare that provides a rational basis to answer these questions, as well as to create the tools to achieve these goals.

The scope of informatics is thus enormous. It finds application in the design of clinical decision support systems for practitioners, in the development of computer tools for research, and in the study of the very essence of medicine – its corpus of knowledge. Yet the modern discipline of health informatics is still relatively young. Many different groups within healthcare are addressing the issues raised here, and not always in a coordinated fashion. Indeed, these groups are not always even aware that their efforts are connected, nor that their concerns are ones of informatics.

The first goal of this book is to present a unifying set of basic informatics principles which influence everything from the delivery of care to an individual patient through to the design of whole healthcare systems. Its next goal is to present the breadth of issues which concern informatics, show how they are related, and to encourage research into understanding the common principles that connect them.

Each area that is covered has been written with three criteria in mind – its possibility, its practicability and its desirability. **Possibility** reflects the science of informatics – what in theory can be achieved? **Practicability** addresses the potential for successfully engineering a system or introducing a new process – what can actually be done given the constraints of the real world? **Desirability** looks at the fundamental motivation for using a given process or technology.

These criteria are suggested in part because we need to evolve a framework to judge the claims made for new technologies and those who seek to profit from them. Just as there is a long-standing symbiosis between the pharmaceutical industry and medicine, there is a newer and consequently less examined relationship between healthcare and the computing and telecommunication industries. Clinicians should try to judge the claims of these newcomers in the same cautious way that they would examine claims about a new drug (Wyatt, 1987) and perhaps more so, given that clinicians are far more knowledgeable about pharmacology than they are about computers and telecommunications.

Overview of the book

The book is organized into a number of parts, all of which revolve around the two distinct strands of information and communication. While the unique character of each strand is explored individually, there is also an emphasis on understanding the rich way in which they can interact and complement each other.

Part 1 – Basic concepts in informatics

Like healthcare, informatics has both theoretical and applied aspects to its study. This first part of the book is focused on developing an intuitive understanding of the basic theoretical concepts needed to approach informatics practice in a principled way. Three fundamental ideas underpin the study of informatics – the notions of what constitutes a model, what is meant by information and what defines a system. Each of these three ideas is explored to develop an understanding of the nature of information and communication systems. A recurring theme in this part will be the need to understand the limitations imposed upon us whenever we create or use a model of the world. Understanding these limitations defines the ultimate limits of possibility for informatics, irrespective of whichever technology one may wish to apply in its service.

Part 2 – Informatics skills

Building on the concepts in Part 1, the second part of the book looks at the practical lessons that can be drawn from informatics to guide everyday clinical activity. Every clinical action, every treatment choice and investigation, is shaped by the available information and how effectively that information is communicated. Five basic clinical informatics skills are explored, each with their own individual chapter:

- **Communicating** effectively is based upon understanding cognitive models of information processing, and is constantly challenged by the limits of human attention, and the imperfection of models;
- **Structuring** information, with a particular focus on the patient record, is shown to be dependent upon the task at hand, the channel used to communicate the message, and the agent who will receive the message;

- **Questioning** others to find information is essential in clinical practice to fill the ever-present gaps in every individual's knowledge;
- **Searching** for knowledge describes the broader strategic process of knowing where to ask questions, evaluating answers and refining questions in the light of previous actions, and occurs in many different settings, from when patient's are interviewed and examined, through to when treatment options are canvassed;
- **Making decisions** occurs when all the available information needed has been assembled using the other informatics skills, and attempts to come up with the best alternative to solve a problem like selecting a treatment, based not only on the evidence from science, but also the wishes and needs of individuals.

Part 3 – Information systems in healthcare

The chapters in this part explore the special character of information systems in healthcare. The clinical record is given many names and is discussed in many different guises throughout the book, and its role and scope are introduced here. Information systems such as the electronic medical record are shown to manage a wide variety of activities. Ultimately, the way that these activities are modelled, measured and then managed is determined by information system design.

Sometimes, leaving things unsaid or informal is more productive than encoding them in a formal computer system. Consequently, the important concept of system formality is also introduced here, since it is not always appropriate to build information systems. Indeed, it can often be counterproductive. Understanding the role of formality helps principled decisions to be made before information systems are introduced. The concept of formality also helps us to understand the different roles that communication and information systems play in healthcare. The final chapter in this part spends some time describing how one sets out to build such systems, and some of the design problems that bedevil that process.

Having laid down these foundational ideas in the first parts of the book, the next two parts turn to focus on two information problems that are specific to healthcare – protocol-based care, and clinical coding.

Part 4 – Protocol-based systems

Clinical guidelines or protocols have been in limited use for many years. The current emphasis on evidence-based clinical practice has made it more likely that healthcare workers will use protocols, and perhaps be involved in their design and maintenance. In this part, the various forms and uses of protocols are introduced. The various roles that computer-based protocol systems can play in clinical practice are outlined. These cover both traditional **passive support** where protocols are kept as a reference, and **active systems** in which the computer uses the protocol to assist in the delivery of care. For example, protocols incorporated into the electronic record can generate clinical alerts or make treatment recommendations. Their characteristic advantages and limitations are also discussed and these are then used to formulate a set of protocol design principles.

Part 5 – Language, coding and classification

If the data contained in electronic patient record systems is to be analysed, then it needs to be accessible in some regular way. This is usually thwarted by the variations in health terminology used by different individuals, institutions and nations. To remedy the problem, large dictionaries of standardized clinical terms have been created.

The chapters in this section introduce the basic ideas of concepts, terms, codes and classifications, and demonstrate their various uses. The inherent advantages and limitations of using terms and codes are discussed. The last chapter in particular looks at some more advanced issues in coding, describing the theoretical limitations to coding, and outlines practical approaches to managing these issues, as well as presenting open research questions.

Part 6 – Communication systems in healthcare

Interpersonal communication skills are fundamental to patient care, but the process of communication has, for a long time, not been well supported technologically. Now, with the widespread availability of communication systems supporting mobility, voice mail, electronic mail and video-conferencing, new possibilities arise. The chapters in this section introduce the basic types of communication services and explain the different benefits of each.

Given that much of the technology is new for many, one chapter is devoted to describing the basics of the various different communication systems now available. The final chapter in this part examines clinical communication and the field of telemedicine in the context of these new technologies. The potential of telemedical systems within different areas of healthcare is described, but the importance of carefully choosing the right set of technologies for a given problem is emphasized.

Part 7 – The Internet

Information systems are starting to become indistinguishable from communication systems, and this convergence is perhaps nowhere more apparent than with the Internet. This part explores in detail the phenomenal rise of the Internet and the World Wide Web, and examines why its technologies have proven to be so revolutionary. The complex way that the Web alters the balance of information publishing and access is explained, along with the consequences of these changes. The full impact of the Internet on healthcare has yet to be felt. Some of the many different ways that it will change healthcare are presented here, from the way communication occurs, through to the change it will have upon the doctor–patient relationship.

Part 8 – Decision support systems

The concluding chapters of the book look to some of the most complex computer systems created so far – those based upon the technologies of artificial intelligence (AI). The early promise of computer programs that could assist clinicians in the process of diagnosis have come to fruition, and they are now in routine use in many clinical situations. AI techniques also permit the creation of systems able to assist with therapy planning, information seeking, and the generation of alerts.

The final chapters in this part look in detail at some of the specialized ways that decision technologies are applied in clinical practice. They find application in creating intelligent patient monitors, and potentially, autonomous therapeutic devices such as self-adjusting patient ventilators. Along with communication technologies, they are essential components of biosurveillance systems. Finally, in the field of bioinformatics, human genome knowledge is harnessed using computer techniques, and reframes many classes of clinical decision as questions of genetics as much as physical clinical science.

PART 1

Basic concepts in informatics

CHAPTER 1

Models

> A message to mapmakers: highways are not painted red, rivers don't have county lines running down the middle, and you don't see contour lines on a mountain. *W. Kent, Data and Reality (1978).*
>
> Man tries to make for himself in the way that suits him best a simplified and intelligible picture of the world and thus to overcome the world of experience, for which he tries to some extent to substitute this cosmos of his. This is what the painter, the poet, the speculative philosopher and the natural scientist do, each in his own fashion … one might suppose that there were any number of possible systems … all with an equal amount to be said for them; and this opinion is no doubt correct, theoretically. But evolution has shown that at any given moment out of all conceivable constructions one has always proved itself absolutely superior to all the rest.
> *Einstein, The World as I See It (1931).*

The study of healthcare is founded upon a few basic ideas such as the cell or the concept of disease. Informatics is similarly built upon the concepts of data, models, systems and information. Unlike health, where the core ideas are usually grounded in observations of the physical world, these informatics concepts are abstract ideas. As a consequence, they can be difficult to grasp, and for those used to the study of healthcare, often seem detached from the physical realities of the clinical workplace.

This is further complicated because we use the same words that describe these informatics concepts in everyday language. It is common to ask for more information about a patient, to question what data support a particular conclusion, or to read a textbook that describes a physiological model. In informatics these intuitive ideas need to be much more precisely defined. Once they are mastered, however, it is then relatively easy to move on to the key informatics issues facing healthcare.

In this first chapter, we begin the study of informatics by exploring the pivotal concept of a **model**. Whether diagnosing a patient's condition, writing a patient record, designing an information system or trying to deliver an efficient health service to the public, we use models to direct our actions. A deep understanding of what it means to create or apply a model underpins the way we interact with the world and how likely we are to be successful in achieving our goals. Models define the way we learn about the world, interpret what we see,

Box 1.1
Therac-25

Between June 1985 and January 1987, Therac-25 linear accelerators operating in the US and Canada delivered massive radiation overdoses to at least six patients, causing death or serious radiation injury. Patients received doses of up to 20 000 rads where 200 rads was a typical therapeutic dose, and a 500 rad whole-body dose will cause death in 50% of cases. These were arguably the worst radiation incidents associated with medical accelerators in the history of radiotherapy.

Medical linear accelerators operate by creating a high energy electron beam. The beam is focused on to a patient to destroy tumour tissue, and leaves healthy tissue outside the beam focus relatively unaffected. The high energy beam produced by these devices is focused through a tungsten shield. This 'flattens' the beam to therapeutic levels, and acts like a lens to focus the beam to a tissue depth appropriate for a given patient.

In the Therac-25 accidents, the tungsten shield was not in place when the radiation dose was delivered, resulting in patients receiving a full dose of the raw 25-MeV electron beam. There were a number of different causes of the various overdoses, but each essentially resulted from modelling errors in the system's software and hardware (Leveson and Turner, 1993).

One critical error resulted from the reuse of some of the software from a previous machine, the Therac-20. This software worked acceptably in the 20, but when reused in the 25 permitted an overdose to be given. This was because a physical backup safety system that was present in the 20 had been removed in the design of the 25. The Therac-20 software was thus reused in the 25 on the assumption that the change in machines would not affect the way the software operated. So, software modelled to one machine's environment was used in a second context in which that model was not valid.

Another problem lay in the measurement system that reported the radiation dose given to patients. It was designed to work with doses in the therapeutic range, but when exposed to the full beam strength, became saturated and gave a low reading. As a result, several patients were overdosed repeatedly, because technicians believed the machine was delivering low doses. Thus, the measurement system was built upon an assumption that it would never have to detect high radiation levels.

All of these failures occurred because of the poor way in which models were used by the designers of the Therac-25. They did not understand that many of the assumptions that were left implicit in the specifications of the device would quickly become invalid in slightly changed circumstances, and would lead to catastrophic failure.

and apply our knowledge to effect change, whether that is through our own actions, or through the use of technology like a computer.

Humans are naturally adept at developing mental models of the world, and manage to use them robustly, despite the inherent weaknesses of the models themselves. When these flexible mental models are transferred into a fixed technological system like a computer, the effects of modelling error can be amplified significantly, with sometimes disastrous consequences (Box 1.1). This is often because much of the knowledge used in creating the model has not been transferred along with it, and as a consequence, the technological system is unable to define the limits of its knowledge. One of the major ideas to be explored in this chapter is that the implicit and explicit assumptions we make at the time a model is created ultimately define the limits of a model's usefulness. The motto for this chapter is 'A map is not the territory'.

A map is not the territory it represents, but, if correct, it has a similar structure *to the territory, which accounts for its usefulness .... If we reflect upon our languages, we find that at best they must be considered* only as maps. *A word* is not *the object it represents ... the disregard of these complexities is tragically disastrous in daily life and science.* (Korzybski, 1958)

1.1 Models are abstractions of the real world

What is a model and what does it do? Models are commonplace in our everyday lives. People are familiar with the idea of building model aeroplanes, or looking at a small-scale model of a building to imagine what it will look like when built. In health, models underlie all our clinical activities. For example, whenever we interact with patients, we use internalized models of disease to guide the process of diagnosis and treatment.

Models actually serve two quite distinct purposes, and both of these are of interest. The first use of a model is as some kind of copy of the world. The modelling process takes some aspect of the world, and creates a description of it. A simple example will make this clearer. Imagine a camera taking a photograph. The image that is captured on the camera's film is a model of the world:

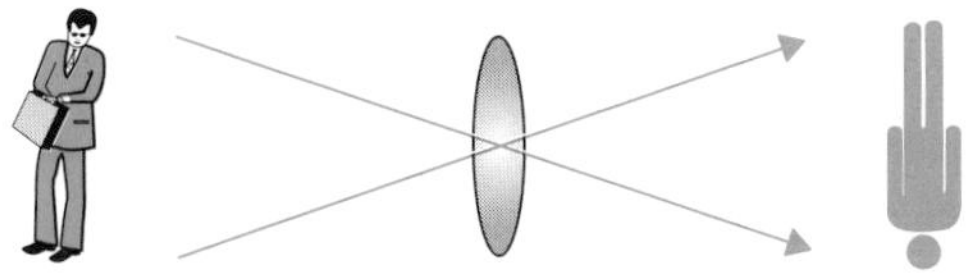

We can generalize from the way a camera lens and film record a physical object to describe the way that all models are created. The process of creating a model of the real world is one of **abstraction**:

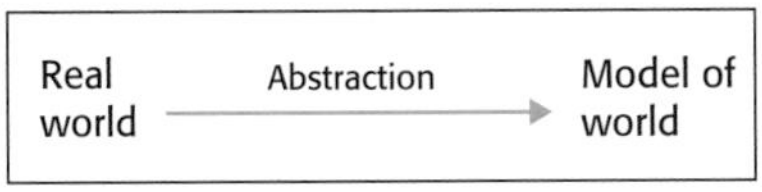
Real world
Abstraction
Model of world

Abstraction
The process of identifying a few elements of a physical object and then using these to create a model of the object. The model is then used as a proxy representation of the physical object.

The effects of the abstraction process are directly analogous to the effects of using a camera. In particular, the image captured on film has four important features that are characteristic of all models.

- Firstly, the image is simpler than the real thing. There are always more features in the real world than can be captured on film. One could, for example, always use a more powerful lens to capture ever finer detail. Equally, models are always less detailed than the real world from which they are drawn. A map, for example, will not contain every feature of the city streets it records. Since models are always less detailed than the thing they describe, data are lost in the abstraction process.
- Secondly, the image is a caricature or distortion of the real world. The three physical dimensions occupied by the photographed object are transformed into two on the film. Through the use of different filters, lenses or films, very different images of the observed world are obtained. None of them is the 'true' image of the object. Indeed there is no such thing. The camera just records a particular point of view. Similarly, abstraction imposes a point of view upon the real world, and inevitably the resulting model is distorted in some way. Thus a map looks very little like the terrain it models. Some land features are emphasized, and others de-emphasized or ignored. In physiology, one view of the heart models it as a mechanical pump. This model emphasizes one particular aspect of the organ system, but it is clearly much more than this. It also has a complex set of functions to do with the regulation of blood pressure, blood volume and organ perfusion.
- Thirdly, as a consequence of distortion and data loss, there are many possible images that can be created of the same object. Different images emphasize different aspects of the object or show different levels of detail. Similarly, since there are a variety of aspects that could be modelled of any physical object, and a variation in the level of detail captured, many models can be created. Indeed, the number of possible models is infinite. Since we all carry different 'lenses' when we see the world, it is no surprise that different individuals see the world so differently. Psychiatrists, for example, might consider the brain from a Freudian or Jungian perspective. Neurologists may model it as a collection of neurones, each with different functions. Physiologists may model the function of a brain on that of a computer. When a clinician meets a patient, do they see a person, an interruption, a client, a task, a disease, a problem, a friend, or a billing opportunity?

- Finally, the camera records a particular moment in time. Thus as the model remains static and the physical object it represents changes with time, the similarity between the model and the physical object it represents degrades over time. The difference between you and a photograph of you as a child increases as you get older. A map of a city becomes increasingly inaccurate as time passes, because of changes to the city's roads and buildings.

As a consequence of these four characteristics of abstracted models, a final one now becomes evident. All models are built for a reason. When we create a model, we actively choose amongst the many possible models that could be created, to build one that suits our particular purposes. For example, the point of view captured in a map is determined by the way the map will be used. A driver's map emphasizes streets and highways. A hiker's map emphasizes terrain and altitude. Thus, one actively excludes or distorts aspects of the world to satisfy a particular purpose. There is no such thing as a truly 'general-purpose' model.

Karl Popper would ask his students to 'observe and describe.' They would be puzzled, and eventually ask 'observe what?' That was his point. We always have to observe something in order to describe something. The notion of pure observation, independent of direction, is a myth (Skolimowski, 1977).

This last point is crucial to much of what will follow in later chapters. It leads on to a related idea, which has already been touched upon. Just as a camera cannot capture a 'true' image of an object, one cannot ever build a 'true' model of an object.

In philosophy, the argument against things ever being inherently correct or true is equivalent to arguing against the Platonic ideal. This is the idea that pure forms of physical objects exist outside the realms of the physical world. Thus, although a physical sphere may always have an imperfection, Plato believed there existed an 'ideal' mathematical spherical form. The arguments against Plato's ideas say that there is no such ideal or objective truth in the world. There can only be our subjective and local point of view or need, based upon the input of our senses.

Even in 'pure' geometry, there is no ideal sphere, just an infinite family of possible shapes that vary depending on the rules of the geometric system you choose. We cannot say that only one of these geometries is correct. Rather, they are different explanations of space, based upon different assumptions. We use the one that gives the most satisfactory explanation of the phenomenon we are interested in. For example, Reimann geometry works best for Einstein's relativity theory, rather than classic Euclidean geometry, since it handles the notion of curved space (Figure 1.1).

This philosophical argument continues into the present century, as the process of scientific enquiry has been debated, and the nature of experimental evidence defined. This is because a scientific hypothesis is nothing more than a model of some aspect of the world, which is to

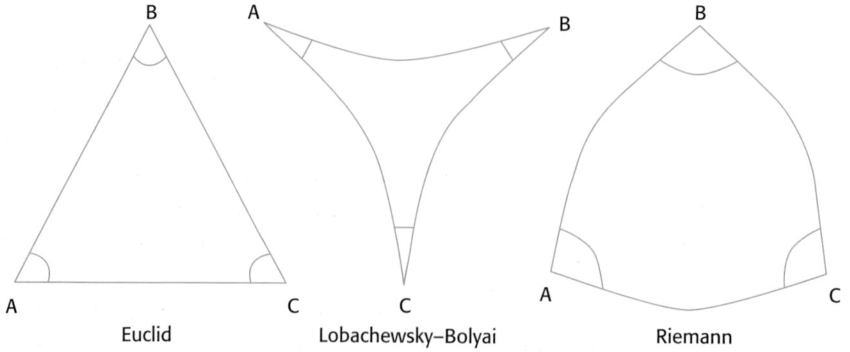
B
A
C
Euclid
A
B
C
Lobachewsky–Bolyai
B
A
C
Riemann

Figure 1.1
There is no 'correct' geometric shape, just an infinite number of possible geometries. The angles in classic euclidean triangles always add up to 180°, but in Riemann geometry they always add to more than 180°, and with Lobachewsky–Bolyai geometry they are always less than 180°.

be tested by an experiment. However, if a model can never be correct and thus objective truth can never be known, then our experiments can never actually **prove** anything to be true. We are never sure that we are right. The best that experiments can do is show us when our models of the world are wrong (Popper, 1976). What remain are theories that are in some way more useful or less useful than others in managing the world.

And though the truth will not be discovered by such means – never can that stage be reached – yet they throw light on some of the profounder ramifications of falsehood. (Kafka, 1971).

1.2 Models can be used as templates

So far, models have been described as copies or images of the world. There is a second way in which we use models that is equally commonplace. Some models, rather than being copies of real things, are used as templates from which a new thing will be created. An architect, for example, creates a set of drawings that will be translated into a building. Economists build mathematical models of a country's economy, and then use these models to predict the effects of changes in monetary policy. An emergency procedure is written down, and will come into effect if a hospital team is called to a major civil disaster.

Again, a simple example will make this second use of models clearer. If we take an image captured on a photographic slide or strip of movie film, a lamp can be used to project a copy of the image on to a screen:

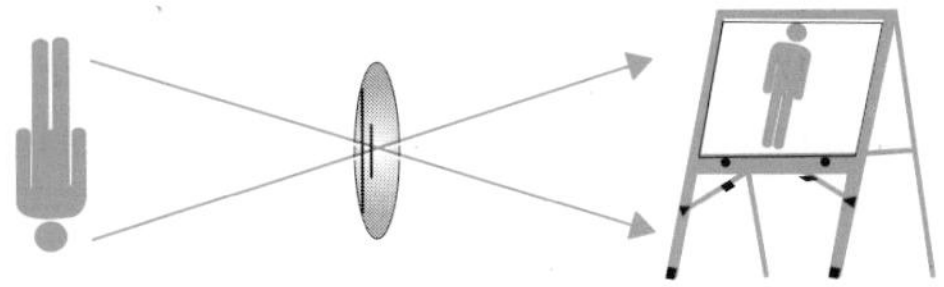

The image stored on the film is a model of the real world. The projection process uses this model to create a second, slightly altered, image. We can generalize from this to understand how models can act as templates. The process begins with the creation of a model. This might be a design, perhaps recorded as a set of blueprints or specifications. This is followed by a process of construction or model **instantiation**. In mathematics and logic, we instantiate the variables in an equation with data values. The equation is a template and it interacts with the supplied data values to arrive at the result. Instantiation uses the model as a template to build an artefact or process that is an instance of the model in the physical world.

Instantiation
The process of building an example or instance of a model, using the model as a template to guide the process.

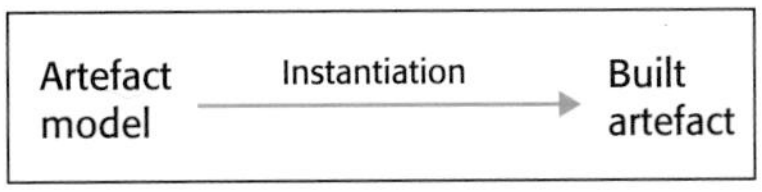
Artefact model
Instantiation
Built artefact

Thus, the process of creating an instance has a variable outcome, and the impact of the instance of a model in the real world also varies. Two very different examples will help reinforce these ideas. Despite having identical DNA, two individual biological organisms are never truly identical. If DNA is a model (see Box 2.1) then the process of DNA transcription results in the 'manufacture' of an instance of an individual organism. Even if we take identical DNA as the starting point, local variations in the process of protein manufacture will introduce minor changes that at some level distinguish the clones.

Similarly, although two patients may be treated according to the same guideline, which is a template for treatment, no two actual episodes of treatment are ever exactly the same.

The features of the specific situation in which a treatment is given result in variations in the way the treatment proceeds and in its final effects on a patient. Variations in the timing of treatments, availability of resources, and the occurrence of other events all can conspire to change the way a treatment is given. Equally, the physical and genetic variations introduced by the patient will result in variations in the effects of a treatment.

The effects of this instantiation process are directly analogous to the effects of projecting a movie image. In particular, the image that is projected is an instance of the image model contained on the film. Many of the effects of the instantiation process are similar to the abstraction process.

- Whereas abstraction loses data to create a model, the process of instantiation adds data to create an instance. The image you see from a projector varies depending upon whether it is projected on a white screen, a wall or the side of a building. The physical surface adds in its own features to shape the final result. The image is the result of the interaction of the projected image and the physical surface it strikes. Thus an artefact is more complex than the model that it came from, because it is situated in the physical world.
- The constructed artefact is thus a distortion of the original template, since we can transform it in many different ways. The projected image can be shaped by the use of filters and lenses to produce a variety of different images.
- No two projected images are ever exactly the same, because of variations introduced by the physical process of construction. No two physical artefacts are identical, even if they are instances of the same template. Even mass-produced objects like light-bulbs, syringes or clay pots have minor imperfections introduced during manufacture that distinguish one instance of an object from another. In contrast, in digital or 'virtual' worlds, where we can guarantee that the exact conditions for creating instances are identical, we can say that no two images **need** be the same.
- The effect of the captured image changes with the passage of time, as the physical world changes. A movie has a greater impact on release than many years afterwards as audiences change. A treatment guideline becomes increasingly inappropriate as time passes and new knowledge indicates that newer methods are better treatment options. Similarly, the effect of an artefact may change although the original template stays the same.

A more general principle follows from these four characteristics of templates. Since the process of creating an instance from a template has a variable result, and the process of doing things in the real world is uncertain because we can never know all the variations that are 'added in' as we follow a template, then there is no such thing as a general-purpose template. All we can have are templates or designs that are better or worse suited to our particular circumstances, and are better or worse at meeting the needs of the task at hand.

As we will see in later chapters, this means that there can be no 'correct' way to treat an illness, no 'right' way to describe a diagnosis, nor a 'right' way to build an information or communication system. There can thus never be an absolutely 'correct' design for a treatment protocol or information system, nor a 'pure' set of terms to describe activities in healthcare. This principle explains why clinical protocols will always have varying effectiveness based upon local conditions, and why medical languages can never be truly general purpose. What we do have are treatments, protocols, languages, information and communication systems that are better or worse suited to our specific purpose than others at any given moment.

1.3 The way we model the world influences the way we affect the world

In the previous sections we saw how models acted either as copies of things in the world, or as templates upon which new things are created. These two aspects of modelling are deeply interrelated. In the photography example, decisions at the moment an image is created influence the way it can ultimately be used.

Assumptions about the purpose of an image will determine how useful it will be when the time comes to use it, since our belief about expected purpose shapes the form and the content of the image. Slides are created with the assumption that they are to be used in a particular type of projector. The value of the projected image in meeting a particular need depends in part on what was originally photographed. A radiograph may be of less value than a CT scan of a skull in the management of a head injury.

When artefacts are created, it is assumed that they too will be used for a particular purpose. If the purpose changes, then a design becomes less effective. Thus, the physical design of the waiting room and treatment areas for a general practice clinic will assume that a certain number of patients need to be seen during a day, and that certain kinds of therapy will be given. If the clinic was bought by radiologists, they would have to remodel the clinic's design to incorporate imaging equipment, and to reflect a different throughput of patients.

Equally, we can consider a particular treatment of a disease written in a textbook to be a template for what should be done to any given patient. If that treatment was based on assumptions about the incidence of diseases in a given population, then it may not work well if attempted in a different one. Treating infant diarrhoea in a developed nation is not the same task as in underdeveloped nations where poorer resources, malnutrition, and different infecting organisms change the context of treatment. Before a model is used, one therefore has to be clear about what has actually been modelled. This is because, when models are created, the circumstances at the time have a strong influence on the final value of the model.

Before the work of the famous physician Galen, it was assumed that the arteries contained air. This was because arteries were observed to be empty after death (Schafer and Thane, 1891). The physicians making these observations had thought they had created a model of arterial function in living humans, but all they had created was a model valid in cadavers. So, the context in which a model is created affects its validity for any other context within which it might be used.

Similarly, a set of rules and procedures might be developed in one hospital, and be spectacularly successful at improving the way it handles its cases. Given that these procedures implicitly model many aspects of that particular institution, one would have to be very cautious about imposing those procedures on other hospitals. Very small differences, for example in the level of resources, type of patients seen, or experience of the staff, may make what was successful in one context, unhelpful in another.

More generally, any designed artefact, whether it is a car, a drug or a computer system, has to be designed with the world within which it will operate in mind. In other words, it has to contain in its design a model of the environment within which it will be used. These specifications constitute its **design assumptions**. Thus there is a connection between the process of model creation, the construction of artefacts based upon such models, and their eventual effectiveness in satisfying some purpose (Figure 1.2).

A few examples should make the cycle of model abstraction and instantiation clearer. Firstly, consider an artefact such as a car. The design blueprints of the car reflect both the purpose of the car, as well as the environment within which it will operate. The car's engine is built on the basis of the not unreasonable assumption that it will operate in an atmosphere with oxygen. The wheels and suspension are designed with the assumption that they will operate on a highway or local street. The car thus carries within its construction a kind of implicit model of the world within which it is designed to work. If the car was put into another physical

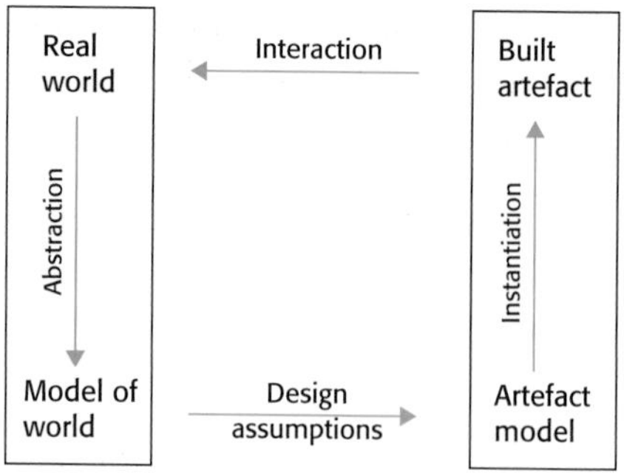
Real world
Interaction
Built artefact
Abstraction
Instantiation
Model of world
Design assumptions
Artefact model

Figure 1.2
Models of the world are used as a basis for creating template models which define how artefacts such as devices or processes will be constructed.

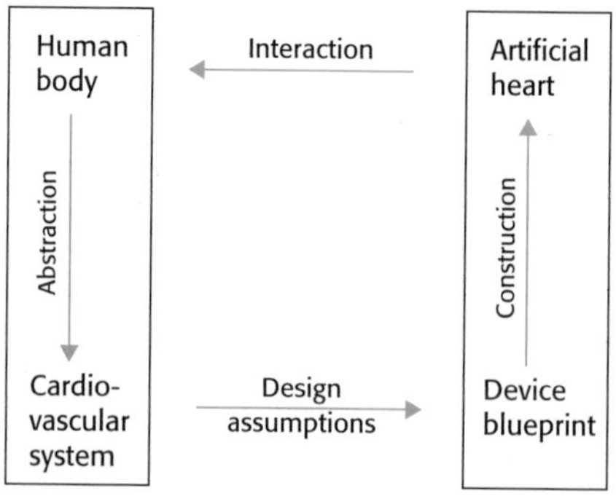
Human body
Interaction
Artificial heart
Abstraction
Construction
Cardio-vascular system
Design assumptions
Device blueprint

Figure 1.3
An artificial heart is based on two kinds of model: first the cardiovascular system has to be modelled, and then a mechanical blueprint is used to model the way the heart will be constructed.

environment – a desert or the lunar surface – it probably would not work very well. Sometimes such design assumptions are left implicit, and only become obvious when a device is used in a way in which it was not intended, sometimes with catastrophic results (Box 1.1).

The human body also makes assumptions about its environment. The haemopoietic system adjusts the number of red blood cells needed for normal function, on the basis of the available oxygen in the atmosphere. As a consequence, the oxygen-carrying system of someone living at sea level is calibrated differently from that of someone living at high altitude. An athlete training at sea level will not perform well if moved quickly to a high altitude because these 'working assumptions' are no longer met.

Finally, consider an artificial heart (Figure 1.3). Such a device must model the heart in some way, since it will replace it within the cardiovascular system. The artificial heart thus is based upon a model of the heart as a mechanical pump, and is designed with the assumption that supporting the pump mechanisms will be beneficial. It is also designed on the assumption that it will need to be implanted, and as a consequence is crafted to survive the corrosive nature of that environment, and to minimize any immune reaction that could be mounted against it.

Conclusions

In this chapter, the basic concept of a model has been explored in some detail. Models underpin the way we understand the world we live in, and as a consequence guide the way we interact with the world. We should never forget that the map is not the territory and the blueprint is not the building.

In the next chapter, a second basic concept of information will be introduced. These two ideas will then be brought together, as we begin to see that knowledge is a special kind of model, and is subject to the same principles and limitations that afflict all other models.

Discussion points

1. 'The map is not the territory'. Why not?
2. Observe and describe. Why?
3. Biologists argue whether nature, expressed in an organism's DNA, or 'nurture', via the physical world, is most important in shaping an organism's development. If 'nature' is the template, and 'nurture' creates instances of an organism, which is more important in shaping an organism, on the basis of the first principles of modelling?
4. In what ways could the limitations of models result in errors in the diagnosis or treatment of patients? Use Figure 1.2 as a template to guide your thinking, if it helps.

Chapter summary

1. Models are the basis of the way we learn about, and interact with, the physical world.
2. Models can act either as copies of the world like maps, or as templates that serve as the blueprints for constructing physical objects, or processes.
3. Models that copy the world are abstractions of the real world:
   - Models are always less detailed than the real world they are drawn from.
   - Models ignore aspects of the world that are not considered essential. Thus abstraction imposes a point of view upon the observed world.
   - Many models can be created of any given physical object, depending on the level of detail and point of view selected.
   - The similarity between models and the physical objects they represent degrades over time.
   - There is no such thing as a truly general-purpose model. There is no such thing as the most 'correct' model. Models are simply better or worse suited to accomplishing a particular task.
4. Models can be used as templates and be instantiated to create objects or processes that are used in the world.
   - Templates are less detailed than the artefacts that are created from them.
   - An artefact is a distortion of the original template.
   - No two physical artefacts are similar even if they are instances of the same template.
   - The effect of an artefact may change while the original template stays the same.
   - The process of creating an instance has a variable outcome, and the impact of the instance of an artefact in the real world also varies. As a consequence, there is no such thing as a general-purpose template. All we can have are templates or designs that are better or worse suited to our particular circumstances and task.
5. The assumptions used in a model's creation, whether implicit or explicit, define the limits of a model's usefulness.
   - When models are created, they assume that they are to accomplish a particular purpose.
   - When models are created they assume a context of use. When objects or processes are built from a model, this context forms a set of design assumptions.
6. We should never forget that the map is not the territory and the blueprint is not the building.

CHAPTER 2

Information

> The plural of datum is not information. *Anon.*

To act in the world we need to make decisions, and to make decisions we must have information that helps us choose one course of action over another. In this chapter, a basic framework will be presented that defines what is meant by information. Whether delivered in conversation, captured in a set of handwritten notes, or stored in the memory of a computer, the same basic principles govern the way information is structured and used. The ideas presented here will build upon the work on models presented in the previous chapter. The simple way that models, data and information interrelate will then be unfolded. At this point it should become apparent that models and information underpin not just the specialized study of informatics, but also every aspect of medicine and the delivery of healthcare.

2.1 Information is inferred from data and knowledge

One can say informally that we have received information when what we know has changed. In some sense this information must be measurable, since intuitively some sources of information are better than others. One newspaper may generally be more informative than others. A patient medical record might be full of new data but to the clinician, who sees the patient every day, contain little new information.

Formally, information has been linked to the concepts of **order** and **novelty**. The more order in a document, the more 'information' it contains. For example, a patient record that is broken up into different sections such as past history, allergies and so forth is more informative than an unstructured narrative that jumbles up patient details. Equally, if what the patient record tells us contains nothing new, then it conveys no new information. One can actually develop statistical measurements for the amount of 'information' communicated from a source using what is known as **information theory** (see Box 4.1). However, statistical measurements of information do not help us much when it comes to understanding information in the way we commonly understand the concept.

Information is constructed by people in a process of perception; it is not selected, noticed, detected, chosen or filtered from a set of given, static, pre-existing things. Each perception is a new generalization, a new construction. (Clancy, in Steels and Brookes (1995), p. 229).

Terms like data, information and knowledge are often used interchangeably in common speech. Each of these terms however, has a quite precise and distinct definition in the information sciences.

- **Data** consists of facts. Facts are observations or measurements about the world. For example, 'today is Tuesday', 'the patient's blood pressure is 125/70 mmHg' or 'Aspirin is a NSAID'.
- **Knowledge** defines relationships between data. The rule 'tobacco smoking causes lung cancer' or 'if a patient's blood pressure is greater than 135/95 mmHg on three separate occasions then the patient has high blood pressure' are examples of knowledge. Such knowledge is created by identifying recurring patterns in data, for example across many different patients. We learn that events usually occur in a certain sequence, or that an action typically has a specific effect. Through the process of model abstraction, these observations are then codified into general rules about how the world works.
- As well as learning such generalized 'truths' about the world, one can also learn knowledge that is specific to a particular circumstance. For example, we can create **patient specific knowledge** by observing a patient's state over time. By abstracting away patterns in what is observed, one can arrive at specific knowledge such as 'following treatment with antihypertensive medication, there has been no decrease in the patient's blood pressure over the last 2 months'.
- **Information** is obtained by the application of knowledge to data. Thus, the datum that 'the patient's blood pressure is 125/70 mmHg' yields information if it tells us something new. In the context of managing a patient's high blood pressure, using our general knowledge of medicine, and patient specific knowledge, the datum may allow us to draw the inference that the patient's blood pressure is now under control.

One can now see how each of these three concepts is related. Using a piece of knowledge, in a given context, data are interpreted to produce information. Another example may make this even clearer. Imagine that someone is speaking to you in a language that you do not understand. You might have received a large amount of data during that conversation, but since you have no knowledge of the language, it is meaningless to you. You cannot say that you have received any information.

Since these ideas are at the very foundation of informatics, we will need to understand their interrelationships in even more depth. To this end, the concepts of models developed in the previous section will be of assistance.

2.2 Models are built from symbols

Knowledge can now be recognized to be the set of models we have built up to understand and interact with the world. Sometimes these models are physical analogues of the real thing. For example, a scale model of a town captures in miniature some physical aspects of the real town. An image captured on film is a direct physical abstraction of the object that has been

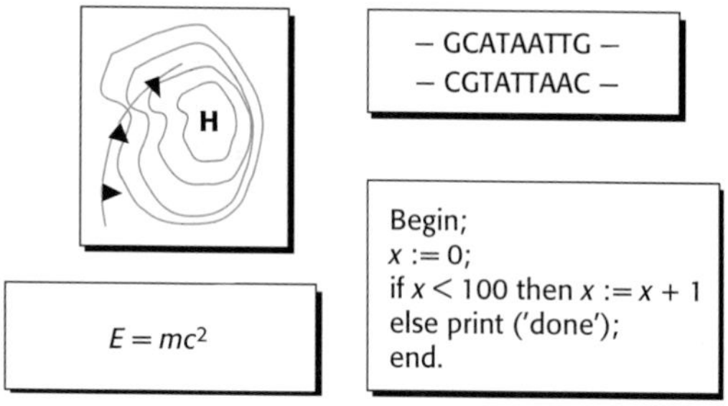
H
– GCATAATTG –
– CGTATTAAC –
Begin;
x := 0;
if x < 100 then x := x + 1
else print ('done');
end.
E = mc2

Figure 2.1
Symbolic models cannot be understood unless the symbol language, and the possible relationships amongst the symbols, are also understood.

photographed. Often knowledge is stored in the heads of individuals. With the development of language and writing, it has become possible for these models to be transferred from being purely mental constructions, to something we can examine and manipulate in the physical world.

A weather map, for example, tries to capture processes that do not look anything like their diagrammatic representation. If we move into the realms of science and mathematics, it is common to create models in the form of diagrams, or equations. These models are all created from a set of symbols, where the symbol is some form of marking that is understood to represent something else. When people talk about knowledge, they are usually referring to this kind of symbolic model, and that is the sense in which knowledge will be used here.

A fundamental characteristic of all symbolic models is that, on their own, they have no intrinsic meaning. To a child, the equation $e = mc^2$ would be meaningless unless each of the letters in the equation was named, and the concept it stands for understood. It would also be meaningless if the child did not understand the mathematical operations that related each of the concepts. A weather map could be equally mysterious.

Terminology
A standard set of symbols or words used to describe the concepts, processes and objects of a given field of study.

Grammar
The set of rules that together specify the allowed ways an alphabet can be put together to forms strings of symbols in a given language.

Symbolic models gain their meaning when we associate concepts with individual symbols. Specifically, symbolic models are built using a recognized **terminology** and a set of relationships or **grammar** between the terms (Figure 2.1). Together the terminology and relationships constitute a **language**. In the information sciences, the languages that are used to create models are usually based upon logic or mathematics.

The terminology contains all the symbols that can be used in building a model, and also maps these symbols to particular concepts. For example, in health we have specific words or terms that stand for observable events like diseases, or for specific treatments. The term 'angina' represents a cluster of data that can be observed in a patient.

The set of relationships we allow among a collection of symbols so that they can be arranged meaningfully together is captured in a **grammar**. In English, for example, our grammar makes sure that when we string together words in a few standard ways, other people recognize the intended meaning of the word sequence.

2.3 Inferences are drawn when data are interpreted according to a model

We use symbolic models to reason about the world. We apply a symbolic model to data that have been acquired from the world to come to some conclusion about how things are. Lawyers examine data in the form of details about a client's case in the light of their knowledge of law to come to conclusions about how likely a client is to succeed in court. Clinicians take data in the form of

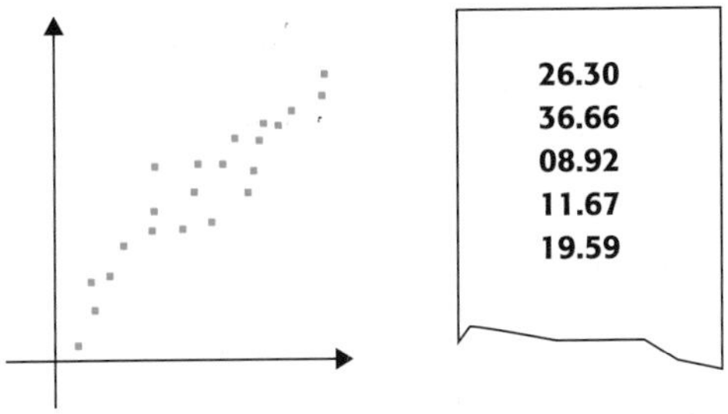
26.30
36.66
08.92
11.67
19.59

Figure 2.2
Data remain uninterpretable in the absence of a language that defines what each datum represents.

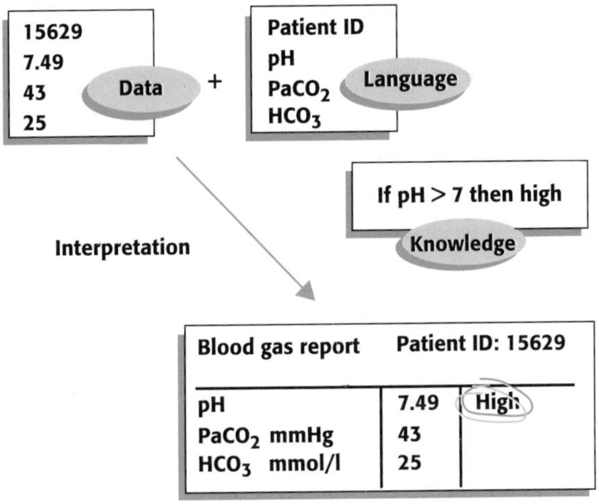
15629
7.49
43
25
Data
+
Patient ID
pH
PaCO2
HCO3
Language
If pH > 7 then high
Knowledge
Interpretation
Blood gas report
Patient ID: 15629
pH
PaCO2 mmHg
HCO3 mmol/l
7.49
43
25
High

Figure 2.3
Data are interpreted with reference to a data model, a knowledge base and rules of inference.

patient observations and measurements, and use their knowledge about disease and therapy to infer what illness a patient may have, and what the most prudent course of action should be.

This process of data interpretation actually requires three different kinds of model. Specifically we need a **database**, a **knowledge base** and an **inference procedure.** Let's look at each of these in turn.

Interpretation commences with a collection of data. The data might be numbers from a laboratory test. The numbers themselves are just symbols, however, and have no meaning on their own in the same way that points on a graph have no meaning without labels on the axes (Figure 2.2). Hence a terminology is needed and each datum is associated with a label or term drawn from the terminology. For example, the number '7.49' is associated with the label 'pH', allowing us to give us the datum 'pH = 7.49'.

This set of labels and relationships is called the **data model** in an information system. Together, a collection of data and their associated data model are called a **database.**

The process of interpretation also requires specific knowledge about the different ways the concepts in the database can interrelate with each other. For example, one might have a laboratory test result for a patient (Figure 2.3).

Rules like 'if the pH is greater than 7.4 then it is abnormally high' or 'if acidosis is present then treat with IV bicarbonate' might be part of a clinician's knowledge of acid–base physiology. A collection of such rules can be thought of as a database containing elements of knowledge, or a **knowledge base.**

Ontology
The set of concepts understood in a knowledge base, and the rules about how concepts can be arranged meaningfully.

Just as a database needs a data model to make the data it holds intelligible, a knowledge base needs a knowledge model, or **ontology**, to make its contents intelligible. In simple terms, an ontology can be thought of as a dictionary of all the allowed concepts in a knowledge base, and of all the allowed ways in which those concepts can be joined together. For example, 'treatment', 'disease', 'pH', 'penicillin' and 'acidosis' might all be known elements in our acid–base ontology. The ontology might also specify that a rule can be of the form 'if *disease* then *treatment*' which would stop us creating nonsense rules like 'if penicillin then acidosis'.

Finally, when the time comes to apply our knowledge to our data, there needs to be a third model which contains the **rules of inference** that specify how we apply the knowledge base to the database to generate the answer. For example, a rule of inference might say that a statement of the form 'if X then Y' means that when we know X is true, we can then also believe that Y is true. This particular example is what is known as logical **deduction** and is one of several different rules of logic that can be used to make inferences (see Chapter 8). There are many different possible methods of inference beyond classic logic. Health epidemiologists make inferences based on the rules of statistics. Lawyers have rules based on precedent established in prior case law.

Technically, we can say that the data model and ontology provide the grammar or **syntax** that defines relationships between terms. The rules of inference are then used to interpret the meaning or **semantics** of the data.

2.4 Assumptions in a model define the limits to knowledge

In the previous chapter, we saw that the assumptions made at the time a model is created affect the way it is used. The way a model is constructed, the context within which it is defined, what is included in it, and the purpose for which is intended, all affect its ultimate usefulness.

This is also the case for the models that define our knowledge of the world. The implication, then, is that the inferences we are able to draw from a model are strongly influenced by the assumptions made when the knowledge in the model was first created.

For example, it is now common for clinical protocols to be used to define a standard way in which a particular illness is to be treated. Such a protocol is a kind of template model that drives the treatment delivered to a patient.

When the protocol is created, the designers have to make many assumptions, not all of which are necessarily obvious to them at the time. For example, the protocol designers might make an implicit assumption that the drugs or equipment they include in the protocol will be available.

What they are actually doing when they make such an assumption is to model the environment within which they expect the protocol to operate. This is usually their own local environment, and it is only when a designer is forced to check with others in very different circumstances that such implicit environmental assumptions are unearthed. This is because a protocol becomes less useful in a context in which some of its implicit assumptions are not valid.

Thus, a protocol created for a well-equipped modern hospital is unlikely to be useful in a primary care clinic. Equally, a protocol might be created with the assumption that a patient has no other significant illnesses. In the case of an individual patient, this implicit assumption might be exposed when the treatment advised by the protocol cannot be used because it interacts with the patient's other medications.

With these examples in mind, we can cast the creation and application of knowledge into the same form as the cycle of model creation and application developed in the last chapter

(Figure 2.4). Firstly, the process of model abstraction is equivalent to the knowledge acquisition process. Observations made of the world are generalized into a model that describes how different parts of the world interrelate. Recall from the last chapter that such models are always limited, and that they emphasize certain observations and omit others.

Next, the knowledge model is applied to data. We can view this process as the construction of an inference, based on a template model that represent our knowledge, and a set of data. As we have just seen, design assumptions made at the time that the model is created affect how it can be used.

One special design assumption associated with a symbolic model is its language. Just as a photographic slide cannot be used unless the right projector is present, a symbolic model cannot be used unless the language and modelling relationships used are also available. In other words, the modelling language becomes a design assumption, which needs to be explicitly catered for when the model is used.

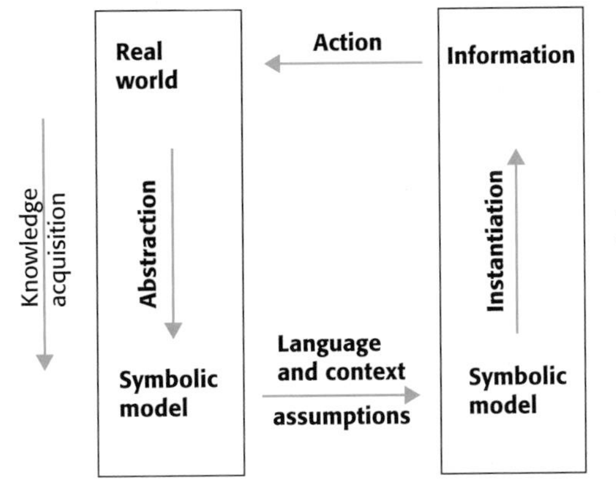
Real world
Action
Information
Knowledge acquisition
Abstraction
Instantiation
Knowledge application
Language and context assumptions
Symbolic model
Symbolic model

Figure 2.4
Knowledge is acquired through the construction of models, and these models are then applied to data, to draw interpretations of the meaning of the data.

Box 2.1
DNA is just data

Conceptualizing an information system into knowledge, data and interpretation components has a certain universality. In biology in particular, there is a strong information paradigm arising out of our understanding of the role of DNA.

Since its structure and function began to be unfolded, DNA has been seen as some form of master molecule, dictating the development of individual organisms. The doctrine of DNA has perhaps reached its most extreme position in the notion of the selfish gene (Dawkins, 1982). Here, DNA is characterized as clothing itself in cells, which allow the DNA to survive and reproduce from generation to generation. DNA, in this view of the world, creates and dictates the development and activity of organisms. The organism phenotype is merely the survival machine used by the genetic sequence.

There is another view that sees DNA as part of a far more complex system. DNA is amongst the most non-reactive and chemically inert molecules in biology. It thus is perfectly designed for its role, which is to store instructions, much like the memory in a computer. DNA is a kind of database, nothing more.

Thus, while DNA stores the models used to create proteins, it is of itself incapable of making anything. It is actually the cellular machinery that determines which proteins are to be made. Although it is often said that DNA produces proteins, in fact proteins produce DNA (Lewontin, 1993).

The symbolic language of DNA, and thus the ability to interpret DNA, resides in the surrounding cellular structures. Without these molecules, there would be no way that we could decode the symbolic meaning of DNA – the data stored in the DNA would be uninterpretable. In other words, an organism's DNA has no meaning outside the context of the cellular structures that contain it.

We can thus regard a complex organism as being the result of a cell's interpretation of the data stored in the DNA database, using a language encoded within its proteins, and within the context of the data provided by the intra- and extracellular environments.

Thus a treatment protocol designer must make assumptions about how the meaning of the protocol will be interpreted. They assume that the people who read the protocol will be capable of understanding the protocol's language, and the instructions built from that language. If a clinician does not recognize the terms in a protocol, and is not familiar with the concepts and principles on which it is based, then they are unlikely to be able to follow the intention of those who wrote it.

2.5 Computational models permit the automation of data interpretation

Acting in the world requires us to make decisions. If the knowledge and data components of a decision problem can be written down, then it can in principle be solved using a computer. Sometimes the actual work of data interpretation for a given problem is shared between human and computer. For example, the computer may organize and consolidate data into a graphical presentation, and the human then examines the processed data to make a final interpretation.

The proportion in which models can be stored either in the computer or as mental models in the head of a human determines where the interpretation takes place. Computer systems thus form a spectrum, from those that have no ability to assist in the interpretation of data, to those that are able to carry out a complete interpretation, within the bounds of a given task (Figure 2.5).

Computers can act as data stores

If a computer is used solely as a repository for data, it acts as a database. The data are organized according to a data model, so that the origin of each datum is recognizable. Medical data often consist of images or physiological signals taken from monitoring devices, and may occupy a vast amount of storage space. As a consequence, the databases that store complex patient data can be huge.

Computers can generate data views that assist interpretation

In contrast to passive databases, a computer can carry out some degree of interpretation by generating a view into a body of data. In this case, given some large data set, the computer

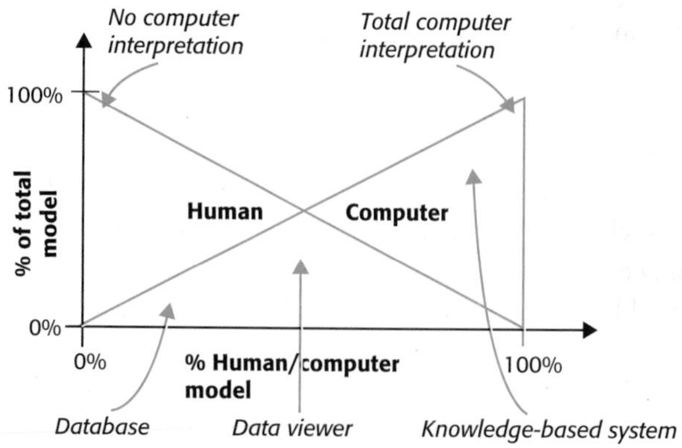
No computer interpretation
Total computer interpretation
100%
% of total model
Human
Computer
0%
0%
% Human/computer model
100%
Database
Data viewer
Knowledge-based system

Figure 2.5
Humans and computers can share the burden of data interpretation. The amount of interpretation delegated to the computer depends on how much of the interpretative model is shared between human and computer.

shows a user only that portion of data which is of immediate interest, and in a way that is best suited to the task at hand.

Consider a database that holds publication data and abstracts of articles from medical journals. Given the thousands of papers published weekly, there would be little value in a researcher simply inspecting each record in the database. It would be practically impossible to locate an article within it. What is required is a way of viewing a relevant subset of the data that matches the researcher's interests.

For a computer system to provide such 'views' of stored data, a model of the user's needs has to be conveyed to the computer. This communication between the database and the human might be provided by what is known as a **query language**. This is a method commonly used to search library catalogues. Using special words like 'and', 'or' and 'not', the user constructs a question for the query system about the things that should be displayed (see Box 6.1). Since it recognizes these special words and their meaning, the query system is able to retrieve those records from the database that match the terms provided by the user.

A patient physiological monitor is also a kind of viewer. A clinician looking at the raw data stream coming from a measurement device such as an ECG would be confronted with streams of rapidly changing digits that would be completely unusable in a clinical setting. It is the monitor's role to present sensor data in such a way that they can be viewed sensibly. In this case, the view might show data as a set of waveforms for a measurement such as the ECG, or as averaged numeric values for a measurement such as the blood pressure. To do this, the computer must have models of the signals, and the kinds of noise and artefact that may corrupt the signals. It also needs a model of the preferred ways of displaying signals to allow humans to carry out the interpretation.

The same process occurs with computer generated images. CT and MRI scanning, for example, are both dependent on complex models that reconstruct raw data into images that can be interpreted by clinicians. By varying the model parameters applied to the data, the imaging systems can produce different views, or 'slices', through the raw image data.

In general, the degree of division of responsibility for data interpretation between human and computer will vary for a number of reasons. It may be that it is inherently difficult to formalize all the knowledge used in the interpretation of data, or it may simply be that the effort involved in modelling is greater than the reward. This is often the case when problems are rare or highly variable.

Computers can be responsible for all data interpretation

As the understanding of how knowledge could be represented in a computer developed, it became clear that computers could be used to perform quite powerful forms of reasoning on their own.

Such computer interpretation can occur in real time. For example, a pacemaker may analyse cardiac activity looking for the development of an arrhythmia. Computers are now often used as backup on reasoning tasks that are performed by humans. For example, in safety-critical situations such as the operation of a nuclear power plant, the human benefits from a computer watching over the complex system with a second pair of fail-safe 'eyes' looking over the operator's shoulder. Computers are also used to interpret data when the task is routine, but occurs with high enough frequency that automation would help. The automated interpretation of laboratory test results is a common example of this use of computers, although typically a human audits the results of such interpretation.

In all these cases, the interpreting computer does not just possess data and the knowledge that will be used to interpret the data. It also needs a model of the way the computer will 'think' about the problem. More precisely, the computer needs a representation of the rules of interpretation discussed earlier. For example, a computer's 'inference engine' may use rules of formal logic – most **knowledge-based systems** are built in this way. Sometimes the systems reason with rules of mathematics, probabilities or other more modern techniques such as neural networks (discussed in Chapter 26).

Conclusions

In this chapter, we have used the idea of a model to help develop an understanding of what it means to have information. In reaching more precise definitions of data, information and knowledge, it has been possible to look at how they interact, and arrive at a rich understanding of everything from the way people draw conclusions to the role that DNA plays in the cell.

These last two chapters have been a prelude to introducing a third fundamental informatics concept – the notion of a system. In the following chapter, the discussion will introduce the concept of systems, and lead on to an exploration of what it means to create an information system. In this way, one can begin to understand the ways in which information systems can be forces for good, as well as understand some of their inherent limitations.

Discussion points

1. Take a patient's laboratory result sheet. Rewrite the information there into a database of facts and showing the data model. If the results have been flagged or interpreted in some way, write out what you think the knowledge base used to make the interpretation was. What rules of inference were applied?
2. Compare your answer to the previous question with someone else. Why might there be differences? (Think back to Chapter 1.)
3. Explain how an individual who reads the same patient's record on two different occasions can find the first reading full of information, and on the second reading find no information at all.
4. The human genome is the Rosetta stone needed to decipher the origin of human disease. Discuss.

Chapter summary

1 Information is based upon data and knowledge.
- Data are a collection of facts.
- Knowledge defines relationships between data.
- Information is obtained by applying knowledge to data.

2 Knowledge can be thought of as a set of models describing our understanding of the world.
- These models are composed of symbols.
- A symbolic model is created using a language that defines the meaning of different symbols, and their possible relationships amongst each other.

3 This process of data interpretation actually requires three different kinds of model. Specifically we need a **database**, a **knowledge base** and an **inference procedure**.

4 Assumptions in the knowledge model affect the quality of the inferences drawn from it.
- Assumptions may implicitly model the context within which the information was created.
- These design assumptions include the language used if the model is symbolic.

5 Knowledge acquisition and application are an example of the cycle of model abstraction and template-based construction.

6 Once a model and data have been sufficiently formalized, the interpretation can be automated using a computer.
- Computers can store data according to data models.
- Computers can provide different views on to data according to user models.
- Computers can interpret data when they have a knowledge base, and an inference procedure.

CHAPTER 3

Information systems

> One doesn't add a computer or buy or design one where there is no system. The success of a project does not stem from the computer but from the existence of a system. The computer makes it possible to integrate the system and thus assure its success. *C. Caceres, in Dickson and Brown (1969), p. 207.*

A system is often understood to be a routine or regular way of working. One can have a system for betting on a horse race, or a filing system for storing and retrieving documents. These systems can be seen as models providing templates for action in the world. In this chapter, we will first introduce the general topic of systems, and identify a few of the key characteristics all systems share. Then the main focus of the chapter follows, which is the introduction of what is formally meant by an information system, and a discussion of how information systems are used to control the way decisions are made.

3.1 A system is a set of interacting components

Just as there is ambiguity with the normal meaning of words such as data or information, the notion of a system is equally complex. Systems pervade healthcare, and there are countless examples of them. In physiology, one talks of the endocrine system or the respiratory system. In clinical practice, we develop systems for questioning and examining our patients. Indeed, the whole of healthcare itself is often described as a system. Each of these examples is very different, but the simplest thing connecting them is that **each system consists of a collection of component ideas, processes or objects**.

We saw in Chapter 1 that models are the basis for building artefacts and interacting with the world. We can use these ideas to understand that the collection of entities we call a system can be one of three things:

- a model acting as an abstracted description of a set of objects or processes observed in the real world

- a model consisting of several interlinked elements acting as a template to action
- an artefact constructed by the process of instantiating such a template in the real world.

So, when you read the words 'the health system', there are three different possible meanings. The 'health system' could be someone's description of how they see healthcare, based upon observation of the world; it could be a proposal or plan for how health should work; or it could be the physical collection of people, buildings and infrastructure that collectively come together to deliver healthcare.

As abstract descriptions of the world, systems help compartmentalize a portion of the world in a way that makes it more understandable. For example, a collection of anatomical structures whose function is closely related might constitute a system. Thus we may speak of the nervous system, and collect within its definition organs such as the peripheral nerves, the spinal cord and the brain.

The collecting together of such elements into a system can be a particularly powerful way of enhancing our understanding of the way things work. For example, when Harvey first proposed the notion of a system of circulation for blood through the body in 1628, he essentially constructed a model that connected together for the first time the arteries, veins and heart into a functioning whole. So powerful was this model that it was adopted despite its inadequacies at that time. It was, for example, not until 1661 that Malpighi finally demonstrated that it was the capillaries that connected the arterial and venous systems together (Schafer and Thane, 1891).

As templates or blueprints, systems allow us to develop clear models of how complex entities will interact. There will be separate blueprints for different systems in a building, including the electrical system, the plumbing system and the air conditioning. The discipline of decomposing a complex structure into elements that might carry out different function simplifies the design process, and makes it more likely that the plan, when carried out, will result in something that is well designed for its intended purpose.

As constructed processes or objects in the real world, systems are a common feature of modern technology. Cars have separate fuel systems, suspension and brake systems, and the separation into different component systems means that each can be maintained and repaired fairly independently of the others.

3.2 A system has an internal structure that transforms inputs into outputs for a specific purpose

Systems have inputs and outputs

Systems usually have a set of **inputs**, which are transformed by the components of the system into a set of **outputs** (Figure 3.1). The inputs to a coffee maker are ground coffee, water, and heat. The output is hot liquid coffee. The inputs to a leaf are water and carbon dioxide, and the photosynthetic system produces as output oxygen and carbohydrates. The inputs to a hospital emergency department are the clinical staff, patients and supplies – the outputs are patients who have been in some way transformed by their visit to the emergency department.

In the process of transforming inputs into outputs, the **state** of a system may change. For example, a car may have as its state a location, and the input of fuel, oil and a driver transforms the state of the vehicle to a different location. An influx of patients may rapidly

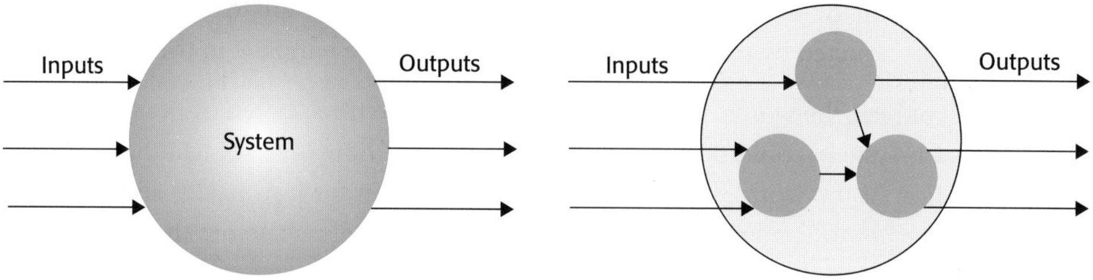
Inputs
System
Outputs
Inputs
Outputs

Figure 3.1
A system is characterized by a set of inputs and outputs and can be internally decomposed into a set of interacting components or sub-systems.

change an emergency department from the state 'able to receive patients' to 'full'. Further, the state of a system may determine just how it will change inputs into outputs. If a human's state is 'physically fit' then they will transform food into energy more efficiently than someone in the state 'unfit', who with the same food inputs may tend to deposit more of the food as fat.

Systems have behaviour

For a system to be distinguishable from its environment, it should have a characteristic behaviour. Thus, a weather system might be a set of related pressure bands, whose collective behaviour stands out and demands attention. One of the behaviours of the vascular system is that it can be observed to contain flowing blood within certain pressure bands. This behaviour distinguishes the vascular system, from say, the nervous system. It is this identification with a particular behaviour that helps conceptually separate a system from other parts of its environment.

Critically, a system's behaviour cannot usually be predicted by an examination of its individual components, but emerges out of the way that the components interact with each other. Thus the behaviour of social groups, communication networks, roads, and neural processes are all emergent properties of the interactions between their components (Box 3.1). The emergence of system behaviour means that the behaviour of anything we build is not directly predictable from an examination of the individual components, but is dependent upon an understanding of how the components interrelate.

Physical systems are embedded in an environment

To be distinguishable from everything else, there must be a **boundary** between a system and the rest of the environment. However, that boundary may be very fuzzy and hard to precisely define. Depending on the completeness of the boundary, three different kinds of system are possible:

- **Closed systems** have no external inputs and outputs, behaving like a black box that is unaffected by the external world.
- **Relatively closed systems** have precisely defined inputs and outputs with their environment.
- **Open systems** interact freely with their surrounding environment.

Except for the rare closed system, which does not interact with its environment, a system can never be completely separated from its external environment. It is for this reason that the emergent behaviour of a physical system is even harder to predict, since that behaviour will in part be determined by the environment in which the system is embedded, and we usually

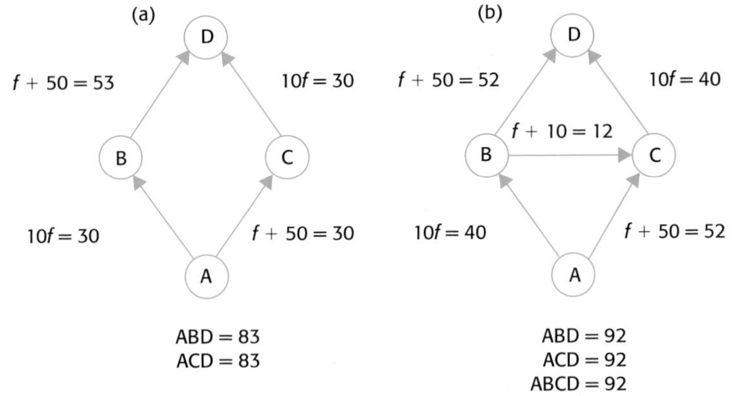
(a)
D
B
C
A
f + 50 = 53
10f = 30
10f = 30
f + 50 = 30
ABD = 83
ACD = 83
(b)
D
B
C
A
f + 50 = 52
10f = 40
f + 10 = 12
10f = 40
f + 50 = 52
ABD = 92
ACD = 92
ABCD = 92

Figure 3.2
The effect of building a new road in a congested system.

Box 3.1
Braess' paradox

Simple cause and effect predicts that putting more resource towards achieving a goal should improve performance, but this is not always the case. The creation of new roads can lead to greater traffic congestion. The installation of new telephone or computer network elements can lead to degraded system performance. Introducing new workers to a team may actually result in a decrease in the team's performance.

To understand these apparently paradoxical results, one needs to examine events from a system view. Studying the effects of new roads on traffic, Dietrich Braess discovered that if a new road is built in a congested system, everyone's journey unexpectedly lengthens (Bean, 1996). He explained this result by examining the behaviour of drivers, who made individual decisions about their journey, and the emergent effects of all these individual decisions upon the whole system. Consider a journey from A to D that can follow several routes, such as ABD or ACD (Figure 3.2).

The delay on any link is a function of *f*, which is the number of cars on that link. In case (a), there are two equidistant path choices. With 6 cars in the system, they will tend to distribute equally, with 3 cars on each path ABD and ACD. If they did not distribute equally, the congestion on one link would over time cause drivers to choose the less congested path. The expected delay is thus 83 on both routes. In case (b), a new link BC is added, creating a new path ABCD. Assuming previous path costs, drivers think ABCD is now the quickest route. Users take the new path to try and minimize their journey (Glance and Huberman, 1994), but the choice hurts the whole system. Equilibrium eventually occurs when 2 cars choose each of the paths ABD, ACD and ABCD. This puts 4 cars on the link AB. Now, the new road has increased the expected delay for everyone to 92.

do not know the exact state of the environment. For practical purposes, we usually restrict the description of a system to include a limited set of elements of the environment that are of immediate interest (see Box 3.2). Thus, one cannot divorce a physical system from the environment within which it exists because, by doing so, the very context for the system's existence disappears and its function will alter.

Systems have internal structure

If a system's overall behaviour arises out of the behaviour of its parts, then it has some internal structure. These components of a system are often decomposed into sub-systems for ease of understanding, manufacture, or maintenance. A health system is decomposed into community and hospital services. A hospital is decomposed into different departments. The amount of internal detail that can be described within a system is probably limitless. The description of the cardiovascular system could descend to the cellular level, or even the molecular level and beyond. The amount of detail one includes in the description of a system is usually determined by the purpose of the description, which is usually to describe its function.

Box 3.2
Penicillinase and the closed-world assumption

The introduction of antibiotics in the second half of the twentieth century heralded a period of optimism. Infectious diseases were soon to be a thing of the past, and every year saw the discovery of new drugs that attacked an ever-wider spectrum of bacteria. Then, as time went on, the tide started to turn the other way, as individual organisms such as penicillinase-producing bacteria developed resistance to specific drugs. Through a process of natural selection, the drugs that were created to kill bacteria were actually selecting individual organisms that were immune to their effects, allowing them to survive and dominate the gene pool. Some organisms now have such widespread resistance that their detection can shut down large sections of a hospital.

Modern medical science is often challenged by critics who cite examples like the development of antibiotic resistance as proof that its methods ultimately do more harm than good. However, this 'fight-back' of natural systems following the introduction of technology is not a phenomenon confined to medicine, but potentially affects every technological intervention made by humans (Tenner, 1996).

From a systems viewpoint, whenever a technology is introduced, the fight-back effect is not so much a fault of the technology as it is an inevitable consequence of the way that we understand systems. When we model the world, we intentionally simplify or exclude whole sections of reality to create a point of view. When a technology is applied, it is aimed at solving a particular problem with a system, with the assumption that its effects are predictable 'everything else being equal'. This clearly is never completely possible.

The assumption that everything that can be known is known is called the **closed-world assumption** in logic (Genesereth and Nilsson, 1988). Its function is to allow reasoning to proceed, even if our knowledge is incomplete. It serves a similar role when a technology is introduced into a system, because without it, we would never be sure we understood all the possible consequences of its actions.

So, rather than being a specific consequence of technology, unexpected outcomes are a result of the imperfect way we in which we understand the world. Our only way around it is to assume, at some stage, that we know enough to try things out. The alternative is to do nothing.

For a system to function each of its subsystems or components have to interact or communicate. This means that they may share inputs and outputs, with the output of one component providing the input to another. Inputs to a factory might be raw materials and energy, and its outputs could be manufactured products such as cars or foodstuffs. These in turn are inputs into the retail sector, which uses them to generate a financial output.

Systems can regulate their output by using feedback as input

A special case of connection of output to input between systems occurs when some or all of the output of a system is taken back as its own input. This is called **feedback** (see Figure 3.3). In this way a system can influence its future behaviour on the basis of a measurement of its past performance. The simplest feedback control system consists of three components:

- a **sensor**, which measures the parameter that is to be controlled
- a **comparator**, which determines whether the measurement deviates from the desired range
- an **activator**, which creates an output which then alters the environment in some way to change the value of the parameter being measured.

Feedback systems can become quite complicated in their design, and are used to create what are known as **cybernetic** or **control systems**, which are systems that are able to adapt their output to seek a particular goal. A closed control system might take its system output and directly pipe it back as feedback into the system. Most feedback control systems are more open and use a measurement sub-system to sample their output and determine what the next

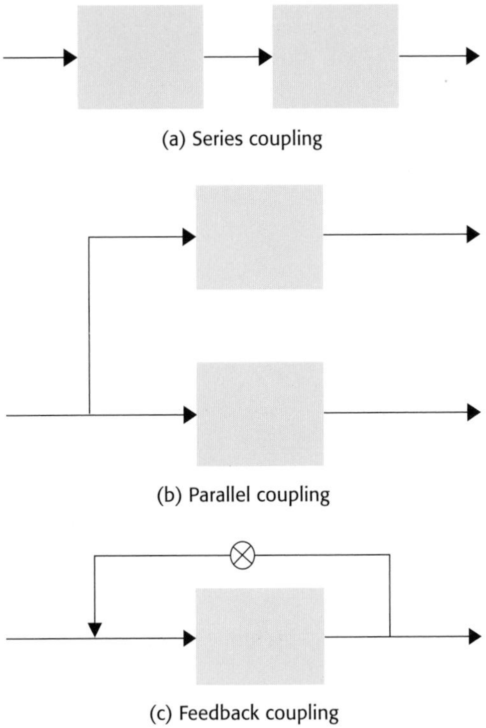
(a) Series coupling
(b) Parallel coupling
(c) Feedback coupling

Figure 3.3
Sub-systems may be coupled by joining their inputs to their outputs. In the special case of feedback, a sub-system takes some of its own output to modify its input.

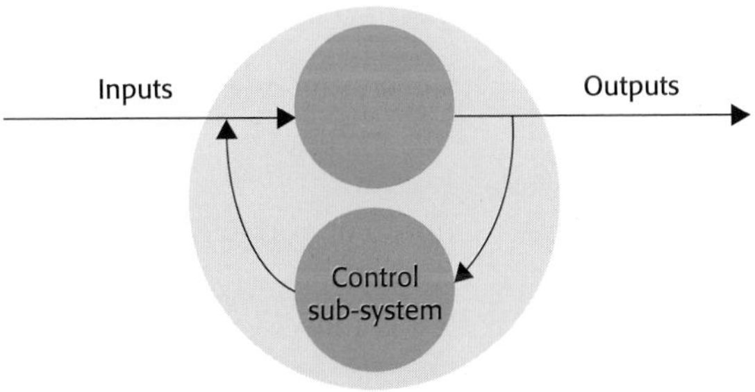
Inputs
Outputs
Control sub-system

Figure 3.4
The output of a system may be regulated by a control sub-system that measures the system's outputs and uses that to regulate the subsequent system inputs.

input should be (Figure 3.4). The extra feedback that is input into the system might come from an external source, but it is regulated by measurement of the system output.

For example, bank account interest is determined by measuring an account value, but the interest money comes from the bank – money sadly does not grow by itself. A thermostat is part of a feedback system for controlling temperature. The thermostat samples the temperature of a room that is being warmed by the heating system. As the temperature rises, the system shuts off when a preset temperature is reached, or turns on when the temperature drops below the **set point**. An insulin-dependent diabetic samples their blood sugar level with a glucometer, and uses the glucose value to adjust the next dose of insulin to be administered, on the basis of a rule or a formula that aims to keep blood sugar within a set range. The input to the diabetic patient 'system' is a dose of insulin and food, and the output is an effect on blood sugar that is then used to alter the next input of insulin and food. The thermostat and the glucometer are both measurement devices that form an integral part of a feedback-controlled system.

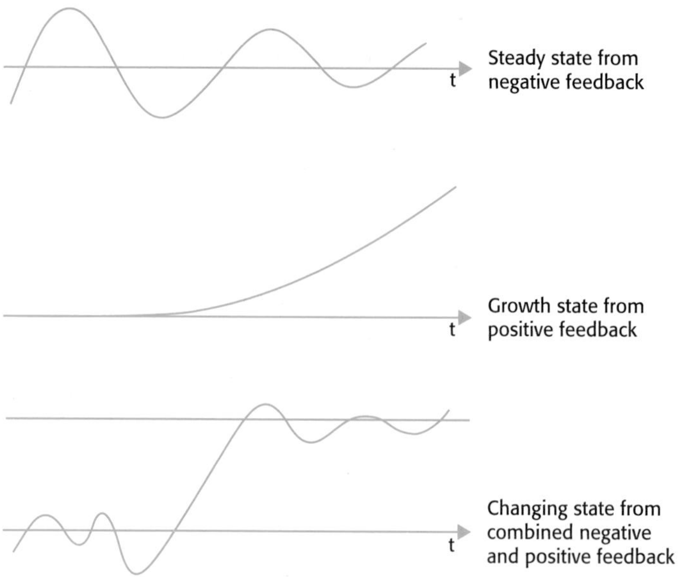
t
Steady state from negative feedback
t
Growth state from positive feedback
t
Changing state from combined negative and positive feedback

Figure 3.5
System states can be maintained or varied, depending on the type of feedback control being used (after Littlejohn, 1996).

There are two basic types of feedback system (Figure 3.5):

- In a **negative feedback** arrangement, the output of a system is subtracted from the next input, with the effect of restricting the system to working within a steady operating range. Physiological systems mostly use negative feedback mechanisms to provide **homeostasis** – the maintenance of a desired pre-set physical state, despite variations in the external world. Homeostatic mechanisms maintain everything from body temperature to the concentration of ions within cells.
- In a **positive feedback** system, the output of a system is added to its next input, resulting in the system output increasing with time. For example, a savings account increases in value if interest is added to it. Even a single deposit 'input' in a bank account will cause the value to increase over time if interest is added regularly, since each interest payment increases the system value and is used to calculate an even larger interest payment the next time.

Positive and negative feedback systems can be combined to allow a system to change from one to another of a number of predefined states. The positive feedback component permits the system to move from one state to another, and the negative feedback comes in to play when the new state has been reached, and keeps the system there.

Systems are arbitrary

We create descriptions of systems to help us understand the observable world. So, by their very nature, systems are completely arbitrary human creations. There can thus never be something called 'the correct' definition of a system, whether one is talking about a description of something in the world or a design to accomplish some function.

There are many possible ways in which one might choose to create a system, and it is often only a matter of convention and practicality that one set of descriptions is chosen over another. Equally, it should come as no surprise that two system descriptions might overlap, and have common elements. Are the pulmonary arteries more properly part of the cardiovascular system, or are they part of the respiratory system? It depends entirely upon one's point of view.

Systems are purposive

This brings us to a key point. Descriptions of a system are constructed with a function or purpose in mind. The reason people developed the modern descriptions of different physiological system was with the intent of treating illness. The reason that one particular system begins to gain common acceptance over another is that it is seen to be inherently more useful for that purpose. Thus phrenology, the study of bumps on the skull, was replaced by a system of thought we now call neurology, as this newer viewpoint proved itself to be a more useful approach to the treatment of illness. So, over time whole systems of thought gradually fall into disuse as newer and more valuable ones appear.

People also tend to develop systematic routines because they find themselves doing the same task again and again. They thus pick out some elements of their actions that recur, and give them some objective existence by calling them a routine. So, with a purpose in mind, a part of the world is labelled, and a system is born.

During the French revolution, a method was devised to create logarithm tables en masse. *Individuals called computers each carried out a small calculation, and as a result the team of individuals was able to carry out a large number of complex calculations. In his seminal treatise* On the Economy of Machinery and Manufactures *(1833), Charles Babbage reasoned that, since such complex calculations could all in principle be broken down into simple steps of addition or subtraction, then these could be carried out by machine. This inspired him to devise his difference engine, which was the first proposal for a general purpose calculating machine.*

3.3 Information systems contain data and models

When the same kind of decision is made on a regular basis, it will require access to the same kind of data and may use the same knowledge. In these circumstances, one can develop a regular process or **information system** to accomplish the task. An information system could thus be anything from the routine way in which a clinician records patient details in a pocket notebook, the way a triage nurse assesses patients on arrival in an emergency department, through to a complex computer-based system that regulates payments for healthcare services.

An information system is distinguished from other systems by its components, which include data and models. Recall from the last chapter that there are several different kinds of information model, including databases and knowledge bases. These different information components can be put together to create an information system. For example, consider a calculator that can store data and equations in its memory. The data store is the calculator's database, and the equation store is its knowledge base. The input to the calculator becomes the equation to be solved, as well as the values of data to plug into the equation. The database communicates with the knowledge base using a simple **communication channel** within the device, and the output of the system is the value for the solved equation (Figure 3.6).

There are many potential internal components that could be included within an information system, including a database, a knowledge base, an ontology, and decision procedures or rules of inference. The different components of an information system are connected together with input/output channels, which allow data to be shifted between the components as needed.

A patient record system is a more complex example of an information system. Its purpose is to record data about particular patients in some formalized fashion to assist in the control

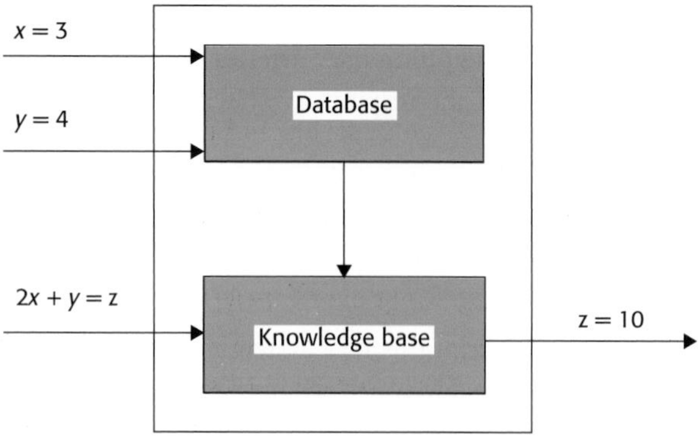
x = 3
y = 4
Database
2x + y = z
Knowledge base
z = 10

Figure 3.6
A calculator with a stored equation is an information system. The inputs are the equation to be solved and the data values, and the output of the system is dependent on the input values.

of patient management. The patient record system is composed of a patient database, organized according to data models which are based upon the way clinicians use the data in their decision-making process. The definition of a patient record system might also include an ontology that stipulates the medical language or terminology to be used in the records. The record system may also contain decision procedures that govern the way that the records are to be accessed and filed, and possibly even which individuals are permitted to use the records. All these elements together constitute the whole of a system which has been created to capture and re-use information about patients to facilitate treatment. The patient information system itself is a component of a bigger system, which might be the particular institution within which it exists, or the health system as a whole.

We saw at the beginning of this chapter that there are actually three different meanings of the word 'system' – a system can be an abstracted description of the real world, a template to action, or an artefact constructed from the real world. Consequently, an 'information system' might be one of three things:

- A simplified description of an existing set of information processes. For example, one could produce a document or diagram cataloguing the different input and output flows of information that connect a number of different organizations.
- A plan for implementing a new set of information processes.
- An actual physical system. The Internet is an information system consisting of computer hardware, software, data such as text and graphics stored as web pages, network connections, and the people using these technologies.

Information systems can be created for a number of reasons. In the main, it is because an information process is very common, very complex or in some way critical. In the first case, the goal of introducing an information system is to reduce the effort of decision-making by streamlining the process. In the case of complex or critical decisions, the information system's role is either to reduce complexity, or to minimize the likelihood of error.

Information systems share all of the characteristics of systems described earlier. We pick out decisions, data and models that are in some way consistent as a group that is of interest for some purpose, and then look upon them as a system. Each information system exists within an environment, and is usually purpose built to interact with the environment. In other words, we want to manage specific activities within that environment, and want to influence their outcomes in a certain way.

Conclusions

We have now reached a point where we can look at an information system in a fairly complex and rich way, on the basis of an understanding of the basic principles of models, information structures, and systems. Through a variety of examples, we have seen how information systems are often designed to be part of a feedback control system used to manage clinical activities. Whenever a decision is important enough, or is made often enough, then an information system is built to manage the process. With this background, it is now possible to move on and look at how information is used to support clinical activities.

In the next section of the book, we will learn how to search for, structure and use information in the support of clinical processes, and in the following section, see how healthcare is structured from an informational viewpoint, and see how information systems reflect and contribute to that structure.

Discussion points

1 Why might a patient object to being considered an input to a 'health system'?

2 What are the inputs and outputs of a patient record system?

3 How many states can you identify for the cardiovascular system, and how does each state change the way the system handles its inputs and outputs?

4 What is the purpose of the health system? What are the components of the health system? What is the purpose of each component?

5 Compare the structure of the health system in the United States and the United Kingdom. If the purpose of both systems is the same, how do you explain the differences in their components?

6 When is a model not a system? When is a system not a model?*

7 Identify one positive and one negative feedback system in the health system. What are the inputs and outputs? Which components act as sensors, comparators and activators? What is the purpose of the system in terms of control?

* If a model has no decomposable parts, no inputs and outputs, then it is not a system. If a system is an artefact or a process in the real world then it is not a model; however, if that system has been constructed, then it is probably an instantiation of a model.

Chapter summary

1 A system is a collection of component ideas, processes or objects.

2 Systems transform inputs into outputs, and may change their state in doing so.

3 A system has behaviour that cannot usually be predicted by an examination of its individual components, but emerges out of the way that the components interact with each other.

4 Physical systems are embedded in an environment: closed systems have no external inputs and outputs; open systems interact freely with their surrounding environment.

5 Systems have internal structure.

6 Systems can regulate their output by using feedback as input: In a negative feedback arrangement, the output of a system is subtracted from the next input; in a positive feedback system, the output of a system is added to its next input.

7 A feedback control system consists of a sensor, which measures the parameter that is to be controlled, a comparator, which determines whether the measurement deviates from the desired range, and an activator, which creates an output to change the value of the parameter being measured.

8 Systems are arbitrary and purposive.

9 Information systems contain data and models, which include databases and knowledge bases that interact via a communication channel.

PART 2

Informatics skills

CHAPTER 4

Communicating

The chart is not the patient. *Gall (1986).*

Every clinical action, every treatment choice and investigation, is shaped by the available information. We can think of this information as the clinical evidence that is used to make a judgement about the right course of action. Clinicians gather evidence through communication with others, either through what is said now, or what has been documented from before.

There are many different sources of clinical evidence that can be used in the routine care of a patient, and these include:

- the patient, who will give information about their symptoms and their problems, as well as demonstrate clinical signs through physical examination
- the clinical literature, which captures past knowledge about disease and treatment
- the patient record, which records the history of a patient's state, based upon clinical observation and laboratory and imaging reports, as well as their various treatments and the impact of treatment on their disease
- clinical measurement devices, from simple things like a blood pressure cuff, through to complex devices such as a glucometer, cardiogram or multiprobe patient monitor in intensive care
- clinical colleagues, who may exchange messages containing information about the state of patients, their opinions, their own workload and needs, or clinical knowledge.

The information contained in these clinical 'messages' comes in a variety of media and formats and can be delivered in a variety of ways including face-to-face conversations, letters, e-mail, voicemail, and electronic or paper medical records.

When this exchange of information works well, clinical care is solidly based upon the best evidence. When information exchanges are poor, the quality of clinical care can suffer enormously. For example, the single commonest cause of adverse clinical events is medication error, which account for about 19% of all adverse events, and the commonest prescription errors can be redressed by the provision of better information about medications or the patients receiving them (Bates *et al.*, 2001). Poor presentation of clinical data can also lead to poorly informed clinical practice, inappropriate repeat investigation or unnecessary referrals, and wastes clinical time and other resources (Wyatt and Wright, 1998).

In this chapter we will look at the communication process and explore how variations in the structure of clinical messages affect the way in which they are interpreted, and therefore affect the quality of care. If the motto for Chapter 1 was 'a map is not the territory' then the motto for this chapter is 'the chart is not the patient'.

4.1 The structure of a message determines how it will be understood

What a message is meant to say when it is created, and what the receiver of a message understands, may not be the same. This is because what we humans understand is profoundly shaped by the way data are presented to us, and by the way we react to different data presentations. Thus it is probably as important to structure data in a way so that they can be best understood, as it is to ensure that the data are correct in the first place.

What a clinician understands after seeing the data in a patient record and what the data actually show are very different things. For example, the way data are structured has a profound effect on the conclusions a clinician will draw from the data. In Figure 4.1, identical patient data are presented in four different ways (Elting *et al.*, 1999). The data show

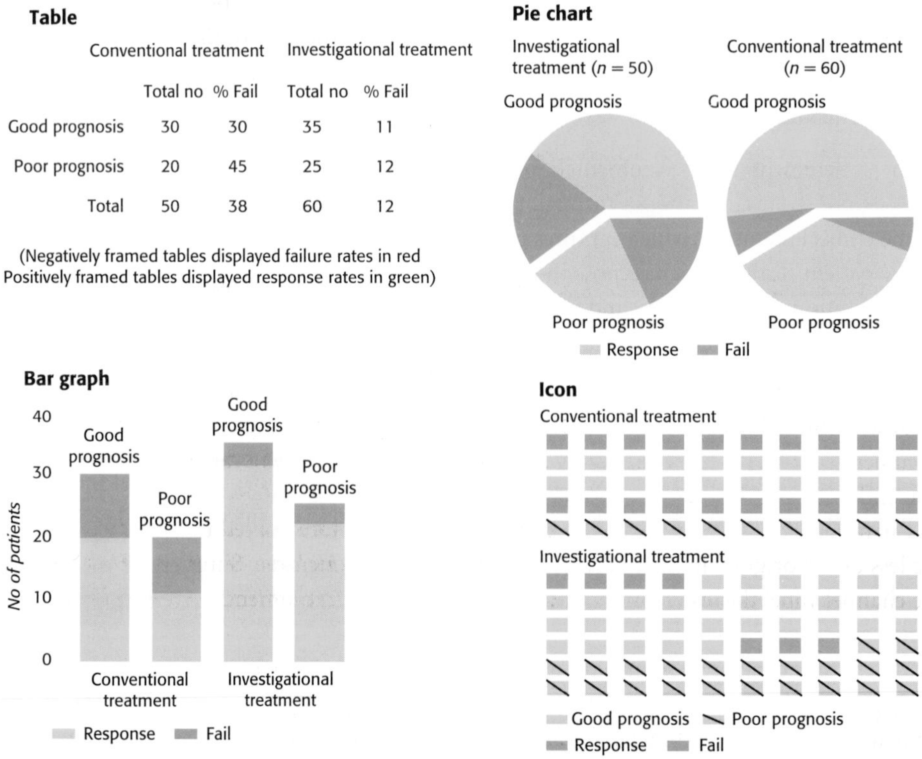
Pie chart
Investigational treatment (n = 50)
Conventional treatment (n = 60)
Good prognosis
Good prognosis
Poor prognosis
Poor prognosis
Response
Fail
Bar graph
40
30
20
10
0
No of patients
Good prognosis
Poor prognosis
Good prognosis
Poor prognosis
Conventional treatment
Investigational treatment
Response
Fail
Icon
Conventional treatment
Investigational treatment
Good prognosis
Poor prognosis
Response
Fail

Table

	Conventional treatment		Investigational treatment	
	Total no	% Fail	Total no	% Fail
Good prognosis	30	30	35	11
Poor prognosis	20	45	25	12
Total	50	38	60	12

(Negatively framed tables displayed failure rates in red
Positively framed tables displayed response rates in green)

Figure 4.1
Table, pie chart, icon and bar graph displays of the same data from a hypothetical clinical trial, each resulted in a different percentage of correct decisions to be made. The icon display (bottom right) was most effective for the decision to stop the clinical trial (from Elting *et al.*, 1999).

preliminary results from two hypothetical clinical trials of a generic 'conventional treatment' compared with a generic 'investigational treatment', both treating the same condition. In an experiment to see if clinicians would decide to stop the trial because the data show one of the treatments was obviously better than the other, the decision to stop varied significantly depending upon how the data were displayed. Correct decisions were significantly more common with icon displays (82%) and tables (68%) than with pie charts or bar graphs (both 56%).

If this example was reflected in actual clinical practice, up to 25% of the patients treated according to data displayed as bar graphs or pie charts would have received inappropriate treatment. Consequently, there is an enormous difference between simply communicating a message to a colleague, and communicating it effectively.

4.2 The message that is sent may not be the message that is received

Messages are misunderstood both because of the limitations of the agents interpreting them, and because the very process of communication itself is limited. To explore the nature of communication, we will develop a general model that describes the process of sending a message between two agents. The agents might be two human beings, or a human and a computer. A communication act occurs between the two agents A_1 and A_2 when agent A_1 constructs a message m_1 for some specific purpose, and sends m_1 to agent A_2 across a **communication channel** (Figure 4.2).

The second agent A_2 receives a message m_2, which may in some ways be different from the intended message m_1. The effectiveness of the communication between the agents is dependent upon several things – the nature of the channel, the state of the individual agents, the knowledge possessed by the agents, and the context within which the agents find themselves.

Communication channels distort messages

A wide variety of different communication channels are available to us, from the basic face-to-face conversation, through to telecommunication channels such as telephone or e-mail, and non-interactive channels such as the medical record.

The message is sent as a signal down the channel, and the message signal may be corrupted because of limitations in the channel bearing the message. For example, faxed or photocopied documents may be harder to read than digitally transmitted documents because of poor resolution and distortion of the transmitted document.

*The **signal to noise ratio** measures how much a particular message has been corrupted by noise that has been added to it during transmission across a channel.*

Channels vary in their **capacity** to carry data, and the more limited the channel capacity, the less of the original message can be transmitted at any one time. Simply put, the thinner the channel 'pipe', the less data can flow through at any given moment.

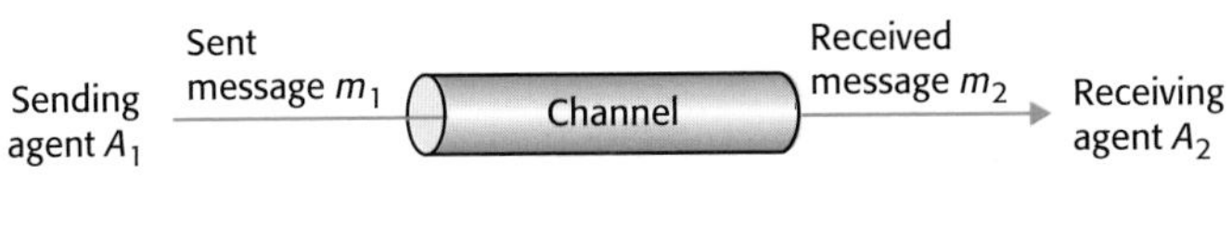
Sending agent A_1
Sent message m_1
Channel
Received message m_2
Receiving agent A_2

Figure 4.2
A communication channel between two agents.

Channels also have different abilities to send a message exactly as it was sent, and often the message is distorted in transmission. This distortion is usually called **noise**. Noise can be thought of technically as any unwanted signal that is added to a transmitted message while being carried along a channel, and distorts the message for the receiver. So, noise can be anything from the static on a radio, to another conversation next to your own, making it hard to hear your partner – one person's signal is another's noise. Standard information theory

Box 4.1
Information theory

Claude Shannon developed the mathematical basis for information theory while working at Bell Laboratories during the 1940s. Motivated by problems in communication engineering, Shannon developed a method to measure the amount of 'information' that could be passed along a communication channel between a source and a destination.

Shannon was concerned with the process of communicating using radio, and for him the transmitter, ionosphere and receiver were all examples of communication **channels**. Such channels had a limited capacity and were noisy. Shannon developed definitions of channel capacity, noise and signal in terms of a precise measure of what he called 'information'.

He began by recognizing that before a message could enter a channel it had to be **encoded** in some way by a transmitter. For example, a piece of music needs to be transformed through a microphone into electronic signals before it can be transmitted. Equally, a signal would then need to be decoded at the destination by a receiver before it can be reconstructed into the original signal. A hi-fi speaker thus needs to decode an electronic signal before it can be converted back into sound.

Shannon was principally interested in studying the problem of maximizing the reliability of transmission of a signal, and minimizing the cost of that transmission. Encoding a signal was the mechanism for reducing the cost of transmission through **signal compression**, as well as combating corruption of the signal through **channel noise**.

The rules governing the operation of an encoder and a decoder constitute a **code**. The code described by Shannon corresponds to a model and its language. A code achieves reliable transmission if the source message is reproduced at the destination within prescribed limits. After Shannon, the problem for a communications engineer was to find an encoding scheme that made the best use of a channel while minimizing transmission noise.

With human verbal communication, the information source is the sender's brain and the transmitter is the vocal chords. Air provides the communication channel, and may distort any message sent because of extraneous noise, or because the message gets dampened or **attenuated** the further the distance between the communicating parties. The receiver in this model is the listener's ear, and the destination that decodes what has been received is the listener's brain.

Although Shannon saw his theory helping us understand human communication, it remains an essentially statistical analysis over populations of messages, and says little about individual acts of communication. Specifically information theory is silent on the notion on the meaning of a message, since it does not explicitly deal with the way a knowledge base is used to interpret the data in a message.

Further reading

van der Lubbe JCA (1997) *Information Theory*. Cambridge University Press, Cambridge.

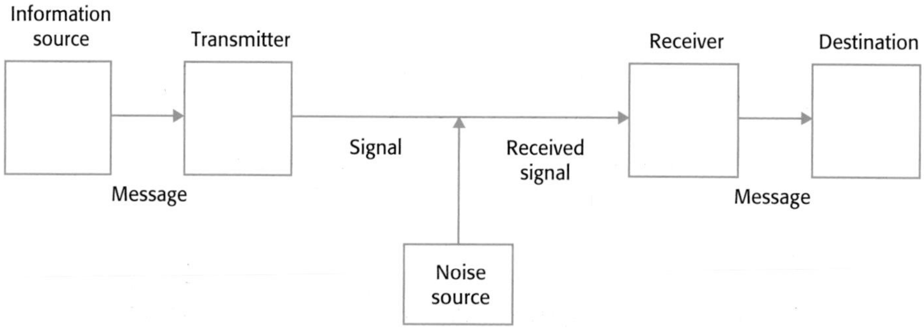
Information source
Transmitter
Receiver
Destination
Message
Signal
Received signal
Message
Noise source

Figure 4.3
Information theory describes how a message is transmitted between two agents.

describes how the outcome of a communication is determined in part by the capacity and noise characteristics of a channel (see Box 4.1).

So, we note that in general, when an agent sends a message, the message may be modified by the channel, and be received as a slightly different message by the receiving agent.

Individuals don't know the same things

In Chapter 2 we saw that the inferences that can be drawn from data are dependent on the knowledge used to make the inference. Since different individuals 'know' slightly different things, they will usually draw different inferences from the same data because of this variation in their individual knowledge. Thus variations in diagnosis and treatment decisions, based upon the same data, may simply reflect the differences in clinical knowledge between individual clinicians.

However, when sending a message, we have to make assumptions about the knowledge that the receiver has, and use that to shape our message. There is no point in explaining what is already known, but it is equally important not to miss out important details that the receiver should know to draw the right conclusions. Thus notionally identical messages sent to a clinical colleague or to a patient end up being very different because we assume that the colleague has more common knowledge, and requires less explanation, than the patient. The knowledge shared between individuals is sometimes called **common ground** (Coiera, 2000).

This explains why individuals communicate more easily with others who have similar experiences, beliefs and knowledge. Intuitively we know that it takes greater effort to explain something in a conversation to someone with whom we share less common background. Conversely, individuals who are particularly close can communicate complicated ideas in terse shorthand. One of the reasons agents create common ground is to optimize their interaction. By sharing ground, less needs to be said in any given message, making the interaction less costly (Box 21.1).

With this in mind, we can now say that each agent possesses knowledge about the world, in the form of a set of models *K*. Critically, the private world models of the two communicating agents in our model, K_1 and K_2, are not identical. Thus agent A_1 creates a message m_1, based upon its knowledge of the world K_1 (Figure 4.4). A_2 receives a slightly different message m_2 because of channel effects, and then generates its own private interpretation of the message's meaning based on its own knowledge K_2. Further, agent A_1 makes a guess about the content of K_2, and shapes its message to include data or knowledge it believes agent A_2 will need to make sense of the message being sent. The effectiveness of the message is dependent

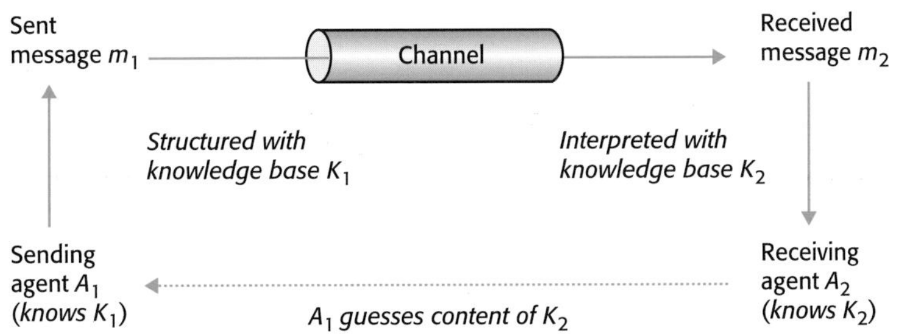
Sent message m_1
Channel
Received message m_2
Structured with knowledge base K_1
Interpreted with knowledge base K_2
Sending agent A_1 (knows K_1)
Receiving agent A_2 (knows K_2)
A_1 guesses content of K_2

Figure 4.4
When a message is sent between two agents, it is built according to a model that we think will be understood by the receiving agent, and is potentially distorted during transmission by the communication channel.

upon the quality of the guess an agent can make about what the receiving agent knows. Usually, agents send more than is needed, because some redundancy in a message improves the chance that what the receiver needs is actually sent.

Messages are constructed according to imperfect models of the world

Sending and receiving messages are model-based processes. Consequently, the process of communication is fundamentally limited in its capacity not just by physical limitations of transmission channels, but by the inherent limitations of modelling which were outlined in Chapter 1.

Model theory tells us that the sender of a message is operating with models of the world that will always be inaccurate in one way or another, and that equally, the receiver must attempt to interpret messages according to models that are themselves flawed in some way. Consequently, communication will never be a perfect process, and misinterpretation is at some level unavoidable.

The process of human communication suffers from some specific limitations that arise from the way humans use models, either to interpret physical symbols from data received by the senses, or to interpret that sense data according to mental models of the world:

- **Perceptual limitations:** We may misperceive the symbols that have been written or said to us. This may simply occur when the symbols are poorly constructed and therefore ambiguous. Drug names are often confused because of illegible handwriting. Further, each of the human senses can be thought of as a communication channel, each with its own unique capacities to carry and distort data. For example, individuals have different abilities to hear or see, and messages may be misunderstood because of sensory deficits. However, at a more fundamental level, the human perceptual system itself distorts sense

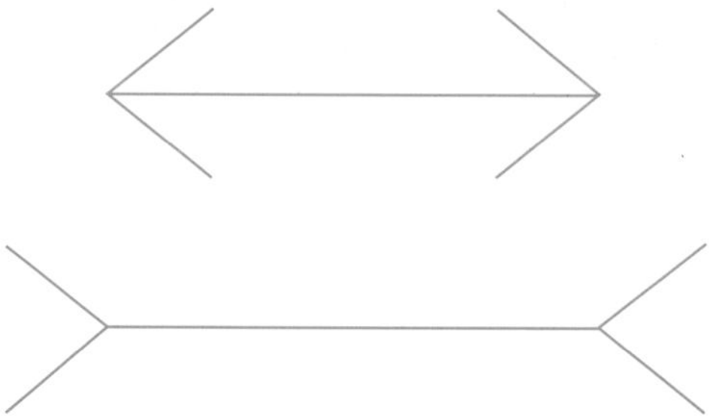

Figure 4.5
The Müller–Lyer illusion demonstrates how human perception distorts sense data. The central lines in both upper and lower figures are actually identical in length, but the lower segment appears to be longer.

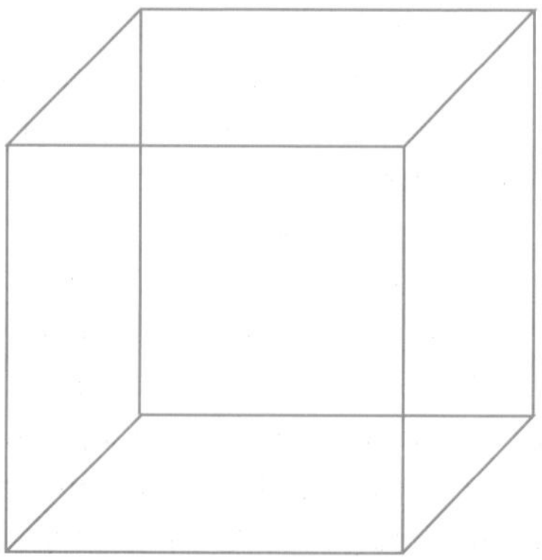

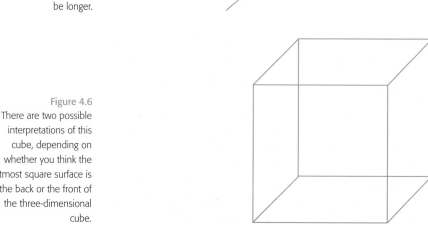

Figure 4.6
There are two possible interpretations of this cube, depending on whether you think the rightmost square surface is at the back or the front of the three-dimensional cube.

data, exaggerating some characteristics and minimizing others. It does this presumably because the brain has evolved to preferentially recognize some patterns over others as more important to survival. Consequently, what we perceive, and what actually exists, are not the same thing (Figure 4.5). Although there is much argument about the exact process, perception is an active process of attempting to map sense data to internal models of the world (Van Leeuwin, 1998). Humans often try and fit what we sense through sight, sound, touch and smell to our pre-existing models of what we think should be there (Figure 4.6).

- **Human attention limitations:** Humans may not pay enough attention to a message, and miss some of its content, or misinterpret the content. This occurs because human attention has a very limited capacity to process items (see Box 8.2). When individuals are distracted by other tasks, they are less likely to have the capacity to attend fully to a message. So, when an individual is receiving a message, the amount of cognitive resource available determines the quality of the inferences they can draw. When a message is constructed, we should therefore consider the cognitive state of the individual receiving the message. For example, in a stressful situation, a clinical flowchart that makes all the steps in treating a patient explicit will require less attention than the same information presented as paragraphs of unstructured text, which require the reader to extract the appropriate steps in the treatment.
- **Cognitive biases:** Humans do not perceive information in a neutral way. We have an inherent set of biases that cause us to draw conclusions not supported by the immediate evidence (see Box 8.3). Put simply, we hear what we want to hear, or think we should hear. For example, recent events can bias us to recognize similar events, even when they are not present. Thus an encounter with a thyrotoxic patient can bias a clinician to overdiagnose the same disease in future underweight patients (Medin *et al.*, 1982). Humans also react to positive information differently to negative information. The way in which treatment results were framed in the experiments shown in Figure 4.1 made a significant difference. Negatively framed tables (those reporting treatment failure rates) resulted in significantly more decisions to stop treatment than positive ones reporting success rates (Elting *et al.*, 1999).

4.3 Grice's conversational maxims provide a set of rules for conducting message exchanges

How is it that agents, whether they are human or computer, manage to communicate effectively given the inherent limitations of message exchange? More importantly from our point of view, given that poor communication can have a profound negative impact on healthcare delivery, what makes a good message?

One of the most influential answers to these questions comes from the work of H. Paul Grice (1975), who took a very pragmatic approach to the mechanics of conversation. Grice suggested that well-behaved agents all communicate according to a basic set of rules that ensure conversations are effective and that each agent understands what is going on in the conversation.

Most generally, the **cooperative principle** asks each agent who participates in a conversation to do their best to make it succeed. Agents should only make appropriate contributions to a conversation, saying just what is required of them, saying it at the appropriate stage in the conversation, and only to satisfy the accepted purpose of the conversation. Grice proposed a set of **four maxims**, which explicitly defined what he meant by the principle of cooperation:

1 **Maxim of quantity:** Say only what is needed.
   1.1 Be sufficiently informative for the current purposes of the exchange.
   1.2 Do not be more informative than is required.
2 **Maxim of quality:** Make your contribution one that is true.
   2.1 Do not say what you believe to be false.
   2.2 Do not say that for which you lack adequate evidence.
3 **Maxim of relevance:** Say only what is pertinent to the context of the conversation at the moment.
4 **Maxim of manner:**
   4.1 Avoid obscurity of expression.
   4.2 Avoid ambiguity.
   4.3 Be brief.
   4.4 Be orderly.

There are some overlaps in the maxims, but they lay out a set of rules that guide how conversations should proceed. Clearly also, people do not always follow these maxims. Sometimes it is simply because agents are not well behaved. At other times, agents break the rules on purpose to communicate more subtle messages. For example, people are often indirect in their answers when asked a question. If someone asked you 'How much do you earn?' a wry answer might be 'Not enough!' or something similarly vague. Such an answer is clearly uncooperative, and violates the maxim of quantity, relevance, and manner in different ways. However, the clear message behind the answer is 'This is none of your business'. The intentional violation of maxims allows us to signal things without actually having to say them, either because it might be socially unacceptable, or because there are other constraints on what can be said at the time (Littlejohn, 1996).

Conclusions

In this chapter, we have used the idea of models and templates to develop a rich picture of the process of structuring and communicating information. Communication is a complex phenomenon that is usually ignored in routine clinical practice, yet getting it right has profound implications for the quality of patient care.

In the next chapter we are going to take this communication model and use it explain the ways we can structure one of the commonest of clinical 'messages' – the patient record.

Discussion points

1 'The chart is not the patient'. Explain why people might confuse the two, perhaps thinking back to Chapter 1, and explain why they should keep the two separate.

2 Marshall McLuhan famously said 'the medium is the message'. What did he mean? Do you agree?

3 The way we interpret a message is shaped by the way a message is constructed. Give examples of the way public figures such as politicians shape their messages to have a specific impact on public opinion.

4 A politician will shape their message differently, depending upon which medium they are using at the time. Compare the way the same message will look on television news, in the newspaper, in a magazine article, or when delivered over the phone or face to face.

5 In the game 'Chinese Whispers' a message is passed along a chain, from one individual to the next. By the time the message reaches the end of the chain, it is highly distorted compared to the original. Explain the possible causes of this message distortion.

6 Within healthcare, a message can be passed down long chains of individuals. What mechanisms do we have to prevent the 'Chinese Whispers' effect distorting critical clinical data?

7 You need to send a copy of a 200-page paper medical record to a colleague in another institution. What is the best channel to use? Consider the impact that urgency, distance or cost might make on your answer.

8 You have a question about your patient's treatment. What is the best channel to use to get an opinion from a colleague?

Chapter summary

1 What a message is meant to say when it is created, and what the receiver of a message understands, may not be the same.

2 The structure of a message determines how it will be understood. The way clinical data are structured can alter the conclusions a clinician will draw from the data.

3 The message that is sent may not be the message that is received. The effectiveness of communication between two agents is dependent upon:
- the communication channel which will vary in capacity to carry data and noise which distorts the message
- the knowledge possessed by the agents, and the common ground between them
- the resource limitations of agents including cognitive limits on memory and attention
- the context within which the agents find themselves which dictate which resources are available and the competing tasks at hand.

4 Grice's conversational maxims provide a set of rules for conducting message exchanges:
- **Maxim of quantity:** Say only what is needed.
- **Maxim of quality:** Make your contribution one that is true.
- **Maxim of relevance:** Say only what is pertinent to the context of the conversation at the moment.
- **Maxim of manner:** Avoid obscurity of expression, ambiguity, be brief and orderly.

CHAPTER 5

Structuring

> Everyone writing in the medical record is an information designer, and is responsible for making the data recorded there easy to find and interpret. *Wyatt and Wright (1998).*

Grice's maxims give us a set of rules for conversational economy. The cooperative principle is actually a bargain between agents that they will not waste each other's time and that they will genuinely try to say what is needed. In healthcare, the stakes are higher because the resources of many individuals are thinly stretched, and time wasting or misleading behaviour will have a negative impact on the efficiency of clinical work and patient care.

Consequently, with health communication, Grice's maxims are not a social nicety, but a professional necessity. When constructing a message, it is therefore insufficient simply to pass on information. It is critical that the intended individual actually receives the information, that they correctly interpret it, and that the effort expended in understanding the message fits within the work constraints of the receiver.

How does one decide what should be put into a message? What is 'sufficiently informative', and not obscure or ambiguous? Using the model of communication developed in the last chapter, we can now set out a process for determining the structure and content of a message.

5.1 Messages are structured to achieve a specific task using available resources to suit the needs of the receiver

A message is a package of data and some of the models needed to interpret the data. As with all models, the message is therefore shaped primarily to accomplish a specific purpose. For example, in a request for a radiological investigation, the request contains the clinical data needed to assist the radiologist in interpreting the image, as well as details of the clinical conditions that need to be specifically excluded. The more specific the request is about the clinician's goals, the more precise the answer from the radiologist will be.

In general, the more that is known about the way a message will be used, the more it can be structured according to the specific needs of that task. For example, information in a telephone directory is produced with the goal of assisting people to locate individuals. Compare the structure of a telephone directory where companies are arranged according to their business type with one where companies are organized according to user tasks. In the former case, which we will call **data-oriented**, phone numbers are organized according to general business types, such as you might find in a 'yellow pages' directory. Businesses might appear under a heading such as 'travel agents'. In contrast, in the **task-oriented** directory, headings might be 'planning a holiday' or 'organizing a wedding'. Under 'planning a holiday' you might find entries for embassies to get a travel visa, and businesses that can help book a flight, arrange accommodation, organize health checks and vaccinations, sell luggage and so forth. The task-oriented directory has collected together all the typical information elements needed to accomplish a task.

The data-oriented directory is optimized for users who are assumed to know all the elements of their task, and just need to find businesses that can help them. Consequently it is very space efficient, since most business will appear under only one heading, but an informed user will need to make multiple accesses to the directory using an index to complete a complex task such as booking a holiday. In contrast, the task-based directory is optimized to assist users to complete a defined task. Users don't need to know all the task elements since they are assembled there and their presence in the directory prompts the user to think of them. However, the task-oriented directory is space inefficient. One business might reappear under many different task headings. A photographer might appear under a wedding listing as well as in the travel section because they take passport photographs. Further, if a user's task is not included in the directory, then it is of little value to them. The data-oriented style directory is suited to handling a wide variety of tasks, many that its creators have not anticipated, since it assumes that users know what they are doing, and therefore can be used in a wider set of situations than the task-oriented directory.

A third approach to directory construction avoids the pitfalls of both. The task-oriented directory can be decomposed into a database, which is the original data-oriented directory, and a separate knowledge base, containing all the task knowledge. Each task description in the knowledge base is a template that describes the different steps involved in completing a task, and contains cross-references into the database, which indicate where to look up the information needed to accomplish the task. So, our telephone directory now would have two parts – a front section structured like a normal yellow pages, and a back section with a set of templates for common tasks indicating which professional groups should be called to accomplish a given task. A user can look up a template, which will guide them through the task, and direct them to the appropriate categories in the data-oriented database.

This **template-oriented** directory is optimum both in terms of space usage, since data duplication is minimized, and in terms of utility, since it can be used whether or not the user's task appears in the knowledge base. A user can choose to use either the database alone (when the templates don't fit their needs), the templates alone (when the database is inadequate), or use them together if they are well cross-indexed and meet user needs. However, a template-oriented message is the most complex information structure, since the database and knowledge base need to be defined as separate entities, and then be cross-linked, and this is a complex and skilled task.

Table 5.1 Costs and benefits of different message classes.

Message class	Predominant content	Space utilization	Cost to build	Receiving agent	Cost to use	Scope of utility
Data-oriented	Data	Best	Least	Knows task	Most	Broad range of tasks
Task-oriented	Data intermingled with task knowledge	Worst	Moderate	Does not need to know all steps in task	Least	Narrow, limited to defined tasks
Template-oriented	Data and task knowledge separate but cross-linked	Moderate	Most	May or may not know task	Variable depending upon task	Broad range of tasks

It would seem from this discussion that template-oriented messages might be the 'best'. However, as with any information structure, we can never make the case that a specific message class is 'best' for all messages (Table 5.1). For example, when the sender and receiver share much common ground, as we might find in a pair of clinicians who work closely together, then much of their work communication is going to be data-oriented. On the other hand, if one is writing a manual to be read by many people, when we know little of what common ground they might share with the authors, then a template-directed approach might be best. In some circumstances, when ease of use is the primary concern, then a task-oriented approach may be best. For example, procedures that are designed to be read during an emergency are probably best to be task oriented.

The Gricean 'bargain' between agents thus does not say that the message is always created to maximize the benefit of only the receiver of the message. Conversational economy means that agents agree to create messages that, on average, satisfy the needs of both sender and receiver. The cost of creating a message is as important a consideration as the cost of receiving it. The point of maximal cost might be borne by the sender, or the receiver, or shared equally, depending upon the nature of the message and the nature of the relationship between the agents.

The channel is selected on the basis of its suitability to the task

The choice to use one communication channel over another is often not considered explicitly in clinical settings, but poor channel choice can have a substantial impact on the quality of a received message. For example, some channels, such as the telephone or radio pager, have the characteristic of immediately interrupting the receiver of the message. Others, such as voicemail or e-mail, are not interruptive but can be accessed at a time of the receiver's choice. Interruptive channels are often called **synchronous** channels because they demand real-time interaction between agents. Non-interruptive channels are called **asynchronous** channels, because the interaction between agents can occur at separate moments over an extended period. Many clinicians use synchronous channels, or even face-to-face interruption 'in the corridor' as their preferred way of communicating, without any conscious attention to the cost of that choice to the receiver.

In fact, the decision to interrupt another individual has an impact on their work, and may result in them forgetting the task they are currently working on, or other tasks in memory (Parker and Coiera, 2000). Although it is often appropriate to choose to interrupt others, for example in moments of urgency, the sender of a message should consider the current situation of the receiver and reflect this in their choice of channel, aiming to minimize its impact on the receiver's tasks.

As discussed earlier, communication channels also have varying message transport characteristics, such as capacity to carry a certain amount of data at any given time, and degree to which data are distorted through noise. Depending on the length of the message or the risk of message degradation through noise, we may prefer to choose one channel to another.

Research has also shown that different types of message are more effective when transmitted with some channels than others. For example, are public health messages better transmitted using mass media like television, or as more personal messages, such as letters? The answer is complex, but seems to relate both to the cost of using a channel by the receiver of it, as well as the benefit the receiver expects to obtain from the message (Trumbo, 1998).

The receiver's knowledge alters the effectiveness of a message

As we saw earlier, different agents know different things, and the sender of a message has to make a guess about the common ground they share with the receiving agent. Specifically, a sender must guess what data a receiver has access to, and what knowledge they have. On the basis of that knowledge, the message will contain what the sender believes the receiver is lacking.

Thus, agents vary in the terminology they are familiar with. Communication is often difficult because of the use of unshared technical terms, or jargon, by one agent. When communicating to patients, it is essential to avoid jargon. In one UK study that looked at educational leaflets about asthma written for patients, they found most assumed a 'reading age' close to secondary school entry level. However, to ensure that most of the population can understand such leaflets, the leaflets should have a much lower reading age, around mid-primary school level (Smith *et al.*, 1998). Since at the time of the study 22% of the UK population were judged to have a low level of literacy, they would have had great difficulty in understanding the content of the health messages contained in those leaflets.

Message complexity and jargon also have an impact on effectiveness of messages aimed at health professionals. For example, clinicians are less likely to comply with clinical guidelines that are written in a complex way (Grilli and Lomas, 1994). Using a measure of document complexity, guidelines with high complexity had a significantly lower compliance rate (41.9%) than those judged to be low in complexity (55.9%).

A common problem with clinician-to-patient communication is not just that they do not share the same training and language, but they do not even share the same goals during the conversation. A clinician may be sending messages based upon their medical model of the purpose of a conversation, but the patient may have very different needs (Mathews, 1983).

Messages should be structured to emphasize key elements to enable rapid and accurate understanding

Note every individual will have the same time to receive and interpret a message. Consequently, the information elements in a message need to be structured in a way that minimizes the cost of receiving it, and ensures that the most important elements of the message are easily recognized. Not every agent will have the time to read through a medical document in detail, and those in a hurry may need a summary or key elements highlighted.

Re: Anne Patient d.o.b 10.10.46
29 Some Road, Sometown, Somecounty SC9 9SC
Node positive carcinoma of the left breast treated by mastectomy, chemotherapy, and radiotherapy

Radiotherapy treatment summary: the left chest wall and draining nodal areas received a dose of 42.9 Gy in 13 fractions treating three times a week with 6 MV photons. Treatment started on 15 September and was completed on 14 October 1995.

The patient will be followed up for one visit at Dr X's clinic and thereafter follow-up will be with Mr Y and Dr Z.

RADIOTHERAPY TREATMENT SUMMARY	
Name: Anne Patient **Born: 10 October 1946, age 49** **Address: 29 Some Road, Sometown, Somecounty SC9 9SC**	
Status before radiotherapy	
Diagnosis	**Carcinoma left breast**
Spread	**Left axillary nodes**
Previous treatment	**Mastectomy, chemotherapy**
Radiotherapy given	
Treatment type	**6 MV photons**
Site	**Left chest wall and draining nodes**
Total dose given	**43 Gray**
Schedule	**3 fractions/week from 15 September 1995 to 14 October 1995 (13 over 4 weeks)**
Follow-up plan	
Radiotherapy department	**One visit – Dr X**
Other departments	**Mr Y (surgery), Dr Z (ICRF clinic)**
Summary date: 20 October 1995	

Figure 5.1 Extract from an actual radiotherapy summary and below it a version revised to improve communication. (Gy = Grays, a unit of radiation measurement). (Based on Wright *et al.*, 1998).

In Figure 5.1, an example of a poor clinical message is shown along with a better version. In the original radiotherapy summary, the data are organized exactly as they were dictated by the clinician and typed by the transcriptionist. Date formats are used inconsistently and important data lie buried within the text. The radiation dose given in the therapy is written as the abbreviation '42·9 Gy', but '43 Gray' would probably be clearer. If the reader had never encountered the Gray as a scientific unit for the measurement of radiation, then the addition of an explanatory note defining the units in non-specialist terms might make the meaning of the report even easier to understand. Using the principles in Table 5.2, the revised format is more structured, allowing clinicians to find data such as the dose or duration of radiotherapy more rapidly, to interpret them more reliably, and non-specialists can understand more of it.

A standard template is used to structure a message when many different people will receive it

In the game of 'Chinese Whispers' a message is passed from one individual to the next along a chain. By the time the message has passed through many different agents, it typically is distorted both in structure and content. In healthcare, messages pass between many different individuals. Patient data, for example, may travel from laboratory to hospital medical record

Table 5.2 Six principles of information design that can aid interpretation of medical record data (Wright *et al.*, 1998).

1 **Set the context**
E.g. give the date and main purpose of the consultation
2 **Write informative headings**
Rather than a generic heading 'Symptoms', use a more specific heading, 'Eating problems', to aid interpretation and future retrieval
3 **Limit the information given under each heading**
Records with more subheadings, and fewer data under each, will be more easily used than the reverse
4 **Include signposts and landmarks within the records**
These can be specific locations for certain kinds of information, or marking of abnormal values or adverse reactions with highlighter or marginal symbol
5 **Organize information to meet the needs of more than one profession**
Visual separators, such as lines or boxes, can distinguish instructions to other professionals, such as clinic nurses, from data
6 **Make the organization of the material visually explicit**
Vertical space between sections and horizontal indents helps to signal the relation between different parts of a medical record

to primary care physician to patient. Indeed, the number of possible pathways a message may travel is enormous, and the combination of agents it may pass through equally as complex.

A common strategy to minimize message distortion is to adopt a public standard against which messages are constructed, and against which agents can interpret a message if they receive it. If a message starts to deviate from the standard, it is a warning to agents that the quality of the message may not be acceptable. For example, there are standard ways to record data obtained from a patient history and examination, such as the use of a 'system review' that methodically categorizes data into different organ systems. Journal articles adopt a common framework of structured abstract, methods and results to ensure studies are reported in a uniform way, maximizing the chance that they will contain the necessary information to understand the study, as well as permitting some form of comparison between different studies. As we shall see in Chapter 16, the use of standard terms means that messages written by humans can be understood by computers, or that computer messages can be constructed into terms likely to be understood by healthcare workers.

Standards work because all agents know they exist, and are therefore motivated to learn the necessary standard structures and terminologies. Standards are a sort of publicly agreed common ground. Standards support Grice's maxims because agents know that if they use them, other agents are likely to understand them. They also know that if they receive a message, they have a good chance of understanding what it means.

5.2 The patient record can have many different structures

Of all the messages the clinicians receive, none receives more attention than the patient record. To ensure the patient record effectively communicates between different healthcare practitioners, it is almost always created according to a standard structure, as would be expected from the previous discussion. There are four common record structures (Figure 5.2):

- **Integrated record:** Data are presented in a strictly chronological way, identifying each episode of care by time and date. Data arriving from an investigation such as radiology

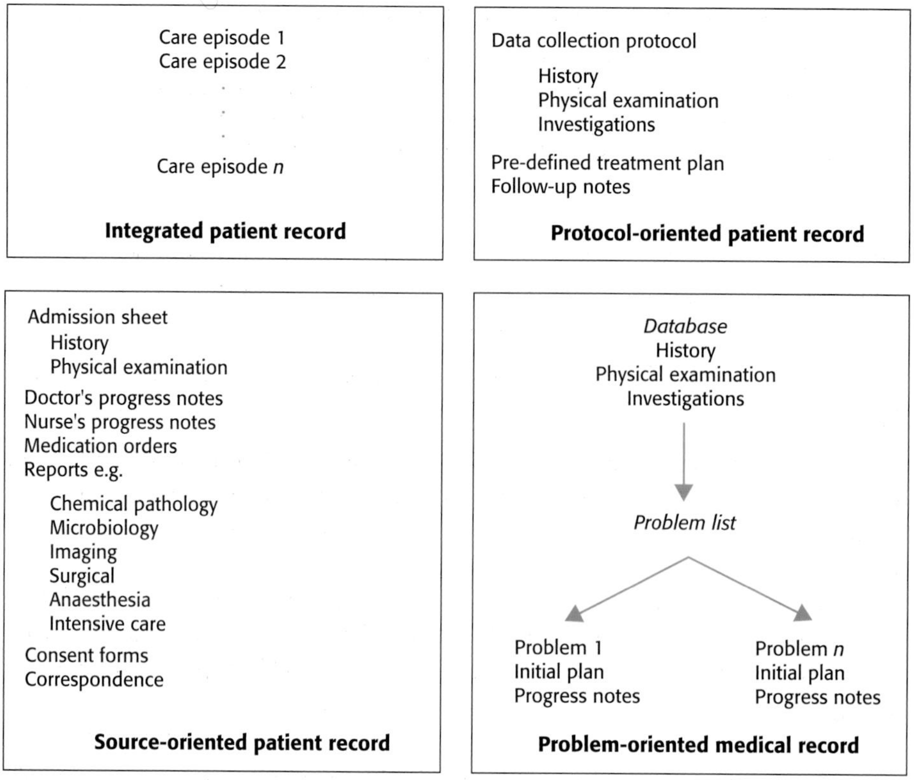
Care episode 1
Care episode 2
Care episode n
Integrated patient record
Data collection protocol
History
Physical examination
Investigations
Pre-defined treatment plan
Follow-up notes
Protocol-oriented patient record
Admission sheet
History
Physical examination
Doctor's progress notes
Nurse's progress notes
Medication orders
Reports e.g.
Chemical pathology
Microbiology
Imaging
Surgical
Anaesthesia
Intensive care
Consent forms
Correspondence
Source-oriented patient record
Database
History
Physical examination
Investigations
Problem list
Problem 1
Initial plan
Progress notes
Problem n
Initial plan
Progress notes
Problem-oriented medical record

Figure 5.2 Typical arrangement of different patient record structures from a hospital admission.

could then be followed by progress notes written by a clinician, a change to medication orders or a laboratory test result. A variation of this is the time-oriented medical record, developed for chronically ill patients, where data are arranged in two dimensions, according to axes of time and data type (Tange, 1996).

- **Source-oriented record:** The source-oriented medical record (SOMR) is organized according to the source that generated the data, typically different hospital departments. There are separate sections for medical notes, nursing notes, laboratory data, radiological results and so forth. Within each source section, data are sometimes further subdivided, for example according to the different types of test, and then arranged chronologically.
- **Protocol-driven patient record:** When a patient is being given a standard treatment for a well-understood condition such as asthma, diabetes or myocardial ischaemia, then a standard template can be used to guide the construction of the medical record. The template or protocol is captured in a pre-structured form that dictates what specific data are to be obtained and recorded by the clinician, and what the treatment plan for the patient will be.
- **Problem-oriented record:** The problem-oriented medical record (POMR) (Weed, 1968) has four components – a problem list, an initial plan, a database containing all patient data, and progress notes. The POMR organizes data according to the list of patient problems, which may be anything from symptoms through to well-defined diagnoses. The problem list is dynamic and is used to name, number and date each problem, and acts as an index to the whole record. The plan describes what will be done for each

Table 5.3 Components of the progress notes in a problem-oriented medical record.

S	Subjective	What the patient states the problem is
O	Objective	What is identified by the practitioner via history, physical examination, and tests
A	Assessment	Conclusion based on subjective and objective data
P	Plan	The method to be used to resolve the problem

problem. All progress notes, laboratory tests, treatment notes and medications are numbered according to the problem they relate to. Progress notes are often written according to the SOAP template (see Table 5.3).

Looking back at the different message types discussed earlier in this chapter it is easy to recognize that:

- The integrated record is a data-oriented message. It provides little to no structure to the data beyond a time-stamp, and consequently guidance is not offered on navigation through the record, nor what elements may be more important than others for a given task.
- The source-oriented record is a variation of a data-oriented record, still strongly focused on presenting data in a simple indexed form, much like a telephone directory. There is no concept of clinical task in the source-oriented record, and it is up to clinicians to extract information that they may need for different tasks.
- The protocol-oriented record is clearly a task-oriented message. It is designed to guide the message creator, as well as anyone who will receive it, through all the necessary steps in the task.
- The problem oriented-record aims to be a template-driven message, since there is clear separation between some of the data, stored in a separate database, and the problem-specific information. However, this structure is not applied uniformly across the whole record. Some data are stored in the progress notes directly associated with individual problems, rather than in the database. Further, although there is a link from problem to different items in the database, it points only one way. There is no link from the individual data items in the database going back to the different problems they relate to. So, at least in its paper-based format, the POMR is a hybrid incorporating features of both task- and template-oriented messages.

No single patient record structure will suit every purpose

It is often claimed that the POMR is the 'best' patient record structure, but as we saw with different message types, this cannot be so for all circumstances. In some settings the POMR may be best, but in others, one of the other structures may be superior.

The integrated record seems particularly weak as a message, since data are not categorized other than by time, and it is therefore hard to integrate data according to the source of the data or patient problem. Yet it may be the best way to present data for patients with complex or long-standing diseases. Patient charts in intensive care are often time-oriented records so that clinicians can look across the time progress of different data sources.

The source-oriented record also makes it difficult to assemble a clear picture of a patient's condition, since data are scattered among different sources. Yet it probably remains the most popular method of structuring patient data, probably because it is a very flexible record structure, and because clinicians know where they can look up specific data very rapidly.

The protocol-oriented record is clearly a very prescriptive document format, but finds favour in highly repetitive situations, such as patient clinics, or the formal trial of new treatments. It not only guarantees that the standard of the record is uniform across different authors, but also tends to be more complete since the pre-defined structure acts as a prompt to remind clinicians to ask specific questions or carry out specific investigations. Even the most skilled clinicians can be overloaded and forget elements of a patient work-up. Clearly a disadvantage of the protocol-based approach is that it is best suited to single-problem patients who have well-defined diseases and treatment pathways. It is not possible to pre-define protocols for every problem a patient has, so sometimes we need a more flexible approach.

While the POMR solves this to an extent, allowing flexibility in defining patient problems, it demands a large amount of time and commitment to write. The POMR is clearly attempting to create task-oriented messages *for the reader* of the document, grouping data according to patient problems, but there are no task-specific guides for the author. Consequently it is up to the author of the POMR to decide what is a distinct problem, and different authors might label the same patient's problems in different ways. In contrast, the protocol-driven patient record pre-defines the task template for common conditions *for the writer* of the document.

The use of distinct problems as a record structure encourages integration of data within the scope of individual problems. However, the POMR also creates barriers to integration of data by clinicians. Compartmentalizing data into separate problems may inhibit a clinician considering how one problem might relate to another, and encourages the thinking that each problem is separate. The end result may be that a patient receives multiple medications each addressing different problems, but that no attention is paid to the total number of medications given, nor a unified dosing schedule optimized to the patient's needs rather than the problems' demands (Feinstein, 1973).

The POMR may have repetition of data entries across different problems, since specific data may be relevant to more than one problem. This has the impact of making the paper version of the POMR large, and this effect itself may obscure trends in data. Thus the POMR is organized to optimize making inferences for particular problems rather than recording and storage of patient data. As a consequence, the paper POMR shows unchanged speed and accuracy of data retrieval compared with source-oriented records, and as a result it has been argued that it does not improve clinical practice substantially (Fletcher, 1974; Fernow *et al.*, 1978).

Many of these problems disappear when the patient record migrates from paper form to a computer version. Computer record systems usually store a specific patient datum only once, and then call up a subset of the data into different 'views' as needed. Thus data are only stored once in the electronic POMR, and then called up when we view the patient database from the perspective of a given patient problem. Indeed there is no reason why in a computer-based patient record we cannot merge the different record types further. When a patient problem is well understood, then a pre-defined protocol could be used, and when not, a clinician-defined problem would appear. If a time- or source-oriented 'view' of data is considered more helpful, then the same data can be reassembled into these different displays. Thus, computer-based patient records have the inherent flexibility to vary their message structure to suit the needs of different clinical tasks.

Table 5.4 Summary of the steps involved in shaping the content of a message.

Determine the specific purposes for which the information will be used.
Break down the information elements needed to achieve the task. What is needed in the database and the knowledge base?
Determine who will be using the information. Is it a named individual, someone in a defined role with specific training, or a general group of individuals?
Determine the capabilities of the receiver to interpret the message. What are you assuming is in their database and their knowledge base?
Determine the context in which the message is likely to be received. How much time will be available to the receiver, how many competing tasks will they have?
Decide if the message should be data-, task-, or protocol-oriented, on the basis of the characteristics of the task(s), the agents and the available resources.
Arrange the information elements in a way to maximize the ease of use, and minimize misinterpretation, by the receiver.
Select a communication channel from those available, on the basis of impact of the channel on the receiver, cost of channel use, and capacity to carry the message (on the basis of message length and risk of noise corruption).

Conclusions

In this chapter, we have used the idea of models and templates to develop a rich picture of the process of structuring and communicating information (see Table 5.4). Communication is a complex phenomenon that is usually not explicitly thought about in routine clinical practice, yet getting it right has profound implications for the quality of patient care. We have also seen that an understanding of the communication process also helps explain the structure of the commonest of clinical 'messages' – the patient record.

Discussion points

1. Should a textbook be source-oriented, task-oriented, or protocol-directed?
2. Look at the two versions of the radiology report in Figure 5.1. Explain how the principles in Table 5.2 were used to transform the first report into the second.
3. Look again at the radiology report in Figure 5.1. Identify two different users of this report and two different ways in which the information in the report is used. Then design two new versions, each one optimized to suit the specific needs of the two different users and their tasks.
4. What do you think about the notion in SOAP progress notes (Table 5.3) that patient-presented data are subjective, and clinician-presented data are objective? What does model theory from Chapter 1 tell us about the notion of 'physician objectivity?'.
5. Try to repeat Question 2, this time using Grice's maxims to explain the changes.
6. Can you justify any of the six principles of medical record design in Box 5.2 using Grice's maxims?
7. Which set of principles, Wright *et al.*'s or Grice's, is more useful? Explain why this might be so, discussing the different roles in which we use a specific set of principle such as those in Table 5.2 and the more general set of Grice's maxims. Hint: Think of each set of principles as a message. Are they more like source-oriented, task-oriented, or protocol-directed messages?

Chapter summary

1 Messages are structured to achieve a specific task using available resources to suit the needs of the receiver:
- **Data-oriented messages** are structured according to the attributes of the data being communicated.
- **Task-oriented messages** are structured according to the attributes of task.
- **Template-oriented messages** have generic task-templates, which can be instantiated by the receiver or through links into a database.

2 The channel is selected on the basis of its suitability to the task:
- Interruptive channels are often called **synchronous** channels because they demand real-time interaction between agents.
- Non-interruptive channels are called **asynchronous** channels, because the interaction between agents can occur at separate moments over an extended period.

3 The receiver's knowledge alters the effectiveness of a message. Agents vary in the common ground they share and the terminology they are familiar with.

4 Messages should be structured to emphasize key elements to enable rapid and accurate understanding. A standard template is used to structure a message when many different people will receive it.

5 The patient record can have many different structures:
- The **integrated record** presents data chronologically, and is data-oriented.
- The **source-oriented record** is organized according to the source that generated the data and thus is also data-oriented.
- The **protocol-driven record** is pre-structured and dictates what data are to be recorded and the treatment plan and is task-oriented.
- The **problem-oriented record** organizes data according to patient problems and has four components – a problem list, an initial plan, a database containing all patient data, and progress notes – it aims to be template-oriented.

6 No single patient record structure will suit every purpose. Computer-based patient records have the inherent flexibility to vary their message structure to suit the needs of different clinical tasks.

CHAPTER 6

Questioning

Knowledge improves patient care. The more we know about our patients, their diseases and treatments, the better the chance that patients receive the best care possible. As a result, patients will require fewer health resources, as they recover more quickly, and with fewer complications than patients receiving less optimal treatment.

In one major study, it was shown that hospitals could save up to 70% in the cost of managing patients with complex illness if clinicians conducted literature searches as part of routine care, looking for new research data on the most appropriate treatment for diseases (Klein *et al.*, 1994). This led the authors of the study to conclude that conducting a literature search was so cost effective that it should become a standard element of clinical care, alongside investigations such as laboratory tests, and should even be reimbursable by insurance bodies.

If searching for and finding knowledge improves patient care, then by implication those not doing the searching are missing key information about patient management. Indeed, researchers of medical problem-solving have found that individual clinicians will vary widely in how well they manage different patient cases, depending upon the knowledge they bring to the problems. This has led to what was initially a quite controversial realization that 'knowledge of content is more critical than mastery of a generic-problem-solving process' (Elstein *et al.*, 1978). In other words, having excellent clinical reasoning skills alone is insufficient to compensate for lack of specific clinical knowledge about patient management.

In the previous century, there was a model that clinicians, and doctors in particular, 'knew best', often meaning that their opinions could not be challenged. Today, we understand that no single individual can know all the evidence to support one course of action over another, and that good medical practice is not so much 'knowing about' diseases and their treatments, but 'knowing where to find out' that knowledge.

Consequently one of the generic skills needed by all clinicians is the ability to formulate questions that will find the answers to the gaps in their knowledge. In this chapter we will explore why asking questions is an essential component of the process of patient management, and examine the sources of knowledge that can be used to answer questions. We will also focus on how questions can be structured to deliver answers that matter.

6.1 Clinicians have many gaps and inconsistencies in their clinical knowledge

Although individual clinicians may be very experienced and widely read, it is unlikely that they will be completely up-to-date in every aspect of their clinical knowledge, nor know which parts of their knowledge base still reflect best practice, and which need updating.

Clinicians' knowledge of treatment decays over time

There is a transfer of knowledge that occurs between the collective published works of clinical researchers, which is contained in journals and textbooks, and the heads of clinicians. After a time, the knowledge in the head of the human has remained relatively unchanged, but the research knowledge continues to grow and change. Consequently, the quality of a clinician's knowledge decays over time compared to the best evidence contained in the latest research sources.

Researchers have shown that the accuracy of a clinician's knowledge is statistically highly correlated with the number of years since graduation, and that younger physicians are more likely than older ones to have an up-to-date knowledge of clinical practice (Evans *et al.*, 1984). This difference has nothing to do with ability, but simply relates to exposure to the latest knowledge, since when the older clinicians are exposed to up-to-date knowledge they quickly match the knowledge of younger clinicians.

The problem of transfer of knowledge becomes increasingly difficult as the volume of research knowledge continues to grow. The number of scientific articles in existence doubles at intervals of 1–15 years, and a new article is added to the medical literature every 26 seconds or less. As a consequence, the growth in the literature is exponential. In one study of the literature related to a single clinical disease over 110 years, it was found that only 3% of the literature had been generated in the first 50 years, and 40% had been generated in the last 10 years (Arndt, 1992). Consequently, it may no longer be possible to simply keep 'up-to-date' by reading the latest literature from time to time, as the volume of published material exceeds human ability to read or understand it all (Coiera and Dowton, 2000).

Clinicians' beliefs about appropriate treatment often do not accord with the facts

We follow a course of action we believe to be the best one. Clinicians' beliefs will thus strongly influence the choices they make about patient management. Even if a clinician is exposed to the knowledge about the best course of action for a particular disease's management, when they hear the 'message' in that knowledge it may be distorted, for any of the reasons discussed in Chapter 4. We also saw that such beliefs are not fixed, but may be influenced by recent experiences, which may include exposure to the opinions of others.

When the best available evidence does not accord with such beliefs, it can result in ineffective or dangerous practices being over-used, or effective practices being underutilized. In one study of the beliefs of general practitioners about the effectiveness of various cancer screening procedures, there was a wide variation between the best available evidence at the time of the study, and the beliefs of the clinicians (Young *et al.*, 1998). On the positive side, the clinicians believed in, and the evidence supported, the value of mammography as a screening tool. However, the clinicians also believed in the effectiveness of many cancer screening approaches that were unsupported by evidence, including clinical skin or breast examination, digital rectal examination and flexible sigmoidoscopy. As worryingly, although the evidence strongly supported the effectiveness of faecal occult blood testing, the practitioners believed it to be relatively ineffective.

Clinicians have many more questions about patients than they look for answers

The degree to which clinicians believe they need to access a knowledge source during patient care will clearly vary according to the individual clinician's knowledge, their beliefs about the adequacy of their knowledge, the patient's problem and local practices.

Several studies have tried to measure the base requirement for knowledge support during routine patient care. In a groundbreaking study, Covell and others (1985) interviewed 47 internal medicine physicians in office-based practice in Los Angeles County. The doctors they interviewed believed they needed information once per week, but the researchers estimated that actually two unanswered questions were raised for every three patients seen (about 0.67 questions per patient) – a very large gap between what is believed and what actually is. Of these questions, 40% were questions about medical facts (e.g. 'What are the side effects of bromocriptine?'), 45% were questions about medical opinion (e.g. How do you manage a patient with labile hypertension?'), and 16% were about non-clinical knowledge (e.g. How do you arrange home care for a patient?'). About a third of the questions were about treatment, a quarter about diagnosis, and 14% about drugs. Most importantly, only a third of questions were answered. The doctors in the study also claimed that when they did search for answers, they used printed materials such as textbooks and journals, but in fact they were actually most likely to consult another doctor.

Many other studies have looked at these questions since (R. Smith, 1996b), mainly focusing on doctors. They show us that:

- Knowledge gaps are routinely identified when clinicians see patients. Doctors can have anything between 0.07 and 5.77 questions per patient encounter, depending upon the study method, how a 'clinical question' is defined and the clinical setting.
- Although doctors are usually aware that they have gaps in their knowledge, they significantly underestimate their needs, or overestimate the quality of their own knowledge.
- In medical practice, many of the questions relate to treatment, and are most often about drug therapy (Table 6.2).
- Further, doctors actually pursue answers to questions in only about one-third of cases (Ely *et al.*, 1999). Doctors are most likely to pursue questions about drug prescription

Table 6.1 Examples of hypothetical disease-oriented evidence (DOE) and patient-oriented evidence that matters (POEM). The number of assumptions needed to apply the evidence to a specific patient decreases from left to right as the evidence becomes more task-specific (after Slawson *et al.*, 1994).

DOE		POEM
Many assumptions needed to ascribe benefit	Some assumptions needed	Few assumptions needed to ascribe benefit
Drug A lowers cholesterol	Drug A decreases cardiovascular disease mortality/morbidity	Drug A decreases overall mortality
Antiarrhythmic A decreases PVCs	Antiarrhythmic A decreases arrhythmia symptom	Antiarrhythmic A decreases mortality
Antibiotic A is effective against common pathogens of otitis media	Antibiotic A sterilizes middle ear effusions in patients with otitis media	Antibiotic A decreases symptoms and complications of otitis media

Table 6.2 The 10 most common question structures asked by family doctors, and the likelihood that once the question was asked, it would then be pursued. Questions of drug prescription are most likely to be pursued (after Ely *et al.*, 1999).

Generic question	Frequency asked (%)	Frequency pursued (%)
What is the cause of symptom X?	9	9
What is the dose of drug X?	8	85
How should I manage disease or finding X?	7	29
How should I treat finding or disease X?	7	33
What is the cause of physical finding X?	7	18
What is the cause of test finding X?	4	40
Could this patient have disease or condition X?	4	14
Is test X indicated in condition Y?	4	29
What is the drug of choice for condition X?	3	47
Is drug X indicated in situation Y?	3	25

(see Table 6.2). Two factors have been shown to statistically predict whether a doctor would pursue a question – whether the doctor believed that an answer actually existed to the question, and the urgency of the patient's problem (Gorman, 1995). If evidence is immediately available, then a clinician is more likely to access it, but when evidence is not readily available, clinicians rarely search for it (Sackett and Straus, 1998).

- Answers are found for between 25% (Gorman, 1995) and 90% (Sackett and Straus, 1998) of those questions that are pursued. Doctors spent about 2 minutes searching for an answer (Ely *et al.*, 1999).
- Of the methods used to access knowledge, most studies also agree that clinicians prefer to ask another human if possible, ahead of accessing formal printed materials such as textbooks and drug manuals. Formal literature searches are rarely performed.
- When questions are answered, it does appear that the evidence found changes the approach of clinicians. Sackett and Straus (1998) found at least one member of a hospital team changed their approach 48% of the time evidence was sought. Accessing evidence seems to change clinical decisions about 13% of the time, initiate it in 18% of the time and confirm existing plans 70% of the time (Haynes *et al.*, 1990).

If keeping your knowledge up-to-date is no longer feasible because the growth in knowledge exceeds your capacity to read it, then searching for changes in clinical knowledge is a basic component of patient care. The difficulty in even keeping textbooks up-to-date has caused some to argue that we should burn all our textbooks, and instead use online information technology to find the answer to clinical questions (Sackett *et al.*, 2000). Thus, the whole notion of ongoing clinical education changes from one of periodic updates to a clinician's knowledge to a 'just-in-time' model where a clinician checks the medical knowledge base, potentially at every clinical encounter (Coiera and Dowton, 2000).

6.2 Well-formed questions seek answers that will have a direct impact on clinical care

Answers to questions should make a difference. They should return knowledge that has a direct impact on the task that initiated the question. Given that most clinicians work in time-pressured environments, and that the range of potential questions that could be asked is enormous, it is essential that the question posed be focused on getting to the key knowledge as directly as possible.

In any field of expertise there are general principles that underpin the discipline. In healthcare these principles include our understanding of the principles of disease and its treatment. In informatics, the basic principles include the theory of model construction, information, and systems. Such knowledge has sometimes been called **background knowledge**, to reflect that the knowledge sits in the background and is brought forward to solve different problems from time to time. In contrast, individual situations might require very specific knowledge that has little application beyond that context. Such knowledge is called **foreground knowledge** (Sackett *et al.*, 2000). For example, a background question might be 'What are the causes of asthma?' and a foreground question might be 'What is the treatment for an episode of severe bronchoconstriction in a child?'.

As a general rule, the number of background questions that arise in a clinical situation probably diminishes as an individual becomes more experienced and builds up their background knowledge base. With experience, the questions asked are more likely to be foreground questions about the specifics of managing a particular situation. However, given that clinical knowledge continues to grow, and that individual clinicians have many gaps in their existing knowledge, there will always be an ongoing need to ask background questions.

Since background questions are about general principles, they are likely to have a smaller impact on the immediate situation, and can therefore probably be asked away from the immediate work setting. For example, answering background questions might require setting aside specific time to study an area. Foreground questions that have a high impact ask for **patient-oriented evidence that matters** (POEM) and should therefore be asked and answered as an integral part of clinical work (Slawson *et al.*, 1994). In contrast, background questions usually ask for **disease-oriented evidence** (DOE).

Typically the medical literature contains much more DOE than POEM. One way to distinguish POEM from the more common DOE is to determine how many assumptions the knowledge requires us to make before it can be applied. For example, if some evidence helps us identify a cancer earlier, then it can be plausibly assumed that doing so will be beneficial. However, until a clinical trial actually reports that identifying cancer causes a reduction in patient morbidity or mortality, or a reduction in resource use, then there is really no verifiable evidence that it actually would occur. The first kind of evidence is disease-oriented evidence that can sit in the background of our knowledge base. The second kind of evidence is patient-oriented and the application of the evidence matters. Consequently it can be directly applied to solving a clinical task. When one studies the type of question that clinicians are most likely to ask, the most frequent questions are all POEM. These generic questions can be thought of as a template and be used as a model when learning to ask clinical questions (Table 6.2). We simply instantiate the generic question with specific data relating to the clinical problem at hand.

Since clinical knowledge is incomplete, it will not always be the case that specific patient-oriented evidence can be located. In such circumstances, it makes sense to turn to the next best-available evidence, which in this case might be disease-oriented knowledge. Using DOE does require the making of assumptions, and sometimes the process of thinking this way is called **reasoning from first principles**. Here, one uses a model of how the mechanisms of a system work, and tries to predict the likely effect of making a change to the system. For example, on the basis of first-principles reasoning, knowing that insulin has the effect of reducing blood levels of glucose, one might conclude that giving insulin to a patient with chronically high blood sugar levels might help reduce the sugar levels. One typically uses first-principles reasoning when exploring novel intellectual terrain, and it is one of the tools of scientific exploration.

6.3 Questions to computer knowledge sources are structured according to the rules of logic

We saw in the previous chapter that a common strategy to minimize message distortion is to adopt a public standard against which messages are constructed, and against which agents can interpret a message if they receive it.

When clinicians ask questions of their colleagues, the questions obviously need to be constructed using familiar technical terminology, and expressed grammatically. The need for standardization becomes much greater when questions are communicated to a publicly available knowledge source such as a computer database.

Typically, questions to a database are expressed using a query language. As we saw in Chapter 2, such a language will have a pre-defined grammar and terminology. For example, we may wish to search a database that indexes recent journal articles, looking for articles discussing the treatment for an episode of severe bronchoconstriction in a child. The query given to the database might use the grammar of **Boolean logic** (see Box 6.1) and look something like:

(treatment and asthma and child and (not adult))

Here the query language uses a grammar that contains pre-defined terms such as **and**, **not** and **or** to conjoin the terms used in the question. The set of terms a database recognizes also includes all the concepts stored in its knowledge base. With a clinical knowledge base these terms represent diseases, treatments and so forth.

Some concepts may be represented by several terms, or synonyms. More powerful clinical databases have the capacity to match a term with its synonyms. Consequently, a question that includes the term **heart** could also return results that contain the term **cardiac**.

As one might expect, the more complex a query language is, the more precise are the questions that can be expressed in that language. Equally, more complex languages will require greater effort to master.

Box 6.1
Boolean logic

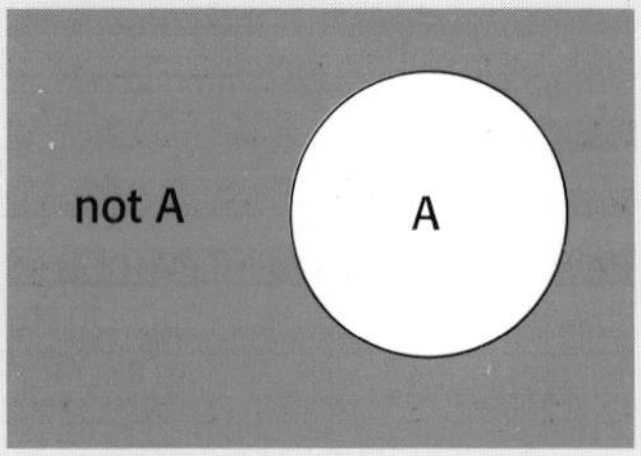
not A
A

A search for concept **A** excludes everything that is **not A**, and vice versa

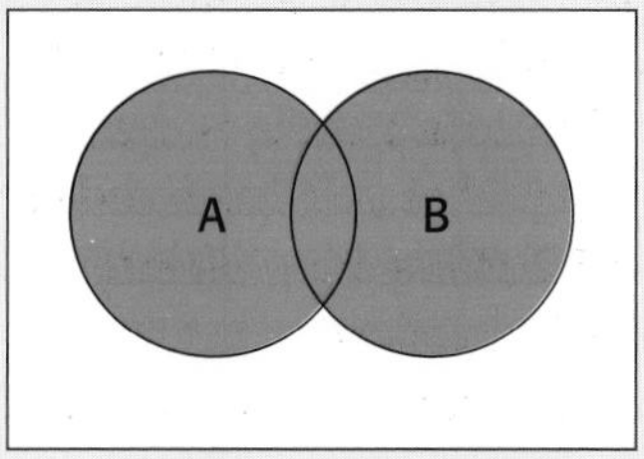
A
B

A search for **A or B** includes everything within either **A or B**

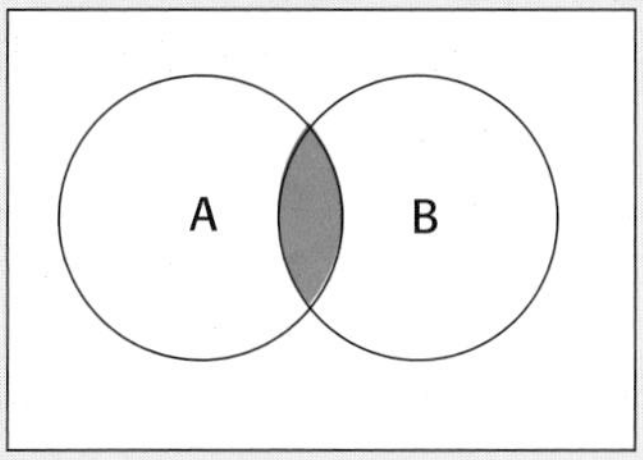
A
B

A search for **A and B** includes only things common to both to **A** and to **B**

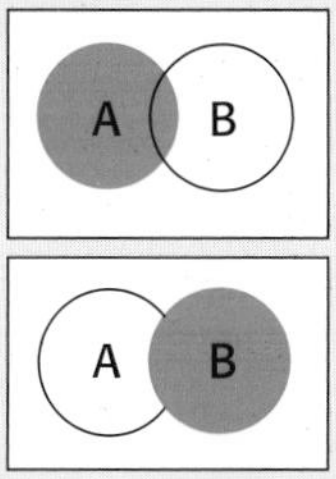
A
B
A
B

A search for **exclusive A or B** includes only either everythings within **A** or within **B** but not both at once

Figure 6.1
Venn diagrams help us visualise how Boolean logic uses the operators **and**, **or** and **not** to identify elements of interest in the database.

In the nineteenth century, Georges Boole formalized the meaning we today attach to the combination of elements using the logical operators **and**, **or** and **not**. When searching for specific items in a database, these logical operators allow us to combine single concepts to express more complex statements in a precise manner. These precise logical statements can be converted directly into a computer search into the database.

In Boolean logic:

- **Not A** is true when **A** is certifiably not true. When searching for elements in a database this search would return all those elements that could be shown to definitely not have **A** in them. We sometimes call **not A** the complement of **A**.
- **A or B** includes everything that is true for either concept **A** or concept **B** and consequently is equivalent to the logical union of both concepts. This search returns the largest number of results as it includes items that have either **A**, **B**, or both **A** and **B** in them.
- **Exclusive A or B** corresponds more closely to normal linguistic use of the term 'or', and includes either everything that is true for concept **A**, or alternatively everything that is true for concept **B**, but not both at the same time. This operator is often written as **xor**.
- **A and B** includes all those elements that are true for both **A** and **B** at the same time, and is thus equivalent to the intersection of the two concepts. Consequently this search retrieves few concepts, since it only looks for those few elements that exist across the union of the two parent concepts.

It is of course possible to build quite complex sentences involving more than two concepts, as well as many combinations of logical operators on those concepts. It sometimes is hard to tell if two complex sentences are similar or not. Many rules exist to transform one sentence into alternative forms, allowing the equivalence of complex sentences to be determined.

These rules include:

- **A and (not A) = 0:** There are no entities which both belong and do not belong to the same thing. This is known as the **law of contradiction**, which says that nothing can both exist and not exist.
- **A or (not A) = 1:** All entities are either related to a concept, or not. This is the **law of the excluded middle**, which says that something must either be or not be. There are no things that can sit in the middle and avoid either being or not being.
- **Not (not A) = A:** a double negative has no effect.

(Contd.)

Box 6.1 (*Contd.*)

One of the most powerful equivalence rules is DeMorgan's theorem, which states that **the complement of the union of two classes is the intersection of their complement**. The theorem can be written simply as:

not (A or B) = (not A) and (not B)

We can visualize the truth of this statement by looking at the diagrams in Figure 6.2, which build this search up from the basic elements.

Figure 6.2 DeMorgan's theorem.

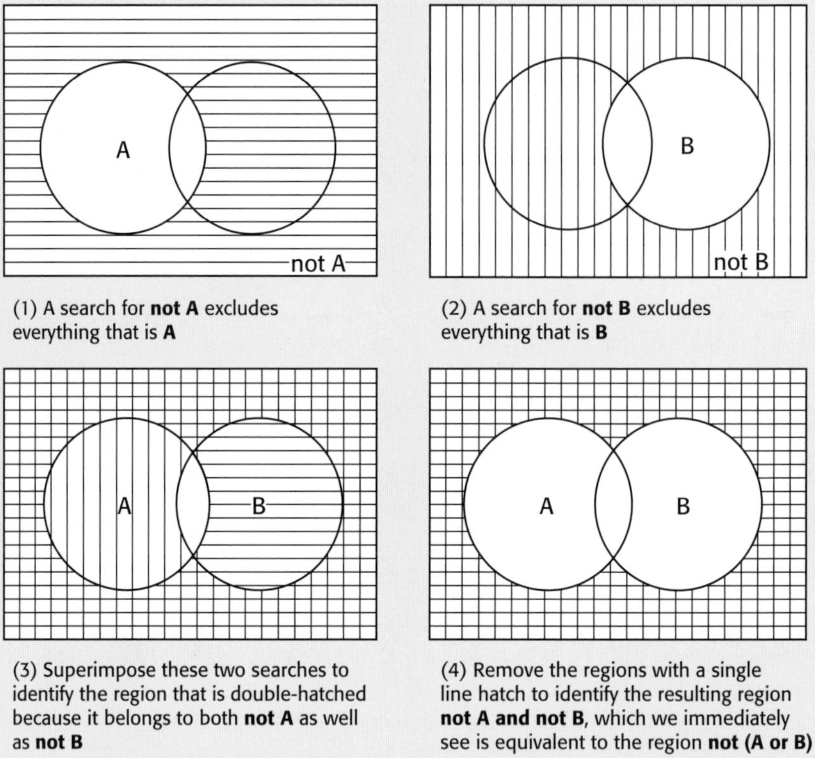
A
not A
B
not B
(1) A search for **not A** excludes everything that is **A**
(2) A search for **not B** excludes everything that is **B**
A
B
A
B
(3) Superimpose these two searches to identify the region that is double-hatched because it belongs to both **not A** as well as **not B**
(4) Remove the regions with a single line hatch to identify the resulting region **not A and not B**, which we immediately see is equivalent to the region **not (A or B)**

Some clinical databases have very rich functionality, and permit very complex queries. One of the most powerful of these databases is **Medline** (see Box 6.2), which indexes the majority of articles published in the clinical journals, amongst other things.

6.4 Well-formed questions are both accurate and specific

Grice's maxims tell us to be as economic and informative as possible when communicating. When asking a question, the answer received will only be as good as the precision of the question asked. Questions can 'miss the target' because they are either **not accurate enough** or **not specific enough** (Figure 6.3).

A statement can vary in how specific or general it is. For example, 'What is the treatment for asthma?' is quite a general question. 'What is the treatment for an episode of severe bronchoconstriction in a child' is much more specific, since it is more precise in identifying the patient, as well as saying more about the problem needing to be solved. Typically, asking

Box 6.2
The Medline database

Medline is a computer-resident database that indexes articles published in the major international biomedical scientific journals, and is maintained by the National Library of Medicine (NLM) in the United States. It is based on three indexes – *Index Medicus*, *International Nursing Index*, and the *Index to the Dental Literature* – and captures about a third of the medical articles that exist on library shelves (Greenhalgh, 1997).

Each published journal article included in Medline is given its own database record, which captures essential bibliographic data about the article, as well as some of its content. Each Medline record has a number of standard fields in which the data are stored. For example, fields exist for the title of an article, its authors, the article abstract, and publication data. There are various public and commercial interfaces that permit users to search the Medline database, but the standard way of constructing queries into Medline is to use Boolean expressions. Articles can be traced in two ways. First, a query can use terms that are likely to appear in the bibliographic fields of the article's record, such as the author's name or keywords that appear in the title.

Secondly, Medline also has a powerful way of categorizing articles according to their content called the Medical Subject Headings (MeSH). For example, an article may contain clinical guidelines for the treatment of asthma, but its title may not include the specific term **asthma**, but refer to **respiratory disease**. To allow a search that uses the term **asthma** to retrieve the article, the Medline record needs to capture the related term **asthma** somewhere. Thus each Medline record contains a field for the MeSH headings associated with an article, and it is here that key concepts contained within the article are recorded. Some of the subject areas captured by MeSH include anatomy, diseases, and chemicals and drugs. MeSH is also useful as a way of capturing synonyms for a specific term. A well-constructed MeSH field will ensure that an article dealing with the management of **bronchoconstriction** can be found by a search that only uses the term **asthma**.

Despite the high quality of the Medline database, it is not always possible to find articles using bibliographic keywords or MeSH headings. The entry of data into Medline records is prone to error both from authors and from editors who select keywords for articles, and those who enter that data into Medline records. In addition, not all sections of a journal may be indexed in Medline. For example, the news section of a scientific journal may not be indexed, unlike the formal scientific papers in the same edition. It has been estimated that 40% of the material that should be listed in Medline can only be accessed by looking through the journals 'by hand' (Greenhalgh, 1997).

Further reading

Hersh WR (2002) *Information Retrieval: A Health and Biomedical Perspective,* 2nd edition. Springer, New York.

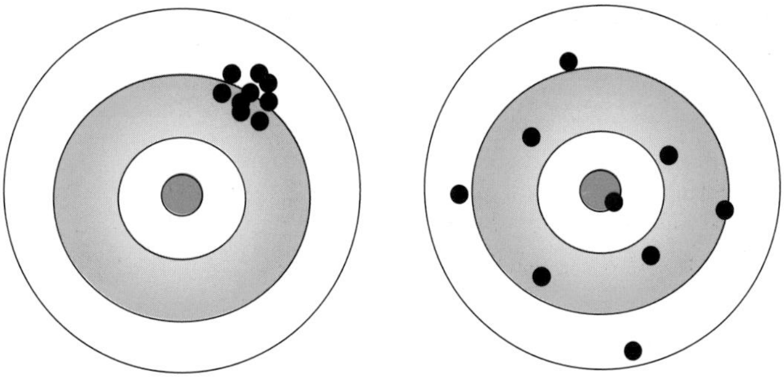

Figure 6.3
A question can be very precise, but because it is inaccurate, miss the target. A question can be too general, and hit a scattering of areas that are wide of the target.

too general a question will result in an answer that contains information that is unrelated to the true target of the question, along with some information that is appropriate. Too specific a question, in contrast, will receive an answer that lacks critical information. Typically if a database query returns too many results the question has been too general, and additional terms may need to be added to narrow down the search. In contrast, if too few or no results are returned it may mean the query is too specific, and that some restrictive terms need to be removed to make the query more general.

Even if a question is very specific, and returns a very specific answer, if the initial question is about the wrong thing it will be wide of the mark. Consequently accuracy in formation of

Table 6.3 The best search terms to retrieve clinically relevant documents in Medline (after Haynes *et al.*, 1994).

Category	Optimized for	Sensitivity/ specificity	Medline query
Therapy	Sensitivity	99%/74%	'randomized controlled trial' [PTYP] OR 'drug therapy' [SH] OR 'therapeutic use' [SH:NOEXP] OR 'random*' [WORD]
	Specificity	57%/97%	(double [WORD] AND blind* [WORD]) OR placebo [WORD]
Diagnosis	Sensitivity	92%/73%	'sensitivity and specificity' [MESH] OR 'sensitivity' [WORD] OR 'diagnosis' [SH] OR 'diagnostic use' [SH] OR 'specificity' [WORD]
	Specificity	55%/98%	'sensitivity and specificity' [MESH] OR ('predictive' [WORD] AND 'value*' [WORD])
Aetiology	Sensitivity	82%/70%	'cohort studies' [MESH] OR 'risk' [MESH] OR ('odds' [WORD] AND 'ratio*' [WORD]) OR ('relative' [WORD] AND 'risk' [WORD]) OR 'case' control*' [WORD] OR case-control studies [MESH]
	Specificity	40%/98%	'case-control studies' [MH:NOEXP] OR 'cohort studies' [MH:NOEXP]
Prognosis	Sensitivity	92%/73%	'incidence' [MESH] OR 'mortality' [MESH] OR 'follow-up studies' [MESH] OR 'mortality' [SH] OR prognos* [WORD] OR predict* [WORD] OR course [WORD]
	Specificity	49%/97%	prognosis [MH:NOEXP] OR 'survival analysis' [MH:NOEXP]

Table 6.4 The accuracy and specificity of a particular search can be measured by looking at how well it performs against benchmark measurements.

True positive rate (sensitivity)	The percentage of elements correctly detected as matching a given attribute by a procedure, out of all the possible correct elements	TP = a/(a + b)
True negative rate (specificity)	The percentage of elements correctly detected as not matching a given attribute by a procedure, out of all the possible non-matching elements	TN = d/(c + d)
False positive rate	The percentage of elements incorrectly detected as matching a given attribute by a procedure, out of all the elements identified by the procedure as correct	TP = c/(a + c)
False negative rate	The percentage of elements incorrectly detected as not matching a given attribute by a procedure, out of all the elements identified by the procedure as incorrect	TP = b/(b + d)
Precision	The percentage of elements correctly matching a given attribute, out of all the elements identified as matching by a procedure	P = a/(a + c)

	Search says is correct	Search says is incorrect
Correct according to experts	True positive (a)	False negative (b)
Incorrect according to experts	False positive (c)	True negative (d)

a question is needed, and this is determined entirely by the original task. For example, asking 'What is the treatment for an episode of severe bronchoconstriction in an adult?' might be very precise, but if the goal is to treat a child, the precise answer will not be helpful, and could indeed be dangerous.

Bibliographic experts have studied the ways questions can be put to databases such as Medline, and have discovered particular conjunctions of keywords will produce answers that are likely to have high clinical relevance (Table 6.3). Technically, a database question can have its performance measured by the number of **false-positive** documents it retrieves and by the number of **false-negative** documents it misses (Table 6.4). The **precision** of a search is the proportion of relevant documents returned by the search. This way of measuring the effectiveness of a bibliographic search is analogous to the way the performance of laboratory tests is measured, where the false positive and false negative rates are used to decide upon the accuracy and specificity of a given test. For large databases it is often impossible to determine all the elements that might match a particular search, so this figure is estimated by performing multiple searches (Hersh, 2002).

Conclusions

Clinicians need to ask questions if they are to deliver safe and effective healthcare. Clinicians have many gaps in their knowledge, and need to consider seeking knowledge to support their practice as a routine part of clinical work, just as much as ordering a laboratory test or conducting a physical examination of a patient. In this chapter we have focused very much on how such questions should be structured to maximize the quality of information received. In the next chapter we take a step back from the specific content of clinical questions, and look at the overall process of searching for information. It's not enough to know what to ask. You also have to understand the process of knowing who to ask, and how to proceed if you are not immediately successful.

Discussion points

1. Will it always be the case that DOE is less useful than POEM?
2. Using Venn diagrams, follow the logic used to demonstrate DeMorgan's theorem for the union of two sets in Box 6.1, to prove the truth of the equivalent law that **not (A and B) = (not A) or (not B)**.
3. Using a similar approach, demonstrate the truth of the **law of absorption** for the union-intersection case: **A and (A or B) = A**; for the intersection–union case **A or (A and B) = A**.
4. What are the advantages and limitations of conducting a Medline search using the predefined clinical queries contained in Table 6.3?

Chapter summary

1. Clinicians have many gaps and inconsistencies in their clinical knowledge because:
   - Clinicians' knowledge of treatment decays over time.
   - Clinicians' beliefs about appropriate treatment often do not accord with the facts.
   - Clinicians have many more questions about patients than they look for answers.
2. Well-formed questions seek answers that will have a direct impact on clinical care.
   - Foreground questions that have a high impact ask for **patient-oriented evidence that matters** (POEM).
   - Background questions usually ask for disease-oriented evidence (DOE).
3. Questions to computer knowledge sources are structured according to the rules of Boolean logic.
4. Well-formed questions are both accurate and specific. Performance is measured by:
   - the number of **false-positive** documents retrieved
   - the number of **false-negative** documents missed
   - the **precision** which is the proportion of relevant documents returned by the search.

CHAPTER 7

Searching

7.1 Successful searching for knowledge requires well-structured questions to be asked of well-informed agents

Searching for knowledge is a conversation between agents. To conduct a search an agent must pose a question, transmit the question to another more knowledgeable agent, and receive an answer. The answer is then evaluated to see if it satisfies the initial question. The more knowledgeable agent might be a human, a computer database or simply printed documents.

The process of search depends upon communicating well-structured questions, as we saw in the previous chapter. Sometimes the question posed may not be accurate enough, or the answer returned not quite what was needed, because of misunderstandings in the communication exchange. Consequently searches often consist of a series of questions and answers, creating a feedback loop where each answer is used as input to modify the next question, until the 'target' task is eventually satisfied.

For a given question, there are many possible agents that could be asked to provide knowledge, and many possible channels that could be used to convey the question. We saw in the last chapter that there are many different sources of clinical evidence, from human agents such as the patient and clinical colleagues, through to published sources such as the medical record, or the scientific literature.

Sometimes we may need to conduct the search by questioning several agents. For example, a search for a piece of clinical knowledge may start with a query to a computer database, and if unsuccessful, continues with a question to a human colleague. Indeed, it has been estimated that searching electronic databases may uncover only half the relevant articles needed

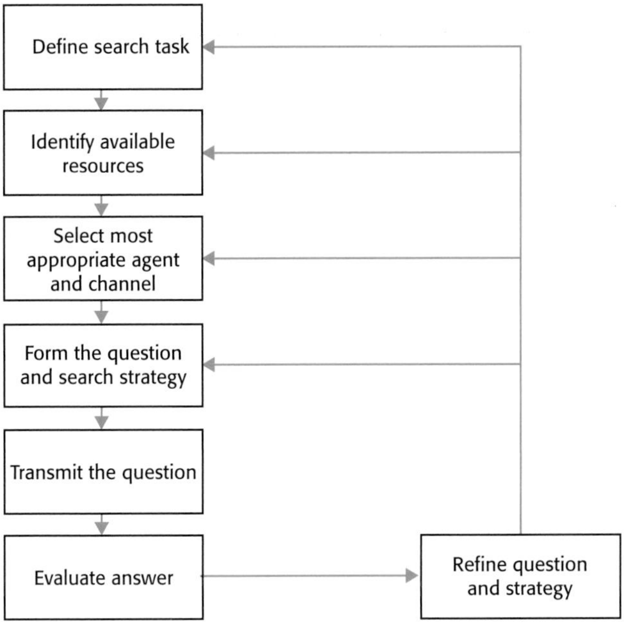
Define search task
Identify available resources
Select most appropriate agent and channel
Form the question and search strategy
Transmit the question
Evaluate answer
Refine question and strategy

Figure 7.1
Knowledge search is a process that starts with a task to fill a gap in knowledge, and then involves the crafting of a question that both satisfies the task need and is understood by the receiving agent. Evaluation of the answer allows feedback to alter the question, the agent being asked, or perhaps even the original task.

to conduct a systematic review of a clinical topic, and that the only way to find the remainder is to ask well-informed humans (McManus *et al.*, 1998). There are many reasons for the incompleteness of electronic databases, including the errors introduced by humans involved in the process of codifying the data, as well as the intrinsic impossibility of any large database being a perfect model of the true state of published knowledge.

The process of search can be reduced to a series of steps involving identifying a task which requires knowledge, choosing the most appropriate knowledgeable agent and channel, crafting a question in a manner suited to the task, receiving agent and channel, and finally sending the message.

Figure 7.1 shows the basic search structure, which builds upon the communication model summarized in Table 5.4, and includes two new elements – a search strategy and a feedback loop where the answer received is evaluated to guide further possible rounds of questioning. In the following section we will examine the process of question formation, search strategy, evaluation and question refinement in more detail.

7.2 Search strategies are optimized to minimize cost and maximize benefit

Asking a question carries an opportunity cost and so we want to make sure that when we ask a question we are likely to get a useful answer. A simple formula for determining how likely it is that a useful answer will be returned from a knowledgeable agent is given by the following formula (Slawson *et al.*, 1994):

$$\text{Usefulness of knowledge} = \left(\frac{\text{Relevance} \times \text{Validity}}{\text{Search effort}}\right)$$

The formula says that the more specifically relevant knowledge is to a given situation, the more value it will have. A general description of the treatment for a disease is less useful than a treatment protocol specifically created for a given patient. Secondly, the more we know that the knowledge is valid and has been through some form of scientific evaluation, the more likely it is to have an impact on our task. A piece of information we find in a systematic review from a peer-reviewed journal is more likely to be useful than a news item in this morning's newspaper.

However, independent of how relevant or valid a piece of knowledge might be, people are still likely to be drawn to knowledge that is easy to access. The harder it is to extract a given piece of knowledge, the less likely it is that the search will be pursued. Consequently knowledge that is easily accessible, has strong scientific validity, and is directly applicable to a specific task, is most likely to be useful.

When humans look for items of information in a document such as a medical record, they usually employ a few simple strategies to find what they want. A clinician who is searching for information may scan many pages rapidly, continuously making some judgement of relevance (search mode). In contrast, if the item of interest is known to be in a particular section, that whole section is read carefully (reading mode) (Nygren and Henriksson, 1992). When asked about their behaviour, clinicians report that skimming the first few words in a paragraph may be sufficient – from their perspective – to make their judgement of relevance. A paragraph judged irrelevant to the search task could be immediately skipped, and when a paragraph seems relevant, they can switch from search mode to reading mode.

In a world where clinical evidence comes from many sources, including electronic databases, the process of searching for answers to questions cannot rely on such simple strategies. Further, even if clinicians say this is how they like to search for information, as we saw in the previous chapter, clinician strategies seem to result in fewer questions being pursued than are actually needed.

In the previous sections we have examined how the search process is dependent upon the quality of the question asked. Since a search may involve an iterative process of exploration, the process of searching for knowledge can become expensive as it consumes time and resources that could always be used elsewhere. Consequently, it is just as important to have a clear search strategy in mind, as it is to have a clear clinical question. In the following sections we will look at how a search strategy is constructed to maximize the chance that useful knowledge will be retrieved.

7.3 The set of all possible options forms a search space

The process of agent and channel selection and question formulation in Figure 7.1 shows that there are many choices to be made in the search for specific pieces of knowledge. The set of all possible sources of knowledge forms a **search space** that has to be explored in the hunt for the answer to a specific question. The search space might be formed by the list of all the likely well-informed agents that could answer a question. We interact with these different agents in the search space through the use of different communication channels. The knowledge base contained within any agent is also a search space that can be drilled down into, to find the specific piece of knowledge we are after.

For example, in seeking the answer to a clinical question raised in the care of a patient, the initial search space might consist of several colleagues, an electronic bibliographic database such as Medline, and some textbooks. Choices need to be made about which agent to ask first, and the way that the agent is to be interrogated, as we explore the knowledge that an agent possesses. The 'search' through the knowledge base of a fellow human requires a different process to the way we ask questions of Medline.

Consider, for example, the way questions are structured and pursued in a legal cross-examination of a witness in a courtroom. Although the lawyer is not constructing well-formed Boolean statements to a database, the process of question formation and sequencing is just as deliberate. Further, a database will be deterministic in its behaviour, returning the same result for a given question time and again. Humans, however, will vary in their responses to a question, as we saw in the last chapter, because of the cognitive biases that might be in operation at a given moment, the cognitive loads limiting their capacity to answer, and the implied context assumed to be in the agent's common ground. Humans will try to shape their answers to match what they believe is being asked of them at a given moment.

7.4 Search strategies are designed to find the answer in the fewest possible steps

For a search to occur, there needs to be a structure or map through the search space to act as a reference point. Otherwise the search is essentially a random process where we hope to eventually bump into the thing we are seeking by chance. For example, a book will have a structure of chapters and subheadings, as well as an index, and these can both be used to guide the search process. We have already met such directory structures in Chapter 4, where they were introduced to explain the different types of message structure. Each of the patient record structures discussed in Chapter 4 is an attempt to create a structured search space to assist data and knowledge retrieval.

A search space is often thought of as a branching tree-like structure, with a hierarchy of nodes corresponding to particular elements in the search space, and the links between the nodes representing the path the searcher must follow from one to the other. The table of contents of a book is a good example of a search space, structured according to a hierarchy of chapters, sections and subsections (Figure 7.2).

The topmost node of the tree, to which everything else connects, is called the **root** node. Sometimes the final nodes at the end of the tree are called **leaf** nodes, the node above

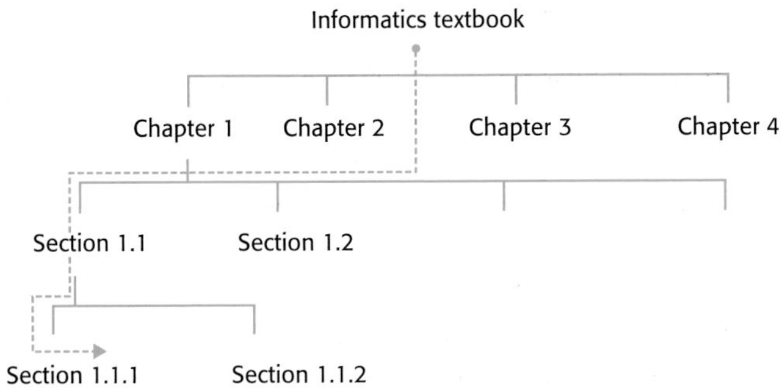
Informatics textbook
Chapter 1
Chapter 2
Chapter 3
Chapter 4
Section 1.1
Section 1.2
Section 1.1.1
Section 1.1.2

Figure 7.2
Search spaces can be represented as a tree, with the entry point to the space at the topmost or 'root' node, which is connected via links to other nodes, eventually terminating in 'leaf' nodes.

another node is called its **parent**, and the node below a parent is its **sibling**, beautifully mixing botanical and genealogical metaphors. The different collections of nodes and links are called **branches**, and the route we take as we 'walk' through the tree the traversal **path**, adding a recreational flavour to the metaphors. In Figure 7.2, 'Textbook' is the root node, and 'Section 1.1.1' is a leaf node. The dotted line connecting these two nodes follows a path that descends the branches of the tree, and 'Chapter 1' is a parent of 'Section 1.2'.

A **search strategy** is the plan that directs the way an agent searches in a space. If the search space is constructed like a tree, then the strategy directs the choices made in walking along the branches of the tree, looking for a node that has the information we want.

Any strategy for navigating through a search tree is constructed from various combinations of three basic actions:

1. Move down a link from a parent node to a sibling node
2. Evaluate a node to see if it matches the search criteria
3. Backtrack up a link, moving from sibling back to parent.

So, for example, a simple strategy might be to:

1. **Start** at the root node
2. **Repeat** the following steps:
   i. **if** the node satisfies the criteria, **then** we can stop the search
   ii. **if** the node does not match search criteria, **then** we continue down the tree moving from parent to the next leftmost sibling that has not been searched
   iii. **if** we have reached a leaf node, **then** we backtrack up one link and continue the process from there.

There are several different classic search strategies that can be followed when navigating a search space (Figure 7.3). We can search the space *systematically*, where we start at the beginning and then keep looking at every item until we find what we want:

- The search strategy described above is a systematic process called a **depth-first search**, since we keep diving more deeply into the search space, until we can go no further, and only then come back somewhat reluctantly, and then resume the dive. Looking for information in a textbook, the depth-first strategy starts at the first chapter, opens it up, and then reads each section, before returning to open up a new chapter.
- A **breadth-first search**, in contrast, will examine a node, and then backtrack immediately if it does not find an answer, continuing to explore all the nodes at the same level. Only then, if it is unsuccessful, will the strategy move on to a deeper level. So, in looking for a section in a textbook, a breadth-first search would first browse all the chapter headings, looking for a match, and only then go down one level and open up a chapter.

Systematic searches are bound to find an answer if one exists in the search space, but might take a long time to get there. When time is short, it makes sense to try and use an *analytic* search strategy, where the searcher uses prior knowledge to focus on areas of the space that are most likely to contain the information being sought:

- A **heuristic search** uses approximate rules of thumb, based upon past experience, to point the search in the right direction. For example, a rule of thumb might be 'if you're looking for the final diagnosis of a patient in their medical record, first look for it in the most recent medical discharge summary'. Table 7.1 lists some commonly used heuristics to track down papers in the biomedical literature.

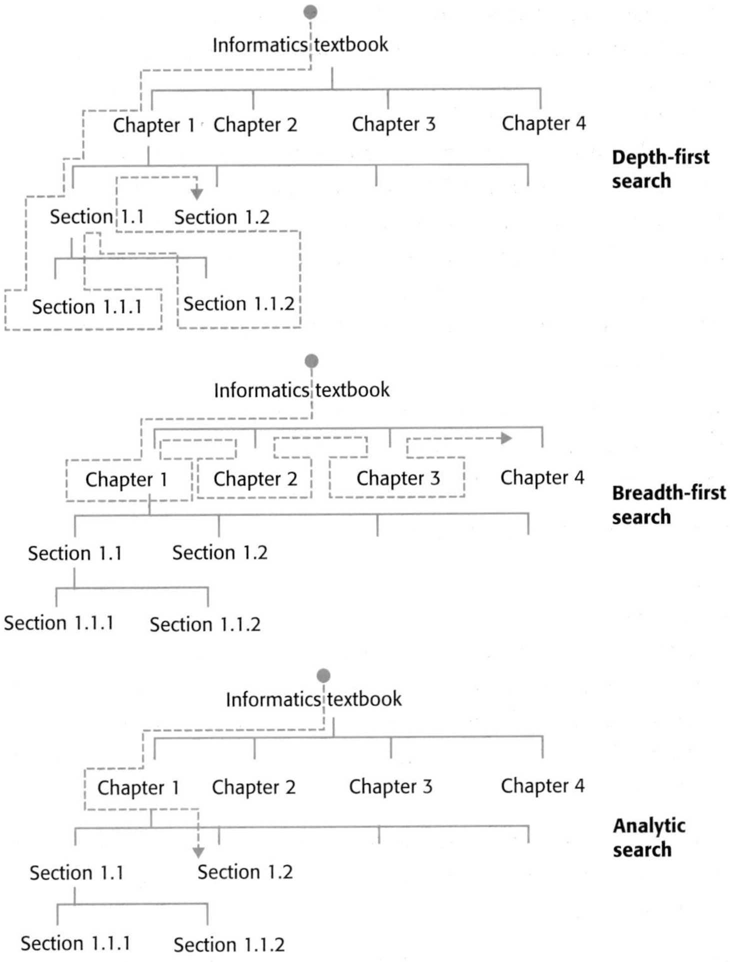
Informatics textbook
Chapter 1
Chapter 2
Chapter 3
Chapter 4
Depth-first search
Section 1.1
Section 1.2
Section 1.1.1
Section 1.1.2
Informatics textbook
Chapter 1
Chapter 2
Chapter 3
Chapter 4
Breadth-first search
Section 1.1
Section 1.2
Section 1.1.1
Section 1.1.2
Informatics textbook
Chapter 1
Chapter 2
Chapter 3
Chapter 4
Analytic search
Section 1.1
Section 1.2
Section 1.1.1
Section 1.1.2

Figure 7.3
A search space can be explored systematically using a depth-first or breadth-first strategy, eventually terminating when the required item is found. When specific knowledge about the location of an item exists, the search can be analytic and ignore parts of the search space, targeting the most likely spots where the item can be found, using heuristics or more complex models.

Table 7.1 Examples of heuristics that may be used to guide a search through the biomedical literature (from Bates, 1990).

Heuristic	Description of search strategy
Journal run	Having identified a journal that is central to one's topic of interest, one reads or browses through issues or volumes of the journal
Citation search	Using a citation index or database, one starts with a citation and determines what other works have cited it
Area scan	After locating a subject area of interest in a classification scheme, one browses materials in the same general area
Footnote chase	One follows up footnotes or references, thus moving backward in time to other related materials
Index or catalogue subject search	One looks up subject indexing terms or free text terms in a catalogue or abstracting and indexing service (online or offline) and locates all references on one's topic of interest.
Author subject search	Having found an author writing on a topic of interest, one looks up that author in catalogues, bibliographies, or indexes to see if they have written any other materials on the same subject.

- A **model-based search** uses a precise model to guide the search. For example, a search party hunting for a lost hiker might use satellite maps, the known direction in which the hikers were heading, and a mathematical estimate of how far they are likely to have walked since they set out, to identify the most likely area to start the search. When looking for evidence, a clinician might use MeSH keywords which model the content of journal articles, along with a limit on publication date to identify the part of the search space that is most likely to contain the documents being sought.

Heuristic search has the advantage that it usually is simple, and, more often than not, will come up with the right answer if the heuristics are based upon real experience. Experts often have the best heuristics because they have refined them over many years of use. Model-based strategies require more calculation and reasoning to identify the target area, and if time is short, they may not be optimal. Neither the heuristic nor the model-based strategies can guarantee success, unlike the systematic search strategies, because analytic methods exclude parts of the search space. Unless we can guarantee that the thing being looked for is within the area defined by the analytic method (and we usually cannot do that with clinical evidence) then there is a chance we are looking in the wrong place.

The process of search is often an iterative one, as shown in Figure 7.1, where the progress of the search process is evaluated in an ongoing fashion. Depending on how well the search process is advancing, it might make sense to keep the current strategy, or if it looks as if the right answer is not going to be forthcoming within an acceptable time, the strategy might be changed.

For complex search tasks, it may make sense to combine different search strategies, to maximize the likely outcomes. For example, when looking for a specific section in a textbook, it may make sense to start with a breadth-first search of the table of contents, knowing that the textbook is hierarchically structured. Once a likely chapter is identified, perhaps using some heuristic knowledge about where the answer is likely to reside, then the reader might switch to a depth-first search of the chapter, combing it systematically until the relevant sections are found. If this does not succeed, then the reader might switch to a different representation of the search space, and use the book's index to identify likely pages.

Database search terms are used to create a working document search space

Sometimes a search space is given to us explicitly, such as a table of contents listing. In some cases, we use tools to create a search space for a specific task. For example, when we are searching a document database such as the Medline database for specific articles, the potential search space is many millions of documents. In such a situation, it does not make sense to begin searching through all the documents individually, since success is likely to be low. In such circumstances, we extract a subset of documents that are most likely to contain the specific documents we are interested in. The process of documents selection is usually driven by supplying the database specific keywords or limits which tell it the type of document most likely to be of interest. For example, we might ask only for documents published in the last 6 months, or documents that match specific keywords.

To start a search with a database, one should try and ask the most specific question possible. For example, rather than using the keyword 'diabetes', the more specific term 'insulin-dependent diabetes' would be used. Once the database query has been made, the database

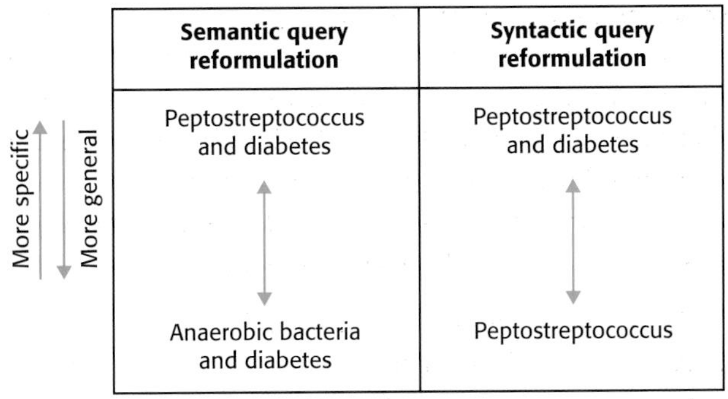
Semantic query reformulation
Syntactic query reformulation
Peptostreptococcus and diabetes
Peptostreptococcus and diabetes
Anaerobic bacteria and diabetes
Peptostreptococcus
More specific
More general

Figure 7.4
When an initial query to a database does not yield results, it may be because the question is either too specific or too general. To improve its performance, the query can be reformulated by altering either its syntactic structure, or the semantics of the concepts being explored.

returns a set of documents, which constitute the working search space the searcher will actually look through. When a tractably sized search space is generated, then the items can be inspected directly to see if they contain the target items.

Since search success is not always immediately guaranteed, the process of search may need to be iterative. As the search progresses, it may thus be necessary to refine the overall strategy. For a given question, there are two overall search space refinement strategies possible:

- **Specific to general enlargement:** If it seems that the target of the search is not present in the search space retrieved, for example because it only contains a very few documents, then the question may have been too specific, and we need to generalize it, which has the effect of enlarging the working search space.
- **General to specific narrowing:** Alternatively if the space is too large, with too many documents, then the question may have been too general, and we may wish to restrict it by becoming more specific in our question.

There are two different ways of changing how specific or general a question is. One way of performing such **query reformulation** is essentially mechanical, where we play with the syntax or structure of the query, and the second is semantic, where we play with the meaning of the query (Figure 7.4).

Syntactic query reformulation

Most queries consist of several words, usually implicitly joined together by the logical operator 'and'. As a rule, the more keywords are given as search terms, the more specific is the search, and fewer items will match the search specification. The fewer the number of terms in a query, the more general it is. Consequently we can make a query more or less specific by simply adding or subtracting terms from the query. For example, in Table 7.2, the query 'anaerobic bacteria and osteomyelitis' can be made more specific by adding on the term 'diabetes', or conversely made more general by dropping a term such as 'osteomyelitis'.

Instead of altering the terms, we can also manipulate the logical operators joining them. For example 'diabetes and osteomyelitis' is a more specific query than 'diabetes or osteomyelitis' (Box 6.2). Some databases allow queries to contain exact phrases such as 'diabetic osteomyelitis' and phrase searches are very specific, since they look for the exact appearance of the phrase. In contrast, breaking the phrase down into its component words to produce 'diabetes and osteomyelitis' only requires that both words appear in the same document or perhaps near each other, and therefore should yield more matches.

Table 7.2 A record of the sequence of actions taken as a clinician searches for an answer to a clinical question by choosing which knowledge sources to interrogate, and by refining the question posed to each knowledge source, based on the success of the query in retrieving appropriate documents.

What anaerobic microorganism is most commonly found in osteomyelitis associated with diabetic foot?

Knowledge source	**Query**	**No. of documents retrieved**	**Query action**
PubMed	anaerobic bacteria AND osteomyelitis	90	First guess
PubMed	anaerobic bacteria AND osteomyelitis AND diabetes	8	Syntactic specification
Medline Plus	anaerobic bacteria AND osteomyelitis AND diabetes	0	Change Knowledge source
Medline Plus	anaerobic bacteria AND diabetes	0	Syntactic generalization
Medline Plus	peptostreptococcus AND diabetes	0	Semantic generalization
Harrisons	peptostreptococcus AND diabetes	6	Change Knowledge source
Harrisons	peptostreptococcus	9	Syntactic generalization

Semantic query reformulation

It is also possible to make a question more or less specific by changing the words used. For example, 'chair' is a more specific term than 'furniture', and more general than 'dining chair'. Similarly, 'peptostreptococcus' is a more specific concept than 'anaerobic bacteria'. Making this type of change to a query requires knowledge of the meaning of the question and the terms in the query. We can imagine that words come from a hierarchy that organizes them conceptually, much like a taxonomy (Figure 16.3), and move up or down the hierarchy to make the term more or less general.

A semantic reformulation can also simply restate the query using synonyms or alternate wording. For example, 'kidney stones' and 'renal calculi' are semantically equivalent expressions. However, if a database is unable to check automatically for such semantic equivalents (for example by using MeSH), then the two searches will potentially retrieve very different document sets. If completely different semantic concepts are chosen in the reformulation, the effect is not to narrow, expand or reshape the existing search space, but to define a new and entirely different space (Figure 7.5).

If, after using such strategies, the item is not found, it may be necessary to reconsider the overall search strategy. It may be that the wrong terms are being used to locate the search items, in which case a complete re-think is needed to describe the search target in other ways. Alternatively, the item may not be in the sources being searched, and it may be necessary to alter the spaces in which the search is being conducted. This may mean looking at different databases, or changing search strategy altogether – for example, consulting an expert for advice on where to look next.

An electronic database such as Medline is sufficiently flexible that it offers multiple structures to search for information, and if one is not helpful, then another can be selected. Medline contains:

- Data-oriented templates in the form of raw bibliographic data about each article in the database.
- Protocol-oriented templates to assist searching for pre-defined classes of question (Table 6.3).
- An implicit template-oriented structure to guide question formation. The template consists of all the MeSH terms, and the Boolean logic that is used to assemble them. Since there are many possible ways the terms can be assembled, MeSH essentially provides

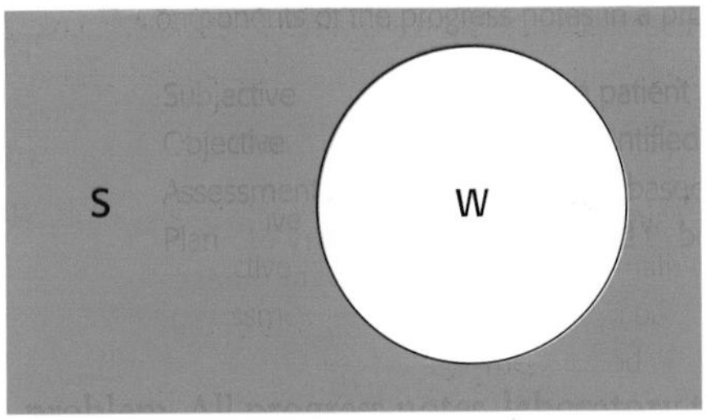
S
W

When searching in a database, we usually retrieve a working subset **W** of the total search space **S** to search through.

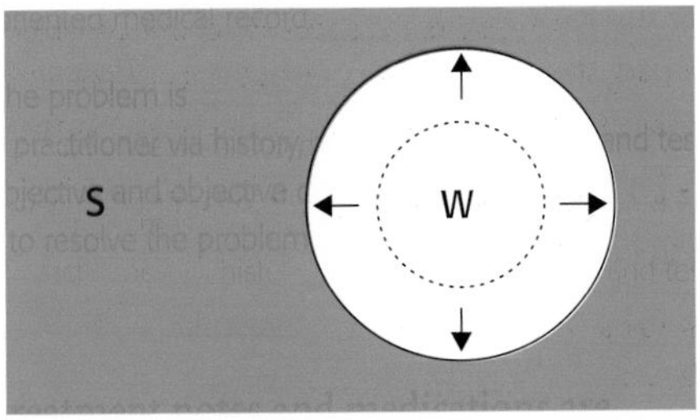
S
W

A strategy of **specific to general** refinement creates the smallest, most specific, working search space, and then expands it until the search is successful

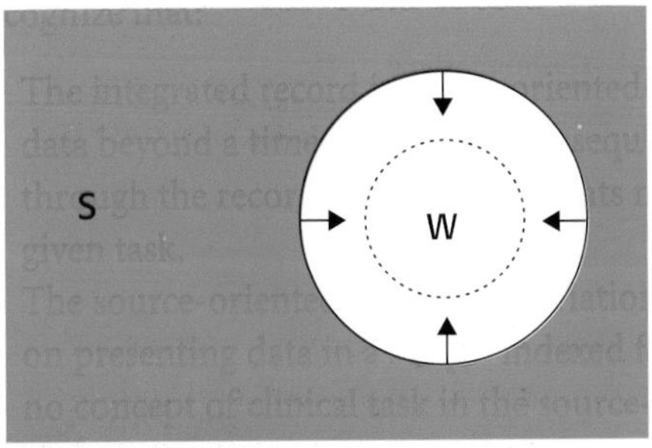
S
W

A strategy of **general to specific** refinement creates the largest, most general, working search space, and then contracts it until the search is successful.

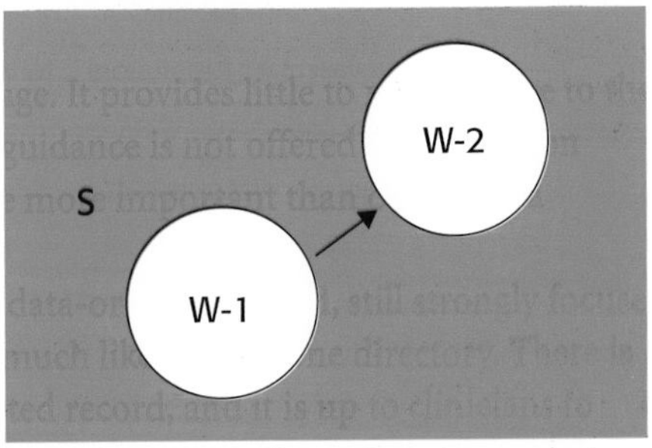
S
W-2
W-1

If the initial working search space is fruitless, a new working search space can be generated using different criteria to select candidate items.

Figure 7.5
When search spaces are large, a subset is usually selected to produce a working search space, W. Using knowledge about the likely location of the search target, there is a good chance the item being looked for will be found in W. W can be modified if the initial working search space is too small, too large, or looks like it does not contain the target of search.

a pre-defined language. The different ways a question can be posed, with variations in use of Boolean operators and different terms constitute their own search space.

Similarly, electronic medical record systems can permit multiple different views into the record databases. Consequently electronic record systems should be capable of supporting information search in a rich manner, just as Medline does.

Patient history-taking and examination combine analytic and systematic search methods

When a map exists, we use it, and when none exists we build our own map, much like leaving a trail of string through a maze. Consequently, when no search structure exists, it is up to the individual asking the question to impose a structure on the search space, which will then act as a reference point to guide the knowledge seeking process.

The process of patient history-taking can be seen as a search for information. No map comes purpose built with a patient's history, so it is necessary to impose a map to guide the search. Taking a patient history is actually a controlled traversal of a search space, structured according to an externally imposed model of organ systems. There are many different ways to take a patient history, but one of the commonest approaches is to:

1 Take a history of present illness (HPI)
2 Conduct a review of systems (ROS)
3 Take a past, family and social history.

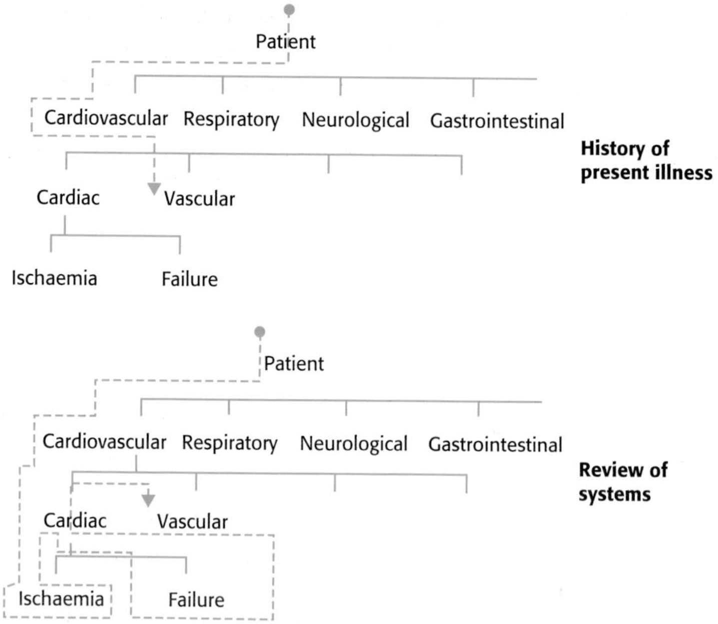
Patient
Cardiovascular
Respiratory
Neurological
Gastrointestinal
Cardiac
Vascular
Ischaemia
Failure
History of present illness
Patient
Cardiovascular
Respiratory
Neurological
Gastrointestinal
Cardiac
Vascular
Ischaemia
Failure
Review of systems

Figure 7.6
Taking a patient history is a process of search with an imposed template to guide the search. The standard review of systems is a systematic process, examining each physiological system in turn, in an approximately depth-first manner. In contrast, taking the history of present illness is much more analytic, requiring the use of knowledge to guide the search to identify specific issues identified by the patient.

Each step approaches search in a different way. The ROS is systematic, in that it forces an exploration of different physiological systems, and ensures the whole search space is covered. It is thus a kind of depth-first search. The ROS is a series of questions that systematically explores body systems in an effort to identify relevant signs or symptoms from a patient. An ROS asks a few key questions for each system that is covered, and will probably examine in turn the cardiovascular, respiratory, gastrointestinal, genitourinary, musculoskeletal, neurological, endocrine, etc. systems (Mikolanis, 1997).

In contrast, taking the history of present illness is an analytic search, and it is here that a clinician's experience, their accumulated knowledge and rules of thumb, help them home in on the key issues presented by the patient. Starting with a chronological description of the present complaint, the clinician then tries to funnel down on what the core problem might be with a targeted set of questions.

By combining the systematic aspects of the ROS with the analytic of the HPI the process of history-taking attempts to be both efficient, homing in rapidly on the most likely issues, but also comprehensive, ensuring key issues that may be hidden to the patient may also be surfaced. The systematic nature of the ROS also ensures that less experienced clinicians have templates to guide their search, and increases the likelihood that relevant patient data is discovered.

In most clinical circumstances there is a trade-off between a comprehensive history-taking process, which is time consuming, and the focused analytic process, which might miss some details, but usually homes in on the key problem. In clinical situations in which time is of the essence, such as an acute asthmatic attack or myocardial infarct, the analytic search will rapidly identify what needs to be discovered, and the systematic ROS will be delayed until the urgency has subsided.

For much of this chapter we have conceived of the search process as one of asking questions of agents who will then provide an answer. In clinical medicine, we may also search in the more traditional way, actually hunting for physical clues. The process of physical examination is thus also a search process, with systematic and analytic components to the hunt for physical signs of disease. Just as with history-taking, when a clinician conducts a physical examination of a patient, there is no map on the patient's body to guide the hunt. Consequently, the search for clinical signs can be conducted in an imposed systematic way, organ system by organ system. Clinicians may also specifically devote attention to key areas where they know they are most likely to find what they are seeking, using a more analytic approach to the search for physical signs.

7.5 The answer is evaluated to see if it is well formed, specific, accurate and reliable

During the process of search, one or more candidate answers are usually found. Before they are accepted at face value, some process of testing or evaluation needs to occur, to make sure the answer is of good quality. In clinical medicine, evaluation is essential, because decisions may be made as a result of the answer that could have an impact on the treatment of patients.

Specifically, we evaluate the answer because it may be either wrong or inappropriate, and there are a number of reasons for that. Recall that search can be thought of as a conversation, where we ask well-formed questions of knowledgeable agents, and that such conversations can fail in specific ways. Different agents have different capacities to answer questions, depending upon what they know, what common ground they share with the enquiring agent, what they understand the question to be, what resources they have available, and how cooperative they wish to be. Recalling Grice's maxims, an answer may be inappropriate because the answering agent:

- has misheard or misunderstood the question
- may be poorly qualified to answer the question
- may be intentionally misinforming
- may only answer a part of the question
- may reply unhelpfully, with irrelevant information
- may reply in excess detail or in terminology that is not understood, or in a manner not appropriate to the context.

An answer can be evaluated at several different levels, depending upon our confidence in the answering agent, the level of quality we require from the answer and the resources we have available to perform the evaluation. Specifically we can evaluate an answer in terms of its **form** and its **content.** We assess form by looking at the following:

- **Syntax:** The integrity of an answer can be quickly checked to see if it is syntactically well structured. If it is garbled or incomplete, then an error may have occurred in transmission, perhaps because of the impact of noise or other interference. Before the details of a laboratory test are assessed, for example, it makes sense to check that the report is complete and well structured.
- **Terminology:** Are the words used in the answer appropriate for the individual that needs the answer? An answer given to a patient will contain different terms from an answer intended for a health professional, who is familiar with technical terms. If the answer contains unfamiliar terms, then it also might be an indication that there is less common ground between the agent asking and the agent responding, which might indicate the question was misunderstood. The use of a shared and standard terminology suggests good common ground.

- **Complexity and structure:** Does the answer's form match the context within which it is received and the constraints on the receiving agent? For example, with a clinical question that requires urgent action, a detailed answer such as a full systematic review is probably less valuable than a short, specific, task-focused answer that makes it clear what action needs to be taken immediately. The amount of detail, complexity of structure and terminology chosen all may make an answer inappropriate to a context, even if it is accurate.

We assess content by assessing the **semantics** or meaning of the answer by looking at:

- **Quality:** How much faith do we put into the information contained in an answer? If the answer comes from a known colleague who is expert in the area of interest, and who has delivered useful answers in the past, then our trust in the quality of the new information is probably high. If the answer comes from a respectable journal, which we know has a rigorous peer review process, then we also have some guarantee that there has been a professional attempt to check the contents of the answer for errors. If the answer comes from a source of which we have little experience or knowledge, then it might be prudent to be slightly sceptical about the answer, and perhaps try to corroborate the information by seeking an answer from another source. When it comes to published information, one way of determining how much trust we can put in the quality of the answer is to assess the methodology used in arriving at the answer, and the amount of evidence that sits behind the answer supporting it (Figure 7.7). For example, if the answer comes from a single case report in a journal, there is less evidence that the case report is valid, than if we find our answer in a **systematic review** of a number of randomized clinical trials. Each **randomized controlled trial** (RCT) has probably involved many patients, testing out a new therapeutic intervention in a very well documented and controlled setting. By pooling together the results of a number of RCTs we increase our trust that the result is generalizable, since it has support from several different groups of researchers, each working independently of each other, and with different populations of patients. Not all documents fit neatly into the levels of evidence structure of Figure 7.7. Specifically, documents designed to support clinical decisions are usually written to make them easy

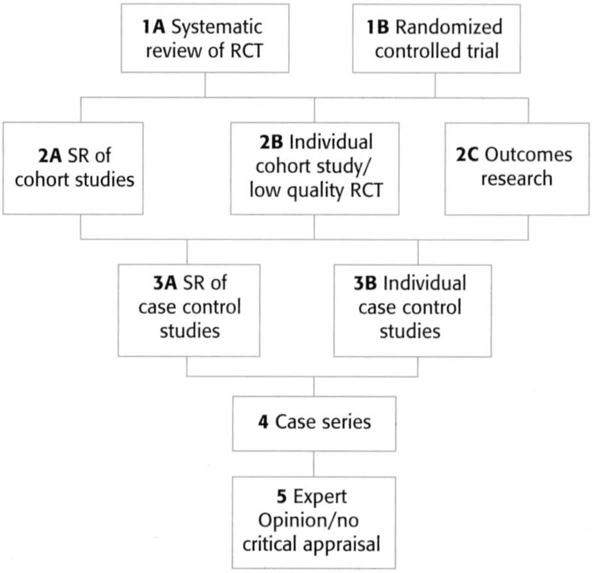
1A Systematic review of RCT
1B Randomized controlled trial
2A SR of cohort studies
2B Individual cohort study/ low quality RCT
2C Outcomes research
3A SR of case control studies
3B Individual case control studies
4 Case series
5 Expert Opinion/no critical appraisal

Figure 7.7 The level of evidence behind an answer assists in assessing its quality. For therapeutic questions, five levels of evidence (level 1 is best, 5 is weakest) may be distinguished. (RCT, randomized controlled trial; SR, systematic review). Adapted from the Oxford Centre for Evidence-based Medicine.

to use clinically, rather than to demonstrate the evidence base behind them. This makes perfect sense if the task is to communicate knowledge effectively to suit the needs of a clinical setting, and indeed, documents such as systematic reviews, which emphasize the evidence base, are often criticized for not being user-friendly in clinical situations. **Clinical guidelines** are documents designed for clinical ease of use, and usually show the steps that need to be taken in a given clinical situation. However, their design de-emphasizes evidence. In such circumstances, the quality of the information contained in the document may not be self-evident. In such cases, people often look for a **quality label** to give some guarantee of the document's pedigree. For example, the document may have the approval of a major professional health group, or well-respected clinical institution. We assume that the process involved in testing whether the document deserves the label was sufficiently rigorous for us to take this at face value. Of course, such guarantees are actually weak certifications of quality, since the evidence on which the labelling decision was made is hidden from the document user.

- **Utility:** In Chapter 6, patient-oriented evidence that matters (POEM) was shown to be more valuable than less specific background or disease-oriented evidence. Consequently, some answers are less useful than others, even though they might be equally true, since the answers do not tell us anything we can usefully act upon.

Conclusions

In this chapter, we have built upon the principle of communication, information structuring and question formation to explain the process of search for knowledge. Searching is an essential core skill in clinical practice, whether we are looking for new clinical evidence to support a clinical decision, or simply gathering all the facts from a patient though their history and physical examination. In the next chapter, we complete the section on informatics skills, by examining how, with all the data and knowledge retrieved through search, clinical decisions are made.

Discussion points

1 Is the search for knowledge a positive or a negative feedback loop?

2 Use the equation of knowledge usefulness to explain why disease-oriented evidence (DOE) is usually less useful that patient-oriented evidence that matters (POEM).

3 What is the search space structure generated by the result of a question to a Web search engine? Discuss search engine results in terms of data, task and template-oriented structuring.

4 Compare and contrast the role and utility of the search spaces created by the different patient record structures presented in Chapter 5.

5 Triage is the process of rapidly selecting patients who are most likely to survive in desperate circumstances such as the battlefield or civilian disasters, where there are many more victims than available emergency workers to help. What kind of search strategy do you think triage is, and why is it appropriate to these circumstances?

6 Discuss the different roles that the system review portion of a patient history takes in both supporting the process of search as well as subsequent communication. Think of the review structure as a task-based template.

7 In what situations is it necessary to impose a search structure on a knowledge source? Think back to Chapter 2 and Figure 2.5, which examined when a computer should or should not provide a model to assist human reasoning.

Chapter summary

1 Search involves identifying an information task, choosing an appropriate knowledgeable agent and channel, crafting a question and search strategy suited to the task, receiving agent and channel, and sending the message. Feedback evaluates the answer to guide further search.

2 Search strategies are optimized to minimize cost and maximize benefit:
- the more knowledge is relevant to a situation, the more value it has
- the more knowledge is valid, the greater its impact on our task
- search is less likely to be pursued if knowledge is hard to extract.

3 The set of all possible knowledge sources forms a **search space** that has to be explored in the hunt for the answer to a specific question.

4 A search strategy is a plan that directs an agent's search in a space.

5 Systematic strategies start at the beginning and keep looking at every item until an answer is found:
- in **depth-first search**, we dive deep into the search space, until we can go no further, and only then come back, and resume the dive
- in **breadth-first search** we examine a node, and backtrack immediately if there is no answer, continuing to explore nodes at the same level; only then will the strategy move on to a deeper level.

6 Analytic strategies use prior knowledge to focus on areas of the space that are most likely to contain the information being sought:
- **heuristic search** uses rules of thumb based upon past experience
- **model-based search** uses a precise model to guide search.

7 For large search spaces, a subset or working search space is selected, and then refined if no answer is found. Refinement strategies include:
- specific to general enlargement
- general to specific narrowing
- search query reformulation may be **semantic** or **syntactic**.

8 Patient history-taking and examination combine analytic and systematic search methods. A review of systems is like a depth-first search ; a history of present illness is an analytic search.

9 An answer is evaluated to see if it is well-formed, specific, accurate and reliable by examining:
- **syntax**, its terminology, its complexity and structure
- **semantics**, looking at its meaning and the quality of that answer.

10 The quality of an answer can be ascertained by the level of evidence used to create it, or if nothing else is available, the existence of a quality label which attempts to guarantee the pedigree of the information provided.

CHAPTER 8

Making decisions

> Evidence does not make decisions, people do.
> *Devereaux and Guyatt (2002).*

Nothing gets done without someone first making a decision. Patients are treated, or not treated, because someone has looked at the facts of the case and the available scientific evidence, thought through the consequences of the different options, and made a choice. Often these clinical choices arise out of mutual agreement between patient and clinician, or between different members of a clinical team.

In previous chapters we saw how a question should be structured and communicated, and how the search for an answer should proceed. Now, we take a step back and look at where questions come from in the first place, and what we do once we have our answers.

Decision-making is rarely a clear-cut affair, and decisions are almost inevitably compromises. Decisions reflect not just 'the evidence', logic and probability, but also our goals, our values and the available resources. Decisions are almost always compromised by uncertainty, and when humans are the decision-makers, by our in-built cognitive biases.

8.1 Problem-solving is reasoning from the facts to create alternatives, and then choosing one alternative

Clinical care can be thought of as a set of problems presented to patients and clinicians. Clinical problems can come in many forms. They might, for example, be diagnostic – 'what is the cause of my chest pain?', therapeutic – 'how do I treat rheumatoid arthritis?', prognostic – 'how long do I have to live?', or about resource management – 'what is the most cost-effective way to run a hospital emergency department?'.

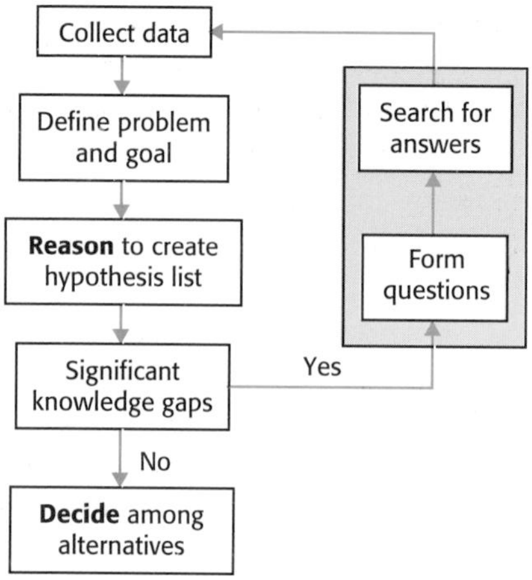
Collect data
Define problem and goal
Reason to create hypothesis list
Significant knowledge gaps
Yes
No
Decide among alternatives
Form questions
Search for answers

Figure 8.1
The problem-solving process is an iterative cycle of discovering data, reasoning from it to form hypotheses, and when no further data would improve the likely outcome, selecting the most plausible hypothesis. The process of search is captured in the grey 'question and answer' box, and can be expanded into the smaller steps shown in Figure 7.1.

The process of problem-solving is essentially the same for most tasks (Figure 8.1) and begins when new data suggest there is a problem. For example, the presentation of new clinical symptoms, or a cash-flow shortfall in a departmental budget, could indicate the presence of a new problem that requires attention.

Once a problem is identified, we next decide what it is to be done about it. For example, if a department will always be given operating funds, whether or not it goes into deficit, then overspending may not really be a problem. If, on the other hand, failure to keep to budget threatens the operation of the organization, then action is needed. Consequently, it is important first to define the exact problem, whether it needs to be solved and its relative importance, as this then determines what happens next. Time is short and resources scarce, and it is probably just as harmful to solve unimportant problems as it is to set out to solve the wrong problem.

The next step in the problem-solving process is to think through what the alternative solutions might be. This is often described as the process of **hypothesis generation** and creates a list of alternatives that need to be selected from. If the problem is a diagnostic one, then the hypothesis list contains potential diagnoses. If the problem is a therapeutic one, then the list contains potential treatments.

At this stage there may not enough evidence at hand to generate a satisfactory list of candidate hypotheses. This is the 'knowledge gap' that we encountered in Chapter 6. As we now know, in such situations, appropriate questions are formed and a process of search commences, looking for answers to those questions. In clinical practice, the evidence surrounding a given case might be obtained from the patient history, physical examination or laboratory investigations. The wider evidence may be contained in knowledge about similar situations that comes from the scientific literature.

A successful search results in the arrival of new evidence that will then be integrated into the problem-solving cycle. The impact of the new evidence might simply be to reduce the number of active hypotheses by eliminating some candidates. New evidence may be sufficiently informative that it allows a choice to be made between different hypotheses, or it might cause the whole problem to be re-evaluated, and new hypotheses to be generated.

Potentially many iterations of this cycle of data gathering and hypothesis generation can occur, until the decision-maker feels that there is enough clarity to move on to choosing between hypotheses. The key to this stage of the problem-solving process is to keep the initial goal in mind. For example, if the goal is to quickly stabilize a critically ill patient who has presented in an emergency department, then the problem-solving goals are not to come up with a detailed diagnosis and therapy plan, which might take many days, but to stabilize the patient. In such circumstances, the problem-solving goal determines a rapid resolution to the process. In contrast, a clinician managing a patient who has presented with a complicated and slow onset autoimmune disorder may need many problem-solving cycles, refining the potential diagnoses as different test results are returned, until a diagnosis with a clear therapeutic goal has been reached.

The final step in the problem-solving process is to make a decision. This involves examining the list of competing hypotheses, supported by the assembled evidence, and choosing the one that is most appropriate. The criteria for making that choice need to reflect the initial goal. For example, a patient may have an incurable disease, and some treatment options may prolong life but make the patient's life unbearable, because of pain and stress. Other treatment options may lead to an earlier death, but through the use of palliative treatments, ensure the patient is relatively comfortable for that time. Clearly in such cases the choice of treatment is not simply one that comes just from the scientific evidence, which might favour the treatment that most prolongs life. The choice is as much one of values and preferences, and in situations such as this there is no right answer, but a spectrum of preferences that results in different individuals drawing different conclusions from the same evidence.

We will now look at the two processes of reasoning from the data, which creates the list of hypotheses, and decision, which selects from that list, in more detail.

8.2 Hypotheses are generated by making inferences from the given data

Problem-solving begins with data, and the need to draw some conclusions from the data. In Chapter 2 we saw that this process of reasoning or data interpretation requires a **database**, a **knowledge base** and **rules of inference.** Rules such as 'if the pH is greater than 7 then it is abnormally high' might be part of a clinician's knowledge base. The **rules of inference** specify how we apply the knowledge base to data. There are many different possible rules of inference, but the two most important from a clinical viewpoint are the rules of logic and the rules of probability.

The rules of logic infer what is known to be true, given the facts

If asked, most clinicians would say that the logical process of diagnosis is most like the process of **deduction,** often associated with the fictional detective Sherlock Holmes. In fact, a diagnosis is obtained by using a logical rule called **abduction**. Along with **induction**, these three together form the basic rules of logical inference (Figure 8.2).

The difference between these three logical rules is straightforward. We start by assuming there is a **cause and effect** statement about the world that we know to be true. For example, assume that 'pneumonia causes fever' is always true. Pneumonia in this case is the cause, and fever is the effect. Another true statement might be that 'septicaemia causes fever'.

We can write these 'rules' in the following way:

if pneumonia **then** fever
if septicaemia **then** fever

For the process of deduction, we are told that a cause is true, and then infer all the effects that arise naturally as a consequence. In this example, having been told a patient has pneumonia, deduction will tell us that the patient will therefore develop a fever.

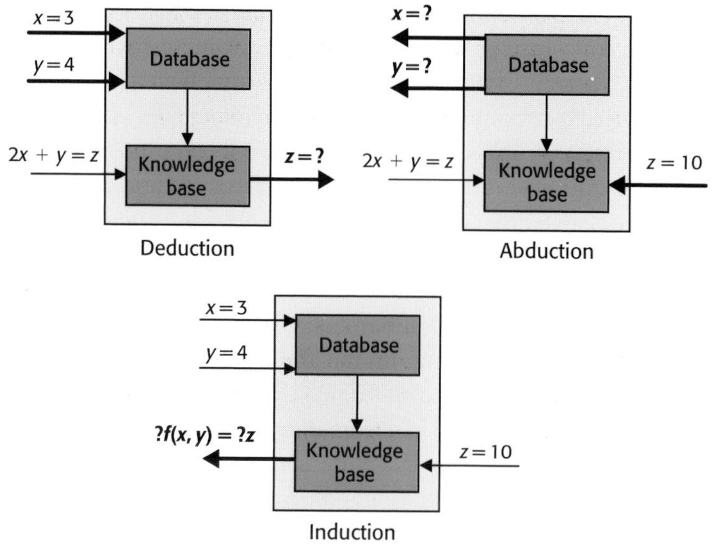
x=3
y=4
Database
2x + y=z
Knowledge base
z=?
Deduction
x=?
y=?
Database
2x + y=z
Knowledge base
z=10
Abduction
x=3
y=4
Database
?f(x, y) = ?z
Knowledge base
z=10
Induction

Figure 8.2
The three basic types of logical reasoning are deduction, abduction and induction. Each method proceeds from a different set of inputs to infer their logical consequences.

In contrast, abduction takes the cause and effect statements we know, and given an observed effect, generates all known causes. In this case, we might be told a patient has fever. Abduction would say that pneumonia or septicaemia are both possible causes.

Abduction allows us to produce a list of alternate hypotheses to explain the given data. Note that whereas deduction produces statements of certainty, abduction produces statements of possibility. To choose between the options generated by abduction, one may need to seek further information that clearly differentiates between the hypotheses. In some cases, the data are so clear that a single hypothesis is confirmed. When the pattern is so distinctive of a disease that it can be nothing else, the pattern is labelled pathognomonic (literally 'naming the disease').

In contrast to abduction and deduction, which use cause and effect statements, the role of induction is to actually create these statements from observations. For example, a doctor may have observed many patients who have had fevers. Some of these die, and postmortem examination shows they all have an infection of the lung, which the doctor labels 'pneumonia'. The doctor then might decide that 'fever causes pneumonia'.

Unlike the other rules of logic, induction is unsound. In other words, it may lead to false conclusions. Thus, when our doctor finds a feverish patient who does not have pneumonia on autopsy, the original conclusion becomes invalid. Perhaps then, the doctor re-uses induction to hypothesize this time the reverse statement 'pneumonia causes fever'. Induction then, is the process of generalization, which creates our models of the world.

The rules of probability infer what is most likely to be true, given the facts

In classic logic, things are either true or they are not. There is no space for imprecision. However, such clarity is often lacking in the real world, and it is more useful to talk about how likely an event might be. A middle-aged smoker with known heart disease and chest pain may have any number of conditions that could plausibly cause their pain, but given our past experience with similar patients, the likelihood is that the pain is caused by myocardial ischaemia. As we saw in the previous section, the rules of logic allow us to generate a candidate list, but in clinical medicine, the full list of possible diagnoses might be very long.

Consequently it makes sense to only consider those hypotheses that are most likely. Statistical rules of inference allow the likelihood that a hypothesis is true to be calculated, and therefore permits the list of candidate hypotheses to be reduced to a manageable size.

Typically a probability is an expression of the frequency of an event in the past. Assigning the event myocardial ischaemia a probability of $p = 0.8$ says that in 8 out of 10 similar past cases the outcome was myocardial ischaemia. In 2 out of those past 10 cases it was not, so the probability of not having myocardial ischaemia is $(1 - p) = 0.2$, since the probability of all events together always sums to 1.

One of the most famous probability theorems used to estimate the likelihood of clinical events is Bayes' theorem, which estimates the likelihood that a patient has a disease, given a certain symptom. For example, the theorem would help answer the question 'What is the probability of a patient having myocardial ischaemia, given that they have chest pain?'. This expression is known as a **conditional probability** and is written $P(ischaemia \mid chest\ pain)$.

Bayes' theorem (Box 8.1) states that the probability of a disease given a clinical finding $P(D \mid S)$ is dependent on:

- The **prior probability** that anyone in the population has the disease $P(D)$, before any information is known about the current patient.
- The probability that the patient has a clinical finding $P(S \mid D)$ given that they have the disease. This is simply the likelihood that anyone with the disease has the symptom.
- The probability that the patient has a clinical finding $P(S \mid not\ D)$ given that they do not have the disease. This is simply the likelihood that anyone has the symptom but not the disease.

Box 8.1
Bayes' theorem

Bayes' theorem can be derived in the following way. First, from Figure 8.3, we note that the conditional probability of a disease *D* occurring, given a sign *S* is:

$$P(D \mid S) = \frac{P(D + S)}{P(S)} \qquad [1]$$

Next, from Figure 8.3, we also note that *P(S)* is simply the sum of the probabilities of those patients who have *S* and *D*, *P(D and S)*, as well as those patients who do not have *D* but do have *S*, *P(not D and S)*. So, we simply replace *P(S)* in the denominator of equation [1] with this new expression to give:

$$P(D \mid S) = \frac{P(D + S)}{P(D + S) + P(\text{not } D + S)} \qquad [2]$$

Next, we need to rewrite the right-hand side probabilities into a form that is more clinically useful. We first note that any *p(X and Y)* is identical to *p(Y and X)*. So we can gently modify the right-hand side of [2] to give us:

$$P(D \mid S) + \frac{P(S + D)}{P(S + D) + P(S + \text{not } D)} \qquad [3]$$

We go back to our first conditional probability equation [1] to rewrite each of the three terms on the right-hand side into the following forms:

$$P(S + D) = P(S \mid D) \times P(D)$$
$$P(S + \text{not } D) = P(S \mid \text{not } D) \times P(\text{not } D)$$

These expanded forms are then substituted back into equation [3] to give use the full version of Bayes' theorem:

$$P(D \mid S) = \frac{P(S \mid D) \times P(D)}{P(S \mid D) \times P(D) + P(S \mid \text{not } D) \times P(\text{not } D)} \qquad [4]$$

Further reading

Hunink M, Glasziou P, Siegel J *et al.* (2001) *Decision-making in Health and Medicine – Integrating Evidence With Values*. Cambridge University Press, Cambridge.

Sox H, Blatt M, Higgins MC, Marton K (1988) *Medical Decision-making*, Butterworths, Boston.

Bayes' theorem states that:

$$P(D|S) = \frac{P(S\,|\,D) \times P(D)}{P(S\,|\,D) \times P(D) + P(S\,|\,\text{not } D) \times P(\text{not } D)}$$

We sometimes call the result of the theorem, $P(D \mid S)$, the **posterior probability**, since it reflects how our belief in the likelihood of an event has changed from the prior probability, given our new information about the state of the symptom in the patient.

Bayes' theorem as presented here requires some very strict assumptions to be true for it to be used, which can restrict its clinical applicability in some circumstances. Specifically:

- Each hypothesis must be mutually exclusive. One hypothesis cannot be dependent on any other candidate hypothesis.
- The symptoms, signs and test results that form the patient data must be independent of each other. No data type should influence the likelihood that another data type will take on a certain value.

The theorem is also often restricted in its practical use because not all the probabilities may be known.

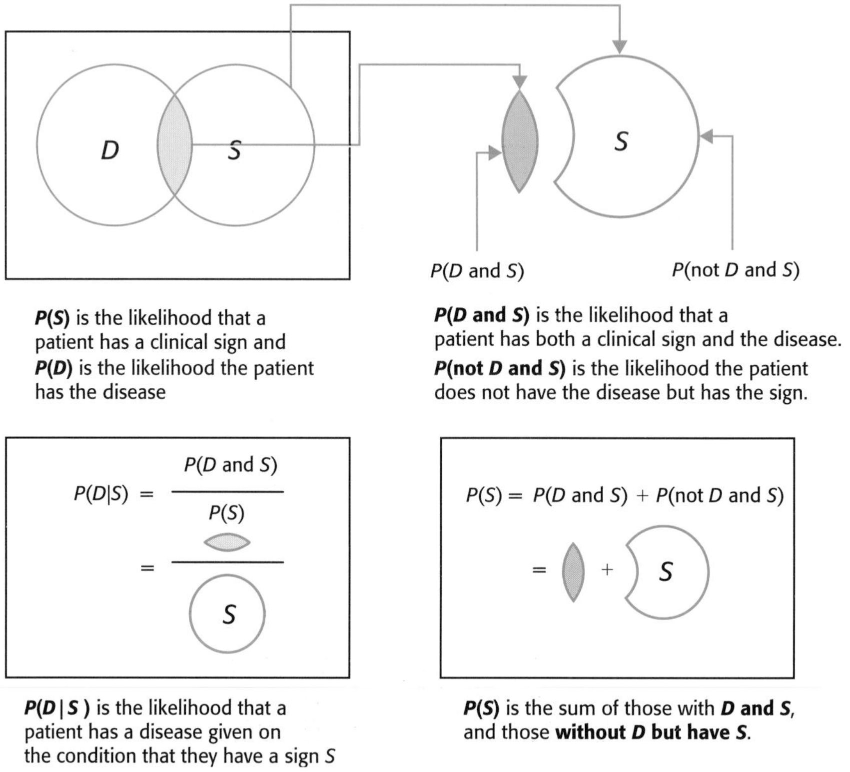
D
S
S
P(D and S)
P(not D and S)
P(S) is the likelihood that a patient has a clinical sign and **P(D)** is the likelihood the patient has the disease
P(*D* and *S*) is the likelihood that a patient has both a clinical sign and the disease. **P(not *D* and *S*)** is the likelihood the patient does not have the disease but has the sign.
P(D|S) = P(D and S) / P(S)
=
S
P(S) = P(D and S) + P(not D and S)
= +
S
***P*(*D* | *S*)** is the likelihood that a patient has a disease given on the condition that they have a sign *S*
P(*S*) is the sum of those with ***D* and *S***, and those **without *D* but have *S***.

Figure 8.3
For a clinical sign *S* and a disease *D* that are not independent, we can derive expressions to calculate the conditional probability of *D* being present, given *S*. The probability expressions shown here are the foundations of Bayes' theorem (Box 8.1).

Bayes' theorem assists in the interpretation of new diagnostic data

Bayes' theorem shows how new evidence changes our belief in the existence of an event. Specifically, our belief in the likelihood of an event depends both on what our belief was prior to the new evidence arriving, and is modified by the likelihood that the new evidence is true. Bayes' theorem can be used to update the belief in the likelihood of a disease given a new test result. When dealing with test results, the prior probability is called the **pre-test probability** and the posterior probability the **post-test probability**.

For example, a patient with chest pain might be asked to take a stress test, to see if exercise causes ischaemic changes in their cardiogram. A positive test will increase the likelihood of disease being present. However, if the pre-test probability of cardiac disease was low in the first place, then the presence of a positive test result, while increasing our belief in cardiac disease, is still much lower than for a patient in whom we had a high suspicion of cardiac disease before the positive test (Figure 8.4).

In Chapter 6 we examined the notion of the accuracy of asking a question, and introduced explicit measures like the true positive rate for information searches. A test can be thought of in exactly the same way, asking a question whether or not a condition is present. The sensitivity and specificity of test results are routinely calculated to give an estimate of how well they perform in identifying a condition.

From Table 6.4, the sensitivity or true positive rate (TPR) is:

$$TPR = \frac{\text{Number of diseased patients with a positive test}}{\text{Number of diseased patients}}$$

The false positive rate (FPR) is:

$$FPR = \frac{\text{Number of non-diseased patients with a positive test}}{\text{Number of diseased patients}}$$

Recall that Bayes' theorem states:

$$P(D|S) = \frac{P(S \mid D) \times P(D)}{P(S|D) \times P(D) + P(S|\text{not } D) \times P(\text{not } D)}$$

Using the TPR or FPR we can easily come up with alternate forms of the equation. If a test result is positive, Bayes' theorem states that:

$$\begin{bmatrix}\text{Probability of disease} \\ \text{if test result is positive}\end{bmatrix} = \frac{TPR \times P(D)}{TPR \times P(D) + FPR \times P(\text{not } D)}$$

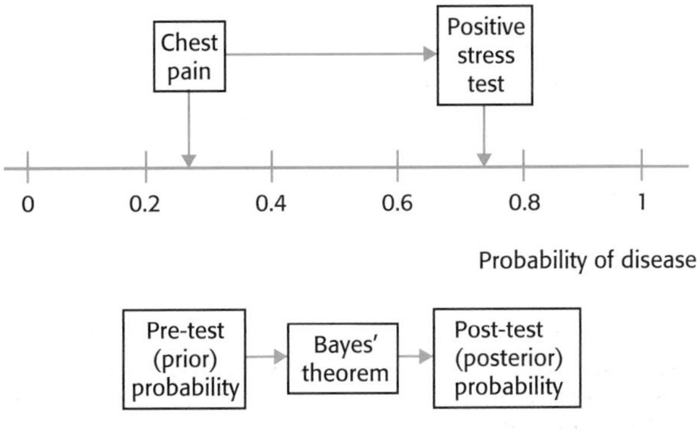
Chest pain
Positive stress test
0
0.2
0.4
0.6
0.8
1
Probability of disease
Pre-test (prior) probability
Bayes' theorem
Post-test (posterior) probability

Figure 8.4
Bayes' theorem calculates the change in likelihood of a disease given new evidence from the discovery of symptoms or signs, or from test results. A positive test result increases the probability of disease, and a negative result decreases the probability (after Sox *et al.*, 1988).

Similarly, if a test result is negative, we want to use the false negative (*FNR*) and true negative rates (*TNR*). However, since all probabilities must sum to 1, we simply note that:

- ***TNR* = (1 − *FPR*):** This says that all the patients who don't have the disease are either correctly identified as such (*TNR*) or mislabelled as having the disease (*FPR*). Knowing one rate therefore allows us to calculate the other.
- ***FNR* = (1 − *TPR*):** This says that all the patients who have the disease are either correctly identified as such (*TPR*) or mislabelled as not having the disease (*FNR*).

We can therefore stick to using the *TPR* and *FPR*, and write:

$$\begin{bmatrix}\text{Probability of disease}\\ \text{if test result is positive}\end{bmatrix} = \frac{(1-TPR)\times P(D)}{(1-TPR)\times P(D)+(1-FPR)\times P(\text{not } D)}$$

Bayes' theorem should be applied with caution to sequences of tests as they may not be independent events

Often a patient undergoes a series of tests to diagnose a disease. For a patient undergoing first an electrocardiogram, and then a stress test, it should now be clear that the post-test probability after the first cardiogram now becomes the pre-test probability before the stress test. As each piece of evidence is added in, our beliefs change in sequence.

However, it was stated earlier that Bayes' theorem makes an assumption that the events under consideration are independent of each other. This also holds for tests, and when a sequence of tests is conducted, typically one has to make the assumption that the *TPR* and *FPR* of one test are not dependent upon the presence of other findings. Such conditional independence does not always hold however. For example, when testing for the presence of coronary artery disease, it can be shown that the results of a positive stress test (exercise electrocardiogram) and a radionucleotide scan are not independent (Sox *et al.*, 1988).

There can be many reasons for such dependence. For example, if a test requires some degree of human interpretation, then the act of interpreting the data to produce the test result may be influenced by prior evidence. So, the expert making the interpretation may already have factored the prior probability of a disease into their interpretation of the test data. In such a situation, the clinician who receives the second test result cannot treat it as a new and independent piece of evidence.

Data about the independence of tests is often not available, and making an assumption that they are independent when using Bayes' theorem is an approximate method. In general, the longer the sequence of tests, the less independent they are likely to be (Sox *et al.*, 1988).

8.3 Decision trees can be used to determine the most likely outcome when there are several alternatives

It is not unusual for a decision problem to have more than one area of uncertainty. Symptoms and clinical signs may introduce uncertainty because their presence is debatable or their meaning unclear. Test results, as we have seen, are associated with uncertainty, and rarely tell us anything without some doubt still attached.

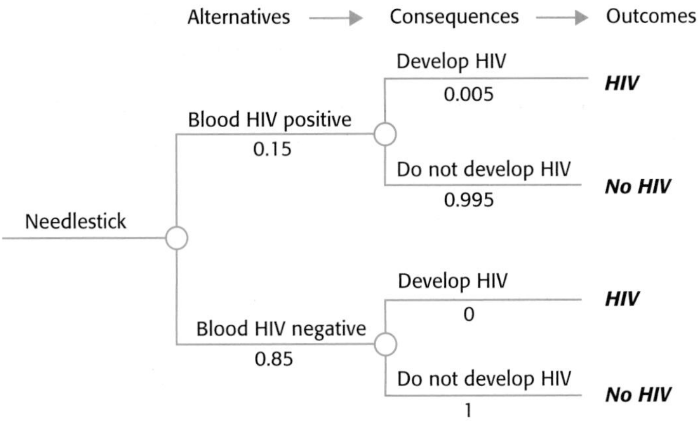
Alternatives → Consequences → Outcomes
Needlestick
Blood HIV positive
0.15
Develop HIV
0.005
HIV
Do not develop HIV
0.995
No HIV
Blood HIV negative
0.85
Develop HIV
0
HIV
Do not develop HIV
1
No HIV

Figure 8.5
A decision tree represents the different alternatives from a chance event, then branches using a chance node to show the possible consequences of each alternative. The leaf nodes of the decision tree are associated with a specific outcome of the event (after Hunink *et al.,* 2001).

A key part of problem-solving is searching for answers to questions, and as we saw in Chapter 7, we can represent a search space as a tree. When making decisions where there are multiple alternatives, each of them with different levels of uncertainty, we can represent the search space as a **decision tree.**

A decision tree takes the individual elements of a decision-making task, and connects them together to show the different possible outcomes. **Chance nodes** represent alternatives and are traditionally drawn as a circle. The events that branch out from a given chance node must be mutually exclusive (they should not overlap) and they should be exhaustive (all significant alternatives must be included). Each path in a decision tree ends in a different **outcome.**

For example, what is the probability of an individual catching HIV after they have had a needlestick injury with a needle from a drug user (Hunink *et al.*, 2001)? We can represent the different outcomes in a simple decision tree (Figure 8.5). The first chance node branches on the likelihood that the blood in the needle came from an individual who had HIV. Let us assume that the probability for having HIV among drug-users is 15%. The second sets of branches represent the conditional probability of developing HIV, given exposure either to HIV-positive blood, or HIV-negative blood. Let's assume that about 5 per 1000 cases of needlestick with HIV-positive blood lead to HIV infection.

The decision tree also allows us to combine the probabilities to determine the overall probability associated with an outcome. The likelihood of a given path is simply the product of all the branches it takes to reach it. To determine the likelihood of HIV we now sum up all the paths that end in this outcome: $(0.15 \times 0.005) + (0.85 \times 0) = 0.001$. Similarly the probability of not getting HIV is $(0.15 \times 0.995) + (0.85 \times 1) = 0.999$. Note that by definition the sum of probabilities of all possible outcomes must always add up to 1.

8.4 Heuristic reasoning guides most clinical decisions but is prone to biases and limited by cognitive resources

Bayes' theorem represents a gold standard for clinical reasoning, and understanding how to use it enhances the likelihood that the hypotheses being considered accurately reflect the given evidence. However, a clinician will not always have access to the necessary probability values, nor know whether the diseases and tests being considered are independent or not. Faced with such uncertainties, decisions still need to be made.

Cognitive psychologists have long studied human decision processes, and have specifically looked at how clinicians formulate a list of hypotheses, and then prune down the list as new evidence comes in. From these studies we can both identify typical mistakes that are made, now that we understand the meaning of Bayes' theorem, as well as identify useful rules of thumb, or heuristics, which can help in the diagnostic process.

The process of hypothesis formation by clinicians has been observed to have the following characteristics (Elstein *et al.*, 1978):

- **Hypotheses are generated early:** Experienced clinicians apparently begin to generate hypotheses early on in their encounter with a patient, rather than deferring hypothesis generation until the history and physical examination takes place. Initial patient data are used to create hypotheses that trigger specific questions or examination, and guide the diagnostic process, eliminating some hypotheses and perhaps introducing others.
- **Only a few hypotheses are considered:** Clinicians have a limited capacity to consider multiple hypotheses simultaneously, regardless of problem complexity, with an apparent upper bound of between five and seven simultaneous hypotheses, which probably reflects the capacity of human working memory (Box 8.2).
- **New hypotheses are generated reluctantly:** Humans are biased to stick to the *status quo* (Box 8.3) and so rather than create new hypotheses, we try to fit the evidence to the existing hypotheses. This may result in errors such as keeping to unduly general

Box 8.2
Human memory

Our knowledge is believed to be stored in notional repositories known as **long-term memory** (LTM). Remembering medical facts or events from childhood all draw upon long-term memory. Most of our knowledge in LTM is inactive and not the focus of immediate attention. **Working memory** (WM) is believed to be where the activated state of information is held and can be equated with our attention. WM actively processes information, including sensory input (for example sounds, sensations or sights currently being experienced) or items from long-term memory. When carrying out a mental calculation, making a plan or recalling a phone number, it is WM that allows the various 'pieces' of information involved to be attended to, integrated and manipulated.

Working memory is extremely limited. The number of items – such as thoughts, sensory impressions and plans – that can be held in WM is very small and is about seven plus or minus two items. Further, items in WM are easily disturbed by each other. This is particularly the case when someone is distracted from thinking about one task by a new one. An intention to carry out an act can be forgotten by the intrusion of another item even when only 10 seconds separates the intention from the intrusion.

Working memory is also severely limited in duration. Without conscious attention to items in WM, their accurate memory persists for no more than about 20 seconds. This decay can be overcome by acts of conscious self-reminder that refresh and reprioritize the items in WM. If there are competing demands upon WM, however, such as the execution of another task, then such rehearsal of intention becomes impossible, and a plan may be forgotten. Considerable empirical evidence exists which demonstrates the powerful negative effects of both interference and diversion of attention upon WM. The process of forgetting is not random. Items that have been longest in WM or most recently added are the most likely to be remembered. Items in the middle of the 'mental list' are most likely to be forgotten.

A further distinction may be drawn within LTM between retrospective and prospective memory. Retrospective memory refers to the factual, autobiographical and 'how-to' knowledge we possess. Prospective memory, by contrast, is the memory for a future act – the memory to remember to do something. Like retrospective memory, prospective memory relies upon WM for its processing work.

The effects of expertise upon memory

With experience, some tasks can be performed automatically. They are sufficiently well learned that once set in train they do not rely on WM, thereby freeing WM for alternative use. This means that the probability of a memory error is greater for less experienced members of staff. Since experts need to rely less upon general attentional resources than do novices, it is probable that more experienced clinicians will suffer less from the effects of interruptions in the performance of specific tasks than will their less experienced colleagues. Experts are also able to create more complex schemas in their long-term memory, as they learn more about a field. Although they may not be able to hold any more items in WM than a novice, the individual items can thus represent far more complex ideas with consequent improvement in their capacity to perform at tasks compared to a novice who may have to reason about the same task from first principles, using more of their WM resources.

Memory errors

Clinicians who work in interrupt-driven environments such as hospitals are likely to suffer failures of WM. As interruptions occur, they interfere with the active rehearsal of what is to be done, and generate new tasks. Consequently prospective plans may be partly or fully forgotten.

When a clinician needs to remember data from one place in a document, for analysis in association with other data, they may make errors of substitution or transposition. Substitution errors replace an item with similar items e.g. eight with eighty. Transposition errors cause problems with sequencing, for example remembering a string of numbers incorrectly – 12345 instead of 12435.

Memory is actively constructed, rather than being a direct record of sensory information. Childhood memories, for example, are often a composite of the original experience interwoven with what other people said about it later. Consequently we can have true memories of events, objects and actions that really occurred. We can also have false memories that we imagine occurred. Confusion between the two is a quite ordinary occurrence, and can lead to clinical errors, with tasks being omitted or repeated. For example, we can confuse the memory to do something with the memory of having done a similar act in the past. If an intention to take a dose of medicine is confused as the action of having done so, a dose will be missed. If the action is mistaken as the intention, an extra dose will be taken. Tasks that are simple, routine and repetitive are particularly vulnerable. Under conditions of high work pressure, when there is insufficient time to perform a reality check, errors may be more readily accepted.

Further reading

Baddeley AD (1982) *Your Memory, A User's Guide*. Macmillan, London.

Parker J, Coiera E (2000) Improving clinical communication: a view from psychology. *Journal of the American Medical Informatics Association* 7: 453–461.

Reason J (1990) *Human Error*. Cambridge University Press, Cambridge.

Box 8.3
Cognitive biases

Despite 'better' solutions existing, people have repeatedly demonstrated that they stick with apparently sub-optimal solutions because the perceived cost of changing is too high.

Cognitive psychologists have examined these decision behaviours and demonstrate that humans make biased rather than rational choices. Kahneman *et al.* (1982) have produced classic results in this area. According to them, humans seem to give greater weight to losses than to gains. Further, they note that a series of losses and gains are always valued independently rather than being lumped together. So, faced with a loss and a gain of equal objective value, each is first weighted unequally before being added. Rather than the effect being neutral, an overall loss is experienced.

Further, a cost that is beyond recovery at the point of decision-making is called a sunk cost and rational economics indicates that sunk costs should therefore be ignored. For a practising clinician faced with a new guideline, the cost of learning existing practices or of setting up existing processes should probably be considered sunk. Only the future cost and benefit of sticking to existing practices should be compared to those associated with shifting to the new practice. However, humans seem to treat such sunk costs as actual losses, and weight them heavily against future benefits. As a consequence of all these decision behaviours, there seems to be a profound bias towards sticking to the *status quo*.

hypotheses that can accommodate inconsistent findings, or disregarding evidence that might require new hypotheses to be generated. Perhaps most often, new evidence is over interpreted, being assigned to support existing hypotheses, rather than used to generate new hypotheses.

- **The quality of hypotheses is more dependent on specific knowledge than general diagnostic competence:** It has long been assumed that ability to reason well in one field means that an individual will do well in others. However, it appears that specific knowledge of a field, such as particular experience with a disease, is more important in determining success than any general problem-solving competence. Although it is good to have general reasoning skills, they alone will not translate into diagnostic skills.
- **Experts may generate a hypothesis by pattern matching rather than reasoning from the facts:** In familiar situations, expert clinicians may circumvent the cycle of generating a list of hypotheses and testing them. Instead they seem to match the pattern of symptoms and signs of the current clinical case against the patterns of similar cases in their past experience (Elstein and Schwartz, 2002). Pattern matching may be a cognitive process of finding the most similar instance to the current case, or of assigning the current case to a category, which is defined by a set of past cases. Expert clinicians apparently only go through a formal hypothesis generation phase when faced with difficult cases or cases outside their experience. In other words, expert clinicians approach hypothesis generation flexibly, using the method most suited to the problem at hand. In contrast, less experienced clinicians rely on hypothesis generation more often, which may explain why experienced clinicians are faster and more accurate in their diagnostic skills, in their area of expertise.

Since probability data are often unavailable, clinicians need to make subjective estimates of the probability of a disease, given the evidence that is at hand. Several heuristics that are commonly, if perhaps unconsciously, used in probability estimation have been identified, and they may be associated with errors (Sox *et al.*, 1988; Elstein and Schwartz, 2002):

- **Representativeness heuristic:** In an effort to estimate the probability that a patient has a disease, one can ask how closely the features of the patient's illness matches the features of the class of patients with that disease. For example, the pattern of the patient's illness is matched to a mental representation of what is typical for a disease, or is matched to a textbook prototype description of the disease. Several errors can be made when using this heuristic. Rare diseases may be considered because they match the patient's features, but given their low prevalence or prior probability, they should really only be considered after more common explanations are eliminated. Sometimes a clinician may have only personally seen atypical presentations of a disease, and therefore have a distorted mental representation of its typical features. Finally, not all the features of a 'typical' disease are equal. Clinicians may assume each feature that matches the prototype increases the likelihood that the patient has the disease. However, some features may all be dependent upon each other, and their appearance together carries little more weight than a single feature – knowing one is present tells no more than knowing all are present (thinking otherwise is called the 'conjunction fallacy'). On the other hand, one or two disease features may be independent, and their absence may be significant.
- **Availability heuristic:** The likelihood of a disease may be measured by the ease with which it is remembered. Since events that are dramatic, vivid or otherwise impressive are

easily recalled, using this heuristic biases us to consider rare or unusual explanations. Recent cases that are still fresh in their memory, or recent articles they have read, may also influence clinicians. The many patients who have had more routine diseases are less memorable as a group, and so their probability is underestimated.

- **Using personal frequency estimates:** A clinician may see many more presentations of a disease than should be expected by chance, perhaps because they have a specialized practice where patients are referred to them. As a consequence, they give the disease a higher prior probability than it deserves, despite its low prevalence in the general community.
- **Presentation bias:** Recall from Chapter 4 that the different ways data are presented affects the way they are interpreted. For example, humans give greater probability weight to more detailed descriptions of events, such as a detailed case history. They also are affected by the order in which evidence is presented, giving greater weight to data that are presented last.
- **Anchoring and adjustment heuristic:** Clinicians may make an initial estimate of a disease's probability (the anchor) and then adjust that with new information, to arrive at a final one, as suggested by Bayes' theorem. However, in using subjective probabilities, the anchor may be set incorrectly because of the impact of any of the distorting factors listed above. Once an anchor is set and new evidence arrives, typically the probability adjustment made after the new information is too conservative, and so its impact is underestimated. This may result in further tests being ordered, for example, when the current evidence using Bayes' theorem would already have made the diagnosis.

8.5 An individual's preferences for one outcome over another can be represented mathematically as a utility

Most decisions have an element of choice in them. Individuals may have to choose between alternatives, and the measures of the likelihood of one event over another are not sufficient to help in making the choice. For example, should an individual who has suffered a needlestick injury with potentially HIV-positive blood choose to be treated prophylactically? As we saw in the example earlier in this chapter, after a needlestick injury contaminated with blood from a drug user, the odds of becoming HIV positive are low. However, an individual in such a situation may nevertheless choose to undergo prophylactic treatment, just in case. This is because, although choosing the treatment may carry some negative consequences, the individual feels the risk or cost of being treated still outweighs the risk of being infected. The individual has expressed a preference for one outcome over another.

The preference for one uncertain outcome against others can be represented with a quantitative value called a **utility**. A utility is a number between 0 and 1, and the outcome with the highest utility is the preferred one.

In Figure 8.6 the decision tree for the HIV needlestick example has been redrawn to show it as a choice of having prophylactic treatment after the injury, or not doing so. These different treatment choices can be represented in a decision tree with a **decision node**, which is traditionally drawn as a box. Two separate branches of the tree are now created. The tree from Figure 8.5 forms the 'no treatment' arm, and we now need to calculate the probabilities for the outcomes if prophylactic treatment is chosen.

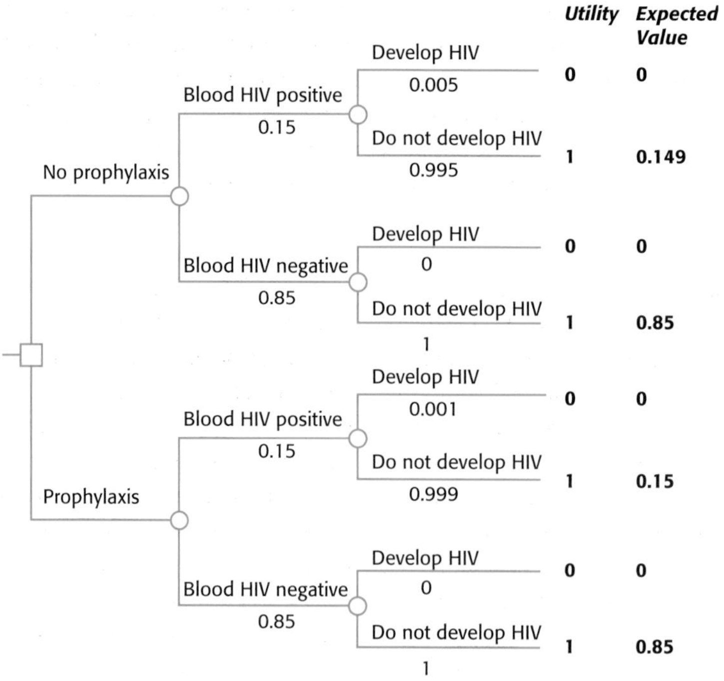
Utility
Expected Value
No prophylaxis
Blood HIV positive
0.15
Develop HIV
0.005
0
0
Do not develop HIV
0.995
1
0.149
Blood HIV negative
0.85
Develop HIV
0
0
0
Do not develop HIV
1
1
0.85
Prophylaxis
Blood HIV positive
0.15
Develop HIV
0.001
0
0
Do not develop HIV
0.999
1
0.15
Blood HIV negative
0.85
Develop HIV
0
0
0
Do not develop HIV
1
1
0.85

Figure 8.6
The expected value of two alternative choices can be determined by summing the individual path probabilities for all possible outcomes of that choice, each probability individually weighted by the utility of the associated outcome. The expected value of prophylaxis after needlestick injury is greater than choosing no treatment (after Hunink *et al.*, 2001).

If we assume that prophylactic treatment after a needlestick injury with HIV-positive blood has an 80% chance of protection, then from Figure 8.5 we know that the chance of developing HIV is reduced from 0.005 to $(1 - 0.8) \times 0.005 = 0.001$ (i.e. only 20% of those treated now go on to be HIV positive). Similarly the probability of not seroconverting to HIV positive now increases from 0.995 to $0.995 + (0.8 \times 0.005) = 0.999$. Finally, our needlestick victim assigns being infected with HIV a utility of 0, and being free of HIV a utility of 1.

The **expected value** of the treatment versus non-treatment choice from the point of view of the assigned utilities can now be calculated. The utility value is multiplied by the different path probabilities to give the expected value of each option. Thus the expected value of prophylaxis is the sum of the expected values of each of the paths in that arm of the tree: $(0.15 \times 0.001 \times 0) + (0.15 \times 0.999 \times 1) + (0.85 \times 0 \times 0) + (0.85 \times 1 \times 1) = 1$. Similarly the expected value of the 'no prophylaxis' arm of the tree is 0.999. In this simple example, the prophylaxis alternative has a marginally greater expected value and would therefore be slightly preferred by the decision-maker.

Utility values can be determined in many different ways

The outcome of a decision analysis is clearly strongly dependent upon the probability values assigned to the chance nodes in the tree, and to the utility values assigned to each different outcome. Two decision-makers working on the same probabilities, but with different utilities, can arrive at very different conclusions.

Probabilities can be estimated from the known frequency of events occurring in the population, and are usually determined by examining the published scientific literature, or by analysis of a statistically significant number of medical records. Utilities can be arrived at using a number of different means, and each method can produce a different set of values. This situation may initially seem unsatisfactory, but we should remember that a utility value in essence is no more than a model of an individual's preference for an outcome, expressed in numerical form, and that the nature of models means that there is no 'correct' utility – only the most appropriate one from the decision-maker's point of view.

The commonest methods used to estimate utilities include (Sox *et al.*, 1988; Hunink *et al.*, 2001):

- **Rating scales:** An individual can simply be asked to assign a subjective assessment of the value of different outcomes. We could ask a question like 'On a scale of 0 to 10, where 0 is the worst possible outcome for you and 10 is the best, what number do you give to being free of HIV infection?'. Repeating the exercise for each different outcome in a decision problem produces an individual's subjective evaluation of the overall value they assign to different outcomes. However, it is unlikely that an outcome assigned a value of 10 is really twice as good as one assigned a value of 5, in an exact mathematical sense, which means that the numbers do not behave in the way mathematicians would like a genuine utility to.

  One way of improving the quality of individual ratings is to ask a large group of people to provide their ratings, using questionnaires called **health indexes**. Such questionnaires need not be limited to asking for a single number for each outcome, but may ask for an individual's ratings for an outcome on multiple attributes. For example, we could ask individuals to classify different health outcomes according to dimensions such as pain, discomfort, mobility, vision, hearing, speech and cognition. Typically each health index will have a method for taking the values assigned by the population and then mathematically transforming them into values that behave much as utilities should.
- **Standard gamble:** In contrast to the ratings scale method, the standard gamble method is considered to be the most theoretically sound way of estimating utilities. The key idea behind the gamble method is to get an individual to express a preference for an outcome where the utility value is unknown as a preference for a gamble between outcomes where the utilities for the outcomes are known. For example, imagine that you have won a free dinner at a restaurant but can't afford to buy any wine to accompany it. What values do you assign to the outcomes of having the dinner with or without the wine? The gamble method asks you to imagine that you have the chance to put your hand in a bag, and if you draw out a red coloured ball you get a free bottle of wine with your dinner, but if you draw out a blue ball you forfeit your dinner and don't get to eat at all. You are then asked to imagine how willing you are going to be to take that gamble, given different probabilities of success. For example, do you take the gamble when there is a 50% chance you will go home without eating, or do you only take the gamble when there is a 1% chance you will go hungry? The probability value you pick where you don't mind whether you do or do not take the gamble is called the **indifference probability**, because you essentially are saying you do not mind which outcome will occur, because the risks balance the benefits.

  Mathematically we know that at the indifference probability, the expected value of both the gamble outcomes together (dinner plus wine vs. going home hungry) is the same as not taking the gamble at all (dinner without wine). With this in mind, given only two utilities, we can calculate the third unknown utility. For example, assume having dinner with wine is the perfect outcome and has a utility of 1, and being sent home without dinner is the worst outcome and has a utility of 0, and the indifference probability you provide for taking or not taking the wine gamble is 0.9. At the point of indifference, we know that the expected value of taking or not taking the gamble is the same, and we can calculate:

$$
\begin{aligned}
\textit{Expected value}(\textit{no gamble}) &= \textit{Expected value}(\textit{gamble})\\
P(\textit{dinner}) \times U(\textit{dinner}) &= P(\textit{dinner} + \textit{wine}) \times U(\textit{dinner} + \textit{wine}) + P(\textit{no dinner})\\
&\quad \times U(\textit{no dinner})\\
1 \times U(\textit{dinner}) &= P(\textit{dinner} + \textit{wine}) \times U(\textit{dinner} + \textit{wine})\\
&\quad + (1 - P(\textit{dinner} + \textit{wine})) \times U(\textit{no dinner})\\
U(\textit{dinner}) &= (0.9 \times 1) + (1 - 0.9) \times 0\\
&= 0.9
\end{aligned}
$$

Intuitively this makes sense since it says that the utility of having dinner is almost the same as having it with wine.

In health settings, patients can be asked to provide their indifference probabilities for different treatment outcomes. For example, if you could take a gamble and be given a magic pill that had a probability that it could cure your disease, but also had a probability that it might kill you, at what probability of cure would you be willing to take the pill? Asking such questions in the form of a gamble allows us to determine a patient's utility for different health states.

- **Time trade-off:** In this method, individuals who have an illness are asked how many years of their life they would be willing to give up, if it meant that they could be in perfect health. For example, an individual with chronic arthritis who is expected to live for 30 years may be just as happy to only live 20 years, but in perfect health. This new figure is a **quality-adjusted life expectancy**.

At the point of indifference between two options, the utility of both is identical. If perfect health lasts for x years and has utility 1, and illness lasts for y years and has utility u, at the indifference point we can say that:

$$
\begin{aligned}
u \times y &= x \times 1\\
u &= \frac{x}{y}
\end{aligned}
$$

Returning to the arthritis example, we now know that 20 years at perfect health with utility 1 is the same as 30 years with arthritis of unknown utility. The ratio of the two times gives us the utility of living with chronic arthritis, which in this case 0.67. We could also say that, adjusted for quality, one year of arthritis is equivalent to 0.67 years of perfect health. This measure is known as a **quality-adjusted life-year (QALY)**.

One of the assumptions in the time-trade-off method is that each additional year has the same value to an individual, but this may often not be the case. For example, the utility of one extra year of life when you have only 1 year to live is probably going to be greater than the utility of one extra year when you have 10 years to live. In such cases the utility u varies with the value of time t, and calculations would need to be adjusted to factor in this effect.

Conclusions

The last five chapters have reviewed the process of clinical decision-making, from interpreting structured data, forming questions and searching for answers, to deciding between alternatives. Communication, with all its complexities and uncertainties, underpins every aspect of these processes, as decision-making is a shared responsibility amongst clinicians and patients. Data that are recorded today may be the basis of someone else's decision-making in the future, and need to be structured with that in mind. The quality of decisions, and as a consequence the quality of clinical outcomes, is firmly determined by how well individual clinicians understand these informatics processes. Informatics skills form the bedrock of clinical reasoning and organizational effectiveness.

Discussion points

1 The problem-solving procedure shown in Figure 8.1 is sometimes called a hypothetico-deductive cycle. Given your understanding of the role of deduction in decision-making, do you agree with this name?

2 Do shortness of breath and chest pain satisfy the condition of independence to allow them to be used as separate pieces of evidence in Bayes' theorem?

3 An apparently healthy patient, with no unusual symptoms or signs, has a chest radiograph as part of an insurance risk assessment. The report that comes back says the patient has pneumonia. How likely is the patient to have pneumonia, and why?

4 How does your answer to the previous question change if the radiography report identified a single mass in one lung, and suggests that the mass could be a tumour? How does your answer change if you knew the patient is a smoker, and has complained of some weight loss and poor appetite, before ordering the test?

5 When ordering the chest radiograph for your smoker with poor appetite and weight loss you fail to include any clinical details in the order, apart from the request for the test. The test comes back identifying the lung mass. Compare the impact on the post-test probability of disease of this positive test result, with the situation in which you gave a full history on the request form to help the radiology department interpret the radiograph. Now explain why, from the radiologist's point of view, it is better to provide as complete a patient history as possible.

6 A patient receiving palliative treatment for a terminal disease suffers a needlestick injury with possibly HIV-positive blood. The patient assigns the outcome of becoming HIV positive with a utility of 0.1, and remaining HIV negative with a utility of 0.6. Recalculate the expected values of the prophylaxis vs. no prophylaxis options in Figure 8.6. Does this change the final decision to start prophylactic treatment?

7 You have a psoriatic skin condition, and there is a new medication that may cure the condition, but might also have an uncommon side effect that causes severe arthritis. You feel that being cured has a utility of 1, but that the current situation is tolerable and has a utility of 0.8. You decide that if the side effect had a probability of 1 in 100, you really couldn't decide whether to take the new medication or not. What utility do you assign to the outcome of severe arthritis?

Chapter summary

1 The problem-solving process is an iterative cycle of discovering data, reasoning from it to form hypotheses, and when no further data would improve the likely outcome, selection of the most plausible hypothesis.

2 Hypotheses are generated by reasoning from the data, and requires a **database**, a **knowledge base** and **rules of inference**.

3 The rules of logic infer what is known to be true, given the facts. There are three basic rules of logical inference:
- **Deduction** takes facts known to be true, and infers consequent effects.
- **Abduction** takes an observed effect, generates all known causes, and is used in diagnosis to generate a list of hypotheses.
- **Induction** creates cause and effect statements from observations, and is the process of generalization used to create new knowledge.
- Deduction produces statements of certainty; abduction produces statements of possibility; induction may generate rules that are later proven false.

4 The rules of probability infer what is most likely to be true, given the facts.
- Bayes' theorem estimates the conditional posterior probability that a patient has a disease, given a certain symptom, based upon the prior probability of the disease, and the likelihood of the new symptom.
- Bayes' requires each hypothesis to be mutually exclusive and symptoms, signs and test results to be independent of each other.
- With test results, the prior probability is called the pre-test probability and the posterior probability the post-test probability. The longer the sequence of tests, the less independent they are likely to be.

5 The process of hypothesis formation by clinicians has the following characteristics: hypotheses are generated early, only a few hypotheses are considered, new hypotheses are generated reluctantly, the quality of hypotheses is more dependent on specific knowledge than general diagnostic competence, and experts may generate a hypothesis by pattern matching rather than reasoning from the facts.

6 Clinicians make subjective estimates of probability using several different heuristics and these may create incorrect estimates.

7 Decision trees are used to determine the most likely outcome among several alternatives. The likelihood of a given path is the product of all branches it takes to reach it. The likelihood of an outcome is the sum of all paths that lead to it.

8 An individual's preferences for an outcome can be represented mathematically as a utility. The **expected value** of an outcome is the product of different path probabilities and their utility.

9 Utilities can be determined in many different ways, including subjective rating scales, the standard gamble and the time trade-off method.

PART 3

Information systems in healthcare

CHAPTER 9

Information management systems

> He will manage the cure best who has foreseen what is to happen from the present state of matters. *Hippocrates, The Book of Prognostics.*

In a complex environment like healthcare, there are many activities that need to be managed, and countless decisions to be made. In Part 1 of this book, we saw that whenever a decision is important enough, or is made often enough, then an information system is built to manage the process.

In this chapter, we will examine how the delivery of healthcare is structured from an informational viewpoint, and see how information systems reflect and contribute to that structure. Two key concepts will be examined. Firstly, the notion of an information management cycle will be introduced. Secondly, it will be shown that it is not always necessary or indeed appropriate to completely formalize an information management system in all its details. To do so may introduce excessive bureaucracy and can be counterproductive, especially when flexibility in decision-making is needed. Consequently, we will see that many information systems are left in an informal state, and as a consequence, are more likely to be supported by communication processes.

9.1 Information systems are designed to manage activities

The main reason an information system is developed is to manage a set of activities. This is true whether one is talking about clinical activities such as the delivery of therapy, or more administrative tasks such as deciding staffing levels for a hospital unit. In every case, information is used to indicate the state of the activity, and decisions are made about that activity on the basis of that information.

For example, consider the case in which we are treating a patient for an acid–base disorder. The goal of management is to maintain the patient's acid–base status in a range that is consistent with good health. Measurements are taken to provide data about acid–base state, such as pH and serum bicarbonate. The model used in this case is physiological. It might include rules that state the relationship between the measured acid–base parameters in health and in disease. On the basis of this knowledge of acid–base disease, one can interpret the measurement data for a given patient (Figure 2.3). Associated with each interpretation, there usually exists a set of management actions that can be taken. In this case, the management actions are a set of therapeutic interventions.

In general, the process of activity management consists of the following steps.

- Define a set of management goals.
- Construct a model of the system.
- Gather measurement data.
- Assess the state of the thing being managed, by interpreting measurements in relation to the model.
- Take actions to alter that state, on the basis of the management goals.

Usually, once an action has been taken, a check then needs to be made to assess the outcome of that decision. For example, if a treatment is given, measurements are subsequently taken of the patient to see if the treatment has been effective. If the outcome is not exactly as hoped for, further action may need to be taken. In this way the result of the first decision feeds back into the next decision-making round, creating a feedback control loop. Depending on the task at hand, the decision-making loop can cycle through its steps many times.

This decision control loop within the information system can be characterized as the **model, measure, manage cycle** (Figure 9.1). It is at the heart of nearly every information system designed to control an activity. 'If you can't measure it', goes an old engineering saying, 'then you can't manage it'. The model, measure, manage cycle defines the function of most information systems. As will become apparent in later chapters, it is the basic way in which computer-based information systems function in healthcare, whether they are concerned with the delivery of clinical care, the administration of services and organizations, or clinical research. Indeed, the relatively complex model abstraction and application cycle that was introduced in Chapter 1 (Figure 1.2) can be mapped directly on to the simple model, measure and manage cycle in Figure 9.1.

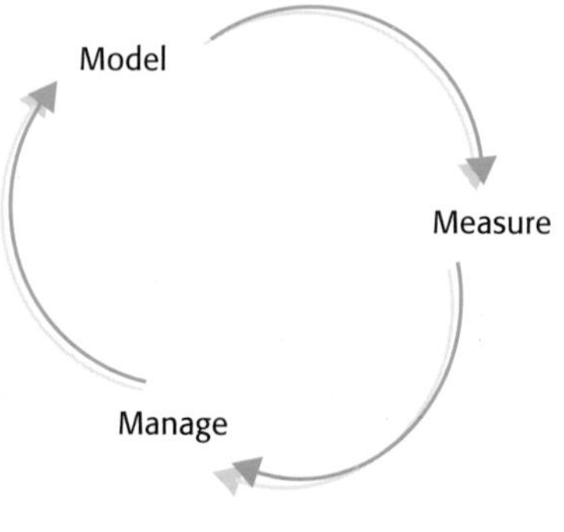
Model
Measure
Manage

Figure 9.1
The model, measure, manage cycle. When the outcome of a management decision is fed back into another cycle, a feedback control loop is formed.

9.2 There are three distinct information management loops

As information moves through a system, it can be used in several quite distinct ways. In particular, it is useful to distinguish three distinct information cycles or loops which reflect different roles for the model–measure–manage cycle. These loops are responsible for the direct **application**, **selection**, and **refinement** of knowledge. Indeed, these information loops exist in some form in most large enterprises, not just in healthcare. Together, they come together to form the **three-loop model** (Phaal, 1994), which describes the main ways that information is used within an organization, or indeed within many other systems requiring informed control (Figure 9.2).

The essence of the three-loop model is to recognize that there is a life cycle for information as it percolates through any complex system. We start by assuming that there is a set of models of the system we want to manage. In the case of clinical medicine, these models correspond to medical knowledge. If we are talking about administering an organization such as a hospital, then the models will capture our understanding of economics, organizational dynamics and so on. The knowledge contained in these models might exist in books and journals, in the programs of information systems, or be in the heads of people.

In the first loop, information is used to directly manage a specific activity, such as the selection of a diagnostic test for a patient. Secondly, as checks are made on the progress of an individual task, changes might need to be made to the models used to manage the task. For example, the model of treatment might need to be changed if a patient does not make appropriate progress. Thirdly, over time the data and models used in one task can be pooled with similar ones to make broader assessments about the quality of decisions. For example, decisions about the cost-effectiveness of a particular test might be made on the basis of the evidence of its use with a large number of patients. Such longer-term decisions can then be used to refine the way tests are selected, and consequently feed back into the original clinical decision process.

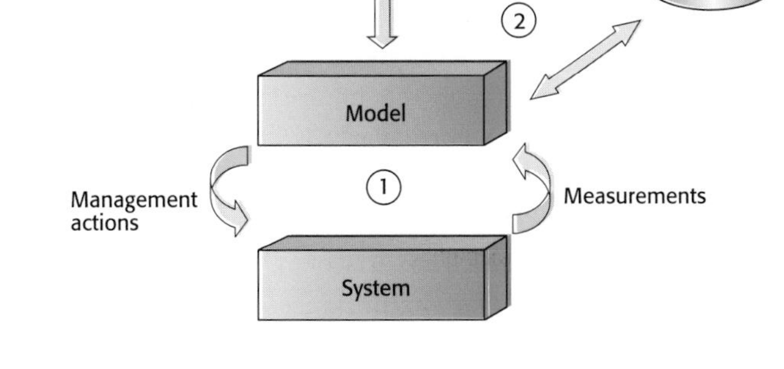
Model assessment and refinement
3
Model library
Model selection and customization
Database
2
Model
Management actions
1
Measurements
System

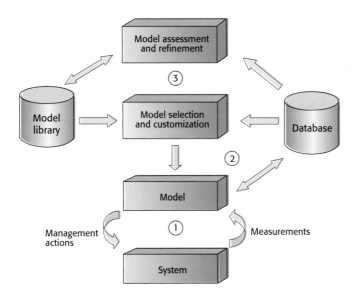

Figure 9.2
The three-loop model. Three separate information cycles interact within the health system. The first and second cycles select and apply models to the management of specific systems. The third information cycle tries to assess the effectiveness of these decisions and improve the models accordingly.

Each loop thus has a different role. Each involves different information sources, and different operations on that information. As a result, each cycle has quite different requirements for the kind of information or communication system needed to support them. We can now examine each loop in some more detail.

Loop 1 defines the direct application of a model to a task

The first loop is all about the application of knowledge to achieve a particular task. Using the knowledge contained in a model, and on the basis of some measurements, actions are taken in a way prescribed by the model, and further measurements are taken to close the feedback loop. This is simply the model–measure–manage cycle.

For example, a clinician may choose an insulin treatment regime for a diabetic patient. Having chosen that regimen, the clinician applies it to the management of the patient's condition. Measurements of the patient's blood sugar levels will be taken, and the dosage of insulin will be varied according to the rules contained in the regimen.

Similarly, in a hospital, there might be a set way of determining the number of nurses required to staff a ward adequately. This might be based upon the number of patients in a ward, and the level of dependency of its patients. For any given day, the nurse manager uses the model to decide staffing levels for different wards, based upon measurements of patient numbers and an assessment of their level of dependency.

Loop 2 defines the way models are selected and customized

In most cases there are a number of different ways in which a task could be completed. This is because there are many possible ways that the world can be modelled, and many ways in which that model can be translated into a prescription for action. One can think of loop 2 as the ongoing process of deciding which models and measurements are most appropriate for a specific task.

In the example of the diabetic patient, the clinician must decide which insulin regimen is the most appropriate one for the patient. This could be based, for example, on an assessment of the patient's disease, and the patient's ability to test their own blood sugar and self-administer insulin. It may be the case that the regimen prescribed will vary many times over the period in which the clinician manages the patient. When the patient is ill, the clinician may prescribe so called 'sick-day' rules that alter the doses of insulin that can be given. These rules constitute a different model of the way the insulin dose is determined.

In a hospital ward, a nurse manager may find that the rules for deciding staffing levels will need to be re-examined depending on the type of ward being considered. A different set of rules might be applied to an intensive care unit, where there are different requirements for staff skills, and different levels of patient dependency, from those on a general surgical ward.

There may not always be a complete set of models to help with a task. Patients have many individual variations in their circumstances that may require the normal treatment to be customized to suit their specific needs. A particularly 'brittle' diabetic may need to be closely monitored and treatment varied because of the unpredictability of their disease. Nursing staff on a ward in a teaching hospital may need to vary the balance of their daily activities if they are expected to train students as well as carry out clinical duties. Sometimes these variations in approach reflect very particular circumstances, and are not frequent enough to be turned into general policy. It is also the case that if a model does not fit circumstances regularly, then it is the model that needs changing. This is the role of loop 3.

Loop 3 is responsible for model creation and refinement based upon the results of application over time

All our knowledge is constantly being re-examined. As a consequence our understanding of the world evolves with time. In loop 3, the knowledge that was used to complete a task is itself examined against the outcome of its application. To make such an assessment, the results from repeated attempts at a particular approach are pooled. When several different approaches have been tried out, these historical data are examined, and over time the most successful approach is adopted.

Loop 3 is thus the place where the scientific examination of existing theories leads to the creation of new ones. The models selected in loop 2 are all regarded as hypotheses about the best way to approach a task. These hypotheses are then examined on the basis of the 'tests' that occur every time they are applied in loop 1. This is the process of inductive reasoning already encountered in Chapter 8.

Thus the many different treatment regimens used in the management of diabetes have all (hopefully) been tested in trials across large numbers of patients. As the outcomes of the treatments are examined, decisions are made about which regimens should be retained, which should be modified, and under which conditions particular regimens should be best applied.

Equally, over time, the way in which hospital units are staffed will be modified when measurements such as patient outcomes, staff retention and satisfaction levels are examined. Those hospitals that perform best on these measurements will be used as role models by hospitals that want to improve in a similar fashion.

9.3 Formal and informal information systems

Just because it is possible to define an information system, it does not follow that it is always reasonable to then build it. If that were the case, then our lives would be regulated in minute detail. What happens in reality is that most organizations, whether they are small groups of individuals or large institutions, try to find a balance between creating formal processes and allowing individuals to behave freely and informally. That balance shifts, depending on the group, and realizes a different set of costs and benefits. Large organizations gain stability through formal processes, but are often criticized for being unduly bureaucratic. Smaller ones, although flexible and able to respond rapidly to change, are often chaotic to work in as a result. The difference between these two extremes lies in the organization's view of the need to formalize its internal systems.

So, while there are clear advantages to structuring processes, including improved reliability, efficiency and consistency, they do not come without cost. There are actually several different costs that need to be considered before a system is formalized.

- Firstly, the creation of a process, by definition, limits flexibility of response. Recall from the discussion on models in Chapter 1 that all models are just views of the world, and a formal process is a kind of model. Consequently, a particular view of how things should be done is captured within the rules, regulations and procedures of any formal process. Alternative views exist, and in some circumstances they would produce better results. The trade-off in adhering to a single view is the hope that the number of times the process produces a good result outweighs the cost of those times when an alternate approach would have been better.

- Secondly, formalizing the information elements that contribute to a process usually requires considerable effort. An explicit model of the process needs to be created, which includes definitions of the data that needs to be collected. In some situations it is too costly to engage in this formalization process, given the likely return.
- Finally, it may just not make sense to contemplate formalization if the situations being dealt with are highly variable. If situations are unlikely to recur, then it would probably be better to come up with a way of handling them from 'first principles' each time, rather than looking to a formal cookbook of solutions.

In the first section of this chapter we saw that there are different cycles of information through healthcare. The way such information cycles can in principle be codified into an information system was demonstrated in Chapter 3. What should now be apparent is that, before a formal information system is created to manage a process, an explicit choice must be made on the basis of a cost-benefit analysis. In many circumstances, the result of that analysis may be that it is preferable to not build the system.

In Chapter 2 we saw that there is a continuum of possible model localization between humans and computer (Figure 2.5). One can imagine a similar continuum stretching between those situations in which everything needs to be formalized, and those where a process can be left completely informal. In between these two extremes, depending upon specific needs, one can formally define some parts of a system, and leave the remaining interactions undefined (Figure 9.3). The proportion that is formalized will depend on the specific needs of a given situation.

Thus a hospital will have many formally defined procedures for managing different activities, but most activity in the organization will be left informal. Similarly, the way patients are managed falls along this continuum of formality. Patients enrolled in a clinical trial have their management completely regimented, to maximize the scientific significance of any results. Patients with common conditions may be treated according to well-defined guidelines, but will have some aspects of their treatment modified informally to match individual needs. At the other end of the spectrum, a patient's problems may be approached in a non-standard

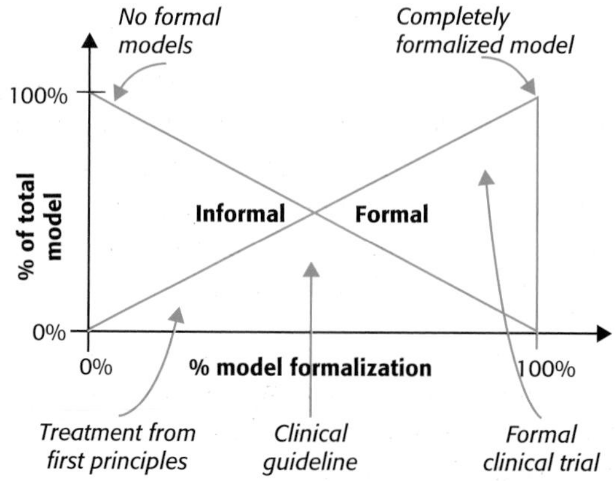
No formal models
Completely formalized model
100%
0%
% of total model
Informal
Formal
0%
% model formalization
100%
Treatment from first principles
Clinical guideline
Formal clinical trial

Figure 9.3
There is a continuum of possible formalization of information systems. Formal and informal models combine together to cover the total modelling needs of a given problem. The degree of formalization depends on the type of problem being addressed.

way, perhaps because of the uniqueness of circumstances. There may be a few general guidelines on how to approach such patients, but most of what occurs has to be created 'from scratch'. This does not mean that such a treatment, if it is repeated over time, cannot slowly become part of the formal treatment of similar patients.

Not all data need to made available for computer interpretation

Since not all processes need to be formalized, it follows that just because data are available, they may not necessarily benefit from being analysed. There clearly are many examples within healthcare when data are collected so that they can be analysed in depth. Data from clinical trials for example, are all defined in precise detail, so that the value of different treatments can be analysed.

Sometimes data are only of short-lived value and do not warrant the construction of a formal model to interpret them. Consider for example, a recorded voice message that is left by a member of a healthcare team for a colleague, containing an update on a patient's progress. The message is likely to be loosely structured, and cover a number of topics that would not normally be predictable in advance. It is also likely that the message will be of most interest only to the individuals who recorded and listened to the message.

Nevertheless the recorded message constitutes data that are stored, perhaps even on a computer system, and clinical decisions may be altered on the basis of the content of the message. Unlike the data that might be written into a patient record, or collected on a hospital information system and used by many people over an extended period, the data in such cases are of interest to a very few individuals and have a limited model–measure–manage cycle.

As a consequence, the message data are treated in a very different way from data that might be formally recorded in a patient record. In such cases, it is unlikely that anyone would want to develop a model that allowed a computer to analyse the message. There is no formal agreement in advance on the content of the message or the ways in which it will be used. Such agreements are at the heart of traditional computer-based information systems, where data formats are specified in advance of system construction.

It thus follows that the model and the interpretation of the data are owned by the recorder and listener of the message. The machine that stores and transmits the data takes on a more passive role. It is used as a data repository, or as a channel between the communicating parties, rather than for any active interpretation it might make.

In general, one can make a distinction between information systems in which data are explicitly modelled and those in which data are left unmodelled:

- A **formal information system** contains an agreed model for the interpretation of data, and data within the system are structured in accordance with that model.
- An **informal information system** is neutral to the interpretation of data, containing no model, and thus imposes minimal structure on any data that are contained within the system. Further, we can say that the model and the act of interpreting the data contained within an informal system are external to that system.

Thus an informal system does not imply the absence of a model or the inability to interpret data in the light of a model. With an informal information system, the model exists externally to it. In practice these models are often kept in the heads of those who create or access the informally stored data (Figure 2.5).

There is thus no sense in which the data in an informal system are less valuable than formally structured data. Such data are used in fundamentally different ways, and in different situations. In general, we can say that informal information systems are used when data are only of temporary value, of interest to a very few people, are complex or the content is not predictable in advance.

Communication systems frequently support informal exchanges

We have already seen that a distinction should be made between organizational procedures that are worth supporting formally, perhaps with a computer-based information system, and those that are best left informal. This does not mean, however, that tools cannot support informal tasks. Some tasks, such as storing and retrieving phone numbers, lend themselves to being formally organized. Other tasks, such as writing quick notes, are impaired by such structured methods. People often use simple tools like pen and paper to manage a variety of unstructured tasks. The key requirement for any tool used to support informal tasks is that it provides a means of managing information that is flexible, and can be used in a variety of ways.

One of the commonest ways of supporting informal processes is to use a communication system to channel data between people. This is because these systems are usually designed to be very informal about the content of the data they transfer. Thus, although usually thought of as a communication system, a telephone is a good example of an informal information system. The models for interpreting the data transmitted across the telephone are in the heads of the parties conversing, and not in the machinery responsible for mediating that conversation.

In fact, communication systems are commonly used to support informal information processes, because they are so flexible. When examining the flows of information through an organization, it would be a mistake to only look at the formal processes in place, since this would give a very skewed picture of what really is going on. There is a complementary, and probably significantly larger, body of information coursing through the informal channels of the organization's communication infrastructure.

An example will make the contrasting roles of communication and information systems in managing information clearer. Consider the information that might pass between a primary care physician and a cardiologist when a patient requires specialist assessment by the cardiologist. While the patient is still with him, the physician could transmit an ECG by fax to the cardiologist for an immediate opinion. In contrast, a more complex system could be set up to capture the ECG signal directly from the cardiograph. Such a system would store the ECG data on a local computer, and then transmit the signal as a data file across the phone line to a computer used by the cardiologist.

Faxing an ECG

In the fax case, the ECG is printed out by the cardiograph and is then sent across the telephone system. The fax system is not configured in any special way to recognize that it is transmitting an ECG. It just as well could be sending text or a photograph. Thus the fax system is informal with respect to the content of the data. The cardiologist who reads the fax image possesses the model for the interpretation of the ECG.

The advantage of using a fax is that it is relatively cheap, easy to use and widely available. For example, the physician could be at a patient's home with a portable cardiograph, and use the patient's own fax machine. Further, it does not need to be in any way dedicated to a particular task such as ECG transmission, since no model will be associated with the data it transmits. These are generally the characteristics of most informal communication systems like the telephone or paper. The disadvantage of using this system is that it requires someone with expertise on the receiving end of the fax to provide the model and interpretation.

Transmitting the ECG signal

If a patient's cardiogram is transmitted directly from a cardiograph to a remote computer in the cardiologist's office, the remote computer can take the original waveform signal and reconstruct the cardiogram. This is because the data are specifically structured according to a data model that allows it to be recognized as an ECG by the second computer system.

The advantages here are largely the inverse of the case with the faxed image. Having data structured according to a model permits flexible manipulation of the data. One could choose to display only some portions of the signal, at different resolutions. Equally, the signal could be automatically interpreted by an expert system, since the waveform data arrive in a highly structured form that is amenable to computer interpretation. The disadvantages of this system are that one requires a dedicated system at the sending and receiving ends to encode and decode the signal.

It is usually the case that there are many more general-purpose systems available than there are complex and specialized ones. Thus at present there are more fax machines in the world than computer systems connected up to an ECG machine. A primary care practitioner who rarely has the need to transmit an ECG would find the cost of purchasing such a dedicated system unjustifiable. A cardiologist, for whom this was a common occurrence, would find the case easier to make.

So, in summary, the fax system can be used on many different tasks, but will perform each of them less effectively than a system that has been formally designed for the task. Like most communication systems, the fax is relatively informal about what data are transmitted. When tasks are infrequent, it is more cost-effective to use an informal solution. In contrast, as a task starts to require formalization because of its frequency or importance, more expensive and specific tools can be brought in to support it.

Discussion points

1 Pick a health service that you are familiar with, and describe its function in terms of the three-loop model.

2 Is the model–measure–manage cycle a positive or a negative feedback system?

3 When is it appropriate to introduce a computerized information system into an organization?

4 Describe the way you might design a diabetes information service for consumers, first using only a computer-based information system, and then using only communication technologies.

5 Clinicians often seem to prefer using communication devices such as mobile phones, or speech-driven devices like dictating machines, rather than computers. Why might that be?

Chapter summary

1 An information system is developed to manage a set of activities, and its functioning can be characterized as repeated cycles of modelling, measurement and management.

2 Three quite separate information loops exist which reflect different instances of the information management cycle.
- Loop 1 defines the direct application of a model to a task.
- Loop 2 defines the way models are selected and are customized.
- Loop 3 is responsible for model creation and refinement based upon the results of application over time.

3 There are considerable advantages to structuring information processes, including improved reliability, efficiency and consistency. There are also costs associated with formalization, including lack of flexibility to varying circumstances, and the effort involved in defining the system.

4 Not all data need to be available for computer interpretation. There is a trade-off that exists between creating explicit models that permit formal information systems to be created, and leaving the system in an informal state, with minimally defined models and data.

5 A formal information system contains an agreed model for the interpretation of data, and data within the system are structured in accordance with that model.

6 An informal information system is neutral to the interpretation of data, containing no model, and thus imposes minimal structure on any data that are contained within the system. The model and interpretation for data contained within an informal system are external to that system.

7 Communication systems are frequently used to support informal exchanges. Information flows through an organization occur both through formal processes as well as through the informal channels of the organization's communication infrastructure.

8 Informal information systems are used when data are of temporary value, of interest to very few people, are complex or the content is not predictable in advance. When tasks are infrequent, it is more cost-effective to use an informal solution. However, if a task requires formalization because of its frequency or importance, more expensive and specific tools can be brought in to support it.

CHAPTER 10

The electronic medical record

> The problems of medical practice and hospital functioning are rapidly approaching crisis proportions, in terms of cost, limited personnel resources, and growing demands. The application of computer technology offers hope, but the realization of this hope in the near future will require a much greater commitment than is presently true of … the medical academic community, and the health services community. *G. Octo Barnett, H. J. Sukenik (1969), p. 268.*

In the previous chapter, we saw that three distinct information cycles govern the operation of the healthcare system. The content of the information coursing within these cycles ranges from staff salaries through to details about the care of patients. The last chapter also explained how some of that information is captured formally, although a large part of it is left informal and communicated without necessarily ever being recorded. The formal aspects of clinical information are largely contained within the patient record, which serves as the single point of deposition and access for nearly all archival clinical data. The patient record is thus one of the primary mechanisms supporting the three information loops.

The medical record is so pivotal a topic in informatics that it makes sense to begin our detailed discussion of healthcare information systems here. Consequently, the remainder of this chapter will attempt to look at the benefits and limitations of existing paper-based systems, and the major functions that could in principle be replaced or enhanced by the electronic medical record (EMR).

Since the functional scope of the electronic record is so broad, the survey will inevitably widen to touch upon information and communication aspects of healthcare that extend beyond the pure record of care. In particular, the need to support communication among healthcare workers, protocol-based care, and the need for controlled medical terminologies will all be introduced here. However, given the importance and complexity of each of these topics, they will be returned to individually in greater detail in later sections of this book.

10.1 The EMR is not a simple replacement of the paper record

The medical record has traditionally had a number of distinct functions, both formal and informal, and not all of these are always immediately recognized:

- The patient record provides a means of communicating between staff who are actively managing a patient. Notes left by staff assist those who work on different shifts, or who are unable to meet up during the working day.
- During the period of active management of a patient's illness, the record strives to be the single data access point for workers managing a patient. All test results, observations and so forth should be accessible through it. The record thus provides a 'view' on data about a patient's illness.
- More subtly, the record offers an informal 'working space' to record the ideas and impressions that help build up a consensus view, over the period of care, of what is going on with a patient. One can view the evolution of such a consensus as storytelling or the development of a narrative about the patient (Kay and Purves, 1996). In this narrative, healthcare workers assemble data into a story that can then be communicated to others. This amounts to the imposition of an interpretation on the patient data, and explains why the patient record is never the patient's own story, but rather the story as told by those who care for the patient.
- Once an episode of care has been completed, the record ultimately forms the single point at which all clinical data are archived, for longer-term use. This might be to assist in later treatment for the same patient, or to be pooled with other data to assist in research.

The amount of patient data stored around the world in this record system is bewilderingly large, complex, and far flung. Every primary care practitioner's office contains patient records. Every hospital has dedicated professional staff whose main focus is to act as custodian and guide through its record store.

This information exists in a multitude of forms, sometimes unintelligible except to those who created the record, and usually not accessible to anyone except those who are caring for individual patients. Often it is not even available to these individuals, as records are misplaced, lost or being used by someone else. One of the purposes of information is to help the growth of knowledge, but with the medical record in such a form, it can only be a poor participant in this wider process.

With drawbacks both at the point of care and outcomes assessment, many have turned away from paper systems to computer-based ones in the hope that they will more closely meet the information needs of healthcare. The computer-based systems that are intended to deal with this formal information are known variously as the **electronic medical record (EMR)**, **computer-based patient record** (**CPR**) or **electronic patient record** (**EPR**).

Without doubt, over the last three decades an enormous amount of controversy, confusion and distress has been associated with the development of clinical computer record systems. At the core of much of this difficulty lie the very different views of individuals about the role and importance of the EMR.

For some, the EMR is simply the computer replacement for existing paper medical record systems. The computer provides mechanisms for capturing information during the clinical encounter, stores it in some secure fashion, and permits retrieval of that information by those with a clinical need.

The advantages that are often cited for moving to such a computer record system include a reduction in storage space, the possibility of simultaneous access to the records by many individuals, and the possibility of using data for a variety of clinical research activities. Individual clinicians, for example, could do rapid searches through their practice records for audit purposes. Data pooled from many patients in a region could be used to study local aspects of the epidemiology of disease.

At the other extreme, for many the EMR represents the totality of information and communication systems that could be made available in the support of clinical activities. The term 'record' starts to become increasingly inappropriate as the functionality expected of the EMR broadens far beyond the computerized duplication of a paper record system. Everything from systems for ordering tests and investigations, digital image archiving and retrieval, the exchange of messages between different workers in the healthcare system, through to the automated coding of patient data for administrative purposes might be included as components of the extended EMR's function.

Indeed in 1991, when the Institute of Medicine (IOM) in the United States issued a highly influential committee report on the computer-based patient record, it intentionally used a broad and inclusive definition of the EMR (Dick and Steen, 1991). The EMR was defined as 'an electronic patient record that resides in a system specifically designed to support users by providing accessibility to complete and accurate data, alerts, reminders, clinical decision support systems, links to medical knowledge, and other aids'.

With such a wide variation in the functions that could be expected from an EMR, it is probably unwise to try to define the EMR in any formal way. It is more fruitful to observe that there are a range of clinical activities that use and communicate information, and that some of these can be supported through the introduction of technology (Figure 10.1). The extent to which that is actually done in any one locality depends entirely on the resources, needs and expertise of those concerned. We saw in the previous chapter, for example, that it is not always appropriate to introduce a formal computer system when a more informal solution might be more effective.

The main recommendation of the 1991 IOM report on the computer-based patient record was that healthcare professionals and organizations should adopt the EMR as the standard method for recording all data related to patient care (Dick and Steen, 1991). The justification for such a recommendation rests as much on people's aspirations for transforming clinical practice as it does on the limitations ascribed to paper-based methods of recording clinical information, for which there is much evidence.

10.2 The paper-based medical record

In one form or another, the method of recording patient data on paper has served clinical practice successfully for centuries. However, although the physical nature of the paper record has remained relatively unchanged, the formal structure of the information contained within the record has undergone much change in the last 50 years. The patient record has moved from being an unstructured chronological record of events, to the problem- or task-oriented structure discussed in Chapter 5 (Tange, 1996).

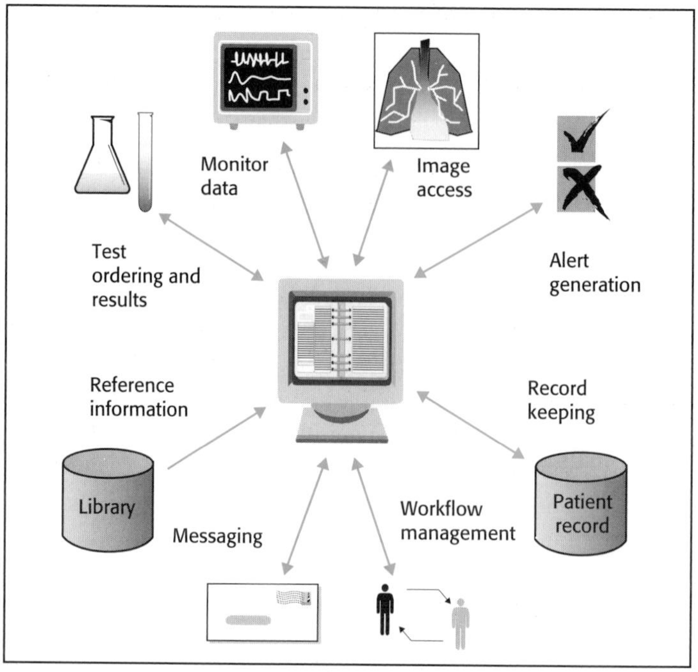
Monitor data
Image access
Test ordering and results
Alert generation
Reference information
Record keeping
Library
Messaging
Workflow management
Patient record

Figure 10.1 The electronic medical record has a variety of potential functions that it can fulfil, requiring different degrees of investment and technological sophistication to implement them.

The notion that a 'computer' record system is inherently better than a 'paper' one is a weak one. If we think of a medical record as a message, then we know from Chapter 4 that the channel of message delivery (in this case a computer) is only one of many factors that affect the ultimate utility of the message on the individual who receives it. Issues like the informational structure adopted for the record clearly have a large impact on a record's effectiveness, independent of the medium of delivery.

There are thus at least two quite separate aspects to the paper record that need to be considered. The first is the physical way, or medium, that individuals interact with paper. The second is the structure and content of the information that is recorded upon it. It is important to make such a distinction, because it is easy to confuse criticisms of existing record systems with criticisms of paper as a recording medium. In many cases, the reason a paper record system is poor has much to do with the chosen structure, the processes in place to support it, and the effort people choose to make when creating a record.

Physical aspects of the paper record

The way paper lends itself to being handled, marked upon and stored is often taken for granted, but has some remarkably rich implications. As a physical system, the paper record thus has many positive attributes.

- Paper is portable, and access is self-contained. Apart from needing a light source, there is nothing preventing notes being worked on in most places. A computer system requires power to be supplied to it, and may require connection to a computer network.
- Paper and pen are a highly familiar method of recording information, and require no special training of medical staff. The educational process has occurred well before individuals come to interact with the paper medical record. In contrast, for many

existing health professionals, use of a computer system may require specific training in the workplace.

- Access to data written on paper can feel very direct. Browsing through a reasonable quantity of notes permits a form of rapid scanning of what is recorded there.

There are also some drawbacks associated with the physical characteristics of any paper system, some of which only become apparent when record systems become quite large.

- A paper record can only be used for one task at a time. If two people want to look at a patient's notes, one has to wait for the other to finish. Thus, a patient's records may be unavailable during a consultation because they are being cared for by a number of different workers. Notes might be lying in a different clinic, in a physician's office or home or elsewhere. Several studies have found that records are unavailable up to 30% of the time in larger institutions (Dick and Steen, 1991). It is also, sadly, the case that records can be lost, with the percentage varying according to the record processing and tracking procedures of different institutions. Even if they are available, the time required for notes to be requested and delivered can be unacceptable, and the process of retrieval may require substantial expenditure of human resource.
- Paper records consume space when large amounts of data are recorded. There are methods of reducing this, for example creating copies on microfiche, but these require additional effort and expense, as well as imposing new barriers to easy retrieval.
- Large records for individual patients can be physically cumbersome, heavy, and difficult to search through for specific information. Patients whose chronic illness spans a number of years of care can generate particularly unwieldy records.
- Paper is fragile and susceptible to damage and, unless well cared for, will degrade over time.
- The production of paper has environmental consequences, related for example to the bleaching processes and forest management.

Informational aspects of the paper record

Somewhat independent of the physical nature of paper is the choice of the structure and content of the information that is recorded upon it. It is thus not necessarily the case that a record is poor simply because it is captured on paper. The quality of a record might have more to do with the quality of data written upon it, or the way the data are structured.

Information entry

One of the great advantages of paper is how little structuring it demands. The way that data can be recorded on paper is quite unconstrained in both its form and content. A paper entry might capture a terse set of laboratory results, a record of physical examination with hand-drawn diagrams, or a long and detailed narrative containing subjective assessments of a patient's mental state. In the terms of the previous chapter, paper is a relatively informal medium, since it imposes few models on the data that are captured. The models that interpret the data captured on paper are contained within the head of the reader. This means that paper is a quite general-purpose tool for capturing data. Everything from the most personal scribbled note to highly standardized forms can be captured on the same medium. Unfortunately, this freedom of structuring is not without its drawbacks.

- Since the structuring used to create a paper record may be very personal, it may be difficult for someone other than the writer to understand what is recorded there. The reader may not possess the model used when the data were captured, making interpretation difficult. This may simply mean that what is recorded is illegible, or that the words are clear, but their intended meaning is not.
- In the absence of any formal structure to guide record creation, there is increased opportunity for errors to occur, for example the omission of relevant data. There has been much study of the quality of patient records over the years, focusing on the amount of missing or inaccurate data. Many of the defects in records are due to the manner in which examinations are conducted and their results recorded, and have little to do with the fact that records are made on paper. The imposition of a formal structure for data capture such as pre-printed forms can certainly improve this situation, at the cost of making the process very directed. It seems fair to say then, that many difficulties with the content of existing record systems are largely due to the processes in place for data capture. In principle, it is still possible for a well-designed set of paper forms to be far more effective in improving the quality of a medical record than a poorly designed computer-based one.

Information retrieval

A very different but equally important aspect of the structuring of information relates to the way one is able to search within a given record, or across a body of records, for specific data. Clinicians use a wide variety of information sources during decision-making, and patient-specific data stored in the record are a major component of that (Smith, 1996b).

There is now clear evidence that clinical workers routinely fail to find pieces of information that they need during a patient consultation from the paper medical record. Tang *et al.* (1994) studied 168 outpatient consultations and found that data were searched for but not found in 81% of cases. In 95% of these cases, the medical record was available during the consultation. The categories of missing information included laboratory tests and procedures (36%), medications and treatments (23%) and history (31%). It is not clear from this study what the effect of the failure to locate data had on the delivery of care or patient outcomes. Nevertheless, the phys-icians in the study expended additional effort pursuing the data they needed. These included searching alternative data sources, making decisions despite the missing data, or relying on the report of patients or their relatives. In another, earlier study, the consequence of missing laboratory data was that 11% of tests in a hospital setting were duplicated (Tufo and Speidel, 1971).

A different type of problem with data retrieval arises when data need to be extracted from a subset of records from within a larger number of records. All substantial record systems, in whatever form they exist, require some form of indexing to allow individual records to be retrieved. Libraries have the Dewey system for the classification and retrieval of books. Medical records are similarly accessed via an indexing system, at a minimum allowing a record to be found according to patient name or identification number.

It is a feature of paper systems that fixed indexes need to be created before such searches can occur. For example, it would not be possible to walk into a paper record office and obtain the notes from every patient admitted with a particular disease over the last 2 years, unless a disease-based index had already been created. The only solution in this case would be to read each record individually to check if it contained the diagnosis in question. This is such a time-consuming process that it not frequently done.

Despite such a large set of shortcomings, the perceived advantages of the paper-based medical record are sufficient to make its continued use attractive in some circumstances. Indeed, there are data that suggest that at least some medical practitioners are quite happy to stick to the paper record for their everyday clinical activities (Tange, 1995).

10.3 The EMR

With so many difficulties associated with the paper record, there has been a growing drive to replace it with a computer-based one for most of the last half-century (e.g. Barnett and Sukenik, 1969). This has resulted in the design and implementation of many different systems, with varying functionality, and variable success. In 1990, one of the most successful implementations of the EMR reported that only about 25% of all patient data in the hospital were available electronically, the remainder residing in the paper system (Kuperman and Gardner, 1990).

Consequently, despite such significant investments in information technology, some today still feel that it is difficult to quantify the explicit benefits of doing so. In several recent reviews of the literature on hospital information systems, the evidence for their cost-benefit was found to still be inconclusive (van der Loo *et al.*, 1995; Lock, 1996). This is partly due to the inherent difficult associated with the evaluation of complex systems, but it may also reflect the lack of clear objective measurements in many studies. It is also the case that for many, the case for the introduction of computer-based systems is 'obvious', and so the need for detailed assessment is not apparent to them.

It is clear that this situation is changing rapidly, as medical informatics develops a more scientific basis. Thus, today it is at least possible to make a comprehensive qualitative assessment of the value of replacing paper with computer, and individual studies that demonstrate specific advantages are increasingly becoming available. Nevertheless, there is still a great need for the development and application of robust formal methods for the evaluation of information technology in healthcare (Friedman and Wyatt, 1997).

In the next sections, some of the advantages and disadvantages of a computer-based medical records and paper-based systems will be discussed. With a constant stream of technological innovation, and changes in the cost of information technologies, many of the traditional drawbacks associated with computer systems are disappearing. It is likely that soon the most profound difficulties will reside in the design and adoption of these information systems, and not their technological implementation.

Physical aspects of the computer-based record

Computer-based systems have a number of powerful physical attributes that make them ideal data capture and storage systems.

- Perhaps first amongst these, and now taken for granted, is the enormous quantity of data that can be stored in a small physical space once data are in electronic form. With continual advances in the technologies of optical storage, and in magnetic particle systems, this capability will continue to deliver ever greater storage capacity for some considerable time to come.

- A second physical implication is the ability to easily create duplicate copies of data, either to allow sharing of data, but more importantly to act as back-up copies for security reasons. The costs and efforts involved in transferring paper records to microfiche, or in scanning them into electronic form, make them much less attractive in this respect. In the worst case, paper records are never duplicated and remain susceptible to physical damage and even loss through disasters such as fire or flooding.
- One of the traditional advantages of paper is its informality. If needed it can support a wide variety of data. In contrast, computer systems have traditionally demanded far more formal data models, and as a consequence, imposed these on their users during data entry (Figure 9.3). It is common to hear comments about the rigidity of the way data have to be entered into a computer, and how much simpler it would be to use paper. Fortunately, this situation is changing for a number of reasons.
  - Firstly, the interaction technologies that define the way data are entered into a computer are becoming less constraining. Rather than forcing individuals to use a keyboard, it is now possible for data to be captured in a number of alternative ways. Raw data can be entered as a dictated voice recording, or as handwritten notes and diagrams using a pen-based computer system (e.g. MacNeill and Huang, 1996). Such data can be stored and left uninterpreted, still permitting subsequent retrieval when the data can be viewed or listened to in their original form. Further, using advanced pattern recognition methods, voice and handwriting data can be converted by the computer system into text. These interpretation methods are variable in their success, depending upon the situation in which interpretation occurs, but can usually achieve recognition levels much greater than 90% accuracy. Ultimately, recognition systems are limited by the way that the meaning of spoken or written language is based upon an understanding of the context within which a word is used (see Chapter 18). This ability to fully interpret natural language requires a computer system to possess some degree of artificial intelligence, and remains an open research problem in computer science.
  - Secondly, as more system designers realize the value in capturing spontaneous and unstructured data as part of the computer-based medical record, they will design features that allow this type of data to be entered. Thus, even without advanced interpretation systems, it is now physically easier to enter unstructured data into computer systems. This move to more familiar methods of data entry will also reduce the discomfort experienced by some individuals who have not grown up with computer systems.
- It was stated earlier that an advantage of the paper record is its portability, as if to imply that this was not an attribute of a computer-based one. This may have been the case in the past, when a computer system consisted of heavy fixed terminals connected to wired hospital computer networks, but it no longer need be the case. It is now possible to provide wireless connections to lightweight portable or handheld computer systems, allowing workers to roam within a hospital, or even widely across much larger regions using cellular radio and satellite technologies (see Chapter 20). As a consequence, data can be accessed or retrieved in a wide variety of circumstances.
- The situation in which records are missing, lost or unavailable because they are elsewhere in an organization does not arise with an electronic system. Database technologies permit multiple individuals to read a record simultaneously, and network

technologies permit these individuals to be geographically separated. If data exist in electronic files, they should be immediately available to those who have access permission.

- Finally, physical access to the computer record can be protected by a variety of different security measures. These are designed to prevent unauthorized individuals accessing the clinical record. Complex schemes involving restricting access to different components of the record, on the basis of an individual's role and need to know, can also be devised. Associated with such advantages is a different set of security risks (Anderson, 1995; Barrows and Clayton, 1996). It is often possible for knowledgeable and determined individuals to 'hack' into computer networks, despite security barriers such as password entry systems. This type of risk can be reduced through the use of data encryption methods that make data unintelligible in the event that unauthorized individuals access them.

Informational aspects of the computer-based record

Many of the advantages of an EMR become apparent when there are a large number of patient records, or when information tasks are complex. One of the most immediate benefits of having data available electronically is that the speed of searching for data is significantly improved. While a computer has searched through thousands of records for specific items, a human will still be leafing through one paper record.

Perhaps even more importantly, as we saw in Chapter 6, the types of search that can be performed across electronic databases can be complex. A primary care physician should be able to use Boolean logic to search through the records of the practice and extract files for patients with specific attributes such as age or diagnosis, and conduct a local audit of care, or search for patients that are similar to a current case. A researcher should be able to conduct retrospective studies of the epidemiology of specific diseases by accessing the records in a region that match specific study criteria. The ability of a computer database to search according to a number of different attributes means that each record is 'indexed' in a large number of different ways – certainly far more than could easily be accomplished by hand-generated indexes. It is possible to move completely away from the notion of creating fixed index structures. In principle every word in a document can act as an index. Many **search engines** use the frequency of appearance of a word in different documents to retrieve those that are most likely to match the search query.

The EMR can actively participate in clinical care

So far, the EMR has been considered as if it were simply a repository of clinical data, which is either added to or looked at, as the situation demands. One might characterize the EMR's role in this case to be a passive supporter of clinical activity. This is the traditional way in which the record has been used during care. Perhaps the greatest advantage of the EMR will ultimately be that it can be used in a more active way, by contributing more directly in the process of clinical care. An active EMR might suggest what patient information needs to be collected, or it might assemble clinical data in a way that assists a clinician in the visualization of a patient's clinical condition.

For the EMR to become more active in clinical care, there must be some mechanism by which the computer system is able to 'understand' what is needed of it. More precisely, the

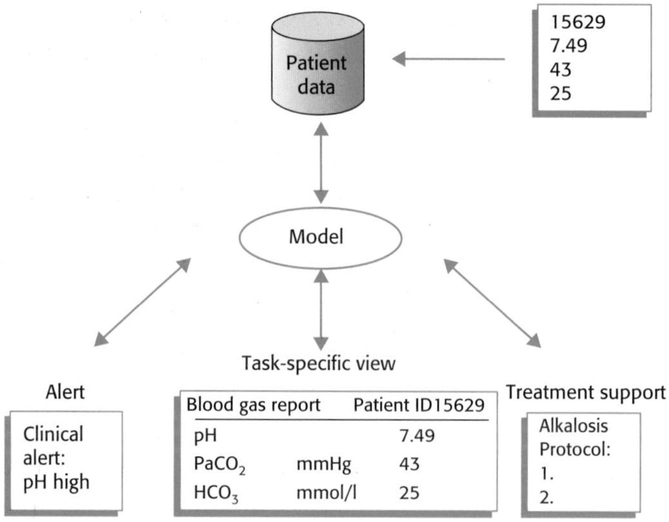
15629
7.49
43
25
Patient data
Model
Alert
Clinical alert: pH high
Task-specific view
Blood gas report Patient ID15629
pH 7.49
$PaCO_2$ mmHg 43
HCO_3 mmol/l 25
Treatment support
Alkalosis Protocol:
1.
2.

Figure 10.2
Using models of clinical tasks, the EMR can actively participate in clinical care, for example by generating specific views of clinical data, by sending alerts or by invoking models of treatment protocols.

EMR must possess some model of the clinical process that allows it to interpret data in a way that is clinically useful. At present, most research into active aspects of the EMR is focused on the generation of clinical alerts and reminders, the construction of task-specific views of data, and the structuring of care around protocols or guidelines (Figure 10.2).

Computer-supported prescribing

Prescribing medications is an increasingly difficult task with the large number of drugs available, and the ever-present risk of drug–drug interactions, dosage errors, and misinterpretation of handwritten medication orders. Indeed, the single commonest cause of adverse clinical events is medication error, which accounts for about 19% of all adverse events

The commonest prescription errors can be redressed by the provision of better information about medications or the patients receiving them (Bates *et al.*, 2001). Prescribing systems can check for the integrity on an individual new set of orders, for example dosage and compatibility. They become more powerful when linked to an EMR where they can check the orders against patient data, for example looking for other existing medications that may interact with the present orders, or detect allergies or pre-existing medical conditions that may contraindicate the new order. Computer-supported prescribing has been shown to reduce serious prescribing errors by 55%, and overall prescribing errors by about 83%. Prescribing errors are reduced through automated checks for dosage, drug–drug interactions, and appropriateness of indication. Although the benefit of computer prescription increases when it is integrated into an EPR system, the absence of such record systems is no reason to delay introducing electronic prescribing.

Alerts and reminders

Many clinical decisions require revision over time, as new evidence arrives, and computer-generated alerts also can be used to inform clinicians about the arrival of new information. Alerts may notify clinicians of errors in their medication orders, new laboratory results or changes in the physiological status of patients attached to monitor equipment. Simple alerts can be generated automatically, for example by laboratory computer systems, or be sent as e-mails that are redirected into the alerting system, for example when a hospital pharmacist detects a medication abnormality during routine patient review.

Even simple alerts and reminders can have a positive impact on care. Computer-generated reminders of the appropriate length of stay for a particular diagnosis have been shown to reduce the median length of stay in hospital (Shea *et al.*, 1995). In a meta-analysis of 16 randomized controlled trials of computer-generated reminders in ambulatory care, there was clear evidence that they improved preventative practices. Clinicians were found to perform better with the reminders on tasks like breast and colorectal cancer screening, cardiovascular risk reduction and vaccination (Shea *et al.*, 1996).

Much more complex reminders can be generated on the basis of data contained within the EMR, including laboratory results and current medications. When physicians were alerted via e-mail to increases in serum creatinine in patients receiving nephrotoxic medications, medications were adjusted or discontinued an average of 21.6 hours earlier than when no e-mail alerts were delivered (Rind *et al.*, 1994). When clinicians were paged about 'panic' laboratory values, the time to therapy decreased by 11% and the mean time to resolution of an abnormality was 29% shorter (Kuperman *et al.*, 1999). The methods used to accomplish this type of interpretation can be quite complex, and this advanced topic will be explored in much more detail in Chapters 25 and 26.

Task-specific views of data

One of the basic roles of the medical record is to provide a 'view' on to all the known patient data, so that they can be used to make clinical decisions. As records grow in size, searching for data relevant to a specific decision becomes increasingly difficult. This problem is not specific to healthcare, but is common to many professions in which large quantities of data need to be searched before a decision can be made. Airline pilots are surrounded by a variety of instruments and manuals in their cockpits, and nuclear power plant operators are similarly beset with data. Computer-based patient records have the inherent flexibility to vary their display structure to suit the needs of different clinical tasks. The same patient data can be displayed in any number of different structures, including source, time or problem-oriented displays. Research into the psychology of engineering systems suggests that the creation of even more task-specific data displays can assist in decision-making by presenting views of only the data that are directly relevant to a decision (Wickens and Hollands, 2000). Such displays both reduce the effort expended in collating data, as well as focusing the attention on important data that might otherwise be ignored.

The creation of task-specific views is also supported by research into clinical behaviour, which suggests that the creation of data displays specific to particular clinical contexts can be of value (Fafchamps *et al.*, 1991). The creation of such task-specific data views requires some model of what the different tasks might be, as well as what data are 'relevant' for that particular task. Such models can be created by system designers, or be specifically designed by the staff that will use the system (Gierl *et al.*, 1995). Most commonly, task-specific views are created around measured data, which might be obtained from laboratory tests or instruments (Figure 10.3).

Protocol-guided care

The problem-oriented medical record is based upon the assumption that care can be best delivered when the record focuses on the management of specific problems. With the EMR,

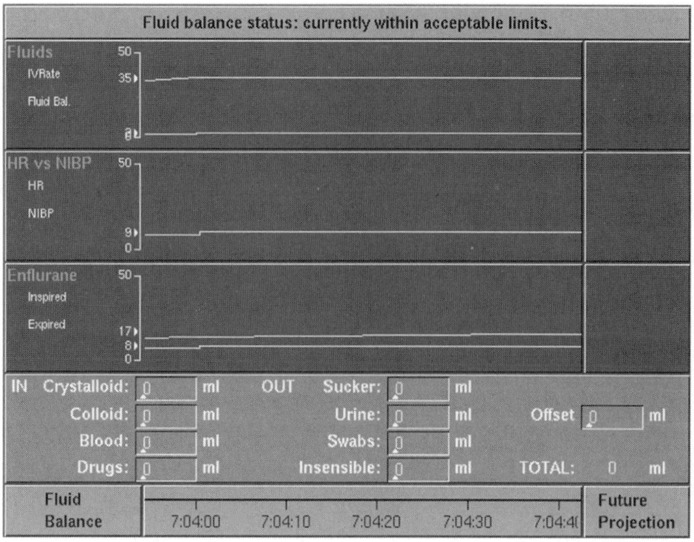
Fluid balance status: currently within acceptable limits.
Fluids
IVRate
Fluid Bal.
HR vs NIBP
HR
NIBP
Enflurane
Inspired
Expired
IN Crystalloid: ml
Colloid: ml
Blood: ml
Drugs: ml
OUT Sucker: ml
Urine: ml
Swabs: ml
Insensible: ml
Offset ml
TOTAL: 0 ml
Fluid Balance
7:04:00
7:04:10
7:04:20
7:04:30
Future Projection

Figure 10.3
Using models of clinical decisions, different views of patient data can be constructed to support distinct tasks. Here data relevant to determining fluid balance during surgery are collected together on one screen as part of an anaesthetic EMR. (© Hewlett-Packard, 1992)

this notion of record structuring around problems can become more active when the EMR has models of the management of different problems. Clinical protocols or guidelines can provide such models, and if integrated into the EMR, could support a rich variety of new functions. Guidelines can be used to ensure that specific data are gathered, to suggest tests that need to be ordered or treatments that could be contemplated.

Clinical audit and outcomes assessment

Patient records contribute not just to the immediate care of individual patients, but can be pooled to assess the efficacy of particular treatments, to determine cost-benefits or to audit the performance of individual care centres. To do this, data often need to be condensed. For some purposes, for example, it may only be necessary to record a patient's ultimate diagnosis. Much of this data condensation is done through the process of **coding**. Here, the treatments and diagnoses of a specific patient are assigned a code from a predetermined list. For example, the World Health Organization (WHO) has a set of epidemiological codes called the International Classification of Diseases (ICD) (WHO, 1993) which are used to track broad global health patterns. Most countries return data to WHO based on their local records. For a long time this has been a manual process, but the data stored in the EMR could be used to partially or completely create such codes.

Conclusions

This chapter has presented a broad survey of the rationale for and potential roles of the EMR. It should now be clear that the role of a computer-based information system in healthcare extends significantly beyond the simple storage and retrieval of patient data. Many of the aspects of the EMR introduced here will be returned to in subsequent sections. In particular, protocol-based care, clinical coding and classification, and the support of communication in a clinical setting will all be examined in much greater detail.

The final chapter in this section looks at the way all such information systems are designed and evaluated. Within the constraints of these design principles, we can understand better how information and communication systems fit into the clinical workplace, and work more comfortably with some of their inherent limitations.

Discussion points

1. What is the purpose of a medical record?
2. Do you think clinical practice will ever be 'paperless'?
3. What is the purpose of an EMR?
4. What do you think might be lost when a clinical practice changes from a paper to an electronic record system?
5. 'Paper record systems can never be better than electronic ones.' Do you agree? Discuss from both a physical and an informational perspective.
6. Compare the different contributions that the medium and the message make to the effectiveness of paper- and computer-record systems. If you wish, use Chapters 4 and 5 as your template.
7. Do you think the problem-oriented medical record is better suited to the paper or electronic medium?

Chapter summary

1. At its simplest, the EMR is the computer replacement for existing paper medical record systems. It provides mechanisms for capturing information during the clinical encounter, stores it in a secure fashion, and permits retrieval of that information by those with a clinical need.
2. For many, the EMR represents the totality of information and communication systems that could be made available in the support of clinical activities. Systems for ordering tests and investigations, digital image archiving and retrieval, the exchange of messages between different workers in the healthcare system, through to the automated coding of patient data for administrative purposes may be components of the EMR's function.
3. There are two quite separate aspects to record systems:
   - the physical nature of the way individuals interact with it
   - the way information is structured when entered into or retrieved from the system.
4. Advantages of the paper-based medical record include its portability, its support of informal and formal data capture, and its familiarity and ease of use.
5. Disadvantages of the paper-based medical record include its poor use of space, its fragility, its limitation to a single user at any one time, the ease with which records can be misplaced or lost and the effort required in searching for information either in large single records, or from collections of records.
6. The computer-based medical record can be used passively as a repository of data, or actively by assisting with the shaping of care. Active use requires the EMR to contain models of care, permitting some degree of interpretation of the data contained in the record.
7. Active uses of the computer-based medical record include electronic prescribing, the generation of clinical alerts and reminders, task-specific views on to clinical data, protocol-guided data entry and action suggestion, and generation of codes for the classification of the contents of the record.

CHAPTER 11

Designing and evaluating information systems

Given that there are limits to resources in healthcare, just because something is possible, it may not be desirable, or indeed affordable. This certainly is the case with information technologies, and the last few decades are littered with examples of healthcare information systems that were ill considered in their design, or in the resources they consumed. Equally, there are many examples of well-conceived projects that have delivered considerable benefit. The difference between success and failure often comes down to the approach taken by the creators of a system.

There are essentially two ways in which a technology can be applied to solve a problem. The first approach is **technology driven**. Here one asks 'What problems will best be solved by using this new technology?' Inevitably, whatever the problem, the answer will always be that the technology is the solution. This approach is often useful when trying to demonstrate the potential of a particular technological innovation.

The second approach to the application of technology is **problem driven,** and asks the question 'What is the best way to solve this particular problem?'. In this approach, all kinds of solutions are explored, from changes in clinical process to the introduction of a new technology. Consequently, sometimes the answer to the problem may be that new technology is not the best solution.

Informatics, when it is focused on building healthcare systems that will be routinely used, should fundamentally be problem driven. It should first and foremost be concerned with understanding the nature of information and communication problems in healthcare. Only then should informatics try to identify if it is appropriate for technology to solve these problems and, if necessary, develop and apply these technologies.

Sadly, however, this is not always the case. It is not uncommon for information system developers to put most of their effort into the technology, leaving problem definition scarcely addressed. One thus sometimes finds clinical information systems that are designed in a way that does not address the needs of the clinicians who will use them. Equally, sometimes informatics research explores exotic technologies that solve problems that could be more easily solved with simpler existing technology, or indeed in non-technological ways. Sometimes, despite the best advice to the contrary, managers are still persuaded to purchase expensive technical solutions because it is 'simpler' and quicker than actually finding out what the real problems are and doing something about them.

So, how does one choose which clinical problems are good candidates for a technological solution? Further, how should one design an information system in a way that maximizes the likelihood that it will actually solve the problem it is intended to? These are complex questions, with many technical ramifications. This chapter will simply try to examine the problem selection and system design processes from a general perspective. In particular, the focus will be on understanding what is theoretically possible, what is technically practicable, and in the context of limited resources, what is desirable.

In the first section, we will define the stages in the development of an information system, covering both design and evaluation. Next, methods of arriving at good problem-driven formulations will be examined. We will see that system design is a sociotechnical issue, and involves modelling both people and technology. Then some key issues that limit what is possible in the design of systems will be outlined, in particular looking at the life cycle of an information system. The final section will look, in a relatively systematic way, at how one arrives at a well-engineered specification of an information system.

11.1 Design and evaluation are linked processes

The life cycle of an information system from initial conception to final implementation has traditionally been broken down into a set of key stages:

- **Requirements analysis:** Definition of the problem the system will try to solve, and specifically capture the needs of the users of the system. It is at this stage that one tries to understand the specific context within which the system will be used and the abilities and needs of users.
- **Functional specification:** Translation of the user requirements into a formal functional description of the information system.
- **Architecture design:** Translation of the functional specification into a software architecture, which defines the individual components of the system, and how they will interact with each other. For example, the software architecture may define which databases will be needed, and the information model within those databases, as well as the flows of data within the system.
- **Software programming:** The software architecture is still a general description, and has to be implemented as a working system. In the programming phase, software and hardware are chosen, and the detailed system architecture is translated into 'code', which specifically controls each step in the actual functioning of the system.

- **Unit test:** Once an information system has been implemented, it must be tested to see if it contains errors. Errors may be introduced at any of the previous stages. For example, software engineers may have made mistakes in the programming, or the software architecture may have had design flaws. Load testing may check to see if the system can handle the number of users or transactions expected at peak times once it is in the real world.
- **System integration:** Many new information systems will be added into a complex environment where there are pre-existing information systems, and usually some form of linking between the new and old systems is needed. For example, the new hospital medical record system may require to be connected to a pre-existing database containing patient names and demographic details.
- **Acceptance test:** Once integrated, the new system needs to be tested out by the system's users for acceptability. It is checked out to see if it performs as expected, if there are any unanticipated problems now that the system has been placed in a real working environment.
- **User training:** Before a system can go into widespread use, significant investment of resources needs to be made in training the user population, as failure to do so will result in the system being poorly or underutilized. In the worst case, frustrated staff that are unable to effectively use a system might reject it, and lead to the system implementation being a failure.
- **Outcomes assessment:** Once a system has been introduced, its performance against the original design objectives can be measured. For example, is the organization more effective or efficient than before? For new technology, it may be necessary to carry out formally designed trials across multiple sites, to see if there is a significant difference between sites with and without the system.

These stages give the impression that there is a nice and linear sequence of system development, but the risks of simply progressing through these stages is that we end up with a system that is rejected at acceptance testing because the initial user needs were not adequately captured. Indeed, software engineering tells us that the best time to modify a program is early in the development cycle. In Figure 11.1 the cost of error removal is shown to grow exponentially during the development of a computer program. Further, the times at which errors are introduced and detected are likely to be different. Thus an error introduced during the initial functional specification of a program is likely to be detected only when the system is completed and in regular use. At this time, the users will suggest ways in which the system's actual functionality, and the functionality they expected, differs. Introducing changes into a mature system thus becomes increasingly expensive over time (Littlewood, 1987).

Consequently the evaluation and development of an information system are intertwined and concurrent processes. It is often more useful to create a series of increasingly complex prototype versions of a system, and take them through the system design steps including user testing. Allowing users to work with or react to simple prototypes reveals flaws in the initial user requirements description or in the architecture or implementation. This iterative approach to system development avoids over-investment in immature systems and 'surprises' when a system is actually deployed in a working environment.

Taking an iterative view of information system development, rather than a linear one, we can conceptually think of all these steps occurring within two different development

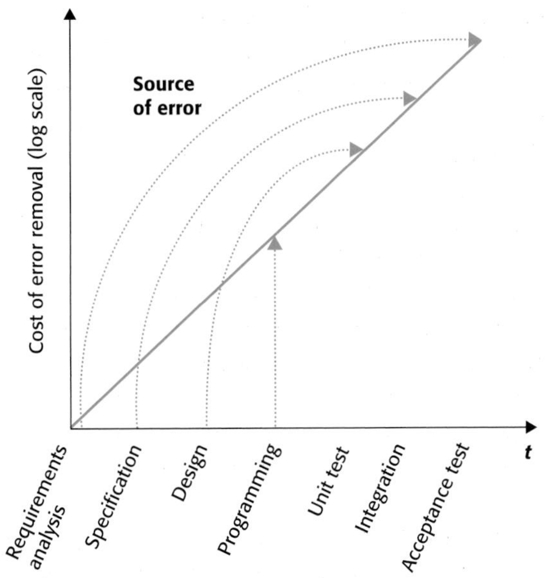
Cost of error removal (log scale)
Source of error
Requirements analysis
Specification
Design
Programming
Unit test
Integration
Acceptance test
t

Figure 11.1 The cost of removing an error in the different stages of software development increases logarithmically. Errors introduced at the beginning of the specification phase are likely to only be detected during the use of the product (after Cohen, 1986).

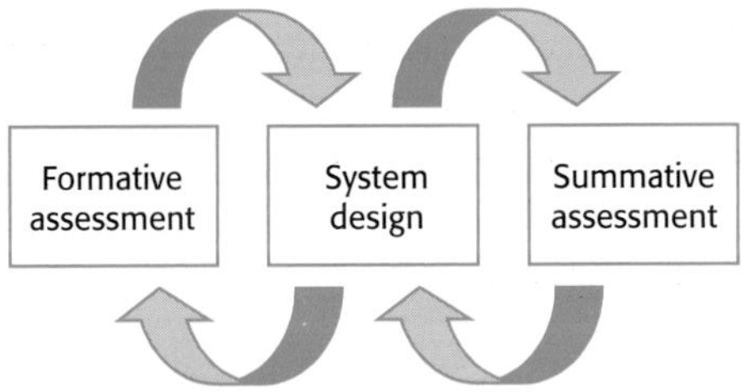
Formative assessment
System design
Summative assessment

Figure 11.2 The process of building an information system is an iterative cycle of forming the system around user needs, designing appropriate interactions between the system and users, and then evaluating the true impact of the system using quantitative studies.

cycles (Figure 11.2):

- **Formative development cycle:** The form that a system takes is iteratively determined by assessing user needs, designing prototypes, and then getting user feedback on system performance.
- **Summative assessment cycle:** Once a system is robust enough for an outcomes assessment, it is put on trial and the summation of system performance results are used to drive the design of the next version of the system.

This view of systems development holds true of most designed systems destined for complex environments, not just information systems. For example, drugs go through a period of drug discovery and testing, in which many versions of a compound are developed and tested in laboratories. This stage is equivalent to the formative assessment cycle. Once the drug is ready for routine use in humans, it goes through the summative assessment cycle, when randomized controlled trials are performed to determine if the clinical performance promised in the laboratory translate to clinical outcomes in the real world.

11.2 The formative assessment cycle defines clinical needs

There is an initial stage in the life of any information system in which its role, costs and benefits are debated. Eventually, this leads on to the creation of a system design that reflects the trade-offs that inevitably will be made at this point. The clarification of the role that a system will play is perhaps the most critical aspect of this process, since it influences everything that will follow.

How does one gain an understanding of the needs of clinical practice, and then convert these into a set of specifications for an information system? There are many approaches, each of which is aimed at understanding what people need. They can be roughly grouped into the following four categories.

- **Anecdotal or individual experience:** At the most superficial level one can draw upon individual experience, or rely on anecdotal evidence from other colleagues, to help pinpoint the tasks with which clinicians need help. This method usually operates within a framework of the existing assumptions about user needs. In other words, it is unlikely that novel needs will be uncovered to challenge the prevailing wisdom.
- **Asking clinicians:** If one wants to be a little more methodical, a survey can be conducted, and ask clinicians about their way of working and their needs. This may seem attractive, but it has its problems. The biggest is that it is unlikely that clinicians really know what they want or need. 'Although users are expert at what they do, they have difficulty predicting what they would like' (Fafchamps *et al.*, 1991).

More specifically, both the anecdotal and survey approaches suffer from a number of methodological difficulties. The problem of attitudinal bias has long been understood in the social psychology literature – people's actions differ from their verbalized responses (Wicker, 1976). We don't necessarily do as we say. Secondly, these methods require a degree of self-reporting. When asked why they made a certain judgement, or how they solved a particular problem, people are capable of providing apparently plausible reports of their mental events. However, asking people to introspect about their behaviour is a contentious investigative method in psychology because verbal reports of influences on behaviour may not be valid. Since there is no method of independently checking the validity of self-reports, the details of cognition remain private to the individual (Nisbett and Wilson, 1977).

- **Non-participatory observation:** The next set of methods does not ask clinicians what they want, but studies the way they work in the field. There are many approaches that one could take, including techniques derived from **ethnography** (Fafchamps *et al.*, 1991), as well as the more traditional software design methods of data-flow and task analysis. Here researchers try to understand the demands made on individuals through detailed observations of them engaged in routine tasks. By making such observations, one is in a position to identify needs that may not be apparent to the individuals being studied.
- **Formal user experiments:** Finally, at the most detailed and scientifically rigorous level, one might have a set of hypotheses about specific aspects of human or system behaviour, and set up controlled studies to test them out. Thus, before a system is built, the impact of different changes to a human decision process could be assessed by trialling then in a controlled laboratory situation. Then, once initial system designs have been prototyped, user responses to the system can be gauged by testing in a controlled user studies

laboratory, where users can be interviewed, or discreetly observed as they react to the prototypes.

Although it may seem that the ideal method of proceeding is to invest in formal laboratory studies, this is not necessarily the case. Laboratory experiments run the risk of studying people carrying out information tasks, independently of the vagaries and interruptions of working life. By their nature, such studies are conducted in laboratory conditions that factor out the interruptions and pressures of the real clinical workplace. In the real world, time pressures mean that short cuts are taken, and that people and events interrupt clinical activities.

What is usually needed is a characterization of clinical tasks as much as possible in the way they **really** occur, as opposed to the way they **should** occur. This will give us the best chance of designing systems for use in working environments, as opposed to designing what would be needed if everything else were ideal. It may be the case, for example, that in an ideal consultation a doctor may want to consult a computer to help with the diagnostic process. However, with the pressures of the real workplace, the bottlenecks to increased performance may be much more mundane and less glamorous. They may, for example, be more closely associated with easy and timely communications between professionals, or even simply reducing the amount of paperwork in the clinical workplace.

This argument strongly favours initially pursuing non-participatory methods in the field, such as the ethnographic approach. Such qualitative research methods are sufficiently formal to allow robust statements to be made about results, and have the advantage of being grounded in the realities of the clinical workplace (Mays and Pope, 1996). Formal experiments will only answer narrow questions and are relatively expensive to conduct. Consequently experiments are more valuable later on in the system development cycle, once there are clear ideas about the role and design of the system.

11.3 Summative evaluations attempt to determine the measurable impact of a system once it is in routine use

Information and communication systems can be considered a health intervention designed to improve the care delivered to patients. As such we should be able to identify the effects of the intervention and measure how large the effects are, just as one would for a new form of treatment like a medication. As with any class of intervention, including pharmaceuticals, success is not guaranteed, and it is likely that some interventions will be less successful than others. A summative evaluation can be made in three broad categories – a user's satisfaction with the service, clinical outcome changes resulting from using the service, and the economic benefit of the service.

- **User satisfaction studies** seek to determine whether users are happy with a service, and as such do not necessarily attempt to compare one service with others. Satisfaction is necessarily a very subjective measure, and many variables may affect it. Consequently simple assessments of satisfaction may not reveal much about the underlying reasons for attitudes to a service. Satisfaction surveys are also prone to positive biases. For example, patients may rate a service positively simply because of the novelty factor associated with new technology, or because they wish to please those providing the service and asking them questions (Taylor, 1998).

- **Clinical outcomes** may often be difficult to evaluate, since one typically requires large randomized trials before any effect can be statistically demonstrated. Some clinical outcomes, such as mortality rates or survival rates, can be directly measured. As we saw in Chapter 8, different clinical outcomes may have a subjective utility value associated with them, and various methods such as calculation of QALYs may be carried out. When final outcomes are difficult to measure, it may be possible to measure intermediate **process variables**, which can act as proxy indicators of the quality of care being delivered. For example, when assessing a prescribing decision support system, we can measure an improvement in patient safety through a reduction in medication errors and adverse events. If we wished to assess the impact of asking clinicians to follow a computerized protocol system that guides management decisions, we could measure process variables such as any improvement in the quality of clinical documentation, changes to a clinician's available time for direct patient care, and increased adoption of recommendations in the clinical guidelines.
- **Economic analyses** determine if there is a cost-benefit in using a new way of delivering a health service. Economic analyses can look at savings that accrue from things such as changes in treatment that favour cheaper but equally effective alternatives, reduction in adverse events or errors, reduction in demand for health services by patients and time freed up for patients or clinicians to attend to other tasks. One specific way of assessing economic benefit is to conduct a utility analysis, which looks at the outcome of using the intervention. For example, if a patient has fewer complications, then a utility can be assigned to that quality of life outcome, and a price can be placed on these utilities. Importantly, one must not only factor in the technical costs of running the service, but also the set-up costs, costs of educating staff, and long-term replacement costs which help determine whether a service is sustainable in the long run. The rapid change in the cost of technology may make it difficult to predict future cost-benefit from the current price arrangements. However, the cost of information technology is never the major component of total costs.

11.4 Interaction design focuses on the way people interact with technology

So far we have examined the overall process of system construction, from the generation of initial specifications, through iterative formative evaluation and refinement of design, to final summative evaluation of performance. We now turn to examine the design process in more detail, to understand how one conceptualizes an information system design, and tries to anticipate the way the system will work, once it is implemented.

The design of information systems can focus on any one of four increasingly complex levels of abstraction (Figure 11.3):

- **Algorithm:** Traditionally information systems are designed around an idealized model of the task that needs to be accomplished, and the result is an algorithm, which is like a recipe, in that it describes each step in a process in an abstract way.
- **Computer program:** For an algorithm to be executable in a specific computer it must be written in a programming language that explicitly instructs the computer in how to

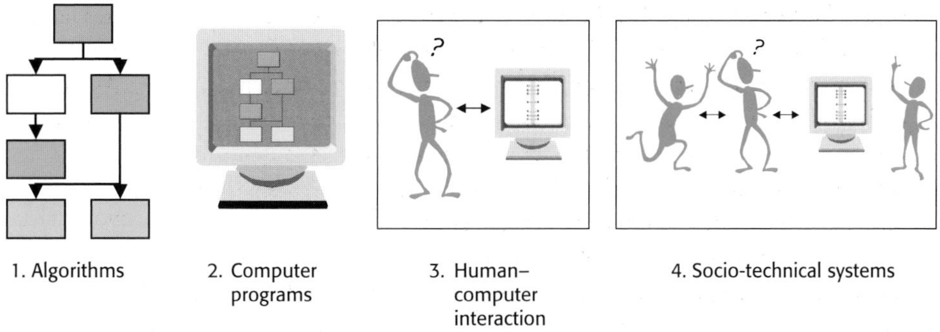
1. Algorithms
2. Computer programs
3. Human–computer interaction
4. Socio-technical systems

Figure 11.3 The four levels of information system design.

carry out each step of the algorithm, defining the data inputs and outputs and the functions that will be used to manipulate the data.

- **Human–computer interaction:** Recognizing that the success of a computer system depends on how usable it is by humans, the human–computer interface and task-flow of the system need to be designed, and to be optimized to maximize usability. Design devices such as icons and windows are intended to make the interaction as natural as possible for the user, unlike the early days of programming, when the interaction was shaped more by how the computer needed to function than the way humans do.
- **Socio-technical system:** The user of a computer system does not operate in isolation, but is affected by other people around them and any other tasks they must also accomplish, all while they try to use the computer system. Consequently the ultimate usefulness of a system is determined by how well it fits the whole organizational structure and workflow, not just the specific tasks for which it was designed.

Thus, in the final analysis, people are part of the system. The web of interactions needed to make anything work in a complex organization always involves humans solving problems with limited resources and working around imperfect processes. We know empirically that the value of any particular information technology can only be determined with reference to the social context within which it is used and, more precisely, with reference to those who use the technology (Berg, 1997; Lorenzi *et al.*, 1997). For example, in one study the strongest predictor of e-mail adoption in an organization had nothing to do with system design or function, but with whether the e-mail user's manager also used e-mail (Markus, 1994).

Further, a highly structured view of human processes sits uneasily with the clinical workplace. It is not just that people have difficulty accepting information technology in a social setting because their interactions are loosely structured. We know that people will treat computers and media as if they were people (Reeves and Nass, 1996). Consequently, they superimpose social expectations on technological interactions.

Designing the technological tools that humans will use, independent of the way that the tools will affect the organization, only optimizes local task-specific solutions, and ignores global realities. The biggest information repository in most organizations sits within the heads of those who work there, and the largest communication network is the web of conversations that binds them.

Together, people, tools and conversations – that is the 'system'. Consequently, the design of information and communication systems must also include the people who will use them.

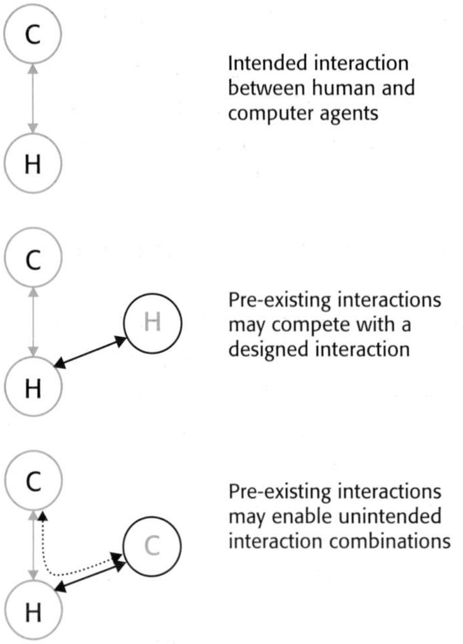
C
H
Intended interaction between human and computer agents
C
H
H
Pre-existing interactions may compete with a designed interaction
C
C
H
Pre-existing interactions may enable unintended interaction combinations

Figure 11.4
When a new interaction is designed it does not exist in isolation but is placed within a pre-existing interaction space. Other interactions that exist in the interaction space impact on the new interaction in a variety of ways, and if they are ignored in the design process may have unexpected consequences when the new interaction is implemented.

We must therefore design **socio-technical systems** that reflect the machinery of human thought and communication, sometimes mediated by communication channels, sometimes in partnership with computational agents.

Interaction design focuses on constructing the ways people interact with objects and systems (Winograd, 1997). As we have already seen, often information system design occurs with a single-task assumption, that the user is going to be wholly focused on interacting with the system that is being designed. Such *in vitro* laboratory assumptions do not translate *in vivo* when individuals use systems in working environments. Since individuals in an organization are working in a complex environment, they may at any one time be carrying out a variety of tasks and interacting with different agents to help execute those tasks. With the exception of environments where there is rigorous workflow control, this means that we cannot predict what interactions will actually be occurring at the same time as any interaction we specifically design.

Although we cannot predict every specific interaction that will occur in the real work environment, the design process can model the typical **interaction space** within which any new system will be introduced. The interaction space can be modelled to include the most important interactions that will be competing with the new designed interaction (Figure 11.4).

An interaction occurs between two agents when one agent creates and then communicates a message to another, to accomplish a particular task. A **mediated interaction** occurs when a communication channel intermediates between agents by bearing the messages between them. For example, e-mail can be used to mediate an interaction between two individuals, just as can an electronic medical record (EMR), which is as much a service to communicate messages between clinical staff as it is an archival information repository.

The first step in modelling the interaction space surrounding a new interaction we wish to design is to note which other agents will be local to the new interaction, and then to examine the likely effects of any interactions they might have on the new interaction that is being contemplated. By doing so we enhance the chance that new interactions will succeed when they are eventually introduced into the intended interaction space.

In general terms the impact of one interaction on another may be to:

- **Compete with another interaction as a direct substitute:** For example, a user could use an online database to seek information, or instead, use the telephone to call a colleague to ask for the same information. The human–human interaction mediated by the telephone competes with the database to meet the user's information needs.
- **Compete with another interaction for the resources of an agent:** An agent has limited resources and if they are expended on one interaction they may not be available to another. For example, an information system may be well received in *in vitro* laboratory tests, but when it is placed in a work environment we may find the users have insufficient time to use the system, because of competing tasks. The new system is then 'rejected' not because it does not do what was intended, but because the impact of the real-world interaction space on its intended users was not modelled. Concurrent interactions can also subvert the execution of a designed interaction. For example, a user may be interrupted in the workplace and take up a new task, and not log off the information system they were using, causing a potential breach of security.
- **Create new information transfer pathways, through a combination of interactions:** Each interaction connects agents, and each new interaction enables novel conversations between agents. If these combinations are not factored into system design, then the introduction of a system may produce unexpected results. For example, consider the interaction between a human agent and an electronic record system or EMR. Computational agents that might co-exist with the EMR could include other applications such as e-mail or a word-processor. If the design process fails to include these additional computational agents, then unintended interactions made possible via these other agents may subvert the original EMR design. For example, it may be possible for a user to copy a section of text from the medical record to a word-processor, where it can be edited, and then re-inserted into the EMR. However, since this interaction with the word-processor is not part of the original design scope, it may introduce problems. A user could inadvertently paste the text into the record of a different patient, and no formal mechanism would be in place to prevent this context-switch error. Similarly, text might be copied from an EMR that has been designed with powerful security features to prevent unauthorized access, and then copied into an e-mail message, which is insecure. In both cases, the co-existence of an unmodelled additional computational agent introduces interactions beyond the scope of the original system design, and permits behaviours which would be prohibited within the designed interaction, but which are permitted in the interaction space.
- **Support the new interaction by providing resources that are critical to its execution:** For example, the designer of a medical record system usually focuses on sculpting the interaction between a single clinical user and the record. However, other human agents also populate the EMR interaction space. The EMR user is often not the sole author of the content that is captured in the record, but is recording the result of a set of discussions with these other clinical colleagues. If the goal of designing an EMR is to ensure the highest quality data are entered into the information system, then it may be even more important to support the collaborative discussion between clinicians than it is to engineer the act of record transcription into the system. Failing to model the wider EMR interaction space means we may over-engineer some interactions with diminishing

returns, when we could be supporting other interactions that may deliver substantial additional benefit to our original design goals.

One of the ways interactions impact each other is to compete for the resources of individual agents. On the basis of cognitive psychological models, we should be able to say something about the cognitive resources available to human agents, the cognitive loads they will typically be under in a given interaction space and the types of errors that may arise because of these loads. Consequently, it should be possible to craft information or communication systems that are tolerant of the typical interaction load our users will be under. There is a rich literature connecting cognitive psychology and systems engineering (e.g. Wickens and Hollands, 2000). Sadly, to date there seems to have been little connection between the design of many clinical information systems, and the work on the cognitive aspects of clinical decision-making.

11.5 Designing for change

Understanding user needs helps determine what a system should do, based upon the constraints of environment in which it will work. The working environment also affects how the system should be constructed. Indeed, we saw earlier that the construction of any object, device or system begins with set of assumptions about the environment in which it will operate (Figure 1.2). Of these assumptions, the intended lifetime of the system is perhaps one of the most fundamental, since it affects the choice of materials and quality of design. Something that is meant to be temporary is engineered in a very different way to something that is intended to stand for many years.

One of the greatest challenges for any designer is arriving at ways of coping with change during a system's lifetime. As the world changes, the design assumptions with which systems are built become outdated. As the effects of these changes accumulate over time, a system becomes increasingly out of tune with the environment for which it was built. There are countless examples of this process of system 'decay' (Hogarth, 1986). Political systems arise out of the needs of a society, only to become increasingly inappropriate as the nature of society changes underneath them. Antibiotics become increasingly ineffective as the bacteria they are intended to attack change their pattern of drug resistance.

The rate of obsolescence of a human artefact is thus directly related to the rate at which its design assumptions decay. Since building an artefact such as a hospital or an information system is often an expensive affair, coping with the process of obsolescence is often critical. This is especially so if the costs of building need to be recouped over an extended period. If the system becomes obsolete before it has paid back the investment in it, then it may fail financially. Consequently, its builders may not be in a position to design and build the next generation of system to replace it.

Time cycles for information systems

An information system is particularly susceptible to the effects of change. We can think of an information system experiencing the effects of change at several different time scales, corresponding to different aspects of its design and construction:

- the user needs that define the role of the system
- the model of user needs, and subsequent system design

- the technology used to construct the system
- organizational resources, including finance and staff availability.

A change in any one of these will affect the performance of the system as a whole. For example, if the original need for a system changes, irrespective of how advanced the technology is, the system as a whole has become obsolete. Equally, technology can change rapidly, and a well-designed system may become obsolete because newer technologies make it seem slow compared to newer ones introduced at a later date.

The time scales over which each of these different aspects of a system age are different, making it very difficult to get any synchronization in replacement cycles. Thus, once it has been built, an information system is probably already obsolete in some respect: its modelling of user needs, its definition of organizational structure or the computer technology used to implement it.

Informal systems are much less susceptible to this sort of obsolescence, since they avoid modelling specific attributes of an organization, and consequently are much more permissive about the information that is being stored or transmitted within them. Consider, for example, how the telephone system in a hospital may undergo little change, while its information systems may go through several revisions or complete change. Indeed, informal systems are often used increasingly during the period that a formal information system becomes out of date, bridging the gap between the deficiencies of the formal system and actual situation.

Withholding design

One solution to this problem of managing replacement cycles in the face of differential ageing is to hold back the introduction of a new design, even through it is appropriate to retire an existing one. This is often the solution chosen when there is a mismatch between the period needed to pay for a system, and the period over which it becomes obsolete.

For example, as healthcare becomes increasingly expensive and the nature of medical practice evolves, the burden of care is being shifted from institutions like hospitals to smaller entities in the community. It is implicit in this change that much of the hospital system as it exists is becoming increasingly obsolete. However, given the huge investment in the hospital system, from the buildings through to the people whose skills are needed to make it work, it is impossible to make the change overnight. The investment in the existing system is too big, and the cost of creating a new one enormous.

As a result, larger hospitals are slowly closing down or changing their function, and staff slowly trickling out to community-based institutions. At the same time, the cost of ramping up the new community-based care system is so large that it also takes time. Change is expensive. The consequence of these costs is that obsolete systems are kept in use well beyond the point at which they could in principle be replaced.

Design modularity

Part of the solution to the problem of designing for a changing world is to construct a system on the assumption that parts of its design will be altered over its working lifetime.

At the heart of designing for change is the concept of design modularity. The designer creates a system in such a way that its different components, or sub-systems, are cleanly separated. In a car, for example, the braking system is designed to be a separate set of components to the suspension. When change demands that a component be redesigned, the effects are contained within that component module. It is redesigned and replaced, and the remainder of the system is left unaffected.

The most useful way of creating modules is to consider the different purposes for which parts of the device's inner structure are intended. Each separate purpose, or function, is then contained within a module. There is a hidden catch to this simple idea. Recall from Chapter 3 that the definition of a system is ultimately arbitrary. In other words, when a designer looks at a system, the decision to separate it into sub-components could be made in many ways. Consequently, there can never be a guarantee that a particular way of compartmentalizing a design will always insulate it from change. What it does achieve is that it decreases the likelihood that changes will affect the whole system – on average using design modularity allows a system's design to gracefully degrade over time.

11.6 Designing the information management cycle

Once a set of user needs has been determined, and constraints of the working environment understood, the next step in the construction of an information system is the formal specification of its design. This specification is used as a blueprint to drive the actual building process.

There are many different methodologies for designing information systems, their popularity changing with time. DeMarco's (1982) influential approach to the software engineering process is a classic example. In this final section, rather than exploring the technical details of any specific design method, the design process will be looked at from first principles. Whether the goal of an information system is to manage the operation of a nursing unit, reduce infection rates or conduct research into basic medical science, the principles determining the successful design of its management cycle should be the same.

The first section of this book examined the general process of creating a model of the world, and of designing artefacts based on that model. The specific interaction of information systems with the world was characterized through the model, measure and manage cycle, containing the following steps.

- defining a set of management goals
- constructing a model of the system
- gathering measurement data from a system
- interpreting the meaning of the measurements
- taking actions based on the interpretation.

For each step, we will now look at the principle issues that affect the design process.

Designing a goal

Goals are the outcomes that a management system tries to achieve. If we are trying to control a patient's cardiovascular system, for example, our goal might be to obtain a blood pressure in the normal range. If we are managing a hospital unit, the goal might be to treat a certain number of patients over a year within a given budget, and with a specified clinical outcome.

Having worked through the first chapters, the prerequisites for a goal to be achievable should come as no surprise.

- The goal should be measurable. If it is not, then there is no way of knowing when it has been achieved. Consider the difference between the goals 'I want to be successful' and 'I want to be a qualified neurosurgeon by the age of 35'.
- The measurements should be interpretable. We should have a model of the system we are trying to influence, and should be able to determine the meaning of the measurements we take in relation to our goal. Thus, for example, we should be able to say whether an action has resulted in a move towards or away from a goal.
- The interpretations should be manageable. We should know what actions to take given a specific interpretation, or at least have a way of finding out what actions to take.

As we saw in Chapter 3, feedback control systems are a very special kind of information management system. Here the goal is called an **equilibrium state**. If the system being controlled is deflected from that equilibrium state, then a controller takes actions to try and reach a new equilibrium state. For example, an IV pump containing drugs that alter blood pressure could be coupled to a blood pressure measurement system. The IV pump would change the dosing rate of the medications on the basis of deviations in the blood pressure from some defined value, always attempting to keep the patient's pressure within some target range.

Designing the model

We already know that for a management goal to be achievable, a model must exist to allow any measurements to be interpretable. For a model to actually fulfil this requirement, there are several things that need to be in place.

- **The model must be sufficiently accurate:** Irrespective of how well we understand any given system, our knowledge of it and the environment within which it exists will never be complete. This means that any management system operating in the real world will never be able to completely guarantee an outcome. As our models of the systems we wish to control improve, so too do our chances of success in managing them. Inevitably, there will always be unforeseen problems that are not included in our models, and for which we will not have developed a plan of management.
- **A model must be sufficiently detailed for the task at hand:** The more closely that model approximates the system in question, the more fine-grained will be our prediction of its response to actions performed upon it. However, it is not always the case that one should use the most detailed model available. Creating and using models consumes resources (Coiera, 1992b). Time, for example, may be limited. If a model is too detailed then it may take too long to work out what is going on, and consequently urgently needed control measures will be delayed. In this case, simple 'rules of thumb' may be sufficient to control a system within a roughly acceptable range. This is often the philosophy taken, for example, in the immediate management of critically ill patients. Rapid assessment and management by simple principles are followed later by a more painstaking assessment, once a patient has been stabilized.
- **The model must be timely:** As we saw earlier, systems in the real world change. Consequently, what has been a good model may over time become less useful – as the

system has changed, the model has remained static. It is thus a good rule of thumb that over time a model becomes increasingly inaccurate – models decay (Hogarth, 1986). The consequences for system control are significant. The system seems to become increasingly unmanageable using the old model. Control actions that once worked are no longer as effective as they once were.

- **The model must be the right one:** A model of the pathophysiology of pneumonia and its treatment will not help to treat cardiogenic heart failure. In effect, a model is a hypothesis about how a system operates, and if the hypothesis is wrong, then it is unlikely that the system can be well managed. If, for example, the treatment goal is incorrect, then so too will be the specific knowledge that is brought to bear in achieving the goal.

Designing the measurements

Measurements provide the data with which we drive our inferences, and represent samples we take from the system we want to control. For example, we examine a patient to obtain physical measurements. These will then be mapped, through a diagnostic process, on to a disease state. In more general terms, we want to map measurement data on to a state description of the system being managed.

For a measurement system to produce data that will be useful to the interpretation process, the following conditions should exist.

- The measurements chosen must accurately reflect the system being observed. Is a patient's core temperature most accurately measured by their axillary temperature or their sublingual temperature? Clearly, the choice of measurement is influenced by the management goals. There is little value, for example, in making a highly expensive and very accurate measurement when a more approximate and cheaper one will do. Further, it is not just the case that some measurements are more accurate versions of others, but some measures may not correspond closely to the elements that are being modelled. Does the number of sick days taken by staff in a nursing unit measure the incidence of illness among the staff population, or does it measure staff morale? When multiple factors affect the value of a measurement, such as total number of sick days, then interpreting the measurement becomes more problematic. Before the interpretation has taken place, we would have to be sure that all the confounding factors affecting its value have been taken into account. For example, surgical waiting times are sometimes used to measure the performance of hospitals. If the hospital waiting lists for surgery at a hospital are long, and patients are experiencing long delays, does that mean the hospital is inefficient, or does it mean that there are more patients to be managed than the hospital has resources to cope with?
- Next, the values of measurements must themselves be accurate. Errors in the determination of the value of a measurement can translate into errors in the management of the system. Errors can occur in several places. They might arise from within the measurement system itself. For example, a thermometer may not be reading correctly, or a CVP transducer might not be placed at the right height. Secondly, the error might arise from the way the measurement system is applied. For example, an incorrect reading of arterial oxygen saturation might be given because of poor positioning of a finger probe.

- If we are measuring a process over time, then we need to measure it frequently enough not to miss any important events. For example, if we are trying to measure the number of days a bed is occupied, then we need to visit the bed with a rate that is more frequent than it is possible to discharge patients. If it is possible for a unit to have two short-stay patients occupy the one bed during a day, then visiting it once per day will miss periods in which the bed is either occupied or unoccupied. In signal processing terms, this problem of missing events because of measurement undersampling is called **aliasing**.

Designing the interpretation

It is usually the case that it is hard to separate the details about the reasoning process used to manage a system from the details of the model being used. Knowledge and inference are inextricably interdependent.

We have already seen that a model should only be as detailed as necessary for the task at hand. Similarly, an interpretation should be as simple as possible given the task at hand. Carrying out complex calculations and deriving an answer to several decimal places of precision is inappropriate if the possible control actions do not have such fine precision.

There are several basic forms of reasoning that are possible with a model. One can try to draw a conclusion about the world based on a measurement of the world. One can try to draw a conclusion about whether the current model is the right one to be using. Finally, one can try to alter the model as new things are learnt about the world. These three types of reasoning correspond to the three-loop model of information use. We shall return to examine these reasoning processes in greater detail in Chapters 25 and 26.

Designing the management actions

Management actions should be chosen to maximally affect the system being controlled, and to minimally affect other systems. In the same way that a measurement may not always accurately reflect the system being modelled, some actions may more directly affect the component of the system being controlled than others. Drugs, for example, are favoured if they treat a condition effectively but have no side effects. Some drugs have an effect closer to the causative mechanism of disease; others are more indirect, treating downstream consequences of a primary cause. For example, in the case of gastric ulceration, the H2 antagonist class of drugs reduce gastric acidity. However, the action that is most direct in controlling the disease process is the elimination of the infection with *Helicobacter pylori* that probably triggered the increase in gastric acidity in the first place.

Discussion points

1. A new computer system has just been introduced into your organization but it immediately causes problems, and the staff decide they don't want to use it. What might have gone wrong?
2. Why should we evaluate information systems?
3. What is the difference between a formative and a summative evaluation?
4. Why might clinical workers not know what type of information system function they need, when asked in an interview or in a focus group?

5 How do social or organizational issues affect the successful deployment of new technologies?

6 Why might an information system that works beautifully when tested with real users in a laboratory trial still fail when it is eventually introduced into a working environment?

7 In what ways can the existing interactions in a work environment interact with a new interaction introduced through a computer system?

8 A working party at a hospital consults widely for 2 years before producing the blueprint for a new hospital information system. After a further 2 years it is finally put into routine use. What kind of problems do you think this delay will produce, and how could they be minimized?

9 The government decides that a clinician in the emergency department must see all patients within 10 minutes of presenting. One hospital meets this measurement target only 70% of the time, whereas a second meets it 90% of the time. Which hospital delivers better clinical care? If the two hospitals initially met the target 70% of the time, what factors might contribute to the 'improvement' in the second hospital's score?

Chapter summary

1 Technology can be applied to a problem in a **technology-driven** or a **problem-driven** manner. Information systems should be created in a problem-driven way, starting with an understanding of user information problems. Only then is it appropriate to identify if and how technology should be used.

2 The formative assessment cycle defines clinical needs and many methods are available: anecdotal or individual experience, asking clinicians, non-participatory observation and formal experiments.

3 Formal experiments will only answer narrow questions and are relatively expensive to conduct. Qualitative research methods relying on non-participatory methods are formal enough to allow robust statements to be made, and also have the advantage of being grounded in the realities of the clinical workplace.

4 A summative evaluation can be made in three broad categories:

- a user's satisfaction with the service
- clinical outcome changes resulting from using the service
- any economic benefit of the service.

5 An information system is susceptible to the effects of change over time at several levels: the user needs that define the role of the system, the model of user needs and system design, the technology used to construct the system, and organizational resources, including finance and staff availability. A change in any one of these will affect the performance of the system as a whole. Aiming for modularity in design will help minimize these effects.

6 Many specific methodologies are available for designing information systems. In general, they are all focused on defining the different elements of the **model, measure, manage cycle**, i.e. defining a set of management goals, constructing a model of the system, defining measurement data for a system, interpreting the meaning of the measurements, and defining appropriate actions based on that interpretation.

PART 4

Protocol-based systems

CHAPTER 12

Protocols and evidence-based healthcare

> But printed flow charts should not be regarded as a problem-solving panacea! They ... serve as recipes for a mindless cook. They are difficult to write, rigid, may inhibit independent thinking, and are often so intricate as to require a road map and a compass.... The good physician generates his own flow chart every time he sees a patient and solves a problem. He should not need to follow printed pathways.
> *Cutler (1979), p. 53.*
>
> Shortly thereafter, I had the last of the 'insights' to be recorded here: a clinician performs an experiment every time he treats a patient. The experiment has purposes different from those of laboratory work, but the sequence, and intellectual construction are the same: a plan, an execution, and an appraisal. Yet ... Honest, dedicated clinicians today disagree on the treatment for almost every disease from the common cold to metastatic cancer. Our experiments in treatment were acceptable by the standards of the community, but were not reproducible by the standards of science. Clinical judgement was our method for designing and evaluating those experiments, but the method was unreproducible because we had been taught to call it 'art' ... *Feinstein (1967), p. 14.*

For those who regard modern healthcare as a rational and scientific endeavour, the contention that the efficacy of much clinical practice is still not validated may come as a shock. The problem healthcare faces is not that it lacks the will or the tools to evaluate treatments. As we saw in Chapter 6, the problem lies in part with the mechanisms that exist for transferring evidence into clinical practice, which are unable to keep up with the ever-growing mountain of clinical trial data (Roper *et al.*, 1988; Wyatt, 1991).

For example, the first trial to show that streptokinase was useful in the treatment of myocardial infarction was published in 1958. Convincing evidence of its effectiveness mounted in the early 1970s, and the first meta-analysis proving its value was published in the early 1980s. However, formal advice that streptokinase was useful in the routine treatment of myocardial infarction only appeared in the late 1980s (Antman *et al.*, 1992). This was a full 13 years after a close examination of the published literature would have indicated the value of the treatment (Heathfield and Wyatt, 1993).

There are many other examples of similar delays in transferring research findings into routine clinical practice. The use of low dose anticoagulants in hip surgery, or inhaled steroids in the treatment of asthma, could both have become routine treatments much earlier than they did. If research into the management of such common and important conditions is so delayed, it is unlikely that less common conditions fare any better. There is thus a bottleneck between the publication of clinical trial data, and its conversion into clinical practice.

Just as there are barriers to research moving into clinical practice, there are barriers that prevent practitioners accessing research findings. With well over 1000 journals being published each week, practitioners with a particular clinical problem can struggle to find the best advice from the mountains of often contradictory research literature. As we saw in Chapter 6, the number of scientific articles grows exponentially, doubling somewhere between every 1 and 15 years. In one study of the literature related to a single clinical disease over 110 years, it was found that only 3% of the literature had been generated in the first 50 years, and 40% had been generated in the last 10 years (Arndt, 1992). This exponential growth in medical knowledge is one of the causes of the many gaps and inconsistencies we find in the knowledge of all practising clinicians.

Finally, as we saw in Chapter 9, one of the key feedback loops in healthcare uses the outcomes from treating past patients to improve the care of future patients. However, this 'loop 3' is still weak. The rigours of formal clinical trials make it hard to conduct them in routine care, and consequently the data from most patients never move beyond the records of their healthcare team. Indeed, since most patient records use varying structures and are often incomplete, even if they were collected it would currently be impossible to carry out useful statistical analyses with them. Usually only the data from patients enrolled in formal trials are analysed scientifically.

These pressures have renewed the interest of many in the use of clinical protocols to guide practice. The hope is that if best-practice guidance can be distilled rapidly from the literature, then it should be convertible into a set of protocols that can be made readily and widely available to practising clinicians. The phrase **evidence-based medicine (EBM)** or **evidence-based healthcare (EBH)** is now used to describe this movement (EBMWG, 1992; Mulrow, 1994). If it is ultimately successful, genuinely evidence-based practice will have the effect of more patients receiving up-to-date treatment, and allow the outcome data from all patients on the same protocol to be pooled for statistical analysis.

Meta-analysis
A statistical method that pools the results from multiple similar experiments, hoping that the improved power obtained from the combined data sets will identify statistically significant patterns that cannot be identified within the smaller sample sizes of individual studies.

There are still many growing pains within EBH. Some are cultural, as a proportion of clinicians argue against such apparent imposition of controls on practice and that much of clinical practice remains an 'art'. Others are technical. Statistical **meta-analysis** for example, is still an unsure tool. Meta-analysis is one of the tools used to combine the evidence contained in the often contradictory studies found in the medical literature. Along with the many notable successes of meta-analysis, such as with the studies of thrombolytics for myocardial infarction, there have also been some failures. For example, meta-analysis predicted that intravenous magnesium would reduce the risk of acute myocardial infarction, but a subsequent large-scale randomized trial failed to find any such benefit (Sim and Hlatky, 1996).

Before the current interest in protocols, they had fallen into relative disrepute for a variety of cultural and technical reasons which we shall return to in later sections. Many of these technical objections can now be circumvented through the application of information technologies. Furthermore, the motivation to establish a more evidence-based practice is now sufficiently strong to overcome many of the cultural objections. With such changes, protocol-guided care now has a clear and critical role in routine clinical practice.

In this chapter, the discussion of protocols in healthcare will begin with a basic introduction to protocols and their uses. In the second chapter of this discussion on protocols, the role that information and communication technology can play in protocol-based healthcare will be explored. In the third and fourth chapters in this part, we will take a look at the issues affecting the design of protocols and the selection of appropriate situations for their use.

12.1 Protocols

A protocol is a set of instructions. These instructions might describe the procedure to be followed when investigating a particular set of findings in a patient, or the method to be followed in the management of a given disease (Figure 12.1). More generally, the notion of protocol permeates most human organizational structures. We talk about following the 'correct' social protocol when meeting a visiting dignitary, or 'having to do things by the book' within an organization. A protocol is thus usually understood to be advice on the 'best' way to carry out some task. It is the way something should always be done.

Alternatively, protocols may simply represent advice on good practice – what should be done in most circumstances. For example, a recipe is a protocol for cooking a particular dish. Following all of the steps in a recipe should guarantee that a reasonable meal will be produced. An experienced cook will know which steps are essential, and which can be varied. In this text we will typically call any set of instructions a protocol, but a variety of alternative terms are in use (Box 12.1).

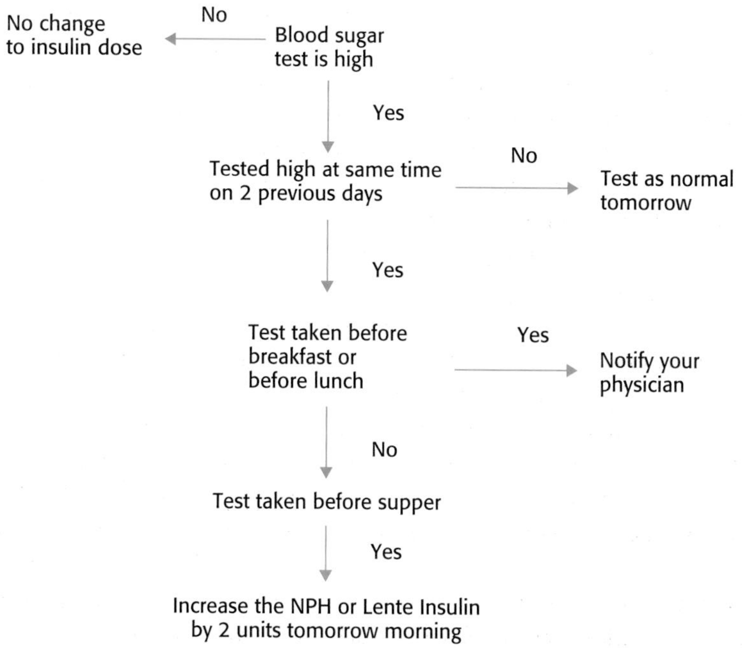
No change
to insulin dose
No
Blood sugar
test is high
Yes
Tested high at same time
on 2 previous days
No
Test as normal
tomorrow
Yes
Test taken before
breakfast or
before lunch
Yes
Notify your
physician
No
Test taken before supper
Yes
Increase the NPH or Lente Insulin
by 2 units tomorrow morning

Figure 12.1
In this sample protocol, a guideline is presented for an insulin-dependent diabetic's self-management of their intermediate-acting insulin regime. Such a flowchart representation of a protocol makes all the choice points and the flow of decision-making graphically explicit, but is space consuming, and for trained individuals may be too rigid.

Box 12.1
A protocol by any other name

The terminology used to describe protocols can often be confusing, as many different terms are often used interchangeably, and sometimes imprecisely. The actual meaning of many terms is however quite specific:

- **Algorithm:** In computer science, a set of instructions to carry out some task programmatically is called an algorithm. In clinical practice algorithms usually, but not always, involve some form of numerical calculation. For example, an algorithm may take as input a patient's data to calculate a cardiac risk index, or a diabetic patient may use an algorithm to calculate the appropriate dosage of insulin on the basis of their blood sugar measurements. Algorithms thus typically carry out small, specific and well-defined tasks within the broader context of a patient's care.
- **Protocol:** Typically a protocol describes all the steps in the management of a clinical condition, and may cover the steps taken to both secure a diagnosis, or to treat the illness. When used as part of a formal scientifically conducted clinical trial, a protocol is a strict set of instructions that must be adhered to for the patient to remain within the trial. Typically a clinical protocol will be based on the latest evidence found in the literature, and often be the product of consensus discussions amongst a panel of experts, who pool their collective skills to resolve any ambiguities found in the literature.
- **Guideline:** Often used synonymously with the term protocol, the term emphasizes that the role of the patient management instructions is to offer guidance rather than dictate a specific course of action. When used outside the clinical trial setting in routine care, most protocols or guidelines are intended to be advisory, and rely on the clinician to use their judgement when the instructions do not seem appropriate for a specific patient.
- **Care pathway:** Pathways are most commonly used in nursing, and describe not just the steps to be taken in managing a patient, but the expected course of the patient's management. A pathway would, for example, describe the whole length of stay for a patient in hospital in terms of expected clinical findings at each stage in the management, and what actions need to be taken at every stage.
- **Practice parameters:** A North American term, used to describe evidence-based clinical guidelines for diagnosis and management of specific clinical conditions. They set measurable parameters that define the acceptable boundaries of safe patient care.

Protocols find uses in most aspects of healthcare delivery

The fundamental value of a protocol is in ensuring tasks are carried out uniformly. It serves as a guide or reminder in situations in which it is likely that steps will be forgotten, are not well known, are difficult to follow, or where errors can be expensive. Consequently, protocols have a wide variety of uses in healthcare.

- **Research:** Protocols have long been an accepted and integral part of medical research. Whenever the efficacy of a treatment is being assessed, a standardized research protocol is drawn up to direct the way that treatment is to be given over the clinical trial period. This maximizes the likelihood that the same thing is being done to each patient, and that the data collected are representative of the effects of that particular treatment. It also provides a basis for comparison with other studies that might have adopted variations in the treatment protocol, and obtained different results.
- **Delegation of responsibility:** There is a strong case to be made for highly trained healthcare staff to delegate the care of minor or routine problems. In the outpatient setting, the routine management of patients with chronic diseases such as diabetes or asthma can be conducted by specially trained nursing staff using protocols, rather than requiring the attendance of more specialized physicians. Patients can be taught to look after themselves at home for a variety of conditions. Everything from insulin administration to ambulatory peritoneal dialysis can be carried out by patients if they

have been given explicit protocols to follow, and instructions on when to follow these and when to seek further advice.

- **Demarcation of responsibility:** A protocol can make clear which tasks are to be carried out by different members of a healthcare team. For example, the roles of a physician, nursing staff and paramedics can all be defined within a protocol for managing a large-scale disaster.
- **Education:** A clinical protocol ensures that, even if there is a variation in ability or training, a certain minimum standard is adhered to in the delivery of care. Thus, when members of the general public are trained in the 'ABC' of resuscitation, they are given a simple recipe to follow.
- **Safety-critical or complex situations:** Even highly trained individuals will use protocols in situations in which errors can have significant consequences. Thus most clinicians will be able to describe step by step the procedures they would carry out in the management of a cardiac arrest. Equally, airline pilots have pre-takeoff checklists that need to be completed to ensure the aircraft is flightworthy. Operators of nuclear power plants have defined procedures for every aspect of controlling their plant. Similarly, when complex machinery is used in clinical situations like the delivery of anaesthesia, checklists may be valuable.
- **Uncommon conditions:** Protocols are also important when they deal with rare conditions, and it is unlikely that the individuals managing a situation have encountered it before.

Protocols have been shown to improve the process of delivering care as well as the outcomes of care

Protocols can have an impact on the way clinicians carry out their tasks – the process of care – or on the effect of that clinical activity on the health of patients – patient outcomes. Before a guideline can have any such impact, it actually has to be used, and some studies measure this adherence rate, or compliance rate, as a marker for guideline uptake. Increased compliance with a guideline should result in decreased variation in clinical practice and the assumption is that this will then translate into improved health outcomes.

Guidelines have indeed been shown to change clinical practice and improve patient outcomes (Anonymous, 2002). Several large-scale evaluations of the impact of guidelines in clinical care have been made over the years, all with similar results:

- In a review of 59 evaluations of clinical guidelines, Grimshaw and Russell (1993) found that all but four studies found significant improvement in the process of care after the introduction of the guideline. The outcome of care was assessed in 11 of the studies, and 9 of these reported an improvement in outcomes.
- In another systematic review of 87 studies (University of Leeds, 1994), 81 examined the effects on the process of care, measured by adherence with recommendations or compliance, and reported significant improvement. Twelve of the studies assessing patient outcomes reported significant improvement.

However, the hypothesis that guidelines will improve health outcomes has not been universally proven and there are significant variations in the impact they have on process and outcomes improvements (Darling, 2002). As we will see later, much of this variation can be attributed, not directly to the evidence contained within a guideline, but to the manner in which the guideline is represented, and the socio-technical environment in which it is delivered. The methods of development, implementation and monitoring of guidelines influence the likelihood of adherence to clinical guidelines. For example, guidelines are more likely to be effective if they take account of local circumstances, are disseminated by an active educational intervention and are implemented by patient-specific reminders relating directly to professional activity.

12.2 The structure of protocols

There are a variety of different ways to represent a protocol, and the structure chosen to represent a protocol will determine how useful it is in different clinical situations. Protocols intended to be used in situations of time pressure or emergency will be designed very differently to ones used in routine practice. Protocols can also vary in their content, depending on the context within which they will be used. For example, the level of detail in the description of steps and the choice of language will vary with the intended user of the protocol.

Entry criteria define a protocol's context of use

Irrespective of its form, every protocol begins with an **entry criterion** that defines the context within which the protocol is designed to be used. For example, 'patient presents with acute retrosternal chest pain' might be one of the criteria that enter a patient on to a protocol for the investigation and management of suspected myocardial infarction. If the entry criteria for a protocol are insufficiently precise, then the protocol might be used in inappropriate circumstances.

It is sometimes argued that protocols are of little value because the decision to use the protocol requires medical expertise (see Box 12.2). Consequently, the argument goes, protocols are of marginal value in permitting non-medical staff to manage serious conditions. The simple counter-argument is that insufficient thought has been put into the design of the protocol's entry criteria. Protocols are valuable precisely in those circumstances in which it is possible to be explicit. If such clarity is not possible, then it is unlikely that the problem is one that is amenable to protocol-directed management.

Protocol form is determined by function

Flowcharts are probably the simplest way to represent a protocol, because they are graphical in nature, and make decision points and the flow of logic explicit (Figure 12.1). Flowcharts can be built up in great detail, especially in areas in which there is a high procedural content to the work, for example in anaesthesia.

A flowchart begins with an entry criterion, for example 'you are a self-managing insulin-dependent diabetic on intermediate acting insulin, and your urine has tested high for blood sugar'. Choice points in the logic are made explicit. Depending on responses to questions,

Table 12.1 The same patient guideline presented in Figure 12.1, this time expressed as a set of rules (adapted from Krall and Beaser, 1989).

If tests are poor 3 days in a row	Do this
before supper	Increase the NPH or Lente Insulin by 2 units on the 4th morning
before breakfast, but good before supper	Notify your physician. You may need an evening dose of insulin
before lunch, but better before supper	Notify your physician. You may need a mixed dose (NPH or Lente + Regular) in the morning

often with simple 'yes' or 'no' answers, the protocol user is guided through a decision-making process. Actions are usually arrived at on the 'leaf' nodes.

Flowcharts are thus a form of the decision tree format introduced in Chapter 8. When the decision process is well understood but uncertain, the protocol can be represented as a full decision tree, incorporating probabilities or utilities when there is uncertainty at a particular decision branch.

Protocols can also be expressed more compactly as a simple set of **logical rules**, structured as if-then statements (Table 12.1). If the rule's precondition is satisfied, then the action in the rule should be carried out. Since rules are more compact, they usually require a little more effort to understand than the same information expressed in a flowchart. For example, the decision tree in Figure 12.1 is identical to the compact set of rules presented in Table 12.1.

Chunking protocols helps manage complexity

As can be seen from the small examples above, protocols for even relatively simple tasks can be complicated. Consequently, capturing the decision-making required to manage a long sequence of tasks can result in very complex protocol structures that may be very difficult to use.

One way to manage this complexity is to break the protocol down into a sequence of smaller chunks, each corresponding to a specific task. Each chunk has entry and exit criteria, allowing one to move from one task to the next. In this way, one is not limited to building protocols that are a simple sequence of tasks, but one can create quite complex pathways.

A simple way to think about such chunks is as a **finite state machine**. A finite state machine is a computer science method that represents processes as a series of different states, and connects them together with links that specify a transition condition that indicates how one traverses from one state to another.

We can think of an ill patient as having a finite number of different states that they can be in during the course of an illness and its management. Each state could correspond to a distinct period in an illness, or a distinct aspect of their management. For example, the states in the management of chest pain might be broken down into initial assessment and management, investigation and treatment (Figure 12.2). Each individual state could be further internally subdivided as many times as needed.

As we saw in Chapter 11, another advantage of breaking a system design down into chunks or functional modules is that it minimizes the effects of design change. Thus, in a well-designed protocol, it should thus be relatively easy to change some detail in a particular protocol segment, usually without affecting other segments.

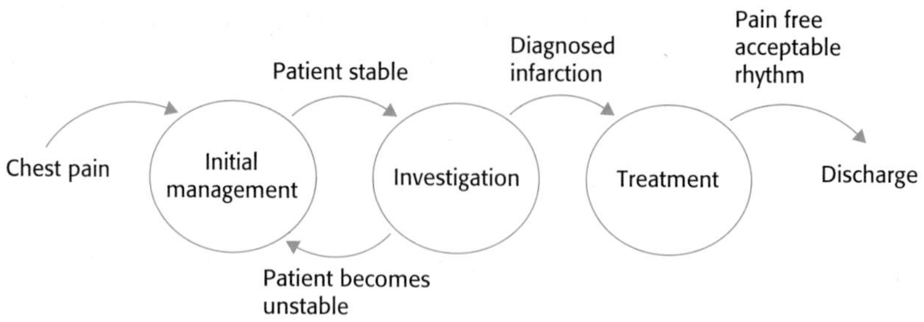
Pain free
acceptable
rhythm
Diagnosed
infarction
Patient stable
Chest pain
Initial
management
Investigation
Treatment
Discharge
Patient becomes
unstable

Figure 12.2 Complex protocols can be broken down into chunks corresponding to different states in a process, or in the progression of a patient's condition. Each state within the protocol is entered or exited when a set of conditions is met. Movement back and forth between states can be permitted if necessary.

Table 12.2 Fragment from a care pathway for the management of a myocardial infarction. Pathways are plotted for each expected problem and plotted out over the expected length of stay, along with expected outcomes. Special difficulties associated with each problem are recorded in the days they are most likely to occur, along with investigations or treatments that need to be scheduled for that day.

Patient problem	**Day 1**	**Day 2**
Myocardial ischaemia	Patient at risk of infarct extension Ix: serial ECG cardiac enzymes Rx: thrombolytics	Patient should be pain free
Cardiac rhythm	Patient at risk of arrhythmia Ix: continuous ECG monitoring	Patient should have stable cardiac rhythm
Cardiac output	Ix: risk of cardiac failure Rx: regular ABP	
Fluid balance		Patient at risk of fluid overload Ix: Check volume status

Ix, investigation; Rx, treatment.

12.3 Care pathways

The process of breaking down treatment into a set of stages or states, each with their own entry and exit criteria, is the basis of care pathways. These protocols are at present especially of interest in nursing, where they are often used to support patient care (e.g. Hydo, 1995).

In a pathway, a patient's care may be broken down into a sequence of days, corresponding to the ideal length of stay in hospital for that condition (Table 12.2). Each day has a set of instructions describing the typical care that should be given to a patient. Each day also has a set of expectations that describe the anticipated clinical state of the patient on that day. For example, 2 days after admission with a myocardial infarction, the pathway might state that a patient should be able to take a short walk. Failure to satisfy these criteria may prevent a patient progressing along the pathway until the conditions are met.

In this way, there is some allowance for individualization of care depending on a patient's rate of recovery, as well as a check to prevent inappropriate treatment being given. Consequently, the protocol begins to be based on the clinical outcome of intermediate steps in a patient's care. This emphasizes the potential for protocols to assist in the process of improving or sustaining quality of care.

Care pathways can have quite complex structures, depending on the nature of the condition being managed. As part of the chunking strategy, the pathway can be decomposed into multiple individual problems that are associated with a condition, and then be used to guide the management of each problem over the period of the patient's stay. For each problem, one can then identify which tasks occur on which days, and what the outcome of those tasks should be. In the previous example of myocardial infarction, problems might correspond to the patient's cardiac rhythm status, cardiac output, fluid and electrolyte balance, coagulation status and so forth.

12.4 The protocol life cycle

In his classic work on clinical judgement, Feinstein (1967) suggested that as much rigour should be applied to the way patients are routinely treated as is applied in medical research. The management of every patient could be considered, at an abstract level, as constituting a scientific experiment. Consequently, the results of that experiment could contribute to the advancement of knowledge.

With the advent of evidence-based practice, we are drawing closer to realizing that vision. If it is possible to treat most patients using protocols, then it should also be possible to close the loop, and use the knowledge gained from each patient's treatment. In effect, every patient treated according to a protocol can be part of a clinical trial.

We are a long way from realizing that vision at present, but at its most abstract, the overall form that the system would take is relatively clear. Indeed it is nothing other than the model–measure–manage cycle introduced in Chapter 9, where the results of protocol application feed into subsequent revisions of the protocol. The wider use of protocols can be understood through the three-loop model also developed in Chapter 9 (Figure 12.3). The information loops are formed around the selection and application of protocols, and the analysis of the protocol's effectiveness.

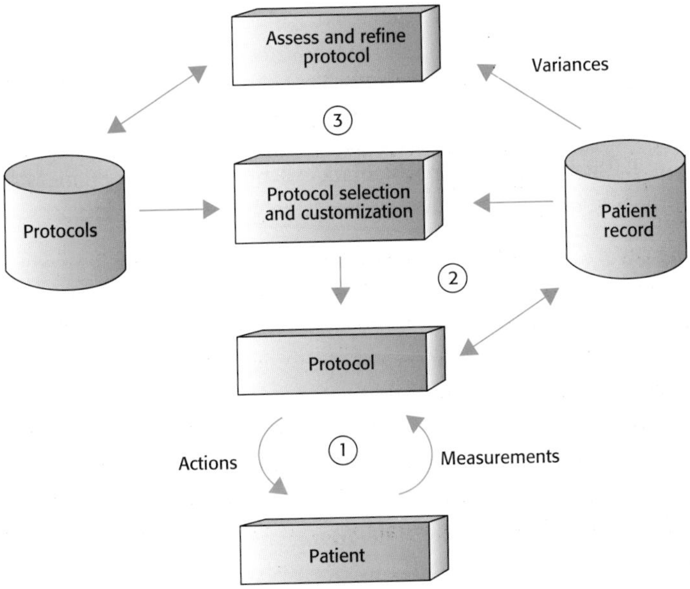
Assess and refine protocol
Variances
3
Protocols
Protocol selection and customization
Patient record
2
Protocol
Actions
1
Measurements
Patient

Figure 12.3
The three-loop model describes the way in which protocols can be used to manage individual patients in a uniform way, and use the results of treatment to advance medical knowledge.

To commence treatment, a protocol is selected in loop 2, based on a patient satisfying some entry criteria. For example, before being admitted on to a thrombolytic protocol, a patient with chest pain may need to have presented within a number of hours, and have ECG evidence of a recent myocardial infarction. Once selected, the protocol drives the treatment of that patient.

Finally, in loop 3, one assesses the outcome of treatment over a statistically significant population of patients. In formal clinical trials, the methodology will involve comparison of variances in outcome comparing the protocol group against a control group treated in a different manner. As a consequence, protocols are refined over time, as evidence suggests ways in which they can be improved.

12.5 Departures from a protocol help drive protocol refinement

A common criticism often voiced of protocols is that patient states are too variable to be amenable to such programmatic care. As we have seen, attention to design can provide some latitude to accommodate individual variation. Sometimes, however, variations will occur that have not been anticipated in the protocol. Such **variances** arise for a number of reasons:

- **Patient condition:** A patient may have an intercurrent illness that makes it difficult to carry out the care designed for a typical patient. Equally a patient may not respond as expected to a treatment because of their background fitness, nutritional status or genetic predisposition to respond to the treatment.
- **Treatment variation:** Treatments may be given that are at variance with the planned protocol, for a variety of appropriate or inappropriate reasons. In any case, such treatment changes may alter a patient's clinical state. Consequently, the likelihood that the patient is able to fit the expectations implicit in the protocol's design may diminish.
- **Resource constraints:** External factors such as the hospital system itself may contribute to variances. For example, it may be that a particular investigation is scheduled to occur on a particular day of the admission. If the laboratory carrying out the investigation is overbooked, then the protocol has to be varied.

Looked at from a systems science point of view, variances can be thought of as signals in a feedback loop. Rather than being problematic, identification of variances can become a central part of the way in which protocol-assisted care is given:

- Firstly, variances are signals to the care team to reassess whether it is appropriate for a patient to be maintained on a protocol, and may indicate that more individualized care is necessary.
- Secondly, when variances from a number of patients are pooled, they act as checks on the way in which care is delivered. It may be that recurrent variances suggest that care delivery is sub-optimal, and that changes need to be made in the way staff or resources are allocated.
- Finally, and perhaps most critically, variances offer an opportunity to assess the appropriateness of the protocol over time. In this case, variances provide a measurement of the effectiveness of a protocol, and consequently can feed a process of continuing protocol refinement in loop 3.

12.6 The application of protocols

The different settings in which protocols can be valuable were outlined earlier. We now examine the underlying principles that can guide us to recognize when it is appropriate to formally structure the care process through the use of protocols.

When should a protocol be used?

The decision tree metaphor captured in flowcharts highlights the analytical aspects of decision-making. It focuses on what information is needed to make choices between alternatives, based on some assessment of the probability and utility of different outcomes. Where people tend to fail, for whatever reason, at this form of analysis, then protocol-based decision support could be helpful. We have already seen such examples, including inexperience of the people making decisions and complex safety-critical situations.

However, it is not always the case that protocols are the best way to improve a decision process (Box 12.2). For example, Klein and Calderwood (1991) argue that formal decision models (of which protocols are one example) are unlikely to be helpful in the following circumstances:

- when clear goals cannot be isolated, and it is dangerous to make simplifying assumptions in order to isolate goals that would allow a protocol to be applied
- when end states or outcomes cannot be clearly defined
- when the utilities of different decisions are not independent of one another
- when probabilities of outcomes or the utility of individual decisions are not independent of the context in which they are made.

Thus, the decision to design a protocol to manage a given situation should not be automatic. There are many situations in which protocol application is at the least difficult, and at worst meaningless.

How should a protocol be used?

Once a decision has been made that the introduction of a protocol for a given situation is desirable, the next step is to determine the way in which the protocol is to be used. The two

Box 12.2
When recognizing is harder than acting

It has been strongly argued that there are many situations in which the attempt to formalize decision models such as protocols is not helpful and may indeed be harmful. Indeed, when decision-making is studied 'in the field' rather than in the laboratory, a very different set of human decision problems is observed.

Faced with complex problems, people may not evaluate more than one course of action at a time (Klein and Calderwood, 1991). Instead, once a situation has been recognized, individuals may just follow the first acceptable plan they consider. This suggests that the main effort that goes into decision-making is in recognizing and classifying a situation, rather than exploring complex plans to manage the situation.

This result is echoed in work on clinical decision-making, in which the order in which data that was presented to clinicians had a significant effect on their reasoning (Elstein *et al.*, 1978). In an analysis of so-called 'fixed-order' problems under experimental conditions, the ability of physicians to generate hypotheses, and to associate data with hypotheses, was significantly affected by the order in which data were presented. In other words, their ability to correctly assess the situation was influenced by the way data were encountered.

The implication of this work is that, if our goal is to improve decision-making, then the focus of decision-support strategies should broaden to improving the ability of individuals to assess situations and not solely on formalizing the decision process that follows once an assessment has been made.

main approaches to protocol use can be divided into **passive** and **active** systems.

- In the **passive** approach, protocols act as a source of information only, and are not formally incorporated into the care process. Protocols might only be consulted as a check, at the end of a decision-making process, or as a reference when an unusual situation is encountered. Healthcare workers might carry the protocols around with them as a set of ready-to-hand guidelines, or might have to consult information sources such as a library, the Internet, or a telephone helpline to access them.
- In contrast, the **active** use of protocols shapes the delivery of care around a protocol. The steps in a treatment are explicitly guided by protocol, requiring the protocol to be consulted at most steps during the care process. Active use of a protocol might suggest what patient information is to be to captured at different stages, what treatment is to given or what tests are to be ordered. In such cases, the patient record system might be crafted around the protocol. In a paper system, specific sheets for the protocol would be created, and data entered according to the sheet's format. A similar approach can be adopted using computer-based systems, albeit with greater potential for flexibility.

The introduction of passive systems is unlikely to cause significant difficulty, since they do not mandate treatment, but just add to the information resources available. One can consider this type of decision support to be **permissive**, in that it permits all courses of action, and only exists as a guide that is accessed as the need arises. In contrast, active systems have the potential to be **prescriptive**, since by definition they are there to actively constrain treatment actions in some way.

Unsurprisingly, the introduction of a new prescriptive process is organizationally difficult, as it inevitably changes the way people work. However, ongoing experience with the re-engineering of corporate information systems suggests that it may nonetheless be more efficient to change work practices. The introduction of a new process is used as the opportunity to redesign and optimize existing systems. The more radical proponents of this approach suggest that 'users must change their ways in order to maximize profits from automation' (Martin, 1995).

As we will see in Chapter 14, such a prescription may be too puritanical, and ignore the realities of human nature. The socio-technical aspects of technological innovation require that compromises be made to reflect the desires, abilities and concerns of those who have to work with new systems, no matter how desirable the changes may be from an organizational point of view – the new system should fit the users and not the reverse.

Discussion points

1. 'Using protocols results in the de-skilling of clinicians'. 'Using protocols improves clinical outcomes'. With which statement do you agree, and how do you resolve the conflict between the two?
2. Can every aspect of medical care be controlled by protocols? Perhaps consider your answer by noting that protocols are models of healthcare.
3. You have just championed the introduction of a new guideline, based on the latest evidence, into your unit. Senior management is concerned about the costs, and wants you to demonstrate that the changes are worthwhile. How will you measure the impact of the new guideline?
4. Under what conditions is the use of a protocol likely to cause harm?

Chapter summary

1. The mechanisms that exist for transferring research evidence into clinical practice are unable to keep up with the ever-growing mountain of clinical trial data, resulting in delays in the transfer of research into practice.
2. Evidence-based healthcare is an attempt to distil best-practice guidance from the literature into a set of protocols that can be made readily and widely available to practising clinicians.
3. A protocol is a set of instructions. These instructions might describe the procedure to be followed to investigate a particular set of findings in a patient, or the method to be followed in the management of a given disease.
4. A protocol can ensure that tasks are carried out uniformly. It can serve as a guide or reminder in situations in which it is likely that procedures will be forgotten, are not well known, are difficult to follow, or where errors can be expensive, for example in the face of rare conditions, safety-critical or complex situations, in clinical research, education, and in task delegation.
5. Protocols have been shown to improve the process of delivering care and the outcomes of care. There are significant variations in the impact which can be attributed to the manner in which a guideline is represented, and the socio-technical environment in which it is delivered.
6. Each protocol begins with an **entry criterion** that defines the context within which the protocol is designed to be used.
7. Protocols can vary in the form of their structure and their content, depending on the context of use. Flowcharts make choice points and the flow of decision-making graphically explicit, but are space consuming. Rules are more compact, but require more effort and training to interpret. Contextual factors affecting design include the patient, treatment goals, local resources, staff skills, local processes and resources.
8. In a care pathway, a patient's care is broken down into a sequence of days, corresponding to the ideal length of stay in hospital.
9. The creation and application of protocols can be characterized as a model–measure–manage cycle, and their overall use in healthcare can be captured within the three-loop model.
10. Variations to treatment that have not been anticipated in the protocol are termed **variances**, which can signal the care team to reassess whether it is appropriate for a patient to be maintained on a protocol. When variances from a number of patients are pooled, they can act as checks on the way in which care is delivered.
11. There are many situations in which the attempt to formalize decision models, such as protocols, is not helpful and may indeed be harmful. These include situations in which clear goals or outcomes cannot be clearly defined, or when probabilities or utilities are not independent of each other or the decision context.
12. Protocol systems can be **passive** or **active**. Passive protocols act as a source of information, and are not incorporated into the care process. Active protocols shape the delivery of care.

CHAPTER 13

Computer-based protocol systems in healthcare

The goal of a computer-based protocol system is to provide a set of tools that allow a clinician to access up-to-date guidelines, and then apply these in the management of patients. In the previous chapter, the nature and role of protocols were explored, and we saw how protocols can either be used as passive resources or contribute actively in shaping the process of care. A consequence of intertwining protocols with active care delivery is that protocols become integral to the design of the electronic patient record.

In this chapter, the role that communication and computer-based systems can play in the delivery of protocol-based care is examined. The discussion covers both passive and active clinical systems, and explores the potential for the Internet to contribute to them. Finally, the complex problems of developing appropriate computational representations for protocols are touched upon.

13.1 Passive protocol systems

A passive protocol delivery system acts as a source of information only, and is not intrinsically incorporated into the care process. The basic goal of a passive system is to make it easy for clinicians to access protocols during routine care, and make it less likely that steps will be inadvertently forgotten or altered. Although they might be accessed as reference material from within a clinical information system such as the EMR, the protocols are not integrated with other modules of the system such as order-entry or results reporting.

There is growing evidence that improving access to clinical protocols through information technology does have a positive impact on adherence to guidelines:

- A randomized controlled trial assessed the impact of providing online evidence to guide the prescription of antibiotics, with the evidence alerting clinicians to the superior effectiveness of a 5-day course of antibiotics over a 10-day course (Christakis *et al.*, 2001). The proportion of antibiotic prescriptions for less than 10 days duration among paediatricians who had access to the evidence rose from 51% before the trial to 70% afterwards. Interestingly, the control group who did not have access to the evidence showed a smaller increase in their use of the recommended dose. It may have been that socio-technical issues accounted for this, specifically the diffusion of the evidence from the members of the control group who were working in the same clinic.
- Vissers *et al.* (1996) explored the value of being able to access guidelines from a computer. In their study, resident staff in an emergency department had access to guidance on the management of fractures, which they could access during their initial assessment of a patient and formulation of treatment plan. In a randomized full-crossover trial comparing access to paper and computer versions of the protocols, several results were apparent. Firstly, the residents did not change their treatments significantly more often between the paper and computer-supported protocols. However, those using the computer had a statistically higher chance that they would change their planned treatment towards the protocol. In other words, the computer system was more likely to cause treatment to move towards the protocol recommendations. Overall, there was a 19% better protocol adherence in the computer-supported trial. Interestingly, this was despite the residents' confidence in the correctness of their own treatment, and their doubts over the value of mandatory protocol consultation.

On the surface, these results are encouraging. They seem to suggest that reminding healthcare workers of the protocol on a case-by-case basis improves protocol adherence, and that computer tools seem to improve upon paper-based reference materials. Yet much still remains unclear. If individuals are not reminded to check a protocol for each case, will the advantages of the passive system remain, or will healthcare workers' performance tend towards that without protocols? More importantly, what is it about the way protocols are accessed on a computer that is so beneficial?

In Chapter 10 we separated out the physical aspects of paper and computer records from the informational aspects such as record structure. The conclusion that a 'computer' protocol is inherently better than a 'paper' one is weak, just as was the notion that an electronic patient record will always be superior to a paper-based record. Since there are so many variables involved in making a computer easy or difficult to use, it is conceivable that a well-designed paper system would outperform a poorly designed computer one. In one large randomized controlled trial to compare the effects of computerized and paper-based versions of guidelines, no significant differences in the consultation practices of recently qualified physicians were found over 3484 patient encounters between the computerized and paper groups (Jousimaa *et al.*, 2002).

If we think of a protocol as a message, then we know from Chapter 4 that the channel of message delivery (in this case a computer) is only one of many factors that affect the ultimate impact of the message on the individual who receives it. We have already seen the role that different representations can play in altering the way a protocol is used, and how the utility of a protocol can depend on variables such as the educational level and experience of the individuals using it. The benefits of using the computer channel will vary with clinical task and setting. For example, in time-critical clinical situations, the speed of a computer system might be a distinct advantage, but in an outpatient setting, other design issues such as the facility to search for evidence using large databases, or the ability to present evidence to patients, might be more significant. The complexity of protocol design is explored in the final chapter of this part, where the multitude of design decisions that can adversely affect a protocol's performance are discussed.

The role of the Internet

We have so far examined how protocols can be made available in a clinical setting. As important as local access is the question of how those protocols are published and distributed by their authors, who may be geographically distant from those who wish to use them.

Increasingly, many see the Internet as the vehicle of choice for the distribution of clinical practice guidelines. Creating World Wide Web sites on the Internet allows anyone connected to the Web immediate access to the guidelines stored there. Placing guidelines on the Web is thus equivalent to immediate global publication. The Internet publication model is just as valid if protocols are being created for local distribution across a campus internal internet (or intranet), as it is if they are being accessed remotely across the global Internet.

As with all things, there are potential drawbacks to using the Internet for protocol distribution. Just as evidence-based healthcare might reap enormous rewards from using the Internet, there are forces at play that could, in theory, have the opposite effect to the one intended. In particular, there are at present no formal controls on what can be published on the Internet, and indeed for many that is its great attraction. This means that while 'centres of excellence' like the Cochrane Collaboration will carefully vet any information they publish, others can publish any material they choose with complete disregard to standards of care. Worse still, unlike academic journals where there is a peer review process, there are no such checks for a would-be protocol author on the Internet. The Web is in its own way contributing to the confusing growth of the medical literature.

Thus, although the Internet offers the technical mechanism for protocol publication and distribution, it does not enforce any particular process. Many have argued that the equivalent of journal peer review mechanisms needs to be established for material that is distributed across the Internet (LaPorte, 1995). In response, several internationally significant Web repositories of clinical evidence and guidelines have been created in recent years, including the US Guideline Clearinghouse, and the Cochrane Collaboration's Web site.

13.2 Active protocol systems

In contrast to passive systems, where clinicians have complete freedom to choose to consult a protocol or not, active protocol systems guide specific actions of clinicians. Using computer representation of a protocol as a template to action, a variety of clinical activities can be supported or automated in some way. These activities range from assisting with recording events into an electronic patient record, to driving medication ordering or test scheduling (Figure 13.1).

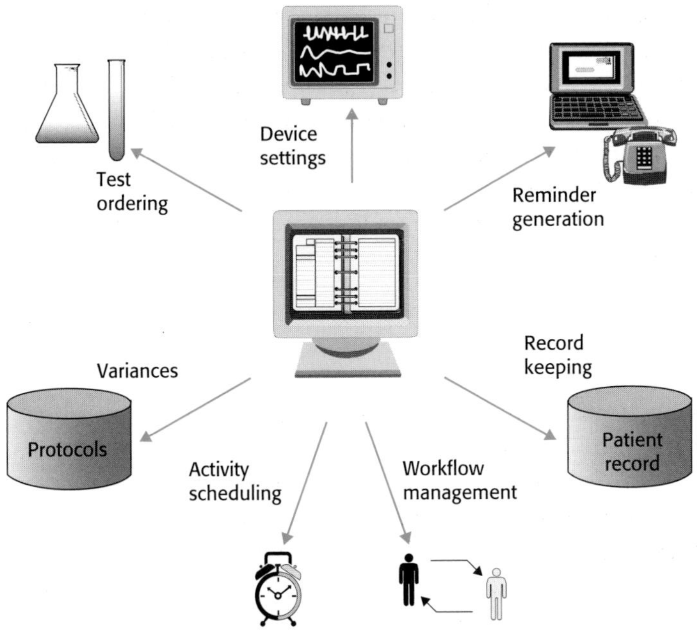
Device
settings
Test
ordering
Reminder
generation
Record
keeping
Variances
Protocols
Patient
record
Activity
scheduling
Workflow
management

Figure 13.1
Protocol-driven information systems can integrate into many different clinical systems, with cumulative benefit. They can for example, guide record keeping, prompt alert generation, and trigger automated order-entry systems and appointment scheduling, as well as providing a mechanism for variance capture.

Consequently an active system may be integrated into a wider organizational information system. Electronic **communication** services are needed to provide the interfaces between active protocol systems and the EMR, and to order-entry functions (Shiffman *et al.*, 1999). Interfaces can also be provided to a variety of other information system components such as pharmacy systems and laboratory results reporting.

In an active system the protocol becomes central to the way care is delivered and care processes are designed around the protocol system. The creation of care pathways, described in Chapter 12, is a good example of the way care processes can be re-engineered to deliver care according to guidelines, as well as capturing variances.

There is a growing literature supporting the benefit that active protocol systems may have in supporting clinical practice. In one systematic review, 25 studies published between 1992 and January 1998 were analysed (Shiffman *et al.*, 1999). All the computer systems provided patient-specific recommendations and in 19, recommendations were available concurrently with care. Their review included 9 randomized controlled trials and 10 time-series correlational studies. Guideline adherence improved for 14 of 18 systems in which it was measured. Documentation improved in 4 of 4 studies. Sadly, few of the studies examined patient outcomes to validate the effectiveness of the systems.

Record keeping can be semi-automated

Protocol-driven record keeping can guide the entry of routine details into the electronic patient record (e.g. Shiffman, 1994). Rather than explicitly describing every action they take in a medical record, a protocol-driven record system allows a user to select which steps in the protocol have been done, and the system can then create a record of activity which automatically contains the action description and the time it occurred. This has benefits both for those creating the record, and for those who will access it subsequently. For the individual recording clinical events, indicating that a step in a protocol has been carried out by checking a box on a screen is quicker than having to enter the details from memory, decreasing time spent in record keeping, as well as acting as a memory prompt to capture all the significant actions that have taken place.

For those who wish to access a patient record, protocol-driven record keeping ensures that records reach a minimum standard of completeness and clarity in three ways:

- Firstly, a well-designed system should be quicker and easier to use than a free input system, thereby increasing the likelihood that an event will be recorded.
- Secondly, by specifying exactly how an event should be recorded, the terms and phrases used in the record can in part be standardized. This becomes especially useful when records are required for clinical audit.
- Finally, by specifying which data are to be recorded, the completeness of the record is enhanced (e.g. Bouhaddou *et al.*, 1993).

Protocol-driven record keeping is thus a good example of a system that delivers direct benefit to those who use the system, by reducing their workload, as well as having long-term benefits because of improved quality of data capture. This contrasts with systems that are designed to code patient events explicitly for audit, but do not improve the lot of those who use them. Systems that are not directly integrated into clinical processes are more likely to cause clinical workers to do extra work, and as a result the system may be poorly accepted for socio-technical reasons.

There are still complexities to be resolved in the design of protocol-driven record keeping systems. For example, it is clear that not all patients will be treated exactly as a protocol specifies. It is thus not possible to exactly specify all the terms that might be used (Heathfield *et al.*, 1995). However, if designed appropriately, such systems should reduce, but cannot eliminate, the amount of free-form data entry that occurs in the patient record.

Recommending and reminding can be situational or alert-based

As with passive systems, a primary role of active protocol systems is to provide healthcare workers with task recommendations and reminders. The scope of clinical recommendations includes appropriate tests and treatments, alerts about at-risk states and reminders of appropriate physical assessments and screening activities (Shiffman *et al.*, 1999). Sometimes active systems provide an **explanation** function that offers background information, definitions and risks as well as the rationale that supported specific recommendations, such as literature citations.

Unlike a passive system, which requires a worker to make a conscious effort to check that their actions are appropriate, protocols in an active system should be a natural part of the workflow. There are two distinct ways in which an active system can remind someone.

- Firstly, an alert can be triggered by a computer-detected event such as a clinician ordering a medication, or the arrival of a laboratory result. The alerts generated by abnormal test results can then be flagged when the electronic record is accessed, or be transmitted via a communication system such as electronic mail or the paging system. The clinical value of such alerts has already been discussed in Chapter 10. Linking clinical pathways or guidelines with order-entry and results reporting systems can increase compliance with guidelines, and has also been shown to reduce rates of inappropriate diagnostic testing. In a randomized trial of antibiotic guidelines, a proportion of clinicians were shown vancomycin prescribing guidelines when they attempted to order this antibiotic using an electronic prescribing system (Shojania *et al.*, 1998). The use of vancomycin dropped by 30% with the guidelines, and when it was prescribed, the medication was given for a significantly shorter duration compared to the control group.

- The second form of reminding is subtler, but just as important, and relies on the protocols being a natural part of the work situation. Active protocol systems can interact with clinicians in simple ways that fit neatly in with traditional work practices. For example, Lobach and Hammond (1997) describe a computerized system that generates a customized management protocol for individual patients using data from the patient's electronic medical record (EMR). The output from the system is then printed on the first page of the paper encounter from where it is immediately visible to clinicians. Its use resulted in a twofold increase in clinician compliance with care guidelines for diabetes mellitus.

If protocols guide record keeping, then the act of generating a record has the side effect of acting as a reminder, since the protocol is visible during recording. Providing a structure to guide the way data are entered into a record has been demonstrated to improve clinical performance. In a study comparing the effects of structured and free-form data entry forms for patients with abdominal pain presenting to a hospital emergency department, it was shown that the diagnostic accuracy of staff rose by 7% over baseline when the structured form was used (de Dombal *et al.*, 1991). There was also a 13% reduction in use of acute surgical beds at night. These improvements were only marginally less than those obtained during the same study by the use of an expert system for abdominal pain.

There are several possible explanations for such results. Firstly, there is a teaching effect that improves the knowledge levels of individuals participating in such studies. This has been recognized by other researchers too. Discussing the use of protocols for ventilator setting adjustment in intensive care, Henderson *et al.* (1992) noted that 'although the protocols were complex, the clinical staff learned to anticipate protocol instructions quite accurately, making it possible for them to recognize that a protocol instruction was based on erroneous data'. Secondly, the ability of individuals to assess a situation may be improved by indicating which data should be collected and the order in which data should be gathered, and presenting them uniformly once gathered (see Box 12.2).

Protocols can drive activity scheduling and workflow management

The facility to enter orders for tests or medications is a basic component of a clinical information system. If such an order-entry function is linked to a protocol, then order generation can in part be protocol driven. For example, as soon as a patient is entered on to a protocol, it should be possible to send requests automatically for the tests or procedures that are specified within the protocol. Thus, you could schedule a stress test several days in advance, at the time a patient is admitted under a myocardial infarction protocol.

The automated management of task scheduling in an organization is more generally carried out by **workflow management systems**. There now exist quite complex and sophisticated computer-based workflow systems that find application in a variety of industries beyond healthcare. The goal of workflow systems is to ensure that work processes are carried out in the most time- and cost-efficient method possible. Workflow systems utilize formal descriptions of tasks, the order in which the tasks are to be executed, and perhaps their interdependencies. For example, a process may require a series of steps to be carried out that involve different departments or individuals. A workflow system can try to balance the work requests that arrive at each point in the process so that the most important tasks are completed, or so that each part of the system works to maximum efficiency. The ability to manage scheduling in a more automated fashion may result in a better use of institutional resources, avoiding peaks in which facilities might be overloaded, or troughs of underutilization (Majidi *et al.*, 1993).

The degree to which the flow of work in an organization can be automated depends on the degree to which tasks can be formalized. At one extreme, we have robot-operated assembly plants which require minimal human intervention, given the high degree of regularity of the assembly process. At the other extreme, if every task in an organization is different, then no workflow automation is possible. Like most organizations, healthcare activities occupy a spectrum in between these two extrema.

The degree to which protocols can drive workflow depends on the sophistication of the protocol care process, and the existence of order-entry and scheduling components in the organization's information system. From the point of view of the care process, it would need to be defined in a quite formal way that lent itself to automation. As we saw in Chapter 9, for some tasks this formalization is not always possible or desirable.

The prescriptive nature of some workflow systems can make them complex to set up, and they may be unduly constraining on staff. However, simple systems that make sure events are scheduled automatically, or that optimize the flow of 'forms' and 'requests' have the potential to yield considerable benefits, if the organization is willing to formalize its processes sufficiently.

Data display can be modified by protocol

The data required to make decisions vary with tasks, and computer system designers often resort to task-specific displays in complex situations (see Chapter 10). If a computer system can be made aware of the current set of clinical tasks – for example, by detecting that a step in a protocol has been executed via a record keeper – then it can prepare itself to generate task-specific data displays.

This is of particular relevance in situations in which large amounts of patient data may need to be filtered, for example in intensive care or anaesthesia. It is also of value in less critical situations, when a large amount of data has accumulated, for example, when patients have long hospital admissions.

Monitor alarms can be set by protocol

If patient-monitoring equipment like arrhythmia monitors or oxygen saturation probes are linked to a protocol system, then they too can be driven in a partially automated manner (Coiera and Lewis, 1994). For example, if anaesthesia is delivered according to computer protocols, then patient monitor alarm settings can be automatically reconfigured, reflecting the changes in alarm bands associated with the different stages of anaesthesia. The computer can detect that a new stage in the protocol has been entered by checking the events noted in the patient record, which can also be protocol driven.

Device settings can vary with protocol stage

Protocols can be used either to advise the settings for biomedical equipment (**open-loop control**), or to control them directly (**closed-loop control**).

- There has been some investigation into open-loop control of ventilators according to standard protocols. For example, protocols have been used to adjust tidal volume and ventilator rate settings for patients with adult respiratory distress syndrome (ARDS) (Thomsen *et al.*, 1993). One system has been reportedly used for over 50 000 hours on 150 ARDS patients (Morris *et al.*, 1994a). In one sub-trial of 12 patients, 94% of 4531 protocol-generated recommendations were followed by staff. Of these patients, 52 met extracorporeal membrane oxygenation criteria (East *et al.*, 1992). These had a 9% expected survival on the basis of historical data, but under protocol-directed care achieved 41% survival, 4 times greater than expected (Morris *et al.*, 1994b).
- Closed loop-control systems are likely to need sophisticated signal interpretation capabilities, as will be discussed in Chapter 27, in addition to protocols.

Variance capture can be semi-automated

Along with a potential to improve record keeping for patient care, protocol systems can also gather broader population data that will contribute to protocol improvement. Whenever a variation in patient management has occurred, it should be possible to include features in the record-keeping part of an information system to record the variance and store it for later assessment.

The successful implementation of active electronic protocols requires attention to a broad spectrum of socio-technical issues

As we saw earlier with passive electronic systems, not all studies have shown active electronic protocol access to be valuable. Eccles *et al.* (2002) evaluated the use of computerized evidence-based guidelines for the management of adult asthma and angina in 60 general practices in the north-east of England. The computerized decision support system prompted clinicians to consider management options in the guideline when it was triggered by data in the electronic patient record. However, it had no significant effect on consultation rates, process of care measures (including prescribing), or any patient-reported outcomes for either condition. Levels of use of the software were extremely low – the median number of active interactions with the computer guideline system was zero for much of the study.

The variable impact of guidelines in improving patient outcomes in primary care has been noted elsewhere (Worrall *et al.*, 1997). As we will see in the next chapter, electronic guideline systems are not simple interventions, but rather function as an embedded component within a complex socio-technical system. The rate of uptake for electronic guidelines in any specific location is influenced by many variables, some of which are local and some more generic. Failure to address any one of these variables may have a significantly negative effect on system adoption and usage.

In the study by Eccles *et al.* (2002) the authors described a number of these variables that might have substantially reduced their system's use and impact:

- Staff had very limited training in the functioning and use of the system, which would have significantly decreased their understanding of the value of the system or how to use it effectively. In contrast, in a similar study that introduced paper-based guidelines and prompts for asthma and diabetes management, the intervention was introduced as part of an educational programme, and resulted in significant improvements in the management of diabetes and asthma (Feder *et al.*, 1995). Provider education, feedback and reminders are all associated with significant improvements in provider adherence to guidelines as well as significant improvements in patient disease control (Weingarten *et al.*, 2002). Without significant time being devoted to interaction with staff during the introduction of protocol systems, it is unlikely that they will be prepared to use the new intervention, nor be able to identify and overcome any social or cultural barriers to system use.
- The primary care physicians were not the only decision-makers in this interaction space, and the system ignored the role of the patient in decision-making. Patients could present with any clinical problem such as arthritis or depression and, despite having asthma or angina, might not wish to discuss the issues raised by the guideline.
- Significant problems were associated with the interaction design of the software. Despite being embedded in routinely used clinical software, the guideline had to be accessed via a separate path within the clinical system, and it was not possible to access all other parts of the clinical system from within the guideline. If the guideline was exited, it was only possible to return to it at the beginning of the pathway.
- The guidelines dealt with the ongoing management of established cases, rather than initial diagnosis or treatment. Clinicians may have a bias to sticking with the *status quo*, or seek evidence only at the beginning of clinical episodes.

The authors of the study concluded that even if the technical problems of producing a system that fully supports the management of chronic disease were solved, there remains the challenge of integrating the systems into clinical encounters where busy practitioners manage patients with complex, multiple conditions.

13.3 Protocol representations and languages

We have already seen in the previous chapter that the representation one uses when writing a protocol has consequences when people come to use the protocol. Decision trees might be useful in some circumstances, for example, but not others. Similar issues arise when a protocol is written for computer interpretation. There is no clear 'best' way of capturing a protocol, and the choice of representational form is dependent on the protocol's intended use.

A prerequisite for developing computer guideline systems is the creation of computer interpretable representations of the clinical knowledge contained in clinical guidelines. In contrast to humans who are able to bring much knowledge to bear when they read a protocol, a computer system does not come with such background knowledge. Recall from Figure 2.5 that the more that is required of a computer, the more knowledge it must be given about the task it is to accomplish. As a consequence, computer protocols need to be specified in considerable detail. One ventilator management protocol needed 12 000 lines of computer code for its specification (Henderson *et al.*, 1992). Consequently, unlike passive protocol representations that are designed for direct human use, computational representations require a richer language that allows protocol designers to direct the internal behaviour of an active system.

Much of the advanced research into protocol languages for computers is aimed at creating ways that ensure that the knowledge is captured in as reliable a way as possible. So, some workers seek to define formal protocol **ontologies** that would then be used to support the writing of specific protocols. An ontology can be thought of as a definition of what is knowable in some context. So, a protocol ontology would capture all the important knowledge about the things being described in the protocol. An ontology about cardiac surgery would include amongst other things, all the tests and procedures that might be of interest. It might also contain rules about the relationships amongst these, which could then be used to prevent some mistakes when the time comes to write a protocol. For example, it makes no sense to write in a protocol that a patient will be treated with a clinical action that the ontology knows is actually a type of test, and not a therapy. It is this need to create ways of automatically checking protocols for errors that has driven the development of such ontologies (Glowinski, 1994).

*Knowledge can be represented either **declaratively** or **procedurally**. In the former, we declare how things relate to one another, but do not specify how we use that knowledge to come up with an answer. In the latter we include the knowledge of how the answer might be derived.*

Several groups are actively developing guideline representation languages, each adopting slightly different approaches. Many of the approaches share a 'task-based paradigm' in which guidelines are decomposed into a hierarchy of component tasks that unfold over time (Fox and Das, 2000). Some of the more significant guideline representation languages include:

- **Arden syntax:** In an attempt to develop a standard method for representing protocols, the American Society for Testing and Materials (ASTM) developed the Arden syntax. This language encodes the actions within a clinical protocol into a set of situation–action rules known as medical logic modules (MLMs). The Arden syntax resembles the Pascal computer programming language, and is procedural in its design. Arden has recognized deficiencies in the type of things that can be described using it (Musen *et al.*, 1995). Further, because it is limited to describing protocols in terms of rules, it has other limitations as far as computers are concerned. Since there is no way to express the knowledge and ideas humans use when they come to read a protocol, there is little tolerance for errors and interdependencies between rules.
- **PRO*forma*:** Driven by concerns that poorly designed computerized guidelines may generate incorrect clinical recommendations, PRO*forma* is designed to emphasize safe and robust guideline creation (Fox and Das, 2000). PRO*forma* is capable of capturing the logical and procedural content of a protocol in the form of a set of 'tasks' that can be interpreted or 'enacted' by a computer. PRO*forma*'s ontology is thus structured around the notion of clinical tasks, which are subdivided into plans, decisions, actions and enquiries (Fox *et al.*, 1996). A distinguishing feature of the PRO*forma* format is the simplicity and intuitiveness of the underlying task model (Figure 13.2). Many PRO*forma*-based systems are in routine clinical use. RetroGram assists in the interpretation of genotype data and decisions for the management of HIV-positive patients (Tura *et al.*, 2002). Other applications include CAPSULE, a system for advising on routine prescribing; RAGs, a system designed to support the assessment of risk of familial breast and ovarian cancer in a primary care setting; ARNO, a pain control system for cancer sufferers, built for St. Christopher's Hospice, London; and MACRO, a system for running Internet-based multicentre clinical trials. Objective evaluations of selected systems have demonstrated their potential to improve clinical practice and resource usage (Humber *et al.*, 2001).

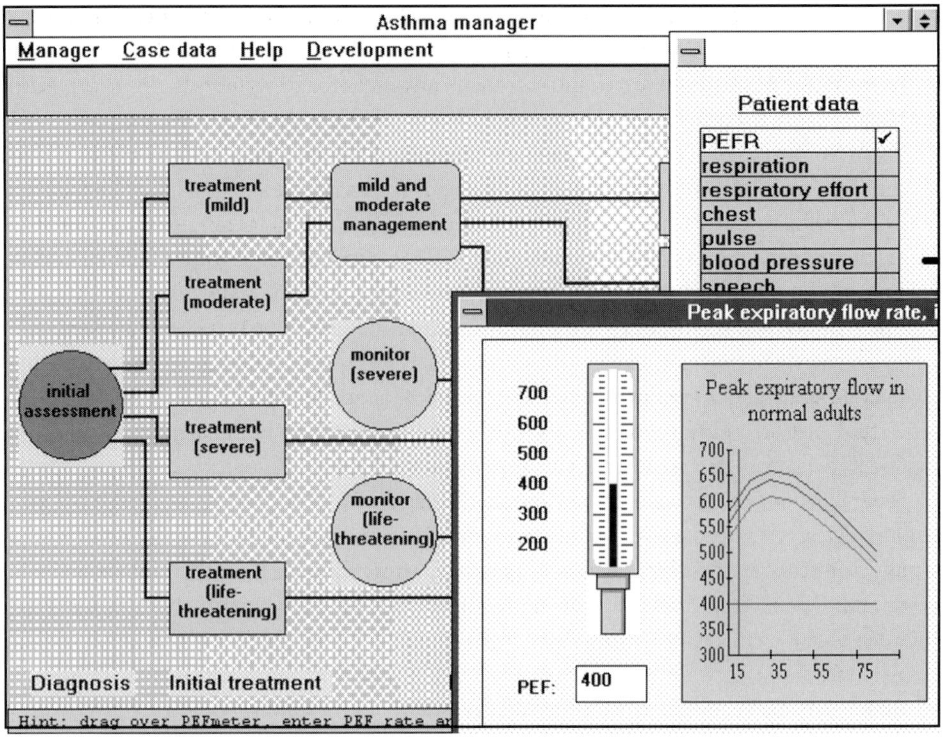

Asthma manager
Manager
Case data
Help
Development
Patient data
PEFR
respiration
respiratory effort
chest
pulse
blood pressure
treatment (mild)
mild and moderate management
treatment (moderate)
monitor (severe)
initial assessment
treatment (severe)
monitor (life-threatening)
treatment (life-threatening)
Diagnosis
Initial treatment
Hint: drag over PEFmeter, enter PEF rate
Peak expiratory flow rate,
700
600
500
400
300
200
PEF:
400
Peak expiratory flow in normal adults
700
650
600
550
500
450
400
350
300
15
35
55
75

Figure 13.2
A user display from a computerized protocol system for managing adult acute asthma built using PRO*forma* (Fox *et al.*, 1996). The asthma manager displays a tree of treatment plans. Other panels show the patient's peak flow data and medical record (square, action; circle, decision; rounded rectangle, plan; arrow, scheduling constraint).

- **Prodigy:** A UK system, Prodigy (**P**rescribing **R**ati**o**nally with **D**ecision-Support **i**n **G**eneral Practice Stud**y**) has been developed to support chronic disease management in primary care (Johnson *et al.*, 2000). Each protocol in Prodigy contains a set of rules, on-screen advice text, patient information and prescribing data relating to one class of disease, e.g. acne, dyspepsia or heart failure (Purves *et al.*, 1999). The main protocol structure is hierarchical, and each protocol is decomposed into **scenarios, therapy groups** and **therapy details**. The **scenario** level subdivides a protocol into specific categories of the disease or different strategies for treatment. For example, the dyspepsia protocol has different scenarios for gastric or duodenal ulcers. The **therapy group** level then offers a choice of types of drug therapy, and the **prescription details** level contains the information necessary to print a prescription (name, formulation, strength, quantity, days supply, user instructions), as well as cost comparison data and regulatory warning status information. Prodigy has had several revisions over the years, and has been running since 1995. It has delivered and maintained over 160 sets of protocols to general practitioners in the UK (Smart and Purves, 2001). Release One of PRODIGY was distributed to all 27 000 general practitioners in England during 1999–2000, although actual uptake is unclear, and several commercial vendors have integrated PRODIGY into clinical information systems for general practitioners (Johnson *et al.*, 2001).
- **Protégé:** Also structured around an ontology of tasks, Protégé has been an ongoing research activity at Stanford University (Musen *et al.*, 1995). Protégé is essentially a protocol design tool that allows a user to build a protocol, guided by an ontology. Once constructed, the protocol is translated into a machine-readable form. As part of the project, a suite of models and software components known as EON was created to

assist in writing guideline-based applications. EON is composed of **problem solvers**, which use clinical guidelines and patient data to generate situation-specific recommendations, **knowledge bases**, which contain the machine-readable protocols, and a temporal **database mediator** which sits between the problem solvers and patient data and provides explanation services for other components. In both Protégé and Pro*forma*, the researchers have spent much effort in developing ways for people to specify a protocol in a simple way. They also needed to develop mechanisms that translated these descriptions into more formal language for computers. They are thus systems that can be programmed using high-level languages understood by humans, but are then translated into a lower-level language understood by computer.

- **Guideline Interchange Format (GLIF):** GLIF is a research system that has not yet effectively been employed in the real world, but was designed with the intention of acting as an interchange format that supported the sharing of guidelines between different institutions and software systems (Peleg *et al.*, 2000). GLIF's developers have now acknowledged that this goal is impractical at present, given the evolving nature and apparent conceptual differences amongst the competing guideline representations (Greenes *et al.*, 2001). GLIF tries to build on the most useful features of other guideline models and to incorporate standards that are used in healthcare. Its expression language was originally based on the Arden syntax, and its default medical data model is based on the HL7 Reference Information Model (RIM).

All computational representations for protocols share similar features

As the commonalities between the different guideline representations become clearer a degree of cross-format standardization may be possible. In a comprehensive review of 11 different formalisms for the computer representation of clinical protocols, all were found to have basic features in common (Wang *et al.*, 2002). Firstly, all of the reviewed protocol representation formalisms contain primitives that represent specific clinical tasks that will be recommended to clinicians (Figure 13.3). In keeping with passive representations such as decision trees (Figure 8.6), these primitives can be classified into two categories:

- **Actions:** An action is a clinical or administrative task that the protocol system recommends should be performed, maintained or avoided, e.g. a recommendation to give a medication. Actions may also result in the invocation of a sub-protocol in the computer system, allowing multiple protocols to be nested within each other.
- **Decisions:** A decision is made when one or more options are selected from a set of alternatives based on pre-defined criteria, e.g. selection of a laboratory test from a set of potential tests.

Unlike passive representations, computer representations also contain primitives that are used by the computer system to record intermediate states during the application of computerized protocols. These intermediate states keep track of the system's understanding of the current situation:

- **The clinical status of a patient:** A patient state records the state that the computer system believes a patient to be in, and is based on the actions that the system knows have already been performed and the decisions that have already been made. For example, a patient who has already received the first dose of an influenza vaccine and is eligible for the second dose could be in the patient state *eligible-for-the-second-dose-of-influenza-vaccine*. Entry and exit conditions on protocols are also examples of patient states.

- **The execution state of the system:** An execution state records the stage of completion of a task, such as an action or decision, during the process of computer guideline execution. For example, a guideline system might record that it is now ready to execute the task *recommend-the-second-dose-of-influenza-vaccine* when a patient has already received the first dose of the influenza vaccine. Finite state machines, introduced in the previous chapter, are examples of protocols driven by representations of a patient's state. State variables determine entry and exit points in a protocol, and drive the transition from one protocol to another.

These representation primitives are used to construct the specific steps in a protocol. The logical connection between the different steps in a protocol are organized using a process model which typically is composed of:

- **Scheduling constraints:** Scheduling constraints specify the temporal order in which representation primitives can be executed during guideline application. The execution of steps may be in a linear sequence, but many systems permit parallel execution if more than one set of actions are required. Most models represent these scheduling constraints either as flowchart-like algorithms or as state transitions. This latter approach is shown to be very useful for the representation of chronic disease guidelines, which typically contain multiple patient scenarios at different encounters and thus could not be represented as linear diagrams with single entry point.
- **Plans or nesting of guidelines:** Nesting of guidelines defines the hierarchical relationship among guidelines during guideline application. Nesting enables multiple levels of abstraction in guideline representation and provides different granularities for the views to a guideline.

In another study that directly compared the ability of six different representations to encode portions of standard guidelines for managing chronic cough and treating hypertension, almost all accurately encoded the knowledge in the guidelines (Peleg *et al.*, 2003). The systems used similar approaches to plan organization, expression language, conceptual medical record model, medical concept model and data abstractions. Differences were most apparent in underlying decision models, goal representation, use of scenarios and structured medical actions. Since all models are essentially task-based constructs, many of the differences among the guideline modelling approaches resulted from their particular classes of intended applications.

Finally, for an active protocol to be applied in clinical practice, it will require access to data about a specific patient's state as well as clinical context data, such as medication orders for a patient. This is ideally provided by integrating the active protocol system into an EMR and an order-entry system. At present there is no standard approach to the definition of patient data, and different representational systems take quite different approaches to solving the problem. Several controlled medical terminologies have been developed as standards to encode patient data. Given the importance of the whole subject of terminologies, and their fundamental relationship with active protocol systems, the next section of the book will examine this field in detail.

Conclusions

In this chapter, some of the different ways a protocol-based system can interact with other components of a clinical information system have been outlined. In many ways, protocol-based systems can provide the glue that can connect these different components together. Since the goal of protocol-directed care is to improve clinical processes, active protocol systems are richly entwined with the delivery of care. As with any such marriage, costs and benefits result from the union. Poorly designed systems can have a significant impact on care delivery. Consequently the emphasis on good design, both of protocols and of the systems that embody them, becomes more critical the more deeply they are used to manage the care process. Striking a balance between prescription and permission, protocol systems need to be only as formal as is necessary to ensure appropriate outcomes, without restricting the permission needed by clinical workers to vary their work patterns.

Discussion points

1. Redraw the decision tree in Figure 12.1 using the guideline primitives shown in Figure 13.3.
2. Compare the peer review process of a major international biomedical journal with that adopted by a major Internet guideline or evidence repository. If there are differences, what explanations can you find for them?
3. How does the representation chosen for a human user of a protocol differ from that used in a computer?
4. Compare the different contributions that the medium and the message make to the effectiveness of paper and computer-based protocol delivery systems. If you wish, use Chapters 4 and 5 as your template.
5. In what way does your answer to the previous question differ to the one at the end of Chapter 10, which examine the paper and electronic record? Hint: Active protocol systems engage in a series of interactions, or dialogue, with their user. Passive systems, as well as strict record keeping systems, usually engage in a one-way interaction. So, consider some of the interaction design differences that may arise.

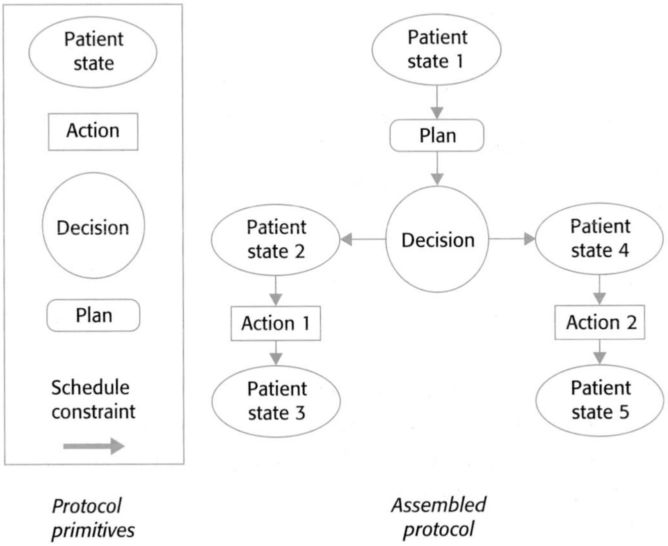
Patient state
Action
Decision
Plan
Schedule constraint
Protocol primitives
Patient state 1
Plan
Decision
Patient state 2
Patient state 4
Action 1
Action 2
Patient state 3
Patient state 5
Assembled protocol

Figure 13.3
Computer protocols typically are constructed from a set of standard primitives, and assembled to produce complete protocols (after Wang *et al.*, 2002).

Chapter summary

1 Computer-based protocol systems can support passive and active protocol usage.

2 There is growing evidence that providing computer-assistance to improve passive access to clinical protocols does have a positive impact on adherence to guidelines.

3 Using protocols as a central template, a variety of clinical activities can be actively supported or automated. These include recording clinical events for the electronic patient record, reminder generation, adjusting settings on monitors or other devices, ordering tests, capturing variances from protocol specifications, scheduling procedures and guiding efficient and effective workflow.

4 The successful implementation of active electronic protocols requires attention to a broad spectrum of socio-technical issues.

5 A prerequisite for developing computer guideline systems is the creation of computer-interpretable representations of the clinical knowledge contained in clinical guidelines.

6 All computational representations for protocols share similar features and are typically constructed from a set of standard primitives, and assembled to produce complete protocols. Primitives include patient states, actions, decisions, nested plans and scheduling constraints.

CHAPTER 14

Disseminating and applying protocols

> ...many of the diseases to which mankind are subject, particularly fevers, smallpox, and other infectious disorders, might be prevented by the diffusion of knowledge in relation to their nature, their causes, and their means of prevention. Were general knowledge more extensively diffused, and the minds of the multitude habituated to just principles and modes of reasoning, such fallacious views and opinions would be speedily dissipated, and consequently those physical evils and disorders which they produce would be in a great measure prevented. *T. Dick, On the Improvement of Society by the Diffusion of Knowledge (1833), 46–48.*

In an ideal world, every clinician would have immediate and easy access to advice on best practice and the supporting evidence. They would have the technology to find the information they need, the skills to understand it and the resources to implement it. In the real world, even if there is a better treatment, not every clinician will know about it or seek it out.

Indeed, the uptake of evidence into clinical practice remains low. Practising clinicians on the other hand complain of being swamped by a growing tide of information. Systematic reviews and guidelines pile up in their offices and proliferate on the Internet, and there seems to be no hope of ever reading, let alone incorporating, the information into their routine pattern of care (Jackson and Feder, 1998).

The Cochrane Collaboration is now perhaps one of the most influential organizations working in the area of evidence-based practice (Goodlee, 1994). It was formed with the intention of creating and distributing evidence-based summaries of best practice, and its first database of systematic reviews covered pregnancy and childbirth research. Yet, despite the relatively high profile of the group, there was a considerable delay in the uptake of the obstetrics digests (Paterson-Brown *et al.*, 1993, 1995).

Further, evidence suggests that, even when clinical protocols are available, clinicians forget to follow them, or deviate from them without clear cause (Renaud-Salis, 1994). Forgetting pre-planned management tasks seems to be especially likely in high-stress clinical situations (Parker and Coiera, 2000).

A further broad area of difficulty is socio-technical and lies within the culture of clinical practice. The introduction of a more regimented approach to care is seen by some, rightly or wrongly, as an intrusion on their clinical freedom to deliver healthcare in the manner they personally consider most suitable.

In this chapter, each of these three areas of protocol dissemination, application and socio-technical barriers will be examined in more detail. We begin by examining the barriers that limit the uptake of guidelines into clinical practice.

14.1 The uptake of clinical guidelines will remain low as long as the costs perceived by clinicians outweigh the benefits

If one takes an economic view, then evidence, whether in the form of a systematic review or clinical practice guideline, is simply an information product, and clinicians are its consumers. Evidence-based recommendations have to compete with every other piece of information that descends on clinicians to gain their attention. For their part, clinicians as information consumers must make decisions about what information seems most useful or accessible to them, in their personal circumstances. The result of this interaction between evidence supply and clinician demand is an **information marketplace**.

As we will see in Chapter 24, information economics may help us understand the apparent low uptake of evidence at a time when evidence has never been more available, and identify strategies that increase the impact of tools such as guidelines in clinical practice. The metaphor of a clinical information marketplace allows us to develop explanations for the current state of evidence-based practice. By all accounts, the global store of clinical evidence is growing rapidly, perhaps exponentially. The current proliferation of evidence by producers, but low

Box 14.1
The dominant design

It is an interesting feature of the marketplace that the introduction of a new class of product at first usually sees a great variety of competing designs enter the market. Each competing design has new features, or different combinations of existing ones. After a period, however, such variety almost completely disappears, and most producers end up creating products which have remarkably similar features.

Thus, the first typewriter was produced by Scholes in 1868, and was followed by a host of competing designs. However, 1899 saw the introduction of the Underwood Model 5 typewriter which has all the attributes of later, more modern typewriters. Soon after its introduction, because of its immense popularity, all other manufacturers found themselves forced to approximate the Underwood design. Indeed, the design persisted well beyond the first half of the twentieth century. It was not until the introduction of electronic typewriters, computers and word-processors that radically different sets of designs and functions were introduced.

The evolution of the modern personal computer followed along the same path, with an initial flurry of different designs. Eventually the marketplace settled upon a set of prototypic features that most people would expect when they bought a personal computer (Figure 18.1).

This stable design point in the history of a product class is known as a **dominant design** (Utterback, 1994). The dominant design 'embodies the requirements of many classes of users of a particular product, even though it may not meet the needs of a particular class to quite the same extent as would a customized design'.

Further, even though a dominant design may after a time become obsolete, its widespread adoption and individuals' investment in learning to work with it make them reluctant to shift to a better design. So, even though there are probably numerous better designs than the QWERTY keyboard, most people exhibit a bias towards the *status quo*. Those who have learnt to use a QWERTY keyboard are reluctant to shift to using a better design. Thus, once in place, the dominant design remains fixed, not because newer designs do not offer benefits, but because changing to them incurs unacceptable costs. Only when the cost-benefit trade-off shifts heavily the other way will a new product class become acceptable.

uptake by consumers, suggests that we are already in a situation of information oversupply. In this case, creating more guidelines will not increase the uptake rate, nor will berating the clinical consumers for not wanting the product.

The consequence for information producers is that their success is increasingly dependent upon their ability to compete for the attention of information consumers. The consequences for consumers of information are just as problematic. The amount of information that can be accessed or 'consumed' is fundamentally limited by the constraints on human attention.

As worryingly, theoretically it should become ever more expensive to find information. In particular, the costs of searching for and evaluating information have the potential to become increasingly expensive over time. If the amount of information is growing exponentially, then the number of documents that match a particular clinical question should also grow. For example, for a given amount of search effort, the probability of finding a document on the Web will decrease with time. In other words, a seemingly inevitable consequence of a global growth in information supply is actually an 'information famine' where we cannot find what we need. For producers of information, the uncomfortable consequence of an ever growing information supply and scarce human attention is an economic Malthus' law of information (Box 24.2) – the fraction of information produced that is actually consumed will, with time, asymptotically approach zero (Varian, 1998).

14.2 The clinical impact of a guideline is determined both by its efficacy as well as its adoption rate

Irrespective of whether the content of a guideline reflects best practice, if it is not used it will have no impact. Consequently, the developers of a guideline should think not only about the contents of a guideline and the evidence behind its advice, but also about the best representational form for the guideline and the best medium for its dissemination.

The implication for those in the business of creating evidence 'products' such as clinical guidelines is that the notion of the 'best' treatment advice needs to be replaced with a more complex notion of the most effective method for disseminating information about a treatment into the information marketplace. Guideline designers need to consider how well their product competes for the attention of clinicians, and the 'market share' that a guideline will ultimately attract. They should also recognize that the level of adoption of any guideline is a reflection of the ease with which their product can be accessed, and its perceived utility amongst clinicians once it is accessed.

One way of understanding these issues is to measure both the change in clinical outcome that a treatment produces if it were to be used, and the actual rate of adoption of the guideline that recommends the treatment. The rate of adoption measures the likelihood that the clinical community will actually discover the information, and the costs and benefits of using it once discovered.

Combining these two measures produces a measure of the actual clinical impact of the guideline. For example, assume we have a disease in which the baseline outcome with current treatments is 50% recovery. Two new competing treatments are introduced into the clinical information market via published guidelines. Treatment A has a 90% clinical success rate and 1% of patients receive it, based upon the adoption rate by clinicians. If B has only an 80% success rate but a 10% adoption rate, which treatment is the most effective? If we take evidence

Box 14.2
Efficacy × adoption rate = clinical impact

Treatment A gives a 90% success rate, and achieves an adoption rate of 1% within the population of patients. The remaining patients use the baseline treatment with 50% success. The overall improvement to population health produced by A is thus:

$$\text{Impact of A} = 0.9 \times 1/100 + 0.5 \times 99/100 = 0.504$$

Treatment B gives a 80% success rate, and is used by 10% of the population. The remaining patients use the baseline treatment with 50% success. The overall improvement to population health produced by B is thus:

$$\text{Impact of B} = 0.8 \times 10/100 + 0.5 \times 90/100 = 0.53$$

The improvement produced by introducing A is thus 0.004, and by introducing B is 0.03. B thus has an impact 7.5 times as great as that of A.

of clinical efficacy, then A is clearly superior. If, however, we measure the impact factor of a guideline to be the product of its improvement in outcome and its level of adoption amongst the population, B is 7.5 times as beneficial as A in terms of improvements to that population's outcome, and is clearly superior (see Box 14.2).

Thus, a guideline describing a treatment that does not have the best clinical outcome may nonetheless be the best when we consider its ease of adoption and consequent impact on the health of the population. Traditional evaluations consider the costs and benefits of new treatments in isolation (Palmer *et al.*, 1999), but the most meaningful cost-benefit analysis is the one that reflects the true impact of a treatment in the community, which is determined by the mode of dissemination. If clinical impact is the measure of success, then designers of evidence products such as clinical guidelines should not only devote their attention to identifying the best treatment; they must also seek ways of ensuring that their information products are adopted widely.

14.3 Strategies for improving the uptake of evidence into practice may alter either actual or perceived costs and benefits

The economic view emphasizes that the costs and benefits of accessing and applying information are at least as important as the costs and benefits of the treatments that the information describes. A substantial body of work now exists in the social and behavioural sciences that examines how personal and systemic changes occur, and these are being used to develop strategies that encourage clinicians to adopt evidence-based practices (Bero *et al.*, 1998; Wyatt *et al.*, 1998). Provider and patient education, provider feedback, financial incentives and reminders have all been associated with significant improvements either in adherence to guidelines or in patient disease control (Weingarten *et al.*, 2002).

In simplistic terms, there are only two ways to increase the uptake of a product:

- The 'cost of ownership' of information can come down, making resource-strapped clinicians more able to access and apply evidence.
- The value of information to the clinician could go up, increasing the benefit to clinical practice. Clinicians should then be willing to devote more resources to accessing evidence than to other activities.

The improvement in the cost-benefit ratio does not need to even be beneficial, it just has to be perceived to be so. For example, it may be that clinicians have a biased view of the value of using evidence (Box 8.3), and simply making the genuine benefits more apparent, or causing clinicians to reassess and discount the costs, alters their behaviour.

Table 14.1 A non-exhaustive catalogue of the costs and benefits of using guidelines in clinical practice for the individual clinician, the patient, and the healthcare system (Dawes, 1996; Haynes *et al.*, 1997; Glanville *et al.*, 1998; Straus and Sackett, 1998; Muir Gray *et al.*, 1997; Guyatt *et al.*, 1999; Haycox *et al.*, 1999; Shaneyfelt *et al.*, 1999; Woolf *et al.*, 1999).

To individual clinician	To patient	To healthcare system
Costs		
Purchase of guideline access technology	Lack of flexible management	Process of guideline construction consumes time and resources
Purchase of or access to guidelines	Population health needs may supersede individual needs	Dissemination of guidelines
Learning EBH skills	Non-guideline treatment may not be reimbursed	Updating guidelines
Time to access guideline	Decreased treatment choice	Investment in technologies for constructing, disseminating and accessing guidelines and evidence
Time to frame clinical question, read guideline and apply to individual patient		Guideline recommendations may be poor
Lack of guideline standardization makes use harder		One policy does not fit all
Effort to resolve mismatch between guideline and clinical problem		Expensive new treatments may be favoured
Learning new practice		Excessive funds may be diverted to subsection of community
Inefficient with new practice compared to old		Commercial interests may use guidelines to disseminate products more rapidly than normal
Decreased clinical discretion		Guidelines may lead to over-utilization of treatments
Guideline does not show all options all options		
Misleading or outdated advice in guideline		
Use of non-guideline treatments generates criticism, litigation or does not attract reimbursment		
Benefits		
Increased protection from litigation	Improved outcomes	Decreased expenditure on treatments
Increased quality of decisions	Increased consistency of care across providers	Support for quality improvement activities
Decreased amount of literature that needs to be read	Being better informed	Increased efficiency Identification of gaps in clinical evidence

Increasing value for individual clinicians

When the costs and benefits of evidence-based practice are summarized (Table 14.1), a number of features are apparent. Firstly, the individual clinician sees a long list of potential personal costs and few personal gains in making changes towards evidence-based healthcare (EBH). Secondly, much of the benefit of EBH is couched in terms of benefit to the healthcare system or to patients, and there has been little emphasis on finding ways to make individual clinicians derive direct benefit. Protection from litigation and the comfort of improved decision-making are amongst the few cited personal benefits of EBH to clinicians. Certainly, an examination of current strategies to encourage EBH reveals a focus on explaining the system rather than personal benefits to clinicians (Bero *et al.*, 1998).

If clinicians are to be induced to use evidence-based resources, then there needs to be clear advantages for the clinician beyond exhortations to the public good. EBH should produce obvious and immediate benefits for clinicians at the point of care. For example, a computer-based record system with evidence-based guidelines embedded in the design has the potential to deliver immediate benefits through automation. Selecting a guideline could automatically generate test orders, pre-prepare prescriptions, schedule tests, create elements of the patient record, call up patient educational materials or even award points that count towards continuing professional education (CPE) programmes.

Decreasing the costs associated with evidence-based practice

Evidence-based practice imposes costs on clinicians in both making the initial change to their practice to become evidence-based, and the effort in maintaining this way of working.

Some of the costs of change are financial, and include the cost of purchasing new technology, redesigning clinical work practice and the consequent need for training. Financial subsidies to assist with such change costs have been shown to increase adoption rates. For example, the Australian Federal Government's Practice Incentives Program enticed general practitioners to computerize at a remarkable rate, with 65% claiming that they used their computers to prescribe electronically in 2000, compared with 15% in 1997 (Kidd and Mazza, 2000).

The costs of evidence-based behaviour continue once they have been adopted. Recall from Chapter 5 that information needs to be appropriately structured to achieve a specific task, using available resources, and to suit the needs of the receiver. The form and complexity of an information artefact such as a guideline will impose costs on those who use it, for example in locating the information, reading it and then interpreting it.

Searching for information imposes a transaction cost on clinicians, at least in terms of their time and mental effort. As the amount of information that needs to be sifted through grows, such transaction costs will also grow. A traditional way that consumers minimize the search costs for goods is to seek out a trusted supplier, such as a department store, that on average delivers a high-quality product at a good price. On the Web, information consumers similarly minimize search costs by constraining their search to areas known to contain high-quality information that usually suits their needs. Such information **portals** act like traditional department stores. Creating and supporting recognized portals containing high-quality evidence will help minimize search costs to some extent. However, more powerful information search and retrieval technologies will be needed as the body of evidence grows, and their development represents a challenge to the field of health informatics.

Well-designed presentations of evidence should also enhance their uptake. For example, if clinical guidelines are unduly complex we know that compliance rates by clinicians are lower (Grilli and Lomas, 1994). Some sacrifice of completeness of information seems to increase the clinical utility of guidelines. Such intermediate descriptions are sufficiently detailed for most uses but are not so detailed that they cover everything. There are also theoretical arguments for choosing intermediate complexity (Coiera, 1992b), which are supported by experimental evidence that the speed and completeness of information retrieval from medical records are best when intermediate levels of detail are used (Tange *et al.*, 1998).

Optimizing evidence to suit the clinical context

The context of care imposes widely different constraints on decision-making. Different user populations have different skill sets, education and resources, and as a result their information needs may demand very different information presentations. One study estimates that up to 50% of the variation in compliance rate by clinicians with guidelines can be ascribed to the clinical setting alone (Grilli and Lomas, 1994).

Context-specific versions of evidence can be created using computerized user models that capture the specific needs of individual groups and permit some automatic tailoring of evidence before it is presented (Pratt and Sim, 1995). Providing access methods that are optimized to local needs can also enlarge the range of clinical contexts in which evidence is used. For example, a clinician faced with an emergency that requires rapid decision-making is unlikely to browse at leisure through information on the Web, although that may be the perfect solution for less time-critical circumstances. The use of small mobile computing and communication devices, and voice-activated rather than text-based services, may help in circumstances where clinicians are mobile, hands are busy or time is limited.

Altering clinician's perceptions of value

Clinician perception is subject to a range of normal human biases that need to be accounted for when the value of EBH is explained to them. Experience in other domains shows that, although 'better' solutions exist, people stick with apparently sub-optimal solutions because the cost of changing is perceived to be too high (Box 8.3). In particular, cognitive psychologists have examined such behaviour and show that humans seem to give greater weight to losses than to gains. For example, if someone is given $10 and it is then taken away, their net outcome is actually neutral, since they are neither better nor worse off financially. However, individuals typically feel negatively toward the transactions, and that they have 'lost' something. Studies have also shown that individuals also give more weight to many small losses than to a single gain (Tversky and Kahneman, 1981).

Thus, faced with the long list of apparent personal costs and few personal gains associated with EBH (Table 14.1), clinician perception may be inherently biased against embracing EBH, independent of the true cost-benefit ratio.

Interventions can be crafted to assist clinicians in making more rational choices about adopting practices by altering the perceived cost-benefit ratio of using guidelines for clinicians.

- **Separate gains:** A higher perceived value is generated when gains can be decomposed into individual items and valued independently. Explaining all the personal benefits of EBM to clinicians explicitly should therefore improve their assessment of its value.
- **Combine losses:** Similarly, perceived losses can be minimized when several losses are lumped into a single item. EBM systems that offer 'all-in-one' acquisition and access, and roll as many purchase and training costs as possible into one, should be beneficial.
- **Avoid valuation of sunk clinical costs:** Presenting costs and benefits of the *status quo* and new practices should always be framed to ignore unrecoverable investments in past practice.

- **Separate small gains from large losses:** This is the 'cash back' effect that makes a consumer item appear more valuable when an expensive ticket price is offset by a small bonus. So, purchasing expensive computer equipment to provide access to guidelines may become attractive with bonuses like electronic prescribing.
- **Combine a small loss together with a larger gain:** By folding a loss within a larger gain, consumers may feel better off than if they were asked to value the loss and gain separately.

14.4 Socio-technical barriers limit the use of evidence in clinical settings

Despite the clear benefits that well-designed protocols can deliver in appropriate circumstances, there is still a wide variation in the level of uptake of protocols, and indeed more broadly, clinical evidence across the clinical community (Gosling *et al.*, 2003). Organizational, social and professional factors have been hypothesized to be at least as important as technical and practical factors in preventing more widespread uptake (Ash, 1997; Kaplan, 1997).

Studies investigating the barriers to the use of online evidence resources have identified a range of factors including insufficient training, both in database searching and in general IT skills (Hersh and Hickam, 1998; Griffiths and Riddington, 2001). Organizational and social factors that promote discussion within the organization and the existence of 'champions' (people who enthusiastically support an innovation) have also been shown to be important predictors of online literature searching (Howell and Higgins, 1990) and the use of point-of-care clinical information systems (Massaro, 1989).

There is also wide variation in the way different professional groups regard clinical evidence and access it. Nurses seemingly place greater value on policies and procedures (Manias and Street, 2000) and have a preference for custom and precedent as a basis for decision-making (Degeling *et al.*, 1998) compared to doctors, who have a stronger emphasis on the role of evidence from the biomedical literature in their decision-making culture (Gosling *et al.*, 2003). In a study of critical care nurses (Manias and Street, 2000), it was found that nurses used policies and protocol to authenticate their decisions and to bring weight to their encounters with registrars and resident medical officers. The preference for nursing procedures and routines even led to neonatal nurses continuing practices they knew to be potentially harmful (Greenwood *et al.*, 2000). This may also be related to nursing culture and professional status within the healthcare system. Other studies have found that lack of organizational support was a barrier to using EBP (Gerrish *et al.*, 1999; Retsas, 2000). Failure to provide support for technological infrastructure or for promoting evidence use and training in searching skills may also limit uptake (Gosling *et al.*, 2003).

Discussion points

1. How does professional culture affect the use of evidence in clinical settings?
2. Can you use the notion of the dominant design from Box 14.1 to explain why clinicians might stick to outmoded practices?

Chapter summary

1 Clinical guidelines are information products, and clinicians are their consumers; the current proliferation by producers but low uptake by consumers indicates an information oversupply.

2 The uptake of evidence will be hampered when the perceived cost of changing to it is too high. At present, most costs are borne by individual clinicians but benefits favour the public good.

3 Just as a citation index measures the impact of a scientific paper within a research community, an evidence uptake index should give a clearer measure of the effectiveness of evidence within the clinical population.

4 Specific strategies to increase evidence uptake include decreasing the 'cost of ownership', increasing the direct or perceived value in routine practice, and the customization of evidence to suit different users, tasks and clinical contexts.

5 Socio-technical barriers limit the use of evidence in clinical settings. Cultural differences between professional grouping accounts for some of these differences, and organizational support through provision of training and infrastructure, and the presence of local champions also have an impact.

CHAPTER 15

Designing protocols

Protocols represent a powerful method for improving the quality of decisions when two conditions can be satisfied:

- It must actually be feasible to prescribe a course of action ahead of time. If the situation in question is novel, constantly changing or in some other way non-deterministic, then it is hard to see how an explicit recipe for action can be predetermined.
- Irrespective of how easy it might be to create a protocol, the conditions at the time of decision-making must make it possible to both access and then apply the protocol.

Failure to meet either of these conditions of **protocol designability** or **protocol usability** will cause difficulties. Understanding when they can be satisfied should increase the likelihood that the use of protocols will be successful.

In the previous chapter, we explored the way a protocol's design can limit its clinical utility, and how the dissemination and uptake of evidence in the form of protocols can be considered a function of the costs and benefits of use. In this chapter, we turn to the task of protocol design, examining the design process and principles of good design.

15.1 Protocol construction and maintenance

Recall from Chapter 1 that in modelling the world, the processes of abstraction, definition of design assumptions and instantiation all influence the final design of an object. When a

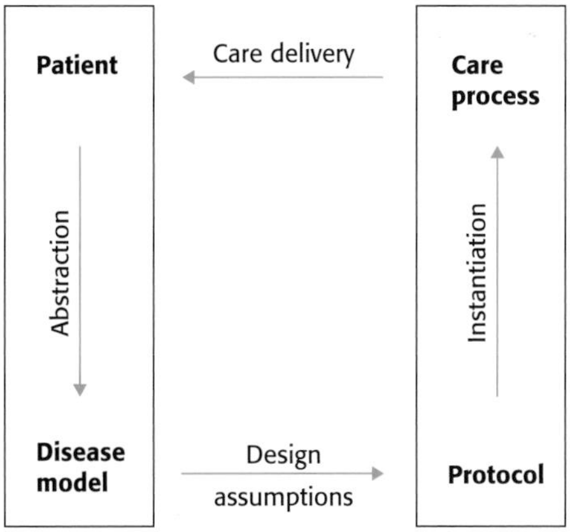
Patient
Care delivery
Care process
Abstraction
Instantiation
Disease model
Design assumptions
Protocol

Figure 15.1
Protocols are designed on the basis of a set of assumptions about the nature of the disease that is to be treated, as well as the context within which the protocol will be used. This context of the care process defines who will be delivering care, their available resources and the local expectations of the goal of care.

protocol is designed, it should be shaped both by an understanding of the best treatments, and by the circumstances in which it will be used. Thus the first step in arriving at such a process is to develop a model of the disease process. Then a set of assumptions is made, based upon an understanding of the context in which the protocol will be used, for example about the level of resource or training of staff. As we have seen, these assumptions have a strong influence on the form and content of a protocol's design. The last step is the construction of a care process around the protocol. The overall process of protocol design, creation and application is summarized in Figure 15.1.

Two key features of the protocol design and maintenance process need to be emphasized:

- Creation of a protocol does not occur at a single moment in time, but is part of an ongoing process that assesses a protocol's performance, and refines it accordingly.
- Creation of a protocol cannot be an isolated event; its form and content must be designed to reflect the context within which it will be used.

Computer-based protocols can be complex. For example, the ventilator protocols developed by Henderson *et al.* (1992), consisting of 25 pages of flow diagrams and 12 000 lines of computer code, required the efforts of 14 physicians and nurses. Unfortunately the cumulative time required from all the team members to build these protocols was not specified. Whether one is envisioning the creation of large global databases of protocols capturing best practice or local databases, probably thousands of protocols will need to be created.

A task on this scale has never been done before. It is also a task that, in all probability, cannot be tackled without either significant human resource, or the use of advanced information and communication technologies. In many respects, then, the uniform and rapid transformation of clinical evidence into clinical process represents not just a major challenge for health, but also a major challenge for health informatics (Coiera, 1996b).

Despite the rewards contemplated by those who advocate mass protocolization, it is by no means yet certain whether it is technically feasible, or even practicable. For informatics the process of protocol creation and application poses a number of significant technical challenges, the solutions to many of which are still the subject of research. Others, thankfully, can be readily solved by the appropriate application of existing technologies.

The degree of technical challenge grows both with the number of protocols contemplated, and with the inherent complexity of individual protocols. For example, a paper-based protocol to help a diabetic patient adjust their insulin therapy is much simpler than an equivalent protocol that is needed to drive a computer to make the same recommendations. The major technical steps in the creation of protocols will now be defined, and their associated challenges explored.

Evidence gathering, pooling and dissemination

The dynamics of the information market means that as the quantity of available evidence grows, good-quality evidence will become harder to find over time. It is relatively cheap to produce poor-quality but attractive information content on the Web, but the cost of generating good material is high. For example, the process adopted by the Cochrane Collaboration is approximately as follows (Wyatt, 1995). To assemble systematic evidence-based reviews for each guideline, a complete literature search has first to be performed. This may involve hand-searching journals from pre-electronic days, as well as doing multiple online bibliographic searches. It may even involve contacting authors for access to data supporting their reported results (Smith *et al.*, 1996).

The simple assessment that we are experiencing exponential growth in the medical literature, but not in the numbers of those available to conduct critical appraisal, means that we will soon need automated means for exploring, collating and disseminating best-practice knowledge. The development of such technological support remains an open and challenging area for computer science and informatics research.

Progress has already been made by biomedical journals through the adoption of standard formats for article abstracts, ensuring that key aspects of a paper are always present. The data gathering process could be further assisted if all papers were available electronically, and even more so if the data used in a study were also available online, for example via the Internet (Delamothe, 1996) (see Chapter 22). There are no technical barriers to such proposals, only organizational ones. Key journals have begun the process that may eventually see all biomedical publication occurring in electronic form in preference to paper (LaPorte *et al.*, 1995).

However, retrieval of published evidence is not only hampered by limited access to the material. In one study, even if barriers to access had been removed, clear information on specific questions for primary care physicians could be obtained from the literature in only about 50% of cases (Gorman, 1993). Finding such information is both time-consuming and complex. For example, there may be variations in the terminology used, or the papers may not come up to appropriate scientific standards because of variations in the quality of peer review. The solution to such problems is probably as much organizational as technological. For example, the adoption of ICD nomenclature in structured abstracts would reduce the effort involved in bibliographic searches.

Just as there are considerable issues to be faced in the gathering of evidence, there are also difficulties associated with the distribution of protocols and guidelines once they have been created. If they are to be used as passive information resources, then the communication of guidelines can be enhanced through publication on the Internet using the World Wide Web (see Chapter 23).

The model for publication on the Web permits updated guidelines to be almost immediately available worldwide. Further, there are no issues associated with multiple editions of a protocol circulating, as is the case with paper-based publication methods. There need only ever be one current version available on the Web, and it can always be regarded as the most current version.

For institutions which have limited communications access, for whatever reason, then regular guideline updates can be delivered on CD-ROM, or other high-capacity computer memory devices. This permits very large databases of information to be easily duplicated and disseminated at very little expense. Especially when the rate of change of information is slow, or communication costs are an issue, then this method of publication may prove to be more than adequate.

Consensus review

Statistical meta-analysis is one of the tools used to decide what constitutes 'best practice' on the basis of published clinical studies. There has to be a consensus process in which individual studies are selected to be pooled for such analysis. Equally, where the literature is equivocal about the best way to treat a condition, then decisions need to be based on other criteria. In both cases, it is important for experts to discuss and reach consensus.

Where discussions occur locally amongst members of an organization, then the process of organizing meetings for consensus review is demanding but not intrinsically difficult. Where team members live in many different countries, then the process becomes more challenging. As we will see in Chapter 21, communication technologies can help minimize the amount of travel that need occur in such circumstances. They can, for example, provide mechanisms for team members to collaborate remotely, through the electronic sharing of information and documents. The Internet is increasingly being used in this way.

As the number of bodies involved in protocol development grows, and the costs of travel and interaction rise, the use of communication technologies will of necessity increase. This will be driven not just by the need to minimize travel, but to speed up the sometimes lengthy process of creating protocols.

15.2 The design of protocols

Perhaps the most common criticisms of protocols are that they are inflexible or rigid, that individual patients do not always neatly fit the guidance recorded in a protocol or that the protocol is too difficult to use. The cause of this apparent rigidity can often be attributed to poor design. We saw in Chapter 11 that designing technological tools independently of the way that the tools will be used is likely to result in ineffective systems. Nevertheless, it is still a commonplace for those designing protocols to spend most of the time 'getting the evidence right' and ensuring the knowledge base of the system accurately reflects the best biomedical evidence, rather than focusing on interaction design and considering how the protocol will work in the clinical setting. Figure 11.1 shows us that there are many development steps at which a protocol can fail, most of which are unrelated to the 'purity' of the knowledge base behind the protocol, and yet can have a significant impact on the performance of the system, and its ultimate impact on clinical outcomes.

In the first chapter in this section, several forms of protocol representation were introduced, and the situations in which one could be favoured over another outlined. We can go further now, and state more general principles about design. In particular, the design of a protocol should reflect two things:

- It should prescribe care according to the best evidence available from clinical research and practice.
- It should be crafted to reflect the context within which the protocol will be used.

The contextual factors include the following.

The patient

Patients are rarely so accommodating as to present a typical pattern of disease. Health would be a simpler and more precise science if that were the case. In reality, patients present at different stages of an illness, with different underlying abilities to recover. They may also have a variety of different concurrent illnesses that mask the appearance of symptoms and signs or alter the course of their illness.

Even if it is clear which illnesses are present, the normal protocol for management of an individual illness may have to be changed because it will have adverse consequences for a particular patient. The potential for drug side effects and interactions are good examples of risks that cause treatment to be varied in individual circumstances. As a consequence, it is often important for a number of treatment options to be included in a protocol. The selection of particular options can then be made to reflect the individual circumstances of a patient.

Treatment goals

The goal of care for the same problem varies with the clinical situation. For example, in disaster situations, triage will be used to ascertain which patients receive immediate treatment, and which are unlikely to survive and should therefore be left untreated. The very same untreated patients may, in the context of a teaching hospital, receive complex and highly intensive therapy. Thus, the immediate circumstances of a situation dictate the goals of treatment. There is thus no absolute 'best' treatment. Notions of best treatment are always constrained by local goals.

Local resources

Local goals are also constrained by the resources available for treatment. Delivery of care in a resource-poor nation will reflect the resources available to it. Thus, there is little point in specifying protocols that cannot be carried out, because either equipment, medications, time, staff, money or other resources are unavailable. The management of diarrhoea, for example, will vary not just to reflect local disease patterns, but the scale of the problem and the availability of medication. A child returning home to a developed nation with possibly infectious diarrhoea will receive very different treatment from a child caught up in large-scale epidemic in a developing nation. The disease is the same, but the circumstances in which treatment occurs are not.

Staff

The skill level of the individuals required to carry out the protocol also affects the form and content of protocols. This affects everything from the words used in the protocol, which would vary for protocols designed for patients or members of the public, to the level of detail and goals of the protocol. In particular, the ability of an individual to recognize that the entry criteria for a protocol have been fulfilled is essential. There is little point in having a set of finely crafted protocols if it is unclear when they should be applied.

Local processes

Local care processes evolve to reflect not just best-practice knowledge, but local resources and goals. A protocol has to be designed with an understanding of how it will be used within such existing processes. Will it simply be looked at as a reference after an initial care plan has been drafted? In this case, protocols might be collected together into a small reference manual. Will it be used to drive every detail of a care process? If so, they might need to be crafted into the basic documentation used to plan and record the delivery of care. In each situation, the requirements for clarity, level of detail and availability are vastly different.

15.3 Protocol design principles

We can now begin to formulate a set of 'good design' principles for protocols, based on an understanding of the need to acknowledge the context of use.

Principle 1 Make any assumptions about the context of use explicit

We have seen that assumptions about the context of use made by a protocol's designer determine its utility in other contexts. The clearer one can be about the context within which a protocol is intended to be applied, the clearer it will be to others in slightly different circumstances whether that protocol can be re-used. Some of the assumptions about the context of protocol use are summarized in Table 15.1.

Table 15.1 A summary list of questions that help identify key assumptions about the context within which a protocol is to be used.

What is the goal of the protocol?
What are the protocol entry and exit criteria, and how will these be determined at the time of use?
Who will decide protocol entry, and who will apply the protocol?
What terminology will be understood by those using the protocol?
How much time will be available to follow the protocol?
What treatment resources are available, including medication and biomedical devices?
Are multiple treatment options to be considered?
How much detail should be included?
Which representation is most appropriate (e.g. flowchart, decision tree, rules)?
Will users wish to, or be able to, access the evidence used in creating the protocol?
How is the protocol to be used in the care process? For example, how is it to be accessed?
How is the protocol's performance to be reviewed, and how are variances to be recorded?
What mechanisms will be available to update the protocol?
How long should a protocol be in use before it is considered to be out of date?

Principle 2 A protocol should not be more specific than is necessary to achieve a specific goal

The more closely a protocol matches a specific local set of conditions, the less likely it is to be generally useful in others. This is an example of a general principle – the more specifically a method models a given situation, the more useful it will be in that situation, but the less useful it will be in others. The converse principle is that very general methods can be applied across many different situations, but will probably have only moderate utility in any one of them.

This, then, is an issue of identifying the appropriate level of detail for the task in hand. Excessive formalization for its own sake does not necessarily deliver any greater return, and may require unnecessary effort (Martin, 1995). It also may cause the disaffection of the staff who are required to use the protocol. Indeed, we know that if clinical guidelines are perceived to be unduly complex, then compliance rates by clinicians are lower (Grilli and Lomas, 1994).

Protocol designers should thus be aware of the degree of generalizability they will require of the protocol, and that the wider the expected adoption, the more likely it is that unduly specific instructions will cause difficulty at sites that have different local practices.

One technique that has been suggested for managing these difficulties is to initially specify a protocol only in general terms, and then instantiate it with local data. The specifics of individual steps are left to be decided on the basis of the details of individual clinical cases. For example, one might specify a treatment goal rather than a specific action. Thus 'establish normal blood pressure through intravenous fluid replacement' might be an appropriate goal for a protocol, rather than specifying exactly how much fluid is to be given. The actual amount of fluid given would be dependent on the specific needs of a patient. This technique is known as **skeletal plan refinement** (Tu *et al.*, 1989), and can be used to create quite sophisticated protocols that are highly flexible to individual patient needs. It is an example of the template-oriented structures introduced in Chapter 5.

Principle 3 Protocol design should reflect the skill level and circumstances of users

The level of description used in a protocol should also match the abilities of those using it. Very simple steps will probably be best for relatively inexperienced users. For example, protocols for first-aid resuscitation taught to the public are kept very simple. Protocols for trained paramedical or medical staff in exactly the same circumstances may be much richer and more complex, despite the similarities in overall goal.

Further, different protocol representations make different demands on those who use them. Mnemonic representations such as the 'ABC' of resuscitation have great value in stressful situations, but may not permit great detail to be recalled. Flowcharts require relatively little reasoning, and can be designed to make the decision logic extremely clear. Thus one might create a flowchart for situations in which the ability to understand the protocol is limited, such as an emergency situation, or when the user has had limited instruction. The flowchart representation can, however, become too complicated for complex decisions. In such cases, a rule-based representation is more likely to be used as a reminder for individuals who are under less pressure of time, or are better trained in the management of the situation.

Principle 4 Protocols should be constantly reviewed

As we saw in Chapter 11, human knowledge tends to decay with time as circumstances change. Part of the difficulty many people have with protocols is that they represent a snapshot in time of what some people consider the best way to carry out a task. Even assuming that there was universal agreement on that method, as time goes by, new ways will be developed that supersede the original protocol.

It is thus a mistake to consider a protocol as a piece of knowledge in isolation. The three-loop model conveys the manner in which protocols exist as part of an ongoing process of improvement. Protocols are simply the intermediaries in this overall process of treatment refinement based upon outcomes. Thus much of the rigidity that some see in the use of protocols lies not in the protocols themselves, but in the failure to update protocols as knowledge evolves over time. Consequently, one kind of protocol rigidity arises out of a failure to adapt over time. Introducing protocols without introducing processes to review the outcome of protocol-based care is a recipe for guaranteeing that protocols will be perceived to be increasingly inappropriate over time.

Discussion points

1. You have joined a working party that will produce expert guidelines in your area of clinical speciality. The team has agreed to devote all the working time to arriving at the consensus guidelines and writing them up for publication, but has allocated no time to thinking about design or dissemination issues. What will you advise them?
2. Design a protocol for a short common clinical process that is to be used by clinicians. Next, redesign the protocol assuming it is going to have to be read by clinically untrained individuals. What issues have guided the design choices you made?
3. Which is more complex – a protocol designed for a human to use, or a protocol designed to be used by a computer? Why?

Chapter summary

1 Protocols are used when a course of action can be prescribed ahead of time and when it is possible to access and apply the protocol. Failure to meet these conditions of **protocol designability** and **protocol usability** will cause difficulties.

2 The rapid transformation of clinical evidence into clinical process represents a major challenge in the following areas:
- supporting evidence gathering, pooling and dissemination, using systems such as the Internet
- facilitating consensus review amongst geographically remote peers through the use of communication technologies
- developing protocol representations and languages that permit large protocol databases to be built with some inherent error checking, and that also support active use of protocols in computer systems.

3 Some design principle for protocols include:
- Make assumptions about the context of use explicit.
- Protocols should not be more specific than is necessary to achieve a specific goal.
- Protocol design should reflect the skill level and circumstances of those using them.
- Protocols should be constantly reviewed.

PART 5

Language, coding and classification

CHAPTER 16

Terms, codes and classification

> By an almost instinctive impulse, similar to that which leads to the use of language, we are induced to collate or group together the things which we observe – which is to say, to classify them … to imagine them combined or grouped in a certain order. … Accordingly, every science and art has endeavoured to classify as completely as possible the things belonging to it; hence, in our field of enquiry, the objects classified are the phenomena and processes of the living body, diseases, remedies, the hundred influences and agencies of external nature, etc. *Oesterlen, Medical Logic (1855).*

Both conceptually and practically, the study of medical language is inescapably central to informatics. Theoretically, medical languages are the building blocks with which we construct and apply our models of health and disease. As such, they exert their influence at the very foundations of medical thinking.

In practice, administrative bodies increasingly require healthcare workers to codify their records using specialized words to permit auditing of their practices. National and international bodies seem to be constantly creating longer lists of words, often in open competition with one another. The support given to individual collections of words sometimes reaches near religious fervour.

So, the languages of medicine and healthcare attract great attention within informatics, and their development consumes much resource. In this chapter, the basic ideas behind terminologies, coding and classification will be explained. The next chapter examines some of the more important terminological systems, their uses and limitations. The concluding chapter in this part critically examines the scientific basis of these coding schemes, outlining the difficulties inherent in creating languages, and reviews the likely avenues for future development.

16.1 Language establishes a common ground

Human beings are designed to detect differences in the world. We distinguish different objects, name them and then categorize them. This process of discovering a difference between two things, and then giving them both names, is basic to the way in which we learn about the world, develop language and proceed to interact with the world (Wisniewski and Medin, 1994).

Unsurprisingly then, language evolves as we interact with the world, discovering new things about it and doing different things within it. However, this growth in language is tempered by the need to communicate with others and share our experiences. When members of different cultures wish to meet, they need to establish a linguistic common ground. To do this there must be some shared language, and agreement on the meaning of that shared language. There is little value in each of us developing a complicated set of words if no one else understands what they are intended to represent. Consequently, the sharing of words and the underlying concepts they represent constitutes an important part of human language development. Thus the natural drive to create new words is tempered by the need to communicate.

The story in healthcare is similar, with a long history of discovery and the creation of new ideas. As a consequence, the words used change both their meaning and their form over time (Feinstein, 1988). A clinician today has a very different understanding of the meaning of the word 'asthma' from one of even 100 years ago. Further, different cultures have different concepts of illness. Even amongst overtly similar western cultures there can be quite different notions of what constitutes a disease and what is normal. Hypotension (low blood pressure) is a routinely treated disease in some European countries, but regarded as within the bounds of normality in others.

Even amongst the different medical 'cultures' there are differences. Different groups of health professionals, from the medical specialities, through to nurses, medical economists and administrators, all evolve slightly different words or jargon.

Healthcare is a practical endeavour, and so in this respect practitioners want to be able to share the same vocabulary so that they can discuss and learn from one another. In an age where communication and travel have combined to unite the global medical community, the need to share knowledge through a common vocabulary has never been so great.

16.2 Common terms are needed to permit assessment of clinical activities

If the need for a common language was solely to permit discussion amongst different groups, then there would probably be little need for organized intervention. Language can be shared informally simply through common usage at meetings and in scientific publications. However, the enormous resources devoted to healthcare provision have made the need to control the delivery of care inescapable. To do this, there has to be some commonality to the way in which illness and care are described.

Consequently, much of the effort devoted to formal medical language development has been for the purpose of epidemiology, resource management and clinical audit. Audit is the process of assessing the outcomes associated with different diseases and their treatments. We can understand the audit process through the model–measure–manage cycle introduced in Chapter 9, which explains the basic process of system control.

To make all such assessments, it is first necessary to make measurements by pooling patient data. Although it is possible to compare patient outcomes on the basis of measurements obtained from instruments, for example serum biochemistry, these are rarely sufficient to describe a patient's state. In healthcare, language itself is often the basis of measurement. Words are needed to describe observed findings such as 'pitting oedema' or 'unconscious' and the diagnoses ascribed to these findings.

Yet the words used by people to describe conditions vary so much that simple analysis of their records is often not possible. Further, the meanings attached to the terms they use may vary. If there was an agreed set of terms to describe the process of care, then data analysis would be much simplified (Ackerman *et al.*, 1994). The goal in developing medical terminologies is to arrive at a consensus on the most appropriate set of terms and the way they should be structured.

Once they have been created, controlled terminologies can also be used in other, sometimes unexpected, ways. For example, if a set of clinical notes was created using standard words, then a computer system could check the words and issue alerts when it detected anomalies. It could check a patient's diagnosis against current treatments, and warn of any potentially dangerous side effects or drug interactions. If a computer system were to try to do the same by interpreting freely entered text, it would need to be a far more complicated system, able to understand the complexities of natural language. Such systems are still the subject of research, and unlikely to appear in clinical practice for many years, whereas the simpler word-based solution could in principle be applied now.

16.3 Terms, codes, groups and hierarchies

Medical terminologies (or nomenclatures), like all languages, start with a basic set of words or **terms**. A term, just like any normal word, has a specific meaning. In this case a term stands for some defined medical **concept** such as 'diabetes', 'tibia' or 'penicillin'.

Most languages permit words that have the same or similar meanings, and this is usually the case in healthcare too. To permit some flexibility, most medical languages allow the same concept to be named in several different ways. However, since several terms may be used for the same concept, it is usual to define a single alphanumeric **code** for every distinct concept in the language (Figure 16.1).

This gives rise to the process of **coding**, where a set of words describing some medical concept is translated into a code for later analysis. Thus a terminology should contain a separate name for each distinct disease entity, as well as any reasonable synonyms. A coding system may collect many such terms into a single code.

The terms and codes in different terminologies vary, depending on how they will be used. For example, if a coding system exists for epidemiological analysis, the concepts of interest are at the level of public health, rather than at the level of a particular clinical specialization.

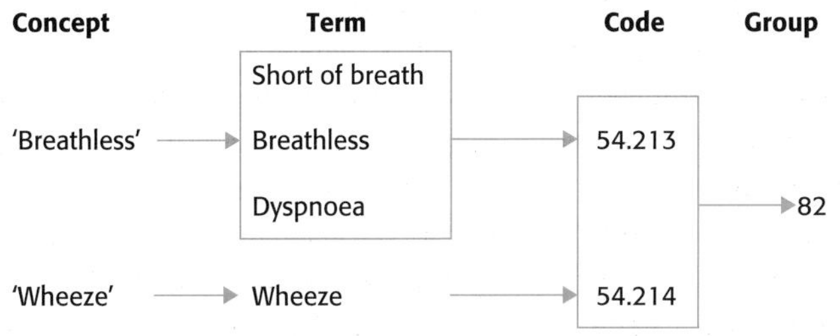
Concept
Term
Code
Group
Short of breath
'Breathless'
Breathless
54.213
Dyspnoea
82
'Wheeze'
Wheeze
54.214

Figure 16.1
Multiple terms may map on to a single numeric code in medical languages. Groups collect together similar codes for more coarse-grained analysis.

The level of detail captured in the codes would be much finer in the latter case, and the concepts would be different.

Terms and codes created at a level of detail that is appropriate for statistical analysis or patient management may be too fine-grained for other purposes. In particular, this information must be pooled to determine the cost of providing care and measure population health outcomes. A **group** thus collects together into a single category a number of different codes that are considered to be similar for the purpose of reimbursement (Figure 16.1).

The process of ascribing terms, encoding them, and then grouping them may seem unduly complex, potentially inefficient, and to some extent *ad hoc*. In the next chapter, where specific systems for each are described, this impression will be reinforced. Driven by practical necessity, terminological systems created for one purpose have been adapted, for example through the grouping process, to other quite different ones.

Classification hierarchies

Once a set of terms and codes are collected together, they can quickly become so large that it is difficult to find individual terms. Consequently, they need to be organized in such a way that the terms can be easily searched through.

Most people are familiar enough with alphabetically organized dictionaries as a way of looking up words. It is often the case that the words used by a person might be different to the terms in a system, or the term may not be known at all. Consequently a straightforward alphabetical listing of terms is of limited value. A terminology needs to be organized in a way that permits concept-driven exploration. For example, it should be easy to locate the word 'pericarditis' knowing that one is seeking a word describing inflammation of the pericardium. Thus, from a user's point of view, a terminology needs to be more like a thesaurus than a dictionary, organizing terms into conceptually similar groupings.

As we saw in Chapter 7, one of the most common ways to assist search is to produce a classification hierarchy. Everything from rocks and minerals, through to the elements and the species, is classified in some form of hierarchical structure. The essence of a hierarchy is that it provides a structured grouping of ideas, organized around some set of **attributes** or **axes**. In this way, the hierarchy begins to provide some meaning to terms through the way they are related to others. For example, in Figure 16.2, it is clear without knowing anything more about the term 'endocrinology', that it is a branch of clinical medicine, and not a part of healthcare administration.

Just as a hierarchy may serve as a map to help locate unknown terms, it can help uncover new relationships between concepts. Here the act of constructing the hierarchy is used to help map out possible relationships. For example, a researcher might try to arrange concepts in such a way that a deeper set of relationships becomes apparent. If this has explanatory power, then the classification system can then be used to direct further research, explain or teach.

The periodic table of elements, developed by Mendeleev, was used in this way. Atomic weights of the elements, along with some of their chemical properties, were the attributes used to construct the initial classification system. Where no elements were known to exist, gaps were left that were later filled as new elements were discovered. Further, the regularity of the table led to a deeper understanding of the underlying atomic structure of the elements. The periodic table is now a standard way of teaching the basics of atomic structure.

Thus, for most people, classification systems are invaluable in imparting knowledge about the relationships between related concepts, and are commonplace in scientific writing and textbooks.

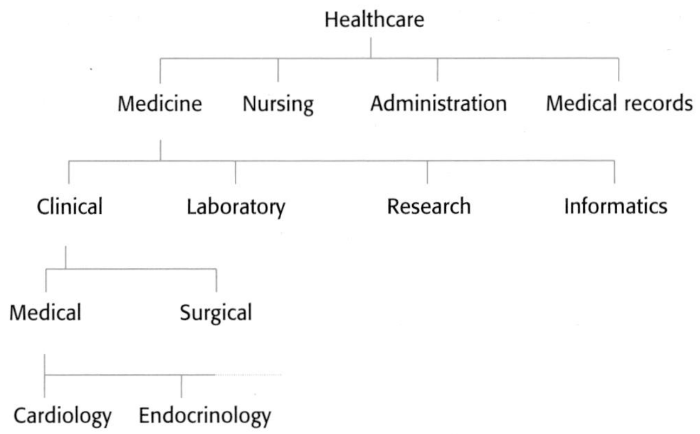
Healthcare
Medicine
Nursing
Administration
Medical records
Clinical
Laboratory
Research
Informatics
Medical
Surgical
Cardiology
Endocrinology

Figure 16.2 Classification hierarchies organize terms in some conceptual structure that gives meaning to terms through their relationship to other terms in the hierarchy.

Box 16.1 The basic level

When people are asked to name objects, they instinctively pick words that describe them at a level that is most economical, but still adequately describes their functionality. For example, people will usually use the word 'chair' in preference to the more general word 'furniture' which loses much sense of function, or the more specific description 'dining chair' which adds little.

This cognitively economic level of description has been called the **basic level** by Elanor Rosch, who developed her classification theory to describe this feature of human cognition (Rosch, 1988).

Rosch proposed that objects in the basic level have the quality that they are prototypic of their class. Such prototypic objects contain most of the attributes that represent objects inside their category, and the least number of attributes of those outside the category. Thus if people were asked to describe 'a chair' they would list a set of attributes that could be used to describe most, but not all, kinds of chair. A stool may be a special kind of chair, even though it does not have a back support which might be considered part of the features of a prototypic chair.

The basic level is thus formed around a natural word hierarchy based upon level of detail of description, coupled with utility of description. The basic level is therefore not absolute, but varies with the context within which a word is used. Sometimes 'dining chair' actually is the most appropriate description to use. Similarly, in some circumstances, it is sufficient to classify a patient as having an 'acidosis'. Clinically however, it is probably more useful to use a description like 'metabolic acidosis', which becomes basic in this context because it is at this level that treatment is determined.

The meaning of terms in a classification hierarchy is determined by the type of link used

There are many ways in which terms can relate to one another in a hierarchy, depending upon which attributes of the concept are of interest. In each case the meaning of the linkage between terms is different. For example, a hierarchy may describe the way a complex structure is assembled (Figure 16.2). Such a **part-whole** description might be used to describe anatomic structures, or the components of a device.

In contrast, in a **kind-of** (or **is-a**) hierarchy, elements are assembled because of some underlying similarity. For example, a drug such as penicillin is a kind-of antibiotic. It is also common in healthcare to use **causal** structures to explain how a chain of events might unfold. So for example, in Figure 16.3, a portion of the possible set of events starting with a plaque in a coronary artery and leading to an arrhythmia is described.

Each of these different types of link allows one term to inherit properties from other terms higher up in the hierarchy. What is inherited depends entirely on the type of link. So, for a part-of hierarchy, terms inherit their location from parent terms higher in the hierarchical tree. In kind-of hierarchies many different properties of parent terms are inherited by their children

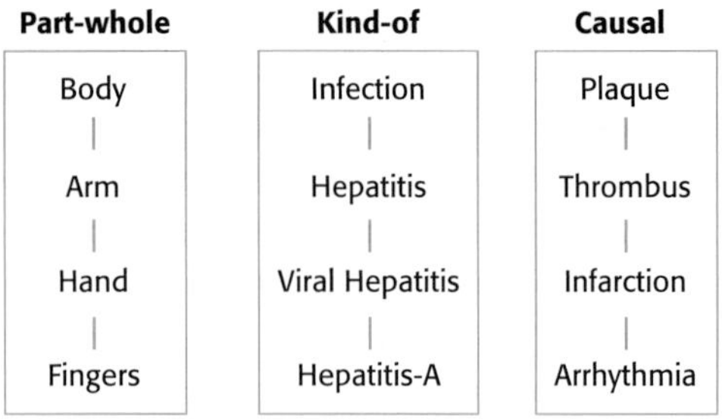
Part-whole
Body
Arm
Hand
Fingers
Kind-of
Infection
Hepatitis
Viral Hepatitis
Hepatitis-A
Causal
Plaque
Thrombus
Infarction
Arrhythmia

Figure 16.3 Depending on the type of attribute used to classify concepts, many different types of hierarchical structure are possible. Each type of link implies a different relationship between the terms in the hierarchy.

terms. Thus there are many chemical and pharmacological properties that amoxycillin inherits from the parent class of penicillins, and that the penicillins inherit from their parent class of antibiotics. Equally, in a causal structure one would not expect that the concept 'thrombosis' to be a kind of 'coronary plaque', but only that it takes its temporal ordering in a chain of events from it.

This leads to an obvious but critical point about classification hierarchies. For the meaning of terms in a classification system to be as explicit as possible, the links between terms should be as uniform as possible. In other words, if one is to be clear what properties a term can reasonably inherit from its parents, then the type of link being used should be clear. Confusion is easy, and it is common to see classifications mixing part-of and kind-of relations. Ideally, to ensure clarity of meaning, an individual hierarchy should either only use one kind of link, or be explicit about the kind of link being used.

Some complex medical terminologies permit multiple axes of classification within them. These **multiaxial systems** allow a term to exist in several different types of classification hierarchy, which minimizes duplication of terms, and also enhances the conceptual power of the system as a whole. So in a multiaxial system a term such as hepatitis could exist both as a kind-of infection, as well as a cause of jaundice.

16.4 Compositional terminologies create complicated concepts from simple terms

Most existing coding systems are **enumerative**, listing all the possible terms that could be used in advance. Terminology builders strive to make such systems as complete as possible, and to contain as few errors or duplications as possible. Understandably, as the numbers of terms in a system rise into the thousands, this task becomes increasingly difficult. Especially when there are many people contributing to a terminology, the natural tendency is to create slightly different terms for similar concepts.

This leads to redundancy in terms, or worse, partial overlaps. Equally, it is difficult to make sure that all the necessary terms in a given area have been produced. As we shall see in Chapter 18, these problems are inherent in the process of terminology creation, and to some extent will always exist. There are, however, ways of improving the situation, and minimizing these types of error.

One approach is to agree on a basic set of primitive terms, and assemble more complex terms from these as they are needed (Rector *et al.*, 1993). For example, 'acute bacterial

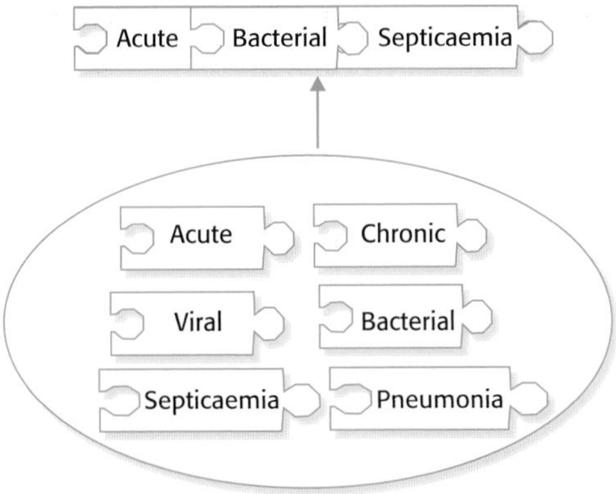
Acute
Bacterial
Septicaemia
Acute
Chronic
Viral
Bacterial
Septicaemia
Pneumonia

Figure 16.4 Compositional terminologies create complex terms from libraries of more primitive ones.

septicaemia' represents a distinct medical concept. An enumerative system would have to have a pre-existing code for this concept. With a **compositional** terminology, the system would generate the complex term from a set of more primitive components (Figure 16.4).

Indeed it should be able to generate many such specific conjunctions. In this way, there is no need to explicitly create all the needed terms in a field in advance, but merely to make sure that all the basic building blocks exist. This helps to minimize incompleteness in a terminology, and eliminates duplication or error in the more complex terms.

Since terms are assembled as they are needed, compositional systems need to try to check that the new compound terms are medically sensible (e.g. Glowinski *et al.*, 1991). For example, 'acute inflammation of the penicillin' is a meaningless term, as is 'viral tibia'. To prevent such composite terms being created, compositional systems need to have rules about the way in which terms can be combined. Suggested combinations are then checked against the rules before they are accepted. An example of such a rule might be that 'only a kind-of body part can be a part of another body part'.

In compositional systems these terms may correspond to concepts such as diseases and drugs, or to **modifiers** or **quantifiers** that describe them. Thus modifying words like 'acute', 'left', or 'proximal' need to be explicitly included in the list of basic terms. It is also necessary to construct rules about the way these modifying terms can be applied, e.g. that a term about duration such as 'acute' or 'chronic' cannot modify a drug. This would exclude a composite term such as 'acute penicillin'.

To do this **type checking**, the terminology builder has to say more about the type of each primitive term than would be needed for an enumerative list. For example, penicillin might be created as a term and the properties that it is a type of therapy, a drug, and a kind of antibiotic would all need to be listed.

Thus each primitive term is classified according to a number of different axes, and this information is used to ensure that any complex terms created from it are sensible. The terminology builder also has to create a library of rules that describes the way terms in the system can combine, which has its own difficulties in terms of completeness and accuracy.

16.5 Using coding systems

The process of using a terminology to generate codes is also complex. In an ideal world, the individual in need of the coded information is actually the person best qualified to assign the code, because there is a certain amount of subjectivity in the coding process. Data in a medical record, for example, needs to be interpreted before a diagnostic code is assigned. The act of interpretation will thus affect the codes selected. To ensure that this process results in codes best suited to the task at hand, those who understand that task should be involved in the code selection process.

Such involvement is not always the case. Medical administrators in a hospital, for example, may wish to code medical data in a certain way for an audit. By the time the coded data have reached the administrator, two different sets of people may have interpreted the data, and potentially introduced distortions into the final codes:

- First, the clinical staff have interpreted what they believe is important to be recorded when they create a record.
- Next, the staff responsible for coding then have to re-interpret this and try and find a set of codes that matches what they have understood the record to contain.

The situation is much improved in a primary care setting, where the coding might occur at the time the record is created. Even more ideally, some of the audit will also be carried out by the doctor creating the record and codes.

We can summarize these observations as follows:

- The quality of coding improves the closer it occurs to the point of information capture.
- The quality of coding improves if the individuals involved in the coding understand the purpose to which the coded data are to be put.
- The quality of coding improves if the staff doing the coding benefit from the coding.

The last point is an important one. If, for example, the burden of coding is shifted to clinical staff at the time of information capture, then they are being asked to carry out an additional task. If this task is for the benefit of others, for example administration, then they are less likely to carry the task out enthusiastically. They would be more enthusiastic if the data were to be used, for example, for a clinical trial in which they were personally involved.

It is one of the maxims of computer system design that if the problem owner is not the same as the user, then there is likely to be reluctance to accept a new computer system. This problem has long been recognized with clinical coding. The chief medical statistician for the World Health Organization's International Classification of Diseases noted in 1927 that

> administrative statistics have no value in the eyes of practitioners, who as a result are completely uninterested in it; whereas unless these practitioners provide exact data, then the scientific value of administrative statistics has to be called into question (Gregory *et al.*, 1995).

It is because of the burden that the coding process imposes that attempts have been made to reduce the effort involved by automating the process. There are actually several different ways that medical information can be converted into a set of coded terms. Each requires progressively less effort from the coder, and more effort from those that design the system supporting the coder.

- **Free code entry, with no support:** This is traditionally how coding has occurred. The coder has access to a list of codes, perhaps in a set of manuals, and access to some information, such as a medical record. It is up to the coder to interpret the content of the

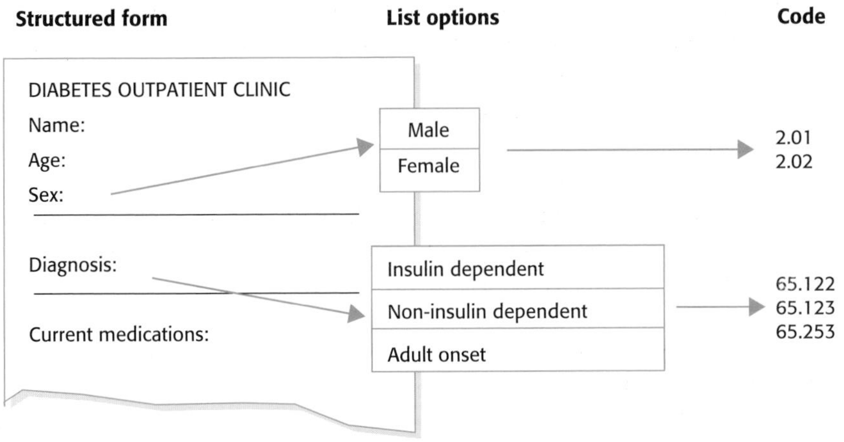
Structured form
List options
Code
DIABETES OUTPATIENT CLINIC
Name:
Age:
Sex:
Diagnosis:
Current medications:
Male
Female
2.01
2.02
Insulin dependent
Non-insulin dependent
Adult onset
65.122
65.123
65.253

Figure 16.5
Structured data-entry forms can offer a predetermined list of acceptable terms for given fields and these can then be converted to codes for later analysis. This minimizes, and to some extent hides, the effort involved in coding.

record, locate codes in the list that seem close to that interpretation and then assign the codes.

- **Free code entry with decision support:** The situation can be improved with tools to help navigate and explore the terminology system. For example, many medical terminologies are enormous, and finding appropriate codes is time consuming. Success is largely dependent upon an individual's experience and knowledge of the particular coding system. If computer tools permitted rapid exploration of a terminology with word searching and graphic visualization, then it is more likely that the coder will access the most appropriate codes (e.g. Hohnloser *et al.*, 1995; Tuttle *et al.* 1995). This can result in a significant increase in the quality of coding (Hohnloser *et al.*, 1996).
- **Semi-structured information entry:** In this approach, the act of coding occurs at the time of information capture. Data are entered on to a structured form, which has fields for the different pieces required. Wherever possible, the list of possible alternatives is specified for each field in the form (Figure 16.5). Thus in a diabetes clinic run by primary care nursing staff, the different types of diabetes would be listed as options against the diagnosis field on the form. Each diagnosis would be a recognized and codable term. Clearly this approach is well suited to computer automation, and different pick-lists of terms can be associated with fields in a form. The benefit of this approach is clear for situations in which there is a clearly defined context, and in which clear procedures are in place.
- **Automatic coding:** In situations in which it is harder to anticipate the type of information that will be captured, or the uses to which it will be put, the structured approach is inadequate. It would be ideal in these circumstances if there were a way to take a piece of text, and automatically encode it, using some type of computer system. To do this the computer coding system would need to be able to work with natural language with all its inherent complexities. It would also need to understand something of the medical context within which the information was recorded, since this too determines meaning. For example, the sentence 'The ventricle was traumatized' changes meaning depending upon whether the patient has had a chest or head injury.

At present, the design of computer systems capable of free natural language interpretation, especially in complex domains like healthcare, is a subject for ongoing research. With the arrival of robust natural language technologies, it may be that the very notion of coding as an explicit task disappears. From the human's perspective, the computer is simply assisting with the completion of the medical record.

Discussion points

1. Is it possible to build an EMR system without an accompanying terminology?
2. Get two people to independently create a short terminology to describe all the words associated with a simple domain like buying a theatre ticket or filling a car with petrol. Describe the similarities and differences between the two terminologies. Why do you think they are different?
3. Should clinicians be asked to code health records as they write them?
4. If coding is so critical to healthcare, why are clinicians so reluctant to assist in coding?
5. Compare and contrast enumerative and compositional terminologies on the basis of message structure (Chapter 5).

Chapter summary

1. Language evolves as we interact with the world, discovering new things about it. This growth is tempered by the need to communicate with others.
2. Medical language develops over time as new concepts emerge. At any one time, medical language varies between different individuals, institutions, specialities, and nations.
3. Most formal medical language development has been for the purpose of epidemiology, resource management and clinical audit. If there is an agreed set of terms to describe the process of care, then data analysis is much simplified. The goal in developing medical terminologies is to arrive at a consensus on the most appropriate set of terms and the way they should be structured.
4. Languages consist of a basic set of words or terms. To permit some flexibility, most medical languages allow the same concept to be named in several different ways. However, it is usual to define a single numerical code for every distinct concept in the language. A group collects together a number of similar codes and can be used for coarse-grained analysis.
5. Classification hierarchies are used to organize terms and codes in a way that permits them to be more easily accessed by those who use them. The type of link used in the hierarchy determines what meaning a term inherits from the terms above it.
6. A terminology can be enumerative, listing all possible concepts, or compositional, allowing complex concepts to be created from a set of more primitive components. In compositional systems, there is no need to create all terms explicitly in advance, but to make sure that all the basic building blocks exist. This helps to minimize incompleteness, and eliminates duplication or error in the more complex terms.
7. Coding of clinical concepts from the medical record can happen in a number of ways. Specialized staff can do the coding, or clinical staff can do it at the time they enter data into a patient record. Computer systems can be used to assist this process, or to automate it partially.

CHAPTER 17

Healthcare terminologies and classification systems

> The terms disease and remedy were formerly understood and therefore defined quite differently to what they are now; so, likewise, are the meanings and definitions of inflammation, pneumonia, typhus, gout, lithiasis, etc., different from those which were attached to them thirty years ago ... It is evident ... that great mischief will in most cases ensue if, in such attempts at definition and explanation, greater importance is attached to a clear and determinate, than to a complete and comprehensive understanding of the objects and questions before us. In a field like ours, clearness can in general be purchased only at the expense of completeness and therefore truth. *Oesterlen, Medical Logic (1855).*

Coding and classification systems have a long history in medicine. Current systems can trace their origins back to epidemiological lists of the causes of death from the early part of the eighteenth century. François Bossier de Lacroix (1706–1777) is commonly credited with the first attempt to classify diseases systematically (WHO ICD-10, 1993). Better known as Sauvages, he published the work under the title *Nosologia Methodica.*

Linnaeus (1707–1778) who was a contemporary of Sauvages also published his *Genera Morborum* in that period. By the beginning of the nineteenth century, the *Synopsis Nosologiae Methodicae*, published in 1785 by William Cullen of Edinburgh (1710–1790) was the classification in most common use.

It was John Graunt who, working about 100 years earlier, is credited with the first practical attempts to classify disease for statistical purposes. Working on his *London Bills of Mortality*, he was able to estimate the proportion of deaths in different age groups. For example, he estimated a 36% mortality for liveborn children before the age of 6. He did this by taking all the deaths classified as convulsions, rickets, teeth and worms, thrush, abortives, chrysomes, infants, and livergrown. To these he added half of the deaths classed as smallpox, swinepox, measles, and worms without convulsions. By all accounts his estimate was a good one (WHO ICD-10, 1993).

Only in the last few decades have these terminological systems started to attract widespread attention and resources. The ever-growing need to amass and analyse clinical data, no longer just for epidemiological purposes, has provided considerable incentive and resources for their development. Further, with the development of computer technology, there has been a belief that such widespread collection and analysis of data are now possible. In parallel, the requirement for clinicians to participate in that data collection has meant that they have had more opportunity to work with terminologies, and begin to understand their benefits and limitations.

In the previous chapter, the basic concepts of term, code and classification were introduced. In this chapter, several of the major coding and classification systems in routine use in healthcare are introduced, and their features compared. Some specific limitations of each system are highlighted. In reality there are a large number of such systems in development and use, and they cannot all be identified here. The systems discussed are, however, representative of most systems in common use, and can serve as an introduction to them. Throughout, a historical perspective is retained, since in this case the lessons of the past have deep implications for the present. The more general limitations of all terminological systems are addressed in the following chapter.

17.1 The International Classification of Diseases

Purpose

The International Classification of Diseases (ICD) is published by the World Health Organization (WHO). Currently in its tenth revision (ICD-10), its goal is to allow morbidity and mortality data from different countries around the world to be systematically collected and statistically analysed. It is not intended, nor is it suitable, for indexing distinct clinical entities (Gersenovic, 1995). The International Nomenclature of Diseases (IND) provides the set of recommended terms and synonyms that correspond to the entries classified in the ICD codes.

History

The ICD can trace its ancestry to the early days of healthcare terminologies. William Farr (1807–1883) became the first medical statistician for the General Register Office of England and Wales. On taking office, he found the Cullen classification was in use, but it had not been updated in accordance with medical advances, nor did it seem suitable for statistical purposes. In his first Annual Report of the Registrar General, he noted:

> The advantages of a uniform statistical nomenclature, however imperfect, are so obvious, that it is surprising that no attention has been paid to its enforcement in Bills of Mortality. Each disease has, in many instances, been denoted by three or four terms, and each term has been applied to as many different diseases: vague, inconvenient names have been employed, or complications have been registered instead of primary diseases. The nomenclature is of as much importance in this department of enquiry as weights and measures in the physical sciences, and should be settled without delay (WHO ICD-10, 1993).

Farr toiled hard at improving the classification, and by 1855 the International Statistical Congress had adopted a classification based on the work of Farr and Marc d'Espine of Geneva. Subsequently steered by Jaques Bertillon, this developed into the International List of Causes of Death. This was adopted in 1893, and continued to develop through the turn of the century and beyond, and ultimately evolved into the current ICD system.

In particular, the system was expanded to include not just causes of death, but diseases resulting in measurable morbidity. This expansion started with the urging of Farr. It was supported by Florence Nightingale, who in 1860 urged the adoption of Farr's disease classification for the tabulation of hospital morbidity in her paper *Proposals for a uniform plan of hospital statistics*. In 1900 at the First International Conference to revise the Bertillon Classification, a parallel classification of diseases for use in statistics of sickness was finally adopted.

Level of acceptance and use

The ICD today is used internationally by WHO for comparison of statistical returns. It is also adopted by many individual countries in the preparation of their statistical returns. Most other major classification systems endeavour to make their systems compatible with ICD, so that data coded in these systems can be mapped directly to ICD codes. ICD thus acts as a *de facto* reference point for many healthcare terminologies.

Classification structure

The ICD-10 is a multiple-axis classification system. At its core, the basic ICD is a single list of three alphanumeric character codes. These are organized by category, from A00 to Z99 (excluding U codes which are reserved for research, and for the provisional assignment of new diseases of uncertain aetiology). This level of detail is the mandatory level for reporting to the WHO mortality database and for general international comparisons.

The classification is structured into 21 chapters, and the first character of the ICD code is a letter associated with a particular chapter (Table 17.1).

Within chapters, the 3-character codes are divided into homogenous blocks reflecting different axes of classification. In Chapter I for example, the blocks signify the axes of mode

Table 17.1 The ICD-10 chapter headings (adapted from WHO ICD-10, 1993).

Chapter	
I	Infectious and parasitic diseases
II	Neoplasms
III	Diseases of the blood and blood forming organs and certain disorders affecting the immune mechanism
IV	Endocrine, nutritional and metabolic diseases
V	Mental and behavioural disorders
VI	Diseases of the nervous system
VII	Diseases of the eye and adnexa
VIII	Diseases of the ear and mastoid process
IX	Diseases of the circulatory system
X	Diseases of the respiratory system
XI	Diseases of the digestive system
XII	Diseases of skin and subcutaneous tissue
XIII	Diseases of musculoskeletal system and connective tissue
XIV	Diseases of the genitourinary system
XV	Pregnancy, childbirth and the puerperium
XVI	Certain conditions originating in the perinatal period
XVII	Congenital malformations, deformations and chromosomal abnormalities
XVIII	Symptoms, signs and abnormal clinical and laboratory findings
XIX	Injuries, poisoning and certain other consequences of external causes
XX	External causes of morbidity and mortality
XXI	Factors affecting health status and contact with health services of a person not currently sick

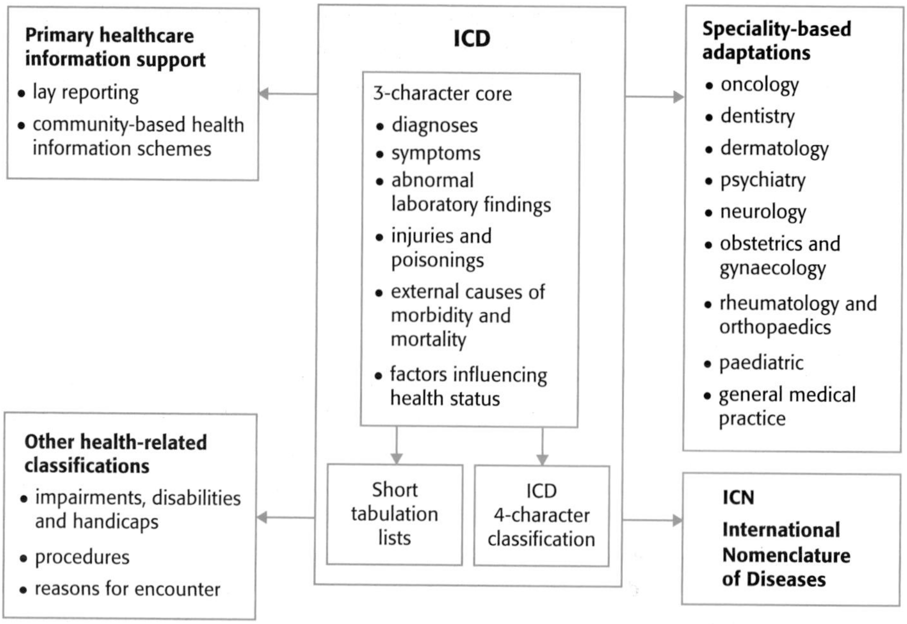
Primary healthcare information support
• lay reporting
• community-based health information schemes
ICD
3-character core
• diagnoses
• symptoms
• abnormal laboratory findings
• injuries and poisonings
• external causes of morbidity and mortality
• factors influencing health status
Short tabulation lists
ICD 4-character classification
Speciality-based adaptations
• oncology
• dentistry
• dermatology
• psychiatry
• neurology
• obstetrics and gynaecology
• rheumatology and orthopaedics
• paediatric
• general medical practice
Other health-related classifications
• impairments, disabilities and handicaps
• procedures
• reasons for encounter
ICN
International Nomenclature of Diseases

Figure 17.1 The ICD family of disease and health-related classifications (adapted from WHO ICD-10, 1993).

of transmission and of the broad group of the infecting organism. Within Chapter II on neoplasms, the first axis is the behaviour of the neoplasm, and the next is its site. Within all blocks some codes are reserved for conditions not specified elsewhere in the classification.

When more detail is required, each category in ICD can be further subdivided, using a fourth numeric character after a decimal point, creating up to 10 subcategories. This is used, for example, to classify histological varieties of neoplasms. A few ICD chapters adopt five or more characters to allow further sub-classification along different axes.

Since ICD continues to be used for ever-wider applications beyond its original intent, the WHO decided in the 10th revision to develop the concept of a family of related classifications surrounding this core set. This 'family' contains lists that have been condensed from the full ICD, and lists expanded for speciality-based adaptations (Figure 17.1). It also contains lists that cover topics beyond morbidity and mortality. For example, there are classifications of medical and surgical procedures, disablement and so forth (Gersenovic, 1995).

The International Classification of Functioning, Disability and Health (ICF) is a more recent member of the ICD 'family'. While ICD-10 focuses on classifying a patient's diagnosis, ICF is aimed at capturing a description of their capacity to function. ICF describes how people live with their health condition and describes body functions and structures, activities and participation. The domains are classified from body, individual and societal perspectives. Since an individual's functioning and disability occurs in a context, ICF also includes a list of environmental factors. The ICF is intended to assist with measuring health outcomes.

Limitations

The ICD has developed as a practical, rather than theoretically based, classification. There have been compromises between classification based on axes of aetiology, anatomical site and so on. Adjustments have also been made to it to meet the needs of different statistical applications beyond morbidity and mortality, for example social security. As such, the ICD exists as a practical attempt at compromise between various healthcare needs. Consequently, for many applications, finer levels of detail may still be needed, or other axes of classification required.

17.2 Diagnosis related groups

Purpose

Diagnosis related groups (DRGs) relate patient diagnosis to cost of treatment (Murphy-Muth, 1987; Feinstein, 1988). Developed in the United States by the Healthcare Finance Administration, DRGs were designed to calculate federal reimbursement for care delivered under the Medicare system. Each DRG takes the principal diagnosis or procedure responsible for a patient's admission, and gives it a corresponding cost weighting. This weight is applied according to a formula to determine the amount that should be paid to an institution for a patient with a particular DRG.

DRGs are also used to determine an institution's overall **case-mix**. The case-mix index helps to take account of the types of patient an individual institution sees, and estimates their severity of illness. Thus a hospital seeing the same proportion of patients as another, but dealing with more severe illness, will have a higher case-mix index. An institution's case-mix index can then be used in the formula that determines reimbursement per individual DRG. Unsurprisingly, different versions of the reimbursement formula favour different types of institution, and case-mix represents an area for ongoing debate and research.

History

In the mid-1970s the Centre for Health Studies at Yale University began work on a system for monitoring hospital utilization review (Rothwell, 1995). Following a 1976 trial of a DRG system, it was decided to base the final system on the ICD-9-CM which would provide the basic diagnostic categories. The ICD-9-CM (clinical modifications) classification was developed from the ICD-9 by the American Commission on Professional and Hospital Activities. It contains finer-grained clinical detail than the old ICD-9 (WHO, 1997), and along with its successor the ICD-10-CM, is intended for healthcare review and reimbursement use.

Level of acceptance and use

DRGs are used routinely in the United States for management review and payment. Given the importance of reimbursement worldwide, DRGs have undergone ongoing development, and have been adopted in one form or another in many countries outside the US.

Classification structure

Patients are initially assigned an ICD-9 CM or ICD-10-CM code. ICD CM is a multiaxial system closely based on the ICD structure. Diagnoses are then partitioned into one of about 23 major diagnostic categories (MDCs) according to body organ system or disease. The aim of this step is to group codes into similar categories that reflect consumption of resources and treatment (Figure 16.1). Codes are next partitioned on the basis of performance of procedures, and then the presence of complications, patient age and extended length of stay, before a DRG is finally assigned (Rothwell, 1995). There is thus a process of category reduction at each stage, starting from the many thousands of ICD codes to the few hundred DRGs:

$$\text{ICD CM} \Rightarrow \text{MDC} \Rightarrow \text{DRG}$$

Limitations

Given the local variations in clinical practice, disease incidence, patient selection, procedures performed, and resources, DRGs and case-mix indices will always only give approximate estimates of the true resource utilization. For example, should a hospital that is developing new and expensive procedures be paid the same amount as an institution that treats the same type of patient with a more common and cheaper procedure? Should quality of care be reflected in a DRG? For example, if a hospital delivers good quality of care that results in better patient outcomes, should it be paid the same as a hospital that performs more poorly for the same type of patient?

As importantly, those institutions that are best able to create DRGs accurately are more likely to receive reimbursement in line with their true expenditure on care. There is thus an implication in the DRG model that an institution actually has the ability to accurately assemble information to derive DRGs and a case-mix index. Given local and national variations in information systems and coding practice, it is likely that institutions with poor information systems will be disadvantaged, unless the information infrastructure across a region is a 'level playing field'.

Developments

DRGs are designed for use with inpatients. Accordingly, other systems have been developed for other areas of healthcare. Ambulatory visit groups (AVGs) have been developed for outpatient or ambulatory care in the primary sector. These are based on a patient's diagnosis, visit status and physician time. Given the increasing age of the population in developed countries, there is a tremendous ongoing cost that comes from the chronic care needed by the elderly. Consequently resource utilization groups (RUGs) have been developed to help determine the usage of long-term care resources. RUGs are based on the time spent by nursing home staff in caring for a patient.

17.3 Read codes

Purpose

The Read codes (now simply called the Clinical Terms in the UK) are produced for clinicians, initially in primary care, who wish to audit the process of care. The Clinical Terms Version 3 (CTV3) is intended, like SNOMED International, to code events in the electronic patient record (O'Neil *et al.*, 1995).

History

The Read codes were introduced in the UK in 1986 to generate computer summaries of patient treatment in primary care. In the subsequent revision Version 2, their structure was changed and based upon ICD-9 and OPCS-4, the Classification of Surgical Operations and Procedures. As Version 2 became increasingly inadequate, the UK's Conference of Medical Royal Colleges, and the government's National Health Service (NHS) established a joint Clinical Terms Project, comprising some 40 working groups representing the different specialities. This was subsequently joined by groups representing nurses and allied health professionals. Version 3 of the Read codes was created in response to the output of the Terms project.

Level of acceptance and use

Use of the Read codes is not mandatory in the UK. However, in 1994 it was recommended by the medical and nursing professional bodies as the preferred dictionary for clinical information systems. The Read codes have been purchased by the UK government and made Crown Copyright.

Classification structure

The Read codes have undergone substantive changes through their various revisions, altering not just the classification and terminological content, but also their structure. In Versions 1 and 2, Read was a strictly hierarchical classification system.

Read Version 3 was released in two stages and was a 'superset' of all previous releases, containing all previous terms, to allow backward compatibility with past versions. Version 3.0 is a kind of compositional classification system. As in SNOMED, a term can appear in several different 'hierarchical structures', classified against different axes. Unlike ICD or SNOMED, the codes themselves do not reflect a given hierarchy. They simply act as a unique identifier for a clinical concept. The 'hierarchy' exists as a set of links between concepts. Terms can inherit properties across these links. For example, 'pulmonary tuberculosis' may naturally inherit from a parent respiratory disorder or a parent infection term.

In Version 3.1, a set of qualifier terms such as anatomical site was added that can be combined with existing terms. When terms are composed, these composites exist outside of any strict hierarchy. To help in the combination of qualifiers with terms, they are grouped into templates. These capture some rules that help describe the range of possible qualifiers that a term in Read can take (Table 17.2).

Table 17.2 Example Read Version 3.1 template showing allowable combinations of terms with qualifier attributes, and attribute values (adapted from O'Neil *et al.*, 1995).

Object	Applicable attribute	Applicable values
Bone operation	Site	Bone, part of bone
Fixation of fracture	Reduction method	Percutaneous, open, closed
Fixation of fracture using intramedullary nail	Reaming method	Hand, powered rigid, powered flexible, etc.
Fixation of fracture using intramedullary nail	Nail type	Flexible, locking, rigid, etc.

The Read Codes Drug and Appliance Dictionary is part of the Clinical Terms and covers medicinal products, appliances, special foods, reagents and dressings. The dictionary is designed for use in software that requires capture of medication and treatment data such as electronic patient records and prescribing systems.

Like other major systems, Read offers mapping to ICD-9 codes to permit international reporting, and in some cases also provides ICD-10 mapping. A set of quality assurance (QA) rules have been developed for the Clinical Terms which are designed to check the clinical, drug and cross-mapping domains between the current and previous versions of the terms and other major terminologies like ICD-10, and for areas of overlap between the domains themselves (Schulz *et al.*, 1998). Each QA rule is written to interrogate the various files that make up the Read code releases and is designed to identify those concepts or terms that violate the basic structure of the Read codes.

Although Read Version 3 does not overtly emphasize axes of classification like SNOMED, both systems allow terms to be linked to each other and to inherit properties across those links. Therefore the underlying potential for expressiveness is the same at the structural level. Differences in the number and type of terms, and the richness of interconnections between them, are probably greater determinants of difference between these coding systems than any underlying structural difference. The presence of a fixed hierarchy, as we find with ICD or SNOMED, carries certain benefits of regularity when exploring the system. It also imposes greater constraints when it is necessary to alter the system because of changes to the terminology. In Read, this burden of regularity begins to be shifted to the rules guiding the composition of terms.

Limitations

The Read templates for term composition are limited in their ability to control combination. A much richer language and knowledge base would be needed to regulate term combination (Rector *et al.*, 1995).

17.4 SNOMED

Purpose

The Systematized Nomenclature of Medicine (SNOMED) is intended to be a general-purpose, comprehensive and computer-processable terminology to represent and, according to its creators, will index 'virtually all of the events found in the medical record' (Côté *et al.*, 1993).

History

SNOMED was derived from the 1968 edition of the *Manual of tumour nomenclature and coding* (MONTAC) and the *Systematized nomenclature of pathology* (SNOP). SNOMED International (or SNOMED III) is a development of the second edition of SNOMED, published in 1979 by the College of American Pathologists (CAP).

Table 17.3 The SNOMED International modules (or axes).

Module designator
Topography (T)
Morphology (M)
Function (F)
Diseases/diagnoses (D)
Procedures (P)
Occupations (J)
Living organisms (L)
Chemicals, drugs and biological products (C)
Physical agents, forces and activities (A)
Social context (S)
General linkage-modifiers (G)

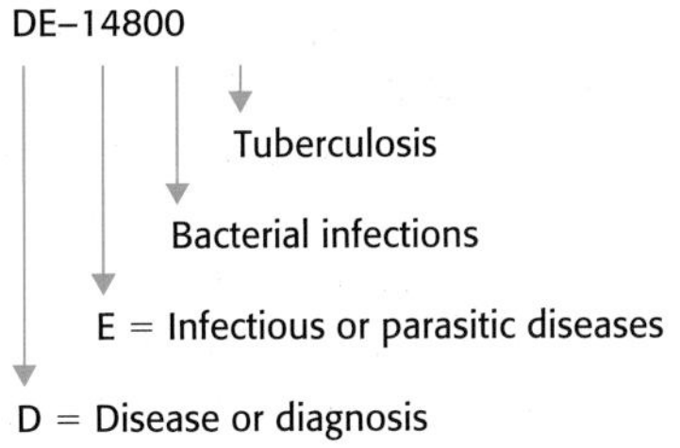
DE–14800
Tuberculosis
Bacterial infections
E = Infectious or parasitic diseases
D = Disease or diagnosis

Figure 17.2 SNOMED codes are hierarchically structured. Implicit in the code, tuberculosis is an infectious bacterial disease.

Table 17.4 An example of SNOMED's nomenclature and classification. Some terms (e.g. tuberculosis) can be cross-referenced to others, to give the term a richer clinical context (adapted from Rothwell, 1995).

	Nomenclature				Classification
Axis	T	+ M	+ L	+ F	= D
Term	Lung	+ Granuloma	+ *M. tuberculosis*	+ Fever	= Tuberculosis
Code	T-28000	+ M-44000	+ L-21801	+ F-03003	= DE-14800

Level of acceptance and use

SNOMED is reportedly used in over 40 countries, presumably largely in laboratories for the coding of reports to generate statistics and facilitate data retrieval. Although CAP is a not-for-profit organization, the cost of SNOMED licence fees may impede its more widespread adoption.

Classification structure

SNOMED is a hierarchical, multiaxial classification system. Terms are assigned to one of eleven independent systematized modules, corresponding to different axes of classification (Table 17.3). Each term is placed into a hierarchy within one of these modules, and assigned a five- or six-digit alphanumeric code (Figure 17.2).

Terms can also be cross-referenced across these modules. Each code carries with it a packet of information about the terms it designates, giving some notion of the clinical context of that code (Table 17.4).

Table 17.5 Comparison between implicitly coded information about 'postoperative esophagitis' in SNOMED III Codes and the explicit coding in SNOMED RT (from Spackman *et al.*, 1997).

Terminology	Code
SNOMED III termcode and English nomenclature:	D5 30150 Postoperative esophagitis
SNOMED III components of the concept:	T-56000 Esophagus M-40000 Inflammation F-06030 Post-operative state
Cross-reference field in SNOMED III:	(T-56000)(M-40000)(F-06030)
Parent term in the SNOMED III hierarchy:	D5-30100 Esophagitis, NOS
Essential characteristics, in SNOMED RT syntax:	D5-30150: D5-30100 & (assoc-topography T-56000) & (assoc-morphology M-40000) & (assoc-etiology F-06030)

SNOMED also allows the composition of complex terms from simpler terms, and is thus partially compositional. SNOMED International incorporates virtually all of the ICD-9-CM terms and codes, allowing reports to be generated in this format if necessary.

SNOMED RT (Reference Terminology) was released in 2000 to support the electronic storage, retrieval and analysis of clinical data (Spackman *et al.*, 1997). A reference terminology provides a common reference point for comparison and aggregation of data about the entire healthcare process, recorded by multiple different individuals, systems, or institutions. Previous versions of SNOMED expressed terms in a hierarchy that was optimized for human use. In SNOMED RT, the relationships between terms and concepts are contained in a machine-optimized hierarchy table. Each individual concept is expressed using a description logic, which makes explicit the information that was implicit in earlier codes (Table 17.5).

Limitations

It is possible, given the richness of the SNOMED International structure, to express the same concept in many ways. For example, acute appendicitis has a single code D5-46210. However, there are also terms and codes for 'acute', 'acute inflammation' and 'in'. Thus this concept could be expressed either as Appendicitis, acute; or Acute inflammation, in, Appendix; and Acute, inflammation NOS, in, Appendix (Rothwell, 1995). This makes it difficult for example, to compare similar concepts that have been indexed in different ways, or to search for a term that exists in different forms within a patient record. The use of description logic in SNOMED RT is designed to solve this problem. Further, while SNOMED permits single terms to be combined to create complex terms, rules for the combination of terms have not been developed and consequently such compositions may not be clinically valid.

17.5 SNOMED Clinical Terms

Purpose

SNOMED Clinical Terms (CT) is designed for use in software applications such as the electronic patient record or decision support systems, and to support the electronic communication

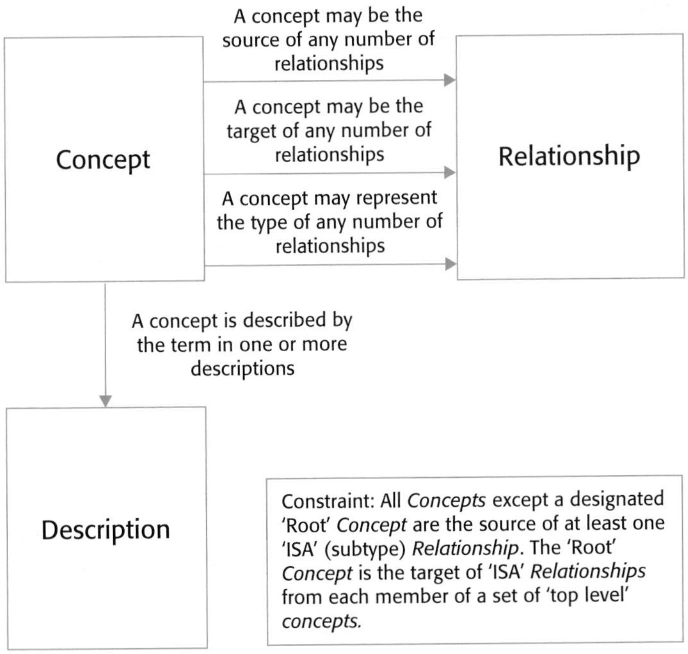
Concept
A concept may be the source of any number of relationships
A concept may be the target of any number of relationships
A concept may represent the type of any number of relationships
Relationship
A concept is described by the term in one or more descriptions
Description
Constraint: All *Concepts* except a designated 'Root' *Concept* are the source of at least one 'ISA' (subtype) *Relationship*. The 'Root' *Concept* is the target of 'ISA' *Relationships* from each member of a set of 'top level' *concepts.*

Figure 17.3
Outline of the SNOMED CT core structure (after College of American Pathologists, 2001).

of information between different clinical applications. Its designer's goal is that SNOMED CT should become the accepted international terminological resource for healthcare, supporting multilingual terminological renderings of common concepts.

History

In 1999 the College of American Pathologists and the UK NHS announced their intention to unite SNOMED RT and Clinical Terms Version 3. The stated intention in creating the common terminology was to decrease duplication of effort and to create a unified international terminology that supports the integrated electronic medical record. SNOMED CT was first released for testing in 2002.

Level of acceptance and use

SNOMED CT supersedes SNOMED RT and Clinical Terms Version 3. It will gradually replace Clinical Terms Version 3 in the UK as the terminology of choice used in the NHS.

Classification structure

The SNOMED CT core structure includes concepts, descriptions (terms) and the relationships between them (Figure 17.3). Like SNOMED-RT and Clinical Terms Version 3, SNOMED CT is a compositional and hierarchical terminology. It is multiaxial and utilizes description logic to explicitly define the scope of a concept. There are 15 top-level hierarchies (Table 17.6). The hierarchies go down an average of 10 levels per concept.

Table 17.6 The top-level hierarchies of SMOMED CT.

Procedure/intervention	includes all purposeful activities performed in the provision of healthcare
Finding/disorder	groups together concepts that result from an assessment or judgement
Measurable/observable entity	includes observable functions such as 'vision' as well as things that can be measured such as 'haemoglobin level'
Social/administrative concept	aggregates concepts from the CTV3 'administrative statuses' and 'administrative values' hierarchies as well as concepts from the SNOMED RT 'social context' hierarchy
Body structure	includes anatomical concepts as well as abnormal body structures, including the 'morphologic abnormality' concepts
Organism	includes all organisms, including micro-organisms and infectious agents (including prions), fungi, plants and animals
Substance	includes chemicals, drugs, proteins and functional categories of substance as well as structural and state-based categories, such as liquid, solid, gas, etc.
Physical object	includes natural and man-made objects, including devices and materials
Physical force	includes motion, friction, gravity, electricity, magnetism, sound, radiation, thermal forces (heat and cold), humidity, air pressure, and other categories mainly directed at categorizing mechanisms of injury
Event	is a category that includes occurrences that result in injury (accidents, falls, etc.), and excludes procedures and interventions
Environment/geographic location	lists types of environment as well as named locations such as countries, states, and regions
Specimen	lists entities that are obtained for examination or analysis, usually from the body of a patient
Context-dependent category	distinguishes concepts that have pre-coordinated context, that is, information that fundamentally changes the type of thing it is associated with. For example, 'family history of' is context because when it modifies 'myocardial infarction', the resulting 'family history of myocardial infarction' is no longer a type of heart disease. Other examples of contextual modifiers include 'absence of', 'at risk of', etc.
Attribute	lists the concepts that are used as defining attributes or qualifying attributes, that is, the middle element of the object–attribute–value triple that describes all SNOMED CT relationships
Qualifier value	categorizes the remaining concepts (those that haven't been listed in the categories above) that are used as the value of the object–attribute–value triples

SNOMED CT incorporates SNOMED RT and Clinical Terms Version 3 (Kim and Frosdick, 2001) as well as mappings to classifications such as ICD-9-CM and ICD-10. It is substantially larger than either SNOMED-RT or CTV3, containing over 300 000 concepts, 400 000 terms and more than 1 000 000 semantic relationships. SNOMED CT also integrates LOINC (Laboratory Observation Identifier Names and Codes) to enhance its coverage of laboratory test nomenclature. Most of the features of the parent terminologies are incorporated into SNOMED CT. For example the Clinical Terms Version 3 templates, although not explicitly named in the new structure, are essentially functionally preserved in SNOMED CT.

Limitations

Since SNOMED CT is a compositional terminology, there is strong requirement to prevent illogical compositions being created, and although a form of type checking is implemented, explicit compositional controls are not evident in the early releases of the terminology.

Reviewing a sample of 1890 descriptions obtained from the initial merging of the two parent terminologies found a 43% redundancy in terms (Sable *et al.*, 2001). Some terms were simply common to both parent systems, but many terms were problematic in some way. For example, some terms were either vague or ambiguous, used the logical connectors 'and' and 'or' incorrectly, had flawed hierarchy links or contained knowledge about disease processes that should have been beyond the scope of the terminology. Many of these problematic terms were identified automatically, but many others required visual inspection and discussion to be resolved. Although the process of merging the two terminologies has substantially improved the quality assurance standard of the resulting terminology, these problems raise many issues fundamental to terminology construction, which are discussed in the following chapter.

17.6 The Unified Medical Language System (UMLS)

Purpose

The Unified Medical Language System (UMLS) is the Rosetta stone of international terminologies. It links the major international terminologies into a common structure, providing a translation mechanism between them. The UMLS is designed to aid in the development of systems that retrieve and integrate electronic biomedical information from a variety of sources and to permit the linkage of disparate information systems, including electronic patient records, bibliographic databases, and decision support systems. A long-term research goal is to enable computer systems to 'understand' medical meaning.

History

In 1986, the US National Library of Medicine (NLM) began a long-term research and development project to build a unified medical language system (Humphreys and Lindberg, 1989).

Level of acceptance and use

Broad use of the UMLS is encouraged by distributing it free of charge under a licence agreement. The UMLS is widely used in clinical applications, and the NLM itself uses the UMLS in significant applications including PubMed and the web-based consumer health information initiative at ClinicalTrials.gov.

Classification structure

The UMLS is composed of three 'Knowledge Sources', a Metathesaurus, a semantic network and a lexicon (Lindberg *et al.*, 1993).

Table 17.7 A comparison of coding for four different clinical concepts using some of the major coding systems (National Centre for Classification in Health, Australia).

Clinical concept	UMLS	ICD-10	ICD-9-CM 4th edition	Read 1999	SNOMED International 1998	SNOMED CT 2002
Chronic ischaemic heart disease	448589 Chronic ischaemic heart disease	I25.9 Chronic ischaemic heart disease	414.9 Chronic ischaemic heart disease	XEOWG Chronic ischaemic heart disease NOS	14020 Chronic ischaemic heart disease	84537008 Chronic ischaemic heart disease
Epidural haematoma	453700 Haematoma, epidural	S06.4 Epidural haemorrhage	432.0 Nontraumatic extradural haemorrhage	XaOAC Extradural haematoma	89124 Extradural haemorrhage	68752002 Nontraumatic extradural haemorrhage
Lympho-sarcoma	1095849 Lymphoma, diffuse	C85.0 Lymphosarcoma	200.1 Lymphosarcoma	B601z Lymphosarcoma	95923 Lymphosarcoma, diffuse	1929004 Malignant lymphoma, non-Hodgkin
Common cold	1013970 Common cold	J00 Acute nasopharyngitis [common cold]	460 Acute nasopharyngitis [common cold]	XEOX1 Common cold	35210 Common cold	82272006 Common cold

The **UMLS Metathesaurus** provides a uniform format for over 100 different biomedical vocabularies and classifications. Systems integrated within the UMLS include ICD-9, ICD-10, the Medical Subject Headings (MeSH), ICPC-93, WHO Adverse Drug Reaction Terminology, SNOMED II, SNOMED III and the UK Clinical Terms. The 2002 edition of the Metathesaurus includes 873 429 concepts, 2.10 million concept names in its source vocabularies, and over 10 million relationships between them.

The Metathesaurus is organized by concept and does not include an over-arching hierarchy. It can be conceptualized as a web rather than as a hierarchical tree, linking alternative names and views of the same concept together and identifying useful relationships between different concepts. This method of structuring UMLS allows the component terminologies to maintain their original structure within UMLS, as well as linking similar concepts between the component terminologies.

Each concept has attributes that define its meaning, e.g. semantic types or categories to which it belongs, its position in the source terminology hierarchy and a definition. Major UMLS semantic types include organisms, anatomical structures, biological function, chemicals, events, physical objects, and concepts or ideas.

A number of relationships between different concepts are represented including those that are derived from the source vocabularies. Where the parent terminology expresses a full hierarchy, this is fully preserved in UMLS. The Metathesaurus also includes information about usage, including the name of databases in which the concept originally appears.

The UMLS is a controlled vocabulary and the **UMLS Semantic Network** is used to ensure the integrity of meaning between different concepts. It defines the types or categories to which all Metathesaurus concepts can be assigned and the permissible relationships between these types (e.g. 'Virus' causes 'Disease or Syndrome'). There are over 134 semantic types that can be linked by 54 different possible relationships. The primary link is the 'isa' link, which establishes the hierarchy of types within the Network. A set of non-hierarchical relations between the types includes 'physically related to', 'spatially related to', 'temporally related to', 'functionally related to', and 'conceptually related to'.

The **SPECIALIST Lexicon** is intended to assist in producing computer applications that need to translate free-form or natural language into coded text. It contains syntactic information for terms and English words, including verbs that do not appear in the Metathesaurus. It is used to generate natural language or lexical variants of words, e.g. the word 'treat' has three variants that all have the same meaning as far as the Metathesaurus is concerned: treats, treated or treating.

Limitations

The very size and complexity of the UMLS may be barriers to its use, offering a steep learning curve compared to any individual terminology system. Its size also poses great challenges in system maintenance. Every time one of the individual terminologies incorporated into UMLS changes, technically those changes must be reflected in the UMLS. Consequently regular and frequent updates to the UMLS are issued, and as the system grows the likelihood of errors being introduced will increase, as we see in the next chapter.

The richness of the linkages between concepts also offers subtle problems at the heart of terminological science. For example, the 'meaning' of a UMLS concept comes from its relationships to other concepts, and these relationships come from the original source terminologies. However, a precise concept definition from one of the original terminologies like ICD or SNOMED may be blurred by addition of links from another terminology that contains a similar concept (Campbell *et al.*, 1998). For example, 'gastrointestinal transit' in the Medical Subject Headings (MeSH) is used to denote both the physiological function and the diagnostic measure (Spackman *et al.*, 1997).

Since UMLS is not designed to contain an ontology, which could aid with conceptual definition, it is difficult to control for such semantic drift.

17.7 Comparing coding systems is not easy

It is beguiling to try to compare the utility of different coding systems, but such comparisons are often ill-considered. This is because it is not always obvious how to compare the ability of different systems to code concepts found in a patient record. For example, Campbell and Payne (1994) reported results of using various systems to code terms found in selected problem lists from US patient records. They assessed that ICD-9-CM and Read Version 2 'perform much more poorly for problem coding' than either SNOMED or the UMLS systems. As a consequence they concluded that 'both UMLS and SNOMED are more complete than alternative systems' when developing computer-based patient records.

Such generalizations are not meaningful. For one reason, term requirements vary from task to task. Indeed, terms develop out of the language of particular groups on particular tasks. It is thus not meaningful to compare performance on one task and deduce that tests on other tasks will have similar outcomes.

As critically, term use will vary between user populations. The terms used in a primary care setting will differ from those used in a clinic allied to a hospital, reflecting different practices and patient populations. Differing disease patterns and practices also distinguish different nations. A system like Read Version 2, designed for UK primary care, may not perform as well in US clinics as a US-designed system. The reverse may also be true of a US-designed system applied in the UK.

In summary, coding systems should be compared on specified tasks and contexts, and the results should only cautiously be generalized to other tasks and contexts. Equally, the poor performance of coding systems on tasks outside the scope of their design should not reflect badly on their intended performance.

Discussion points

1. How likely is it that a single terminology system will emerge as an international standard for all clinical activities?
2. Take the two terminologies created from the discussion section of the previous chapter, and now merge the two into one common terminology. As you go, note the issues that arise, and the methods you used to settle any differences. Explain the rational (or otherwise) basis for the merger decisions.
3. You have been asked to oversee the transition from ICD-9-CM to ICD-10-CM at your institution. What social and technical challenges do you expect to face? How will you plan to deal with them?
4. Many countries will take a major terminology such as ICD and customize it to suit their local needs. Discuss the costs and benefits of this approach from an individual country's point of view. What might the impact of localization be on the collection of international statistics?

Chapter summary

1. The International Classification of Diseases (ICD) is published by the World Health Organization. Currently in its tenth revision (ICD-10), its goal is to allow morbidity and mortality data from different countries around the world to be systematically collected and statistically analysed.
2. Diagnosis related groups (DRGs) relate patient diagnosis to cost of treatment. Each DRG takes the principal diagnosis or procedure responsible for a patient's admission, and is given a corresponding cost weighting. This weight is applied according to a formula to determine the amount that should be paid to an institution for a patient with a particular DRG. DRGs are also used to determine an institution's overall case-mix.
3. The Systematized Nomenclature of Medicine (SNOMED) is intended to be a general-purpose, comprehensive and computer-processable terminology. Derived from the 1968 edition of the *Manual of Tumour Nomenclature and Coding*, the second edition of SNOMED International is reportedly being translated into 12 languages.
4. The Read codes (or Clinical Terms) are produced for clinicians, initially in primary care, who wish to audit the process of care. Version 3 is intended, like SNOMED International, to code events in the electronic patient record.
5. SNOMED Clinical Terms merges Read codes and the SNOMED Reference Terminology (RT) and is intended by its designers to become the international standard clinical terminology.
6. The Unified Medical Language System (UMLS) provides a map between 100 individual terminology systems.
7. Coding systems should be compared on specified tasks, and results should only cautiously be generalized to other tasks, and populations. Equally, the poor performance of coding systems on tasks outside their design should not reflect badly on their intended performance.

CHAPTER 18

The trouble with coding

> The problem was that every system of classification I had ever known in biology or in physical science was designed for mutually exclusive categories. A particular chemical element was sodium, potassium or strontium, but not two of those, or all three. An animal might be a fish or fowl, not both. But a patient might have many different clinical properties simultaneously. I wanted to find mutually exclusive categories for classifying patients, but I could not get the different categories separated. They all seemed to overlap, and I could find no consistent way to separate the overlap. *Feinstein, Clinical Judgement (1967), p. 10.*

Terminological systems such as those described in the previous chapter are usually created with a specific purpose in mind. ICD was created to collect morbidity and mortality statistics. The Read codes were initially developed for primary care physicians, and SNOMED was originally developed to code pathological concepts. As these systems grow in size, and as their use becomes widespread within their intended domain, it becomes increasingly tempting to re-use them for other tasks.

As a consequence, some terminological systems have been redeveloped to become general-purpose coding systems. It is often a declared intention in the evolution of such general-purpose systems that they become complete and universal healthcare languages. Systems like SNOMED or Read should be able, for example, to describe all the necessary concepts that might be found in a patient record.

Recent advances in terminological research, as well as evidence from related disciplines, do not support such a goal. As we will see in this chapter, current thinking suggests that the goal of constructing a complete and universal thesaurus of healthcare terms is ill-posed. Terminology evolves in a context of use, and attempting to define a general-purpose or context-independent terminology is ultimately implausible. Coupled with this view comes the pragmatic understanding that any terminology we build will always be imperfect.

Each of these important issues deserves to be examined in some detail. This chapter first looks at the theoretical limitations facing all terminology constructors. It then moves on to examine how, given these limitations, terminological systems can be built that perform acceptably and at a reasonable cost.

18.1 Universal terminological systems are impossible to build

The ideal terminological system would be a complete, formal and universal language that allowed all healthcare concepts to be described, reasoned about and communicated. Some researchers have explicitly asserted that building such a singular and 'correct' language is their goal (Cimino, 1994; Evans *et al.*, 1994).

This task emphasizes two clear requirements: the ability for the terminological language to cover all the concepts that need to be reasoned about, and the independence of the terminology from any particular reasoning task. A further goal occasionally articulated is that, where alternative terminologies exist, they must be logically related so that one can be translated into the other. For example, if a set of clinical codes is extracted from a patient record, those codes could then be translated into ICD codes or DRGs.

Despite the enormous healthcare investment devoted to achieving these goals, current evidence indicates that they are not possible. There is no pure set of codes or terms that can be universally applied in healthcare. There is consequently no universal way in which one healthcare language can be mapped on to another.

There are two fundamental and related obstacles to devising a universal terminological system. The first is the **model construction** problem. Terminologies are simply a way of modelling the world, and as we saw in Chapter 1, the world is always richer and more complex than any model humans can devise. The second is the **symbol grounding** problem. The words we use to label objects do not necessarily reflect the way we think about the objects, nor do they necessarily reflect defined objects in the real world (Norman, 1993). The cumulative evidence from recent thinking in cognitive science, computer science and artificial intelligence provides a formidable set of supporting arguments. Each of these major issues will now be examined in a little more detail.

Terms are subjective

It is perhaps intuitive to think that the words we use correspond to objective and clearly definable parts of the world. Words should clearly correspond to observable objects. However, cognitive studies of the way people form word categories have shifted us from the view that categories exist objectively. Research suggests that concepts are relative, and are structured around probabilistic prototypes.

These concept prototypes at the **basic level** are the product of pooling many examples observed from the world (Box 16.1). They capture aspects common to all the examples. Equally, they exclude aspects that are not universally shared. Thus the qualities of prototypical categories are only generally true of the examples they classify (Figure 18.1). For example, most people would happily say that flight was a property of birds, and cope with the fact that some birds are flightless. The category 'bird' has no pure definition. By implication, the same must be true of the words used by people in healthcare. Thus the term 'angina' actually corresponds to a wide variety of different presentations of pain. Students will be taught the classical presentations of angina, but will with clinical experience quickly learn that there are many variations to the general case.

Concept creation is thus a process of generalization from example. The creation of concept prototypes is an ongoing part of human activity, as language tracks changes in our way

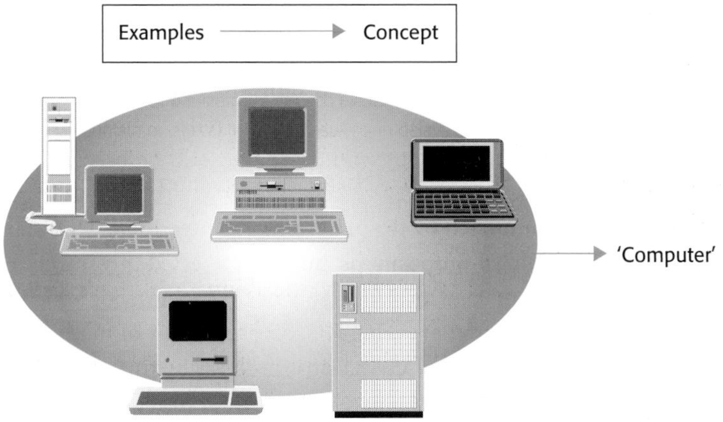
Examples
Concept
'Computer'

Figure 18.1
Word concepts are created to describe classes of objects that have similar but not identical characteristics. Individual examples of the concept may have unique properties that are not shared by other examples that also fall into their class.

of viewing the world. The way in which people use resemblances amongst a group of examples to create general categories remains an area of ongoing research (e.g. Ahn and Medin, 1992). We also saw in Chapter 16 that different hierarchies can be created, depending on the attributes used to link the terms. Selecting a different set of attributes from the same object will probably result in a different categorization structure. Categories may also overlap, and objects might fit into several different categories.

From the point of terminological construction, this means that there can be no clean set of terms that clearly demarcate different concepts. Concepts overlap, and so do terms. There thus can be no objective classification model. Many artificial intelligence researchers agree, arguing that there is no objective model of clinical knowledge. Much of this is based on their experiences in constructing and maintaining knowledge-based systems (Clancey, 1993a, 1993b).

Terms are context-dependent

A consequence of this process of category formation is that there is no stable notion of the 'correct' category for objects or events. The best category to describe an object depends entirely on the context within which it is applied. Thus patients might be categorized as 'elderly' if they are over the age of 70. If a woman is having her first child, however, the term 'elderly' primpara might be given to her if she is over 35. The notion of elderly varies with the context within which one operates. We thus choose attributes of an object or event that are of interest to us in a given context, and use these to place it in a category.

Context-dependence has several implications. Firstly, automatically extracting coded terms from a patient record will be difficult. This requires the ability to understand the wider context surrounding a term. Is a 'ventricle' in the heart or the brain? In the sentence 'I spoke to him' the meaning of the word 'him' depends on information that exists outside the sentence.

As a result, a computer system would need to have a considerable amount of knowledge about healthcare and language before it could successfully interpret much of the patient record. Secondly, if a term is used in a variety of different contexts, then the term may have a different meaning across these contexts. Pooling data coded by terms thus might risk grouping together quite different things.

Terms are purposive

We have already seen that categories can be quite indistinct things, and that category assignment varies depending on context. Both these issues are reflections of the underlying principle that words are created with the intention that they will be used in a particular way. Language is created for a purpose.

This perspective was illuminated by the philosopher Wittgenstein, who started his career searching for pure philosophical propositions, but soon rejected this search. He was unable to conceive of concepts or language independently of the purpose for which they were created. He thus came to understand that even fields like philosophy or mathematics were actually sets of techniques. They were not collections of objective truth, but knowledge about ways of doing things. It followed that their words were no less subjective.

He invented what are known as language games, in which a language was created for some tightly defined purpose. The essential point of these games was that one could not describe the language without mentioning the use to which it was put. Wittgenstein used these games to help free us from considering language in isolation from the purpose for which it was created (Wittgenstein, 1953; Monk, 1990).

Healthcare, unlike mathematics or philosophy, has always been an applied field. Here, more than in most areas of endeavour, it should be clear that our technical terms and words are created to be applied.

Even the apparently most precise clinical concepts usually have edges that are demarcated through use. The concept of a bone fracture, for example, may seem to be a quite distinct concept, but the dividing line between a normal and a fractured bone is quite unclear. As we move from X-rays to CT and MRI scans, the ability to categorize a bone as being fractured increases. The limit of definition is thus actually dependent on the limit of detection.

Further, the lengths we go to in the detection of a fracture depend entirely on the purpose at hand, which is usually to treat. Thus, if cellular studies of bone activity could detect fine fractures that were not visible by other means, would patients investigated in this way be classed as having a fracture? If their management were different, then they would probably be categorized in a quite different way.

In healthcare, one way to deal with this lack of clarity is to create artificial definitions of disease concepts with a purpose in mind. For example, 'hypertension' might be defined as 'the measurement of a blood pressure greater than 140/90 mmHg, on three separate occasions, with the reading taken with the patient having been at rest for 5 minutes'. The purpose of such definitions is to identify patients with clinical conditions that can be treated. These definitions are usually based on observations or measurements. They are constructed in such a way that, on the basis of statistical studies, most patients with the condition will be included within the definition. In this way, healthcare is seen to replicate in a formal way the innate human process of category formation, which is also founded on some quasi-probabilistic basis.

The implication here is that terminologies are most likely to be of value if they are created with a specific purpose in mind. Consequently, a general-purpose terminology will always fail to meet many of the specific needs of different situations, because these cannot be anticipated without specific examination of individual uses.

This is true both of the kinds of concepts represented in a terminology, as well as the level of detail of terms. In general, people choose categories to describe events or objects at a level of description that is most appropriate for thinking about them in a given situation (Rosch, 1988).

A general-purpose terminology will thus always have difficulty matching its level of detail to that needed in specific situations.

This also means that general categories are of little use. It is understood from the field of knowledge representation that the more general a concept is, the less it says about the world, and the weaker its descriptive power. The corollary is that more specific concepts have a much greater power of description. Consider the difference between describing a patient as being 'sick' or as 'hypertensive'. Both might be correct, but the one that is most specific to the patient is the most useful. The general category of 'sick' would describe most patients, and so carries very little descriptive power with it.

Consequently it does not make sense to think of terminological systems developing independently of a context of use. Even those who seek to build a canonical health terminology are forced to select a clinical application to set a context before they can meaningfully proceed (e.g. Friedman *et al.*, 1995).

Terms evolve over time

The terms used in healthcare have evolved over many years and are subject to the same process of cognitive evolution that affects all human language. Disease entities exist for as long as they are useful mental constructs, and are replaced as better concepts emerge. There is no static body of healthcare knowledge.

Not only are new concepts added; often the very structure of clinical knowledge changes as concepts are internally reorganized (Clancey, 1993b; Feinstein, 1988). Many diseases that were commonly discussed a century ago would not be recognized by healthcare workers today. Indeed, since the first ICD was created at the turn of the century with several hundred concepts, the growth in clinical knowledge has expanded the current ICD to contain over 6000 concepts. More recently the process seems to have accelerated. ICD-9 and ICD-10 are substantially different systems, partly because of the changes in healthcare over the 15-year period in which ICD-10 was built (CCC, 1995).

A consequence of the changing state of clinical knowledge is that any attempt at modelling clinical knowledge by the imposition of a structure on its terms will decay in accuracy over time (see Chapter 11). As soon as a terminology is created, knowledge begins to evolve away from that structure (Hogarth, 1986; Tuttle and Nelson, 1994).

Different systems may not correspond directly

Equally, there is no reason to expect that there is any uniform mapping between terminological systems developed in different contexts of use (Glowinski, 1994; Tuttle, 1994). Should one expect, for example, that every concept in ICD should naturally find a corresponding concept in Read or SNOMED? Although there are often clear correspondences, the mapping is never complete. The greater the difference in purpose for which these systems are created, the greater is the mismatch.

The reason that the ICD seems to serve as a common reference system is that it is created at a relatively general level of description. Other systems such as Read or SNOMED tend to be more fine-grained in their terms. Consequently it is more likely that one can find a general ICD category that matches a more specific category within these other systems. Such a translation from specific to general will lose some of the detail and meaning from the original term. As long as this suits the purpose of the translation, it is tolerable. For example, if one wanted to convert a detailed coding of a patient created for clinical purposes into more general ICD categories to create a morbidity report, then the loss of detail is appropriate.

However, even when the systems are of similar construction, problems are encountered when one tries to translate knowledge expressed in one form into another. The authors of one study concluded that sharing knowledge between terminological systems 'does not seem to be easily achievable' (Heinsohn *et al.*, 1994).

18.2 Building and maintaining terminologies is similar to software engineering

Although coding systems can never be truly canonical, they still provide a practical basis for managing the language of healthcare. However, it has to be understood that they define a limited and consensual language that will continually have to be modified. This modification is a predictable consequence of the subjectivity of knowledge. Whenever a knowledge base is applied to a task outside its intended use, it will require change (Clancey, 1993a).

SNOMED, for example, was initially developed to classify pathological items. It has now been expanded to produce a general-purpose system for all of healthcare. However, a study of SNOMED's utility in coding nursing reports found it coded only about 69% of terms, with the implication that the missing terms would need to be added (Henry *et al.*, 1993). Such additions are required every time a terminology is applied to a new area, making the task of updating problematic (Cimino and Clayton, 1994).

Eventually, as a terminology is continually expanded into new areas, its fundamental organizational structure will be altered to reflect the different structure of these new areas (Clancy, 1993b). The process of growth and alteration of terminology introduces huge problems of maintenance, and the very real possibility that the system will start to incorporate errors, duplications and contradictions.

If we simply think of terminologies as computer programs then we already know that continued modification is a poor development strategy. Software engineering tells us that the best time to modify a program is early in the development cycle. In Figure 11.1 the cost of error removal is shown to grow exponentially during the development of a computer program. Further, the times at which errors are introduced and detected are different. Thus an error introduced during the initial functional specification of a program is likely to be detected only when the system is completed and in regular use. At this time, the users will suggest ways in which the system's actual functionality, and the functionality they expected, differs.

Introducing changes into a mature system thus becomes increasingly expensive over time (Littlewood, 1987). As a corollary, maintaining a terminological system will become increasingly expensive over time. Consequently, we have probably reached the stage where uncontrolled addition of terms to existing large thesauri will soon no longer be acceptable. Those who pay for their maintenance will be faced with ever-increasing costs. To manage these costs, one would need to measure the performance of a thesaurus on a particular task, and then determine whether proposed additions or alterations will improve that performance, and at what cost.

18.3 Compositional terminologies may be easier to maintain over time despite higher initial building costs

In the longer term, new approaches are needed. Most existing coding systems are enumerative, listing out all the possible terms that could be used in advance. In the compositional approach introduced in Chapter 16, terms are created from a more basic set of components that may be more practical to build, maintain and use (Rector *et al.*, 1993; Glowinski, 1994).

There are two broad hypotheses behind the compositional proposal. The first is an engineering hypothesis – that compositional systems are easier and cheaper to maintain and update than enumerative ones. The second one is that compositional systems somehow represent a deeper form of knowledge. The first hypothesis has merit, but the second is somewhat more contentious. Each of these claims will now be examined in some more detail.

Maintenance costs may be lower for compositional terminologies than for enumerative systems

As we have seen, terminological systems continually require extensions and alterations that will, over time, introduce inconsistencies to the system. As an enumerative terminology gets bigger, the cost of finding and repairing these inconsistencies increases.

Any change in a concept must also be reflected throughout the enumerative system. For example, if a disease entity is redefined into two related diseases, then every term that exists for the original disease will need to be changed. In contrast, most terms in a compositional system are generated from simpler ones. Thus, one may only need to change the core terms associated with the disease. These alterations can be immediately reflected in any new term generated. As a consequence, fewer changes will be required in a compositional system (Figure 18.2).

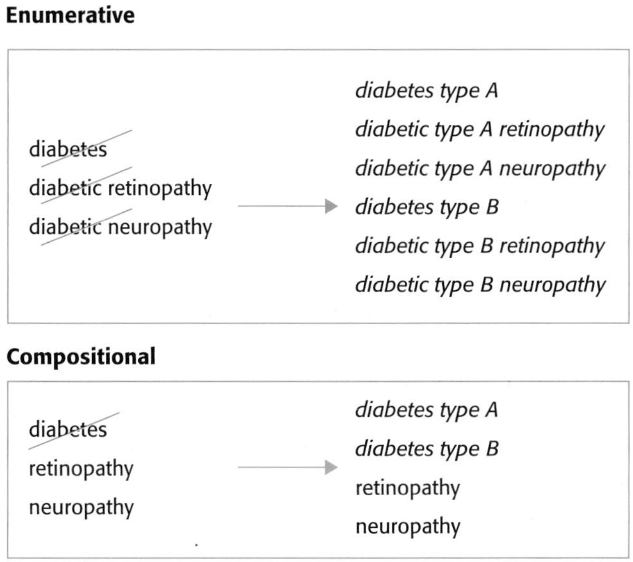
Enumerative
diabetes
diabetic retinopathy
diabetic neuropathy
diabetes type A
diabetic type A retinopathy
diabetic type A neuropathy
diabetes type B
diabetic type B retinopathy
diabetic type B neuropathy
Compositional
diabetes
retinopathy
neuropathy
diabetes type A
diabetes type B
retinopathy
neuropathy

Figure 18.2
The number of changes required when altering a concept is greater for an enumerative terminological system than for a compositional system.

The initial investment in a compositional system may be higher than for an enumerative system

The costs of maintaining a compositional system, as measured by the number of changes needed, should theoretically be lower over time. In contrast, the initial stages of building a compositional terminology are actually much more complex than building an enumerative one. The compositional approach starts by defining a core set of terms, and the rules about the way those terms can be combined. It thus requires more information about individual terms and the ways they could combine.

No such burdens are imposed upon the builder of an enumerative system. Here the cost will be paid later on, as the number of terms grows. In theory, then, the investment in the compositional system is initially higher, but begins to pay off over time, as it requires less effort to maintain and enlarge (Goble *et al.*, 1993a; Glowinski, 1994). Eventually a point is reached where the total investment in the compositional system becomes less than for a comparable enumerative one (Figure 18.3).

However, the cost of maintaining a system does not just come from the need to update the system as knowledge changes. For any large system, it is usually the case that it will contain errors that are introduced when terms are created. The cost of detection and correction of such errors, as we have already seen, is high and grows as a system matures. Current research suggests that this cost of error checking may be reduced in compositional systems (Goble *et al.*, 1993b). Since each term needs to be defined in some detail to permit checking when terms are assembled, this information can also be used to check for errors. Checking rules can be constructed to look over the database of terms whenever new terms are introduced, to make sure that the addition does not introduce new inconsistencies.

There are computational and search costs when using terminologies

Another cost with any terminological system is associated with the time and computer resource needed to retrieve a term from the system. This can be broken down into two broad costs.

- The first is the cost of searching the terminology for a term. Clearly, as the terminology grows it will take longer to search it. The more expressive and complete an enumerative system is then, the slower it is to use (Heinsohn *et al.*, 1994). In this respect, since

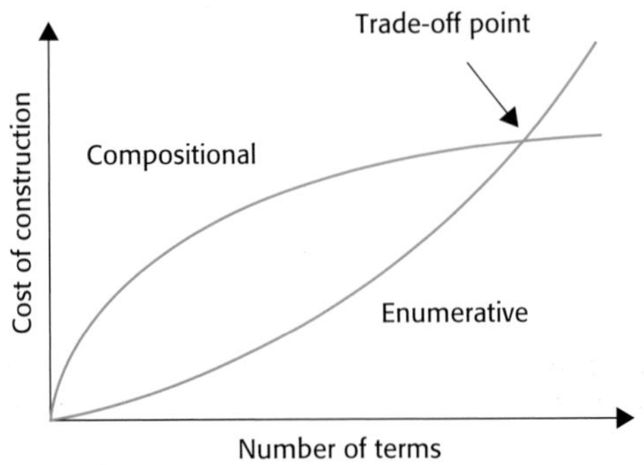
Trade-off point
Compositional
Cost of construction
Enumerative
Number of terms

Figure 18.3 The cost of constructing and maintaining a compositional system may initially be higher, but as the number of terms grows, the enumerative approach may become more expensive. This graph is illustrative only, as the actual shape of these cost functions still remains to be determined.

a compositional system should have a smaller set of terms it will be quicker to search through than an enumerative one.

- However, there is a second cost that is related to the computation needed after searching. There is no such cost associated with an enumerative system. Once a term has been found no further work needs to be done. In contrast, the cost of using a compositional system is that each answer has to be derived from 'first principles'. Simple terms have to be assembled into complex ones, and then checked against rules to see if these constructions are reasonable.

Both searching and composing require computer time, and their effect on usability of a terminology depends on the performance of the computer system used. One of the engineering trade-offs to be explored in the future will be to decide whether a compositional system is quicker to use than a larger enumerative one. The current hypothesis is that, as enumerative systems grow too large, the enumerative search costs should outweigh the compositional computation costs.

Evidence from other disciplines supports the contention that the compositional approach will eventually be fastest. For example, in computer engineering, so-called reduced instruction set computer chips (RISC) have a small set of basic operations that can be combined to do more complex operations. These chips are much faster than traditional ones that have a large enumeration of operations to cover many eventualities.

Mapping across terminologies may be easier if they are compositional

The fundamental difficulties with mapping between terminologies and coding systems have already been described. Although there seems to be no fundamental solution to this general problem, there may be ways of minimizing it through term composition. By definition, since compositional terms are generated from the same core terms and the method of generation is known, they should map on to one another logically.

This means that if terms are created for quite different purposes, but come from the same compositional system, then it should be possible to create a mapping between them (Figure 18.4). However, the degree of success possible from such an approach is still unmeasured.

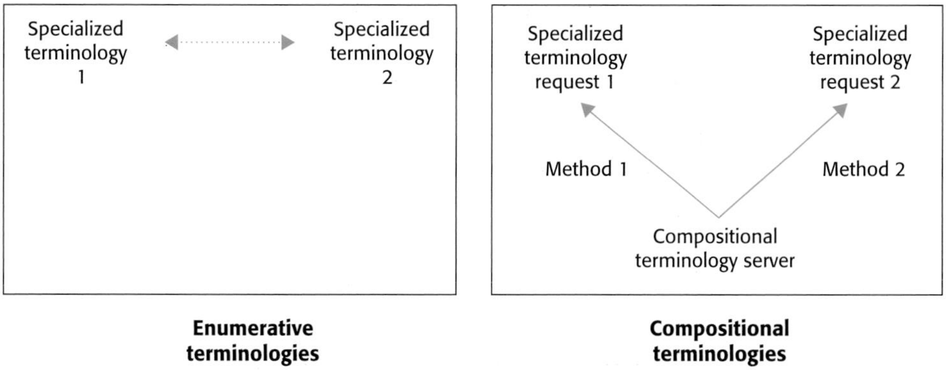
Specialized terminology 1
Specialized terminology 2
Enumerative terminologies
Specialized terminology request 1
Specialized terminology request 2
Method 1
Method 2
Compositional terminology server
Compositional terminologies

Figure 18.4 Enumerative terminological systems are developed independently of each other. Compositional systems try to use basic terminology building blocks along with specialized methods to generate terms for specialized needs. Mapping between specialized terms is not uniformly possible with enumerative systems, but inherent in the design of compositional systems.

It should theoretically be better than customized mappings that are individually developed between independently created terminologies.

Depth of knowledge

The second major compositional hypothesis is a scientific one and is more controversial. It states that there exists a 'deep' set of healthcare knowledge upon which the core terms can be based, and from which new terms can be composed (Friedman *et al.*, 1995).

The quest for 'deep' knowledge has been a focus for considerable effort within the artificial intelligence research community, especially in relation to the construction of expert systems (see Chapter 26). The term 'deep' has now fallen into disuse, as it has become clear that it provides little value in distinguishing knowledge (Coiera, 1992a). As with all models of the world, it is more useful to characterize the differences in knowledge bases on the basis of their level of detail, generality or point of view.

Thus compositional systems, like their enumerative counterparts, are only models of the world. They suffer the same issues of model fidelity and subjectivity. They intrinsically capture a richer set of relations between terms than in an enumerative system, but there is no greater 'depth' to the knowledge they encode. It is either just more detailed, more general or different in point of view.

18.4 The way forward

It should be clear by now that the task of creating, using and maintaining healthcare terminologies is a highly complex endeavour. It should also be clear that, although it is deceptively easy to start to create a terminology, one soon encounters some of the most subtle and difficult problems at the heart of philosophy, language and knowledge representation.

Nevertheless, in the short term administration agencies are keen to obtain aggregate clinical data and so are driven to adopt existing systems, even if they are imperfect. This has led to much debate about the merits of competing systems (e.g. Tuttle and Nelson, 1994).

What is really needed to help rational choice in the longer term is impartial empirical research, comparing the cost and efficacy of different systems in support of well-defined tasks and contexts. For example, in a recent study comparing the utility of different coding schemes in classifying problem lists from patient records, none of the major systems were found to be comprehensive (Campbell and Payne, 1994).

The Board of Directors of the American Medical Informatics Association have suggested that it is not necessary or desirable to have all codes coming from a single master system. They suggest that one should embrace several existing and tested approaches, despite their imperfections, to progress quickly. A first-phase system could be created by borrowing from the different existing code systems, each created for and therefore better suited to, different subject domains (Ackerman *et al.*, 1994).

The longer-term need will be to introduce more maintainable and extensible systems, as the cost of supporting existing systems becomes unsustainable. We have seen that the introduction of compositional terminologies may be the next step in achieving such a goal.

Further on, a solution based in part on multiple compositional systems might be feasible. Since any general healthcare terminology will cover only a small part of the specific vocabulary of any clinical speciality, separate systems may need to be developed for use between and within specialities. 'Vocabularies need to be constructed in a manner that preserves the context of each discipline and ensures translation between disciplines' (Brennan, 1994). Vocabularies developed in this way will be openly based upon the specific needs of specialities. They can more naturally reflect the context and purpose behind specialist terms.

Indeed, over a century ago when Farr constructed the classification system ultimately resulting in ICD, he noted that

> Classification is a method of generalization. Several classifications may, therefore, be used with advantage; and the physician, the pathologist, or the jurist, each from his own point of view, may legitimately classify the diseases and the causes of death in the way that he thinks best adapted to facilitate his enquiries (WHO ICD-9, 1977).

Compositional systems could thus be constructed to agree on a restricted subset of terms necessary for the passage of information between specialities – an Esperanto between different cultures. Work on such communication standards is at present still in its infancy (e.g. Ma, 1995) and more substantive work should be expected in the future. At present, terms for some of the larger terminologies are being created without explicit tasks in mind in the hope that all unseen eventualities will be served. As we have seen, this is a risky strategy, and inter-speciality systems would probably need to be tightly task based to ensure maximum utility.

It is at this point that the importance of evidence-based healthcare also becomes very clear. Treatment protocols are constructed with an explicit task and context in mind. They are written by experts within a speciality, who arrive at a consensus on the management of a specific condition. In the process of doing so they have to define their terms. The communication of information to another speciality can also be defined in the same manner – in the context of a patient on a protocol, what information is needed by an allied specialist? It is clearly the case that good terminologies could be needed to construct computer-based protocol systems (Glowinski, 1994). Equally, the discipline of writing protocols could constrain the terminology problem sufficiently so that a well-defined and relevant set of terms can be agreed upon.

Such a strategy will permit languages to be developed in a way that is optimized for those that will use them. It is still unclear what strategies will best handle the evolution of language once a terminology has been constructed. Not only will terminology developers want to extend and refine a system as it proves inadequate, they will also want it to reflect changes in knowledge. Even if systems are built for narrow specialities with tasks in mind, this imperfection of classification will always remain.

One knowledge acquisition strategy is to accept that terms are created in a given context, and should thus only be used within that context. In the **ripple-down rules** methodology, experts add knowledge to an expert system every time it fails to perform its task (Compton and Jansen, 1990). The new knowledge that 'repairs' the system's performance is attached to the portion of the classification tree that failed. Thus, this new knowledge is placed within the context of the failure of the old knowledge. Over time the classification system grows, always driven by use rather than abstract principles of form. As one would expect, eventually some parts of the system are used less and less, as new classification 'paths' replace more obsolete ones. Despite a process that seems to produce quite large and messy classification systems, ripple-down systems are much easier to build and maintain than normal expert systems, and perform just as well (Compton *et al.*, 1992).

Such an approach might well be suited to terminology construction, where terms are added when the existing system fails to provide an appropriate term. Whenever this happens, the reasons for the failure are noted and kept with the new term, which is then placed in the portion of the classification hierarchy that failed. When the system is used next, this contextual knowledge allows the utility of the new term to be judged against the given need. If it suits the need, then it can be used. If it does not, then another new term can be created and added to the system.

Another benefit of the ripple-down method is that it does not require great panels of experts to debate the knowledge that will go into a system. Since it is created in an ongoing fashion as a result of the way it is used, individuals can themselves own this process. Absolute notions of knowledge being right or wrong are replaced by appropriateness to the circumstances at hand.

Such an idea may seem modern in its embrace of controlled anarchy, but as with all such ideas, has been anticipated long before.

> And since, for all the reasons above adduced, our language and forms of expression scarcely admit of any further fixation, explanation, or definition, without risk of greater danger than utility, it appears more advisable to give a clear, searching *history* of each of these expressions – e.g., of fever, inflammation – of the names of several disorders, and the like. In this way, our ideas of these matters might be most thoroughly fixed and elucidated, by showing how these expressions were first arrived at, and why they must now be received in a sense different from that which was originally attached to them, and why in this sense and no other (Oesterlen, 1855, p. 330).

Discussion points

1 A leading vendor tells you that their terminology system is universal and complete, covering all the concepts that may appear in the health record. Do you believe them?

2 Explain why every major terminology provider issues regular updates to their products.

3 Which do you think is greater over the lifetime of a clinical terminology system: the original cost of purchase, or the cost of upgrades and maintenance to the terminology, as well as the interfaces between the terminology and other clinical information systems?

Chapter summary

1 There is no pure set of codes or terms that can be universally applied in healthcare. There is consequently no universal way in which one healthcare language can be mapped on to another.

2 There are two fundamental and related obstacles to devising a universal terminological system. The first is the **model construction** problem – terminologies are simply a way of modelling the world, and the world is always richer and more complex than any model humans can devise. The second is the **symbol grounding** problem. The words we use to label objects do not necessarily reflect the way we think about the objects, nor do they necessarily reflect defined objects in the real world.

3 Terms are subjective, context-dependent, purposive and evolve over time.

4 The process of terminology growth and alteration introduces huge problems of maintenance, and the very real possibility that the system will start to incorporate errors, duplications and contradictions. Introducing changes into a mature terminological system becomes increasingly expensive over time, and as a consequence maintaining a terminological system will become increasingly expensive over time.

5 Compositional terminological systems are intended to be easier and cheaper to maintain and update than enumerative ones. Early on in their construction, the cost of building a compositional system will be higher than for an enumerative one, but over time will be lower as maintenance costs are comparatively smaller.

PART 6

Communication systems in healthcare

CHAPTER 19

Communication system basics

> It is through the telephone calls, meetings, planning sessions … and corridor conversations that people inform, amuse, update, gossip, review, reassess, reason, instruct, revise, argue, debate, contest, and actually constitute the moments, myths and, through time, the very structuring of the organization. *Boden (1994).*

It has long been recognized that good interpersonal communication is an essential skill for any healthcare worker. Indeed, as we saw in Chapter 4, effective communication is central to the smooth running of the healthcare system as a whole. The care of patients now involves many different individuals, in part due to increasing specialization within the professions. This change is also partly due to an increase in patient mobility, which means that individuals no longer live in the same area for the whole of their life. Clinical encounters are supported by the efforts of many others who work away from patients, from laboratory and radiology staff through to administrators. These trends, amongst others, have significantly increased the need for healthcare workers to share information about patients and to discuss their management.

A recurring theme throughout this book is that the specific needs of a given task drive the choice of technology used to assist with that task. This is just as important when considering the application of communication technologies to healthcare. It is clearly inappropriate in an emergency, for example, to send a letter in the post when a telephone call would be a better choice.

Until recently, the scope for such choices has been relatively limited. Consequently, most people still tend to devote limited attention during their working day to the consequences of choosing one communication option over another for a given task. However, the range of available communication options has now become quite rich. Computer networks, satellite links and mobile telephony, for example, are now commonplace. In contrast, our understanding of the specific roles they can play in healthcare lags behind. As a consequence, there is an apparent delay in the widespread adoption of the newer communication options within healthcare. Although there is some significant advanced research in highly specific areas such as telemedicine, the adoption of even simple services like voicemail or electronic mail is still not commonplace in many health services.

Two things are needed to permit the informed use of any set of technologies: an understanding of the basic problems that need to be solved, and a solid understanding of the available solutions. In this chapter, the basic components of a communication system are explained. The fundamental concepts of a communication channel, service, device and interaction mode are presented first. Several different communication services such as voicemail and e-mail are then examined, along with more traditional forms of communication like the telephone. The next chapter in this section examines some specific communication technologies, explaining their technical operation and identifying their benefits and limitations. The final chapter in this section examines the specific types of communication problems that arise in healthcare, and suggests ways in which communication technology in the guise of telemedicine might be able to improve matters.

19.1 The communication space accounts for the bulk of information transactions in healthcare

We can conceive of all the information that gets exchanged in healthcare as forming a 'space'. The **communication space** is that portion of all the information interactions between people that involves direct interpersonal interactions. For example, face-to-face conversations, telephone calls, letters and e-mail all generate transactions that would fall into the communication space.

There are few studies that have attempted to directly quantify the size of the communication space. Those studies that do exist all paint a similar picture. Covell *et al.* (1985) reported that colleagues rather than document sources met about 50% of information requests by clinicians in clinic. In a similar study, Tang *et al.* (1996) found that about 60% of clinician time in clinic is devoted to talk. Safran *et al.* (1998) reviewed the information transactions in a hospital with a mature computer-based record system, and still found about 50% of information transactions occurred face-to-face between colleagues, with e-mail and voicemail accounting for about another quarter of the total. Only about 10% of the information transactions occurred through the EMR. In some specialized clinical units like the emergency department, where a large number of staff are physically collocated and engage in teamwork, the communication space can account for almost all information transactions. In one study, communication between staff represented almost 90% of all the information transactions that were measured in two emergency departments (Coiera *et al.*, 2002).

The sheer scale and complexity of these interactions within the healthcare system puts a heavy burden on the process of communication. Miscommunication can have terrible consequences. Not only is the communication space huge in terms of the total information transactions and clinician time, it is also a source of significant morbidity and mortality. Communication failures are a large contributor to adverse clinical events and outcomes. In a retrospective review of 14 000 in-hospital deaths, communication errors were found to be the lead cause, twice as frequent as errors due to inadequate clinical skill (Wilson *et al.*, 1995). Further, about 50% of all adverse events detected in a study of primary care physicians were associated with communication difficulties (Bhasale *et al.*, 1998). If we look beyond the raw numbers, the clinical communication space is interruption-driven, has poor communication systems and poor practices (Coiera and Tombs, 1998).

At the administrative level, the poor communication of information can have substantial economic consequences. It is now clear, for example, that the healthcare system suffers enormous inefficiencies because the communication systems that are in place are often of poor quality. One recent estimate suggested that the US health system could save $30 billion per annum if it improved its telecommunication systems (Little, 1992).

So, in summary, the communication space is apparently the largest part of the health system's interaction space. It contains a substantial proportion of the health system information 'pathology', but is still usually ignored in our informatics thinking. Yet it seems to be where most of the information in the clinical workplace is acquired and presented. The biggest information repository within healthcare lies within the people working within it, and the biggest information system is the complex web of conversations that link the actions of these individuals.

19.2 A communication system includes people, messages, mediating technologies and organizational structures

A communication system is a set of processes or components assembled to provide support for interpersonal communication. For example, hospitals have paging systems that provide a mechanism for contacting specified individuals. Alternatively, at the end of a hospital shift, nurses assemble to hand over their patients to the next team, and we can equally conceive of the formal handover process as a different type of communication system, this time governed by the formal structure of the communication and the physical setting.

Even such apparently simple communication systems reveal significant complexity when decomposed. The number of possible conversations that could take place at any one time is determined by the number of individuals who may have a need to communicate (Lang and Dickie, 1978). For example, if there are three members in a clinical team, then we can imagine three separate conversations that might take place between any two individuals. If we increase the size of the team to five individuals, the number of possible conversations increases disproportionately to 10, and for a team of 10 the number of possible conversations blows out to 45 (Figure 19.1). This is because the number of possible conversations is determined by a combinatorial formula:

$$\text{Number of conversions} = \frac{n!}{r!(n-r)!}$$

where n is the total number of individuals, and r is the number of individuals involved in a single conversation.

Given the number of individuals who might be involved in the care of a single patient, even for a single episode, it becomes clear why communication is so complex, and can be so difficult. For example, consider the case of a hospital doctor who prepares a medical discharge summary for a patient who has spent a period in hospital (Figure 19.2). As part of its routine communication system, the hospital sends the document to the patient's general practitioner. We can identify the different agents that could be involved in this simple communication system by looking at the different roles that individuals might take. During the process of preparing and

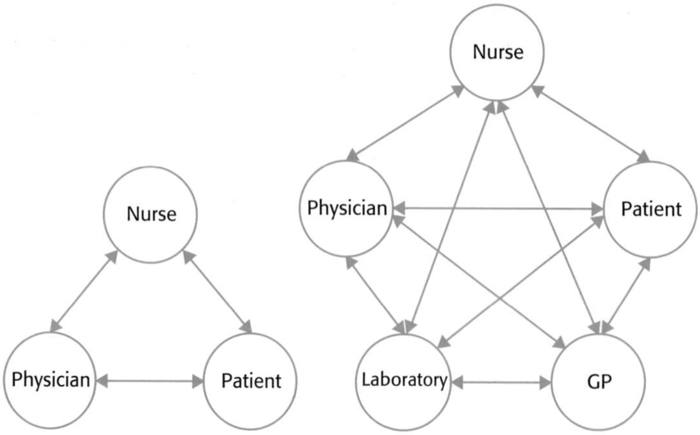
Nurse
Physician
Patient
Nurse
Physician
Patient
Laboratory
GP

Figure 19.1
The number of possible conversations increases combinatorially with the number of individuals who need to communicate (after Lang and Dickie, 1978).

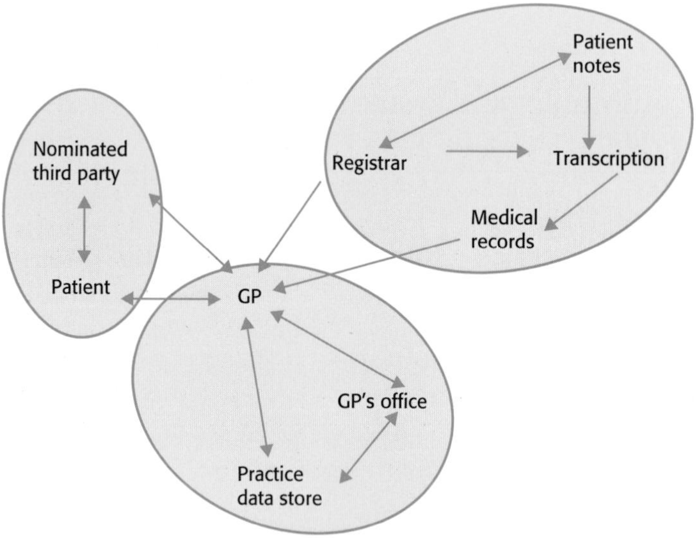
Patient notes
Nominated third party
Registrar
Transcription
Medical records
Patient
GP
GP's office
Practice data store

Figure 19.2
Some of the possible transactions and data flows associated with a discharge summary from a hospital.

then acting upon the discharge summary, the following individuals all might have legitimate roles:

- **Patient roles:** Patient, and patient-nominated additional party roles: patient relative/executor, consulting clinician, insurance company, federal agency (e.g. immigration, etc.).
- **Hospital roles:** Medical registrar, specialist, ward clerk and medical transcriptionist.
- **General practitioner office roles:** General practitioner, practice nurse, office clerk, and information system manager.

Figure 19.2 shows some of the most likely interactions that can occur between these agents, but many others are possible within this system. For example, the general practitioner's office might contact the hospital's medical records department to chase up a discharge summary that has not arrived. Some of the possible conversations that could occur between these different individuals are unlikely because of real world constraints. For example, some conversations are constrained by policies such as privacy rules that determine who is allowed to have access to the contents of a medical record. Each of the possible conversations in the example could occur using a variety of different means. The discharge summary could be sent by post, fax or e-mail. Alternatively, the general practitioner could be updated on the contents of the summary over the phone simply by talking to the discharging doctor from the hospital.

With this example in mind, we can now see that a communication system involves people, the messages they wish to convey, the technologies that mediate conversations, and the organizational structures that define and constrain the conversations that are allowed to occur. Consequently communication systems can broadly include several of the following components:

- **Communication channel:** As we saw in Chapter 4, a wide variety of different communication channels are available, from basic face-to-face conversation, through to telecommunication channels like the telephone or e-mail, and computational channels like the medical record. Channels have attributes like capacity and noise, which determine their suitability for different tasks.
- **Types of message:** Chapter 5 introduced us to the three different types of message structure – data-, task- and template-oriented. Messages are structured to achieve a specific task using available resources to suit the needs of the receiver. Examples of different formal messages include hospital discharge summaries, computer-generated alerts and laboratory results. Informal messages include voice and e-mail messages.
- **Communication policies:** A communication system can be bounded by formal procedure rather than technology, as we saw with the handover example. A hospital may have many different policies that shape their communication system performance, independent of the specific technologies used. For example, it might be a policy to prohibit general practitioners to obtain a medical record directly from the records department without the permission of a hospital clinician.
- **Agents:** A communication system can be specifically constructed around the agents involved in the different information transactions. For example, in a busy clinical unit, one could devise a system where a ward clerk can be tasked to field all incoming telephone calls. The clerk's specific communication role is thus an organizational structure created in support of a policy to minimize interruption to clinical staff, who might otherwise have to answer the phone. Agents have attributes such as their understanding of specific tasks and language. The efficiency of communication between different agents is shaped by their common ground, as we saw in Chapter 4.
- **Communication services:** Just as computer systems can run a number of different software applications, we can think of a communication system providing a number of different communication services. Thus voice communication is only one of the many services available across a telephone line (Figure 19.3). Fax transmission of documents is an entirely different kind of service that uses the same underlying channel. A mobile phone may provide voicemail and text messaging.
- **Communication device:** Communication services can run on different communication devices. Examples of devices include the telephone, fax machine and personal digital assistant (PDA). Different devices are suited to handle different situations and tasks. Communication devices are a source of continuing innovation, and will continue to evolve. One area of recent interest has been the area of wearable computing, where devices are small enough to become personal accessories such as wristwatches or earrings.
- **Interaction mode:** Interaction design, as we saw in Chapter 11, determines much of the utility of different information systems, and this is just as true for communication systems. Some modes of interaction, for example, demand that the message receiver pays attention immediately, such as the ringing tone of a phone, whereas others can be

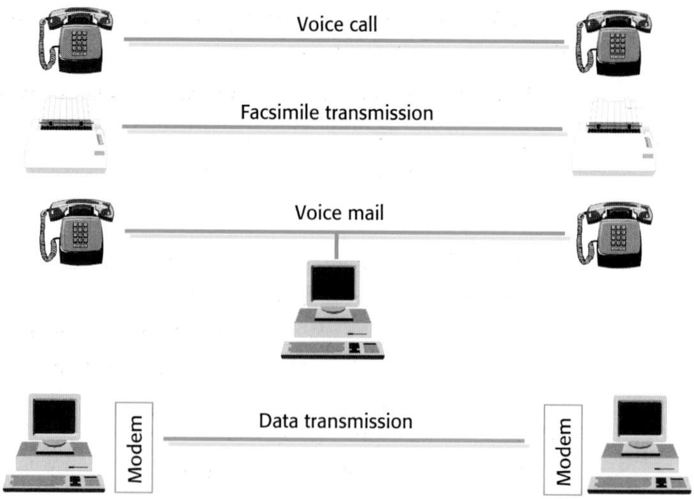
Voice call
Facsimile transmission
Voice mail
Data transmission
Modem
Modem

Figure 19.3
A communication channel can support many kinds of communication service. Public switched voice circuits support voice transmissions, but through the use of additional components can support many other services like fax, voicemail and e-mail.

designed to not interrupt. A service that is inherently not interruptive, like e-mail, may still be designed with an interruptive interaction mode, such as the ringing of a computer tone when a message arrives, altering the impact of the service on the message receiver.

A communication system is thus a bundle of different components and the utility of the overall system is determined by the appropriateness of all the components together. If even one element of the system bundle is inappropriate to the setting, the communication system can underperform. For example, sending a radiograph to a small PDA is unlikely to be useful, both because the size of the device may limit the view of the image, and because the size of the image may exceed the capacity of the wireless channel used by the PDA.

Finally, as with information systems, socio-technical variables will also have a large impact on the benefit of a communication system. For example, failure to adequately train staff to recognize the importance of good communication will no doubt result in a poor outcome, independent of the amount of money spent on new technology.

19.3 Shared time or space defines the basic contexts of communication system use

The benefit of a given communication system is largely determined by the needs individuals have at the time they need to communicate. In other words, the value of a system depends upon the context within which it is used, and the task to which it is put.

The simplest way to model the different contexts in which communication acts can occur is to note that individuals can be separated either by time or by distance. The nature of the separation changes the characteristics of the exchange, and in part defines the type of channel and service that is needed (Table 19.1).

Same time, same place

A face-to-face conversation is the most obvious example of communication benefiting from shared location and time. The participants in the dialogue are able to both hear and see each

Table 19.1 Communication needs can be characterized by the separation of participants over time or distance (after Johansen *et al.*, 1991).

	Same time (synchronous)	Different time (asynchronous)
Same place	Face-to-face meeting	Local message
Different place	Remote conversation	Remote message

other, and share whatever materials they have to hand. Because they can see and hear so much of each other, the opportunity for exchanging complex and subtle cues is high. In whatever other situations communication occurs, we often seek to replicate the effectiveness of face-to-face communication. Consequently, the strengths and weaknesses of alternative channels can be weighed up against this gold standard.

Despite the richness of face-to-face conversation, devices are often still used to augment the interaction. Everything from slide projectors in an auditorium to shared computer workspaces in classrooms can provide additional channels to enhance immediate communication.

Same time, different place

Separated by distance, conversations can nevertheless occur in the same time. When two parties exchange messages across a communication channel at the same time, this is known as **synchronous communication**. Telephone lines provide perhaps the commonest example of a two-way synchronous channel. Broadcast television provides a unidirectional synchronous channel, which prevents it being used interactively in support of a conversation.

It is the nature of synchronous communications that they are interruptive, and interruptions may have a negative impact on individuals who have high cognitive loads (Box 8.2). For example, a busy clinician may forget a clinical task because they have been interrupted while they are busy.

When conversations occur across large distances, there is less likelihood that the parties will be involved in frequent face-to-face conversations. This means that in these circumstances the channels and services bear the full brunt of the communication burden. In such cases, channels may be chosen that support richer communication interaction. Voice telephony is usually sufficient for most conversational needs, but in some circumstances it might be necessary to see the faces of the participants. In this case, video images can be transmitted along with voice to permit a video-conference. The interaction can be enhanced further with data services. For example, one can work remotely on a common document, or use shared electronic white boards. One can thus use a combination of media from sound, image and data, depending on the specific needs of the communication task. The use of such multimedia is still an area of ongoing investigation, as the specific advantages of individual mediums for given tasks is identified.

Different time, same place

In contrast to synchronous communication, when individuals are separated by time they require **asynchronous** channels to support their interaction. Since there can be no simultaneous discussion, conversations occur through a series of message exchanges. This can range from sticky notes left on a colleague's desk to sophisticated electronic messaging systems.

One of the benefits of asynchronous communication is that it is not inherently interruptive, and if a communication is not urgent asynchronous channels may be a preferred way of communicating with otherwise busy individuals. However, as we saw earlier, an asynchronous service like e-mail may still be designed to have an interruptive interaction mode, which negates some of the benefit of using this type of service.

The object of such communication might, for example, revolve around the coordination of a group of individuals all working at the same location but working different shifts. For example, a team of physicians working in a hospital might meet only once during the day as a group, and communicate non-urgent information for the remainder of the day through written messages, voicemail or e-mail. It is a common characteristic of these local message exchanges that they are often brief, since they represent ongoing conversations between working colleagues who also have other opportunities for face-to-face conversation.

Different time, different place

In many ways, this is the most challenging of the four quadrants, since neither location nor time are shared by the communicating parties. Asynchronous messaging is clearly needed in this circumstance. Message services are often provided across computer networks, and are sometimes also known as **store-and-forward** systems. For example, a radiology image stored in a radiology department computer system can be forwarded along with a report to the requesting physician, who reads it at a convenient time.

If the correspondents do not often meet in the same location, there is a potential need for richer services than simple message exchange. For example, messages may need to contain complex documents with text, voice or video records.

Services vary in the media they employ

The time and place classification separates synchronous and asynchronous services. Services can also be understood in terms of the different media they employ. Some for example, are designed only for voice; others may carry images or data (Table 19.2).

Unsurprisingly, the value of one medium over another is also context dependent (Caldwell *et al.*, 1995). The nature of a particular task, the setting in which it occurs, and the amount of information that a medium can bear all seem to have effects on human performance on

Table 19.2 Communication services can be classified according to the media they support, and whether they are asynchronous message based systems, or operate synchronously in real time.

	Sound	Image	Data
Synchronous	Telephony	Video-conferencing	Shared electronic white boards, shared documents
Asynchronous	Voicemail	Letters and notes, computer image store and forward	Paging, fax, e-mail

a communication task (Rice, 1992). For example, relatively information-lean media such as e-mail (Rice, 1992) and voicemail (Caldwell *et al.*, 1995) can be used for routine, simple communications. In contrast, it seems that for non-routine and difficult communications, a richer medium such as video, and preferably face-to-face conversation, should be used.

This may be because, in routine situations, individuals share a common model of the task and so need to communicate less during an exchange. In contrast, in novel situations a significant portion of the communication may need to be devoted to establishing common ground (Clarke and Brennan, 1991).

In simple terms, since the participants do not share a common model of the task at hand, they are unable to interpret all the data passing over the channel (recall Figure 4.4). This means that during the conversation, there are additional demands on the channel to also support the transmission of task models. Since this is a complex communication task, individuals may need to check with each other repeatedly throughout the conversation that they are indeed understanding each other.

19.4 Communication services

We have now seen that the context of communication affects the choice of channel and service. In this section, several basic combinations of service and medium are examined in more detail, with an emphasis on the type of communication they are best able to support.

Voice telephony

Undoubtedly the backbone of any organization's communication system, the apparent simplicity of voice telephony, belies the richness of the communication it can support. In contrast to asynchronous systems, real-time interaction allows problem-solving and negotiation to take place. Voice is also a rich enough medium for many of the subtle cues needed to develop a shared understanding to be exchanged (Clarke and Brennan, 1991).

Perhaps because it is so commonplace, voice telephony is often taken for granted, and people do not look for new or innovative ways with which it can be used. However, innovative use of the telephone can make significant improvements to the delivery of care. For example, patient follow-up can often be done on the telephone, in preference to bringing patients into the clinic (Rao, 1994).

Undoubtedly the biggest change in voice telephony in recent years has been the expansion of mobile telephony. Mobile communication reduces the effort required to locate and speak to people. The combination of mobile telephony and paging systems can reduce the 5–10 minutes out of every hour many clinicians spend answering pagers (Fitzpatrick and Vineski, 1993).

It is important to recognize that even a service like voice telephony is not ubiquitous. In many developing countries it is not guaranteed that an individual will have ready access to a telephone. In the mid-1990s it was often quoted that up to half the world's population had never made a telephone call, nor lived within 3 miles (5 km) of a telephone. With the enormous investment in telephone infrastructure in recent years, it is likely that the number of individuals with telephone access is now much greater, and continuing to grow. Nevertheless, equity of access to basic communication services remains an issue in many nations.

Video-conferencing

The addition of video to voice telephony is seen by many as one of the next major advances in mass telecommunication. It is perhaps surprising, then, that despite being available in one form or another for quite some time (the videophone was first launched by AT&T in 1971) it has not yet entered into common use. This is partly related to the costs associated with delivering video services, and to the benefits video brings over and above voice-only communication.

The channel capacity needed to deliver real-time images cannot be supported by the voice circuits in place in most public telephone networks. Consequently, video-based systems can only appear after a significant investment in higher-capacity networks. However, the costs involved in this process mean that video seems relatively expensive for the extra benefit it gives the average consumer. As cable television services to the home become commonplace, this should change, since fibre-optic cables are capable of supporting the much higher data capacity needed for video. Video over high-capacity mobile phone systems is also increasingly available in many developed nations.

Video-conferencing permits face-to-face interactions when participants are geographically separate. This allows for a richer interaction than is possible by voice alone. However, interactions are not necessarily 'natural'. There may be time lags between events being shown or discussed, depending on the capacity of the channel being used, and the amount of image data that is sent.

It remains unclear in which situations the increased cost of using video delivers a proportionate increase in benefit (Whittaker, 1995). For most conversations, for example, it may be that voice is a sufficiently rich channel that little extra benefit is conferred through the addition of video. Indeed, video-conferencing seems to be more similar in its characteristics to audio-only channels than to face-to-face conversation (Williams, 1977).

One study suggests that the ability to see lips in addition to hearing voice makes only a modest improvement to understanding of meaningful communication. However, it significantly improved an individual's ability to disambiguate meaningful sentences from garbled or anomalous ones. The addition of gestures to face and voice seemed to not help further with meaningful conversation, but slightly improved the handling of anomalous data (Thompson and Ogden, 1995).

More recently, the 'video-as-data' hypothesis suggests that one of the main benefits that video brings is the depiction of complex information about shared work objects, creating a shared physical context for conversations (Whittaker, 1995; Ramsay *et al.*, 1996).

E-mail

E-mail is typically used to send short textual messages between computer users across a computer network. It is one of a number of electronic data exchange services available to those with access to a computer network (Figure 19.4).

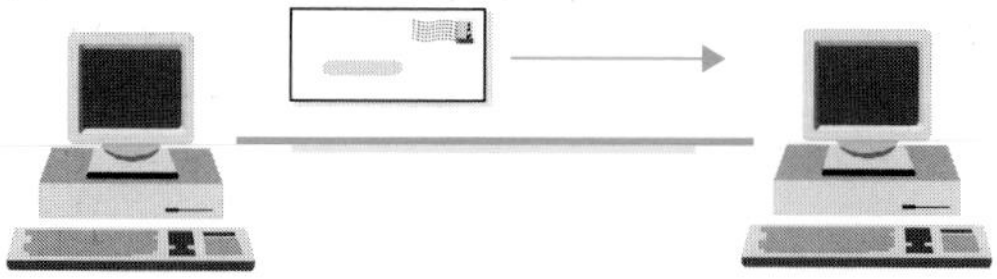

Figure 19.4
E-mail is used to send messages to specified addresses of individual users on a computer network.

E-mail systems can be confined to local computer networks, for example covering a university or hospital campus. However, when separate local networks are connected, messages can be exchanged across much wider areas. As we shall see in Part 7, the Internet permits local networks to join on to an international network, giving electronic mail services a global range.

In some populations, access to e-mail via the Internet is high. Fridsma *et al.* reported that already in 1994 in California about 46% of their patients at a clinic used e-mail, 89% of which was through their place of work. Figures for e-mail uptake vary from country to country, but continue to increase.

E-mail can be used in a variety of ways. It can, like voice telephony, be used for personal communication. It can also be used for the distribution of information. For example, a central resource such as a laboratory can use e-mail to distribute test results, and associated alerts or warnings. The benefits of such exchange need not be confined to large institutions like hospitals, but can be used to communicate information within smaller groups, such as primary care groups. E-mail is also a simple but effective means for communicating between different sectors in healthcare. For example, patient data can be sent from hospitals to primary care physicians after discharge. Drug alerts can be communicated by regulatory bodies to the medical community at large.

E-mail continues to evolve in sophistication, and it is now common to find e-mail programs that allow complex messages. For example, it is possible to use many different media – voice, still images or video – when composing a message. Thus an e-mail could contain a brief explanatory text note, along with a file containing documents from a medical record, a dictated voice message and some images.

Voicemail

Similar in concept to e-mail, voicemail allows the asynchronous exchange of recorded voice messages. The commonest use of voicemail is to collect messages when a phone is unanswered. Unlike a simple answering machine attached to an individual telephone, a voicemail system permits relatively complex message handling:

- It acts like a collection point for many different individuals, each of whom might have a private 'mailbox' on the system. This is possible because voicemail systems are created and operated on computers connected to the telephone system, for example through an organization's switchboard.
- Messages can be tagged with different levels of urgency, forwarded to others with additional information or stored for later review.

Inexpensive voice messaging can deliver simple but powerful services over existing telephone networks. For example, voicemail has significant potential for improving the process of care

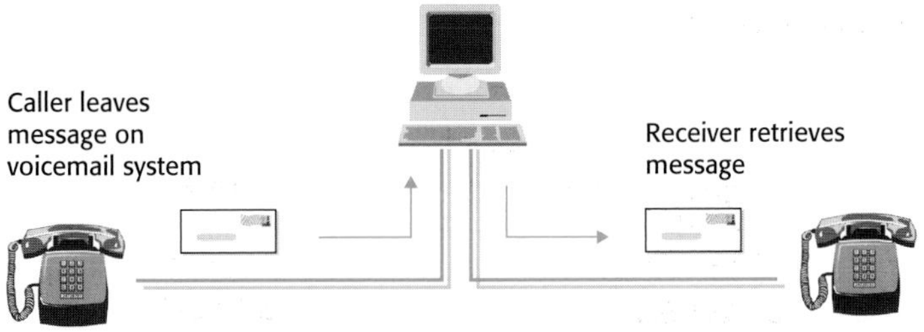
Caller leaves message on voicemail system
Receiver retrieves message

Figure 19.5
Basic voicemail allows a caller to leave a recorded voice message. The receiver calls up the voicemail system, accesses their own private mailbox and retrieves any messages put there.

(Constable, 1994). It can be integrated into many existing processes; for example, it is common for many radiology or pathology reports to be prepared by dictation, then transcribed and committed to text. Eventually much of the transcription will be automated through computer voice-recognition systems. In the absence of that, the dictated reports could be distributed to the ordering physician by voicemail, long before it could be transcribed and arrive through a paper-based mail system.

Quite sophisticated functionality can be incorporated into telephone services based on voicemail. For example, an answer message can incorporate call logic that offers a preprogrammed range of options to the caller. The caller can interact with the system, and indicate preferences. This interaction can happen by collecting information from the caller using the tone created when different digits are pressed on a telephone (called dial tone multifrequency or DTMF). Computer-based voice recognition systems can look for specific words in the caller's response to determine their preferences.

From such seemingly simple elements, many different services can be constructed. For example, a patient could call in to a health information line that begins by playing a prerecorded voice message. Depending upon the information needs of the caller, the system then plays different messages on a variety of health topics. If the recorded information is insufficient, the system could either allow the caller to record a message registering a more specific request, or put them through directly to someone who is able to answer their questions.

The term 'voicemail' is thus in some ways a misnomer, since these systems can do much more than send and capture messages, and can be programmed to provide a variety of information services. They also can be designed to capture and exchange more than voice recordings. For example, DTMF is a simple way of exchanging data across the voice channel.

Conclusions

We have briefly covered some of the basic elements of communication and the way in which technologies can be used to support it. In the next chapter, we delve more deeply into the specifics of current and emerging communication technologies. It may often appear that simply introducing technology will quickly improve poor communication processes, but this is not necessarily the case. Socio-technical variables will always have a large impact on the success of any technical intervention. Taking a broad view, communication systems including people, messages, technologies and organizational structures will assist in deciding which technologies are most appropriate in a particular setting, and help identify which social, cultural and organizational changes may be needed alongside the technology. This is a theme we return to in Chapter 21, where we examine specific ways that technology can and cannot help the process of communication in healthcare.

Discussion points

1 Choose a simple episode of care, for example a patient visiting their general practitioner. Determine all the possible individuals who might be involved in that episode, and sketch out all the conversations that could take place, describing the different channels and services that could be used in support of the different conversations.

2 Now take the diagram from the previous question and add to it all the information systems that could also be involved in information transactions, starting with the medical record.

3 A colleague drops a letter on your desk and tells you that you have mail. Was the letter a synchronous or an asynchronous communication? Break down the system into its components, including your colleague, and determine which components were synchronous.

4 Is a pager synchronous or asynchronous?

5 A pager or bleeper is designed to have an interruptive interaction mode. Can you conceive of ways in which the paging service behaves asynchronously? In what circumstances would such a service be useful, and in which circumstances would it be dangerous?

Chapter summary

1 The communication space is the largest part of the health system's information space and contains a substantial proportion of the health system information 'pathology'.

2 The number of possible conversations that could take place at any one time increases combinatorially with the number of individuals who need to communicate. Even simple communication systems on analysis involve many different individuals and possible exchanges.

3 A communication system involves people, the messages they wish to convey, the technologies that mediate conversations, and the organizational structures that define and constrain the conversations that are allowed to occur. System components include: channel, message, policies, agents, services, device and interaction mode.

4 Many different communication services can be provided over a channel. For example, voice and fax transmission are both available over a telephone line.

5 Communication systems can support communication between individuals separated either by time or by distance.

6 Channels that support communication in real time are known as **synchronous** channels. Channels that support communication over different times are known as **asynchronous** channels.

7 Voice telephony forms the backbone of an organization's synchronous communication system. This is now enhanced through routine use of mobile telephone systems, and the addition of video capabilities that can permit video-conferencing.

8 E-mail is an asynchronous data service available over computer network channels, typically used to send short textual messages between computer users across a computer network. It can be used for the exchange of messages and distribution of information. For example, a central resource like a laboratory can use e-mail to distribute test results, and associated alerts or warnings.

9 Voicemail allows the asynchronous exchange of recorded voice messages. It can be integrated into many existing healthcare processes. For example, dictation radiology or pathology reports can be distributed by voicemail in advance of being transcribed.

10 Video-conferencing adds video to voice telephony. It remains unclear what benefits this additional video brings, since video-conferencing is more like using a telephone than having a face-to-face conversation.

CHAPTER 20

Communication technology

> The simple contrivance of tin tubes for speaking through, communicating between different apartments, by which the directions of the superintendant are instantly conveyed to the remotest parts of an establishment, produces a considerable economy of time. It is employed in the shops and manufactories in London, and might with advantage be used in domestic establishments, particularly in large houses, in conveying orders from the nursery to the kitchen, or from the house to the stable … The distance to which such a mode of communication can be extended, does not appear to have been ascertained, and would be an interesting subject for inquiry. Admitting it to be possible between London and Liverpool, about seventeen minutes would elapse before the words spoken at one end would reach the other extremity of the pipe.
> *Charles Babbage (1833), p. 10.*

In the previous chapter, a broad view of the different communication channels and services was presented. In this chapter, some of the different technological options for communication system construction are discussed in more detail. In this respect, this material is a departure from the content of other chapters, which have sought to de-emphasize technology, and focus on its principled application. However, it is at present difficult to get a concise description of the basics of communication technology. Tanenbaum (2002) provides a comprehensive introduction to the area of computer networks, which will only be touched upon here. This chapter should thus serve as a technological introduction for those who need a deeper understanding of this area. Those without such an interest can move directly to the final chapter in this section, where we shall turn to examine communication problems in healthcare, and assess the roles that particular technologies can play in solving them.

20.1 Machine communication is governed by a set of layered protocols

For communication to be effective, both conversing parties obviously need to understand the language spoken by the other. As we saw in Chapter 4, well-behaved agents also need to

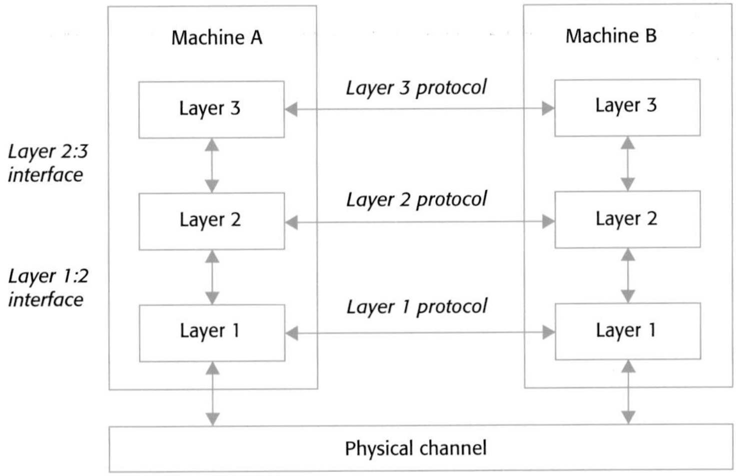
Machine A
Machine B
Layer 3
Layer 3 protocol
Layer 3
Layer 2:3 interface
Layer 2
Layer 2 protocol
Layer 2
Layer 1:2 interface
Layer 1
Layer 1 protocol
Layer 1
Physical channel

Figure 20.1
When two machines communicate, the conversation is regulated by a series of layered protocols, with defined interfaces insulating one protocol from the others. While data are in reality transferred across a physical channel, notionally the individual layers only talk to each other (after Tanenbaum, 2002).

communicate according to a basic set of rules such as Grice's maxims, to ensure that conversations are effective and that each agent understands what is going on in the conversation. The set of rules governing how a conversation may proceed is called a **communication protocol**, and the design of such protocols is central to understanding the operation of communication systems and computer networks. When two machines communicate with each other, the communication protocol defines amongst other things how a message is to be constructed, how its receipt is to be acknowledged, how turn-taking should occur in the exchange and how misunderstandings or errors might be repaired.

Typically communication protocols require significant complexity to ensure rapid and reliable interaction between machines. To simplify the design of communication protocols, they are typically decomposed into a number of different layers, each of which accomplishes a different task. Protocol layers are organized hierarchically, with the bottom layers carrying out tasks that then can be forwarded up the hierarchy to be processed by higher layers (Figure 20.1)

One of the advantages of such decomposition is that individual layers do not need to understand how others actually work, but simply need to know how to interact with a layer. Thus each layer has a defined interface with layers below and above, which in effect defines the input and output that will occur between layers. Together the layers form a **protocol stack**, and at the bottom of the stack lies the physical medium that acts as the channel that transports the data between machines. Although layers in practice pass messages down the stack, to eventually pass along the physical channel between the machines, we can notionally consider that any layer *n* on one machine in effect is able to communicate directly with its counterpart layer *n* on the other machine.

The International Organization for Standardization (ISO) has developed the open system interconnection (OSI) model that is used almost universally as a template to define the protocol layers for communicating between heterogeneous computers. The OSI model consists of seven separate layers, and the different real-world protocols we encounter operate at one or more of the OSI layers (Table 20.1). The OSI layers commence at layer 1, which is directly concerned with translating digital data into a signal that can travel across a channel. Level 1 is therefore interested in managing physical phenomena like voltage variations across wires. At the topmost layer, OSI level 7 is concerned with defining how complex services or applications such as e-mail can be written in a way that the application can operate independently of the machinery of sending bits between machines, which is the concern of the lower layers.

Table 20.1 Summary of the seven OSI protocol layers.

OSI layer		Function	Example
Layer 7	Application	Supports applications that run over the network, such as file transfer and e-mail	Telnet, FTP, e-mail, HL7
Layer 6	Presentation	Sometimes called the syntax layer, translates from application to network format. Encrypts data	HTTP/HTML
Layer 5	Session	Establishes, manages and terminates connections between applications	NetBIOS, RPC
Layer 4	Transport	Responsible for end-to-end error recovery and flow control. It ensures complete data transfer	TCP/IP, NetBIOS/NetBEUI
Layer 3	Network	Responsible for establishing, maintaining and terminating connections. Provides switching and routing by creating logical paths or virtual circuits	IP
Layer 2	Data link	Encodes and decodes data packets/frames into bits. Is divided into two sublayers: the media access control (MAC) layer and the logical link control (LLC) layer	ATM
Layer 1	Physical	Concerned with transmission of unstructured bit stream over a physical link, e.g. electrical, photon or radio signals. Defines cables, cards, and physical aspects	ISDN; Fast Ethernet, RS232, and ATM protocols have physical layer components

Often a communication system is actually built up from several different components, each spanning a different subset of layers, but together providing complete coverage of the communication behaviour implicit across the span of OSI layers. From our point of view, OSI provides a reference framework for understanding some of the different technologies that are used in communication systems, especially those that use advanced communication services beyond simple voice telephony.

20.2 Communication channels can be dedicated or shared

A communication channel provides a connection between the sender and the receiver of a communication. The simplest way to create such a channel is to completely dedicate a physical wire to the transmission. Local telephone systems work in this way, with each telephone number having a dedicated telephone cable running from the telephone unit to the local exchange. Systems like these are called **circuit-switched**, since they make connections by establishing a completed circuit between the communicating parties.

A circuit-switched system is not a very efficient way of transmitting data. If the dedicated circuit is used only infrequently, it results in inefficiency during the idle periods. If there are many people who want to use the same circuit, a bottleneck is created, since once a circuit is in use it is unavailable to others.

Common channels can carry data packets

One solution to this problem is to try to share the resources on a circuit. This can be achieved by allowing a channel to carry packets of data that may come from a number of different sources. Such systems are called **packet-switched** systems.

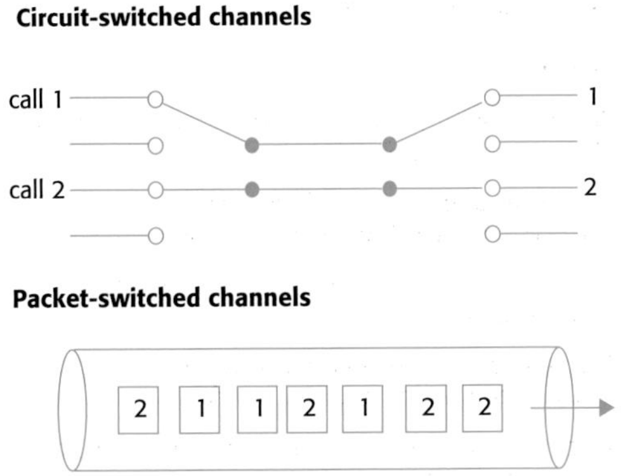
Circuit-switched channels
call 1
call 2
1
2
Packet-switched channels
2
1
1
2
1
2
2

Figure 20.2
Dedicated lines connect communicating parties in a circuit-switched system. In contrast, lines can be shared by exchanging data packets from different conversations across a common channel.

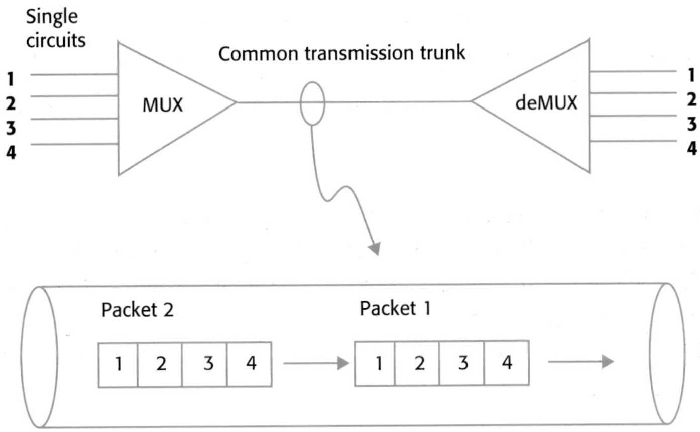
Single circuits
1
2
3
4
MUX
Common transmission trunk
deMUX
1
2
3
4
Packet 2
1
2
3
4
Packet 1
1
2
3
4

Figure 20.3
To increase the efficiency of transmission, the signals on single telephone circuits are concentrated on to common trunk lines. The concentration is achieved by assigning each circuit a time slot on data packets or frames, which are sent down the line. This concentration of signals is performed by a multiplexer (MUX).

Here a message is broken down into a number of discrete packets, and these are sent one after the other down the channel's circuit. On the circuit, the packets mingle with packets from other messages. Each such packet is small, and contains the address of the place it is being sent. In this way many packets, each destined for different locations, can pass down the same wire over the same period (Figure 20.2). When the packets reach a switching point in the communication network, the address is read, and the packet is then sent down the right part of the network towards its final destination. By and large, all computer networks are packet-based.

In telephone networks common channels are multiplexed according to time or frequency

A similar general principle is used in voice telephony. Since a segment of voice from a conversation is reducible to digital data, it too can be broken down into a number of packets. As long as the packets are sent and reassembled in a short enough time, then the speaker and listener will not realize that they do not have a dedicated circuit to themselves.

Once voice data have travelled down a dedicated circuit from a customer's premises to a local area exchange, the data are shipped along a high capacity common trunk. Each packet is passed along the trunk using a technique called multiplexing (Figure 20.3) which is another method for combining a number of calls in order that they may all be transmitted along the same single cable (Lawton, 1993).

One way of multiplexing a number of different conversations is to time the arrival of data, and to divide time into a series of repeating 'slots'. Each call is pre-assigned a different time slot on the same circuit. The receiver of the multiplexed signal knows which conversation occupies which specific time slot, and reconstructs individual conversations as their specific packets are taken from their time slot (Figure 20.3).

The second way in which a number of calls can be multiplexed together is to allocate each a frequency slot rather than a time slot. This is possible because, for analogue channels, there is a spread of possible signal frequencies that can be used to transmit data. The band of possible frequencies is broken up into a number of smaller bands, which then becomes a call slot. Each individual call is then allocated one of the frequency slots on the channel (Figure 20.4). Thus, in contrast to a time multiplexed system, each frequency slot carries its information at the same time down the common channel. The call is limited to occupying a few of all the possible available frequencies on the common channel frequency band.

This explains why one measure of a channel's capacity to carry data is called its **bandwidth**. The wider the range of frequencies available on a channel, the greater the opportunity to break it up into separate bands, each of which is able to carry data independently. Channel bandwidth is calculated in Hertz (Hz), which is a frequency measure (cycles per second); the wider the bandwidth, the greater the channel's capacity to carry signals. In contrast to an analogue channel, the capacity of a digital channel to carry data is measured by the number of data bits per second that can be transmitted by the channel. It is possible to relate a channel's bandwidth to its data rate. For example, a normal telephone line can carry up to 64 kbytes per second, assuming a 3.4 kHz voice requirement for the transmission of intelligible speech (Lawton, 1993). In contrast, a common trunk on a telephone network may handle between 1.5 and 2 Mbits per second.

The current explosion of services in the communication industry is as much a product of the increase in capacity and variety of channels, as it is due to the emergence of innovative ways of using their capacity. These channels can be created either by establishing connections through wired physical circuits, or by establishing wireless links.

The great number of different systems competing in the telecommunications sphere can make this a difficult area to understand. Each system usually offers slightly different technical and economic advantages over its competitors, and the basis for choosing one system over another is rarely straightforward. One may need to compare attributes such as bandwidth, cost, reliability, flexibility, call set-up time and so forth. As a consequence, only some of the major and emerging communication systems can be reviewed here. The discussion

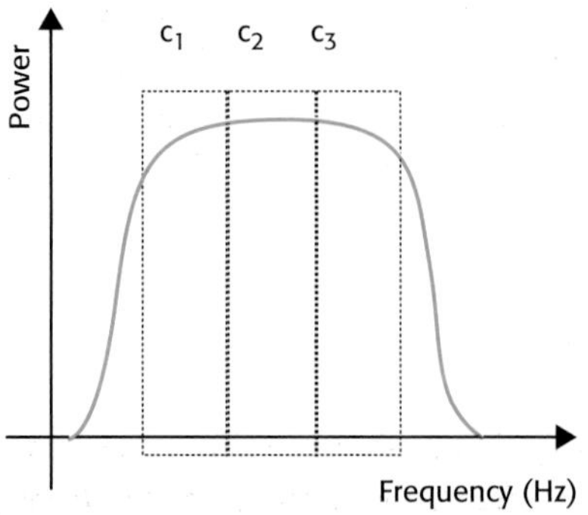
Power
c1
c2
c3
Frequency (Hz)

Figure 20.4
Channels can combine multiple calls by allocating each call a different slot from the frequencies available on the common channel.

should give a clear indication of the types of technologies now available, and their varying ability to support communication.

20.3 Wireline communication systems

Most of the world's communication infrastructure is based on physical 'wire' networks, whether they are made of copper wire of fibre-optic cable. Just as important as the difference in the transmission characteristics of these physical media is the method used to transfer information across them. We saw earlier that using a circuit-switched network meant that only one 'call' could use a wire at any one time. Packet-switched and multiplexed systems, in contrast, because they handle information exchange in a different way, result in a more efficient sharing of network resources.

Consequently, when discussing the capacity for information carriage over any particular system, both the physical attributes of the system and the type of protocol used to carry data over it contribute to the eventual data rate achieved. The technical details of these specific protocols are well beyond the scope of this discussion. However, two in particular – ISDN and ATM – will be introduced, given their importance in telecommunications.

Integrated Service Digital Network (ISDN)

We have already seen that the public switched telephone network was initially developed to carry only voice, but is now also used to carry fax and data. As the desire to provide ever more intricate services across the telephone network grows, it has become increasingly clear that the existing system, developed over the last 100 years, is now reaching its limits.

ISDN, unlike normal telephone circuits, provides direct digital connection between a subscriber and the telephone network. Thus, although on a normal analogue telephone line one needs a modem to carry data across the voice channel, no such device is needed when using ISDN. (A modem converts data into a series of tones that are carried across the voice channel, and then are converted by another modem back into digital format.)

Secondly, ISDN provides two independent data channels to a subscriber (Figure 20.5). One channel could be used to carry a voice conversation, while data are transmitted across the second. Thus, for example, one could be discussing a patient on the telephone, and simultaneously transmitting and sharing data about that patient. A third signalling channel allows the user's equipment to communicate with the network, allowing for rapid call set-up and exchange of other information (Lawton, 1993). For example, caller identification information can be transmitted and read before deciding to accept a voice call.

ISDN services are now available in many countries. Their adoption has been slow, partly because of the costs to users, and partly because the need for the higher speed data services of ISDN to the home has only recently arisen, especially with increased home connection to the Internet (see Part 7).

Asynchronous transfer mode (ATM)

Although ISDN represents a significant improvement on existing telephony, it has a relatively limited bandwidth – roughly twice that of a normal 64 kbit/s telephone line. For some tasks,

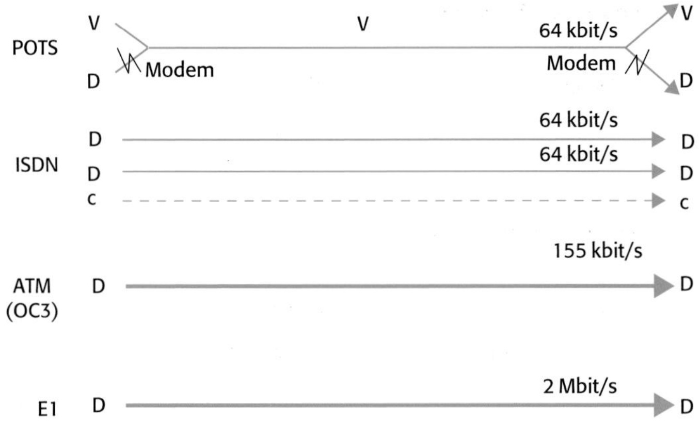
POTS
V
D
Modem
V
64 kbit/s
Modem
V
D
ISDN
D
D
c
64 kbit/s
64 kbit/s
D
D
c
ATM
(OC3)
D
155 kbit/s
D
E1
D
2 Mbit/s
D

Figure 20.5 Wired channels: plain old telephony services (POTS) across public telecommunication networks are the basis for most communication. Integrated services digital network (ISDN) provides a digital connection with twice the bandwidth of POTS. Asynchronous transfer mode (ATM) systems are designed for high bandwidth computer networks. When higher bandwidths are needed private trunks like E1, provide guaranteed connections. (V – voice, D – data, c – control.)

such as the transmission of high-resolution moving images, this is insufficient. In anticipation of a need to provide such high-bandwidth channels, the **B-ISDN** or broadband ISDN system has been developed. Along with the anticipation that there would be a consumer need for such transmission rates, B-ISDN has also been driven by the development of fibre-optic channels. These are able to sustain high-bandwidth transmission, up to several hundred Mbits/s.

One of the main criteria in shaping the design of the B-ISDN was the realization that the demand for data capacity would be highly variable from different customers. Recall that in normal telephony, a channel can be created by assigning a specified time slot in a sequence of packets that are transmitted down a common channel. This is an example of a **synchronous transfer mode**. For largely voice-based systems, because there is a fixed demand on capacity for each given channel, this synchronous system suffices.

If the network is used for other forms of data such as video, then another approach is required. The irregularity with which a user might need to transmit large volumes of video data means that a synchronous method becomes inefficient for broadband services. This is because the large dedicated packets needed to accommodate video might often remain relatively underutilized if they were used for voice. As a consequence, rather than assigning fixed-capacity communication slots, an asynchronous system based on the transmission of data packets (or cells) is needed. The method for transmitting these packets is called the **asynchronous transfer mode** (ATM) (Figure 20.6).

In ATM, each packet is filled with information from different channels in an irregular fashion, depending on the demand at any given time. Since each packet contains information about the specific channels it is carrying data for, they can be reassembled on arrival. In other words, ATM allows a communication system to be divided into a number of arbitrarily sized channels, depending on demand and the needs of individual channels.

Confusingly, ATM is an example of an **isochronous** system because, although packets are sent irregularly, there is a service guarantee that they will arrive within a certain time frame (Table 20.2). Thus ATM can guarantee a specified data throughput as data flow steadily down the network, guaranteeing delivery at a certain minimum rate. Isochronous transport with a guaranteed bandwidth is required for time-dependent services such as the transmission of

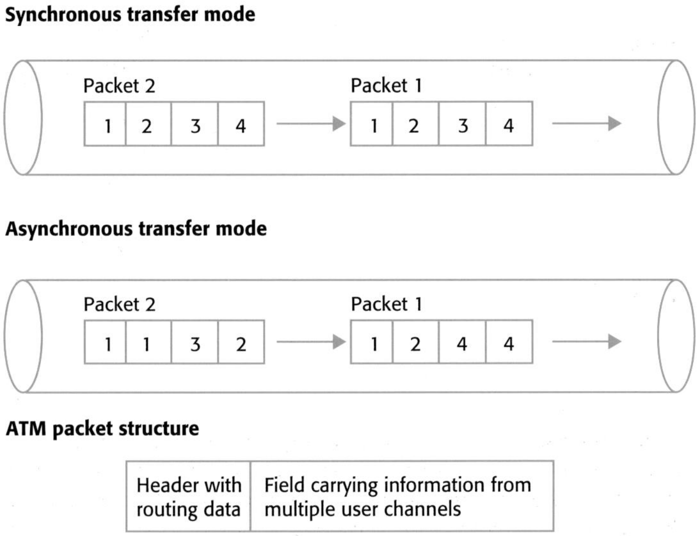
Synchronous transfer mode
Packet 2
1 2 3 4
Packet 1
1 2 3 4
Asynchronous transfer mode
Packet 2
1 1 3 2
Packet 1
1 2 4 4
ATM packet structure
Header with routing data
Field carrying information from multiple user channels

Figure 20.6 Asynchronous transfer mode (ATM) transmission uses a packet transmission system by variably assigning different channels to a given packet, based on the requirements of individual channels at any given time. Each ATM packet (or cell) carries information in a header segment that describes its particular contents, which are located in the main body of the cell.

Table 20.2 Communication protocols can be defined according to the coordination of messages between sending and receiving parties.

Synchronous	Events that are coordinated in time. Technically, a synchronous process is dependent on other processes, and runs only as a result of another process being completed or handed over, e.g. communication that requires each party to respond in turn without initiating a new communication
Asynchronous	Events that are not coordinated in time. Technically, an asynchronous process operates independently of other processes, e.g. sending a communication that does not require a party to respond
Isochronous	Events that occur regularly in time. Technically, an isochronous process operates at a regular interval to provide a certain minimum data rate, e.g. sending a communication with a guaranteed regularity

live video and audio data. ATM is thus well suited for applications where a steady data stream is more important than accuracy. A good example is video-conferencing where irregular small 'blips' in the data stream are tolerable but long pauses are not. Network protocols such as IP, Ethernet and Token Ring are truly asynchronous protocols because their packets are transported over the network on a demand or first-come, first-served basis. If the network is busy, packets are delayed until traffic subsides. An isochronous service is thus not as rigid in its timing requirements as a synchronous service, but not as lenient as an asynchronous service.

As the demand for broadband services like high-quality video image transmission, or video-telephony grows, the economic case for the widespread deployment of ATM will become stronger. The deployment of ATM is also dependent on the rate with which high-capacity fibre-optic cabling is laid in the community, since it cannot run across the existing smaller capacity circuitry. The upper transmission rate for ATM will vary, depending on the network interface standard chosen, but typically is 1.5 Mbits, with upper limits of 2.4 Gbits/s cited.

For many in the telecommunications field, healthcare is an example of an area that could adopt ATM, because it is perceived that telemedical video services will be of high benefit (e.g. Cabral and Kim, 1996). Whether this is an example of a technology seeking problems to solve, or an appropriate solution for healthcare communication needs, is an issue we return to in the next chapter.

20.4 Wireless communication systems

Wireline networks have been developing over an extended period, and now provide affordable voice and data communication channels, but developments in wireless communications systems have been somewhat more recent. The goal of any wireless system is to provide individuals access to voice, video and data channels, irrespective of their location or mobility. The technical requirements that these channels must meet vary according to the data rates expected of them, the mobility patterns of those using the system and the reliability expected of the system. For example, a cordless telephone system that will only be used within a home can be built to far less demanding specifications than a mobile telephone system designed to be used across a continent, in a moving car or to support simultaneous calls.

Radio provided the first wide-area wireless communication technology, followed later by the provision of television services over broadcast radio channels. Over the years the exploitation of the radiofrequency spectrum has continued relentlessly. Microwave and satellite communication links are now commonplace replacements in situations where the laying of cable connections is inappropriate or expensive. Radio technology, in the form of mobile analogue and digital cellular telephony, is now freely available to the public at relatively low cost in most developed countries and many developing countries.

In contrast to this wide-area use of wireless channels, one can also exploit wireless communication at very short distances. In these circumstances, the wireless system might be providing channels for local telephony and paging. It can also be used to provide wireless links for computer terminals. For example, a hand-held computer terminal can connect to a hospital local area network over a wireless link. This allows the user to move over the local area freely, but still be able to interact with information on the network. For very short-distance communication within a room, or between individuals in close proximity, one can exploit the infrared light spectrum. Infrared links can be used, for example, to allow devices such as a computer and printer to communicate with each other.

Of all of these areas, the rapid growth in mobile telephony has been the most spectacular and significant, in terms of adoption rates. Some cellular telephone systems have experienced staggering growth rates of between 35% and 60% per annum in recent years (Cox, 1995). There are several competing standards for the provision of mobile telephony arising from Europe, Japan and the United States, and arguments over the benefits of these systems are as much driven by political and economic imperatives as by technical issues. All these systems deliver more or less the same basic set of services, including voice communications, data communications, and messaging or paging functions (Padgett *et al.*, 1995). Over the last couple of years the GSM system has been widely adopted on a global scale. For this reason, it will be reviewed here in some detail.

The global system for mobile communications (GSM)

GSM was initially developed in Europe, but has in recent years been adopted across much of Asia-Pacific, and in some sections of the United States. The digital nature of GSM allows it to service many more users in a local area than is possible with older analogue mobile systems. The GSM system was initially intended to be deployed around the 900 MHz radio band. It is now also deployed at 1.8 GHz, where it is called DCS 1800 (Digital Cellular system 1800) or Personal Communication Networks (PCN).

One of the obvious advantages of the widespread adoption of the GSM system is that it offers the ability to roam widely while still using the same handset. Thus a mobile telephone registered to a GSM network in the United Kingdom can be turned on and used on a GSM network in Australia. This contrasts with the situation in some countries where roaming with a network is only possible within the boundaries of a city, because adjoining networks are based on different technologies.

The GSM system provides users with several digital channels (Figure 20.7). One synchronous channel is available for voice communication, and one for data communications offering a 9.6 kb/s data rate. In addition, an asynchronous packet data channel, known as the short-message service (SMS), provides a form of e-mail or text messaging for GSM users. In addition, services such as fax and voicemail are supported over the synchronous channels.

This combination of channels and services makes a digital system like GSM quite powerful. The SMS system, for example, can act as an e-mail or paging system. Combined with a voice-mailbox on the network, this gives individuals a significant set of channels through which they can be contacted. The mobile data channel allows a GSM telephone to be connected to a mobile computer. Whilst mobile, one can send and receive fax messages over the GSM system. Equally, one could use it to connect to a computer network while being remote from the site. This would, for example, permit a doctor to retrieve patient data or gain access to Internet services.

Since the GSM system encrypts the data over its channels, it is also a relatively secure system. Unlike analogue systems, it is not possible to listen in to GSM conversations.

There are still several problems that may affect routine use. For many, battery life between recharges remains an issue, but there is steady progress in improving this aspect of handset design. Perhaps more importantly, use of GSM indoors is limited. The geometry of walls and ceilings means that radio signal reception may not be good. In such circumstances, alternative local systems may be more appropriate. In particular, modern cordless telephony systems such as CT2 (Cordless Telephony 2) and DECT (Digital European Cordless Telecommunications) can offer superior in-building performance, but at the cost of installing the whole network privately on a campus (Padgett *et al.*, 1995).

Like any other cellular system, a GSM network is created by dividing up a geographic area into a number of 'cells'. Each cell has its own radio transmitter to receive signals from handsets, and to transmit these to the network's control centre. As a user moves out of one cell, the

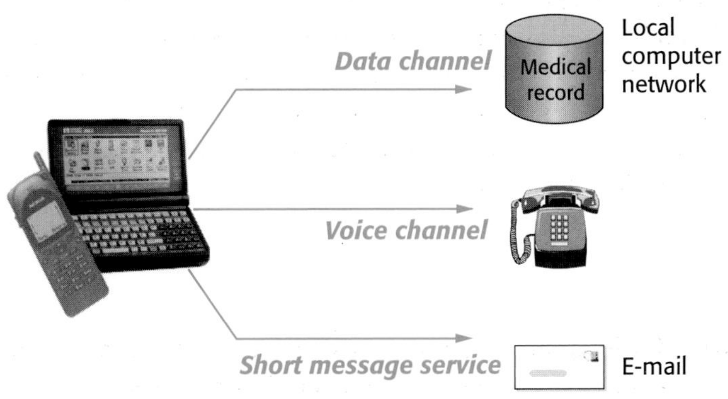
Data channel
Medical record
Local computer network
Voice channel
Short message service
E-mail

Figure 20.7
The GSM mobile digital cellular system provides channels for voice and data connections. The data link allows a mobile computer to connect remotely, via the mobile telephone, to local computer networks. An asynchronous short-message system provides a mobile text-based e-mail service.

call is handed over to the nearest cell with the strongest reception of the handset. Thus, the territory over which GSM can be used is limited by the size of the local networks. If radio base stations have not been installed to create cells in a given region, then no network coverage is possible in that area.

Especially for sparsely populated areas, GSM coverage may thus be problematic. Indeed, as GSM systems are deployed, it is routine to first establish cells in major cities and along transportation routes like highways. Then, over time, coverage is rolled out to less densely populated regions. Consequently, when coverage is an issue, as it is in territories without dense GSM networks, satellite-based mobile telephone systems may provide a useful alternative.

Bluetooth

GSM envisions a single personal device carrying out multiple functions such as voice telephony, messaging and data-oriented applications. However, many individuals work with a combination of personal devices such as notebook computers, mobile phones, PDAs and digital cameras. Bluetooth is designed to allow many such devices to interact using short-range wireless communication. For an individual, it means all one's personal devices may connect together to create a **personal area network** (PAN). For a group of individuals who are physically collocated, it means they can form a temporary *ad hoc* network to share information.

Bluetooth is an ongoing program that was first announced in 1998 when five companies (Ericsson, Nokia, IBM, Toshiba, and Intel) grouped to develop a licence-free technology for universal wireless connectivity in the handheld market. Bluetooth is named after the Danish King Blaatand ('**Bluetooth**') who lived from 940 to 981 and brought Denmark and Norway under common control.

Bluetooth permits individual devices to perform the functions they have been designed for, but allows them to combine in useful ways. For example, a notebook computer in your briefcase can receive an e-mail, but the message alert can be given by your mobile phone, or a new electronic business card could automatically be lodged into the address book on a notebook computer and into the telephone number register on a mobile phone.

A set of Bluetooth devices sharing a common channel is called a **piconet**, in which the device at the centre performs the role of master and all other devices operate as slaves (Figure 20.8).

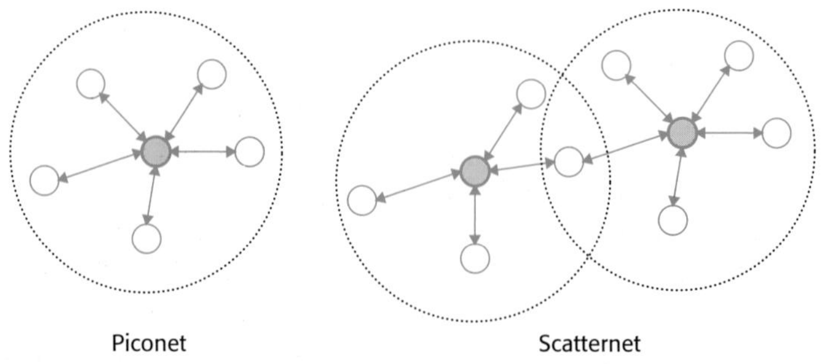
Piconet
Scatternet

Figure 20.8 Bluetooth allows a device to act as a master, connecting together a number of slave devices to form a piconet. Several piconets can be combined to form a scatternet. A device that joins two piconets is called a bridge node. (After Bhagwat, 2001)

Bluetooth also defines a structure called **scatternet**, which is formed by interconnecting multiple piconets to allow communication between them.

Bluetooth communication is packet based and packets have a fixed format with the 'payload' field that contains the data being up to 2745 bits in length. The piconet channel is divided into 625-microsecond slots. To transmit real-time voice, an application must reserve a slot in both directions at regular intervals, called a synchronous (SCO) link. In contrast, asynchronous data link (ACL) slots are allocated on demand instead of being reserved for the duration of the communication.

Bluetooth includes a communication protocol stack specification and supports the integration of an analogue radio front end, signal-processing elements and baseband controller on to a single physical Bluetooth chip, which can then be integrated into the design of personal devices (Bhagwat, 2001). The 2.4-GHz band in which Bluetooth operates is available globally for licence-free use, but is shared by other equipment such as microwave ovens. Transmission range between devices is dependent on their antenna power, but varies from 10 metres up to 100 metres using an antenna with power of 20 dBm. Data are transmitted at a maximum rate of 1 Mb/s, but protocol overheads limit the actual rate to about 721 kb/s.

There are a number of technologies competing with Bluetooth wireless technologies including IrDA, which is an infrared interface standard. The disadvantages of IrDA are its limitation to two parties in a connection, and its need for line of sight.

20.5 HL7 defines standards for the electronic exchange of clinical messages

HL7 is an international standard for electronic data exchange in healthcare, and defines the format and content of the messages that pass between medical applications (Heitmann *et al.*, 1999). For example, HL7 can define the exchange of messages between an EMR and a laboratory system, so that a test can be ordered for a patient via the EMR and then be sent to and be understood by a different laboratory system; or a laboratory result can be transmitted back and be understood by the EMR and incorporated into a patient's notes.

The HL7 standard covers messages for patient admissions/registration, discharge or transfer, queries, orders, results, clinical observations, billing and master file update information. By adopting HL7 as the message format for an information system, system developers hope that their system will be able to interoperate more easily with systems developed by others.

HL7 is an abbreviation of 'Health Level Seven', indicating that it defines a protocol within OSI layer 7 (Table 20.1). Thus HL7 does not specify how messages will be delivered between the applications, and other network protocols such as TCP/IP or FTP file transfers will be used to deliver messages. Equally, HL7 does not describe what is done to a message after it has been received, as this is the domain of the individual applications.

There is no single HL7 standard, but an evolving set of standards that are released by the HL7 organization, Health Level Seven, Inc., which was founded in 1987 and is a not-for-profit standards developing organization. It has over 2200 members representing over 500 corporate members, including 90% of the largest information systems vendors serving healthcare. HL7-sanctioned national groups exist in many countries including Australia, Germany, Japan, the Netherlands, New Zealand and the United States. The wide uptake of HL7 Version 2 has made it *de facto* the international standard for healthcare messaging.

The HL7 messaging standard defines:

- **message triggering events**, which initiate message exchanges between systems, e.g. the act of admitting a patient on a hospital EMR
- **message structures**, which define a limited form of message semantics using a restricted terminology of recognized data types, i.e. how different types of data are to be labelled and arranged so that their meaning is understood
- **encoding rules**, which define message syntax or grammar, i.e. how data structure is to be actually presented, for example the use of different special ASCII characters to delimit the data types defined in the message structure.

There are a number of different message types in the HL7 specification, including ACK (General Acknowledgement Originator), ADT (Admission, Discharge and Transfer), ORM (Order Message Originator) and ORO (Order Response Originator). The HL7 message structure is simple and hierarchical, being built up from **segments**, **fields** and **composites** (Figure 20.9).

Each message is first broken down into a sequence of defined segments, each carrying a different piece of data (Table 20.3). For example, the **PID** segment of a message is defined to always carry patient identification data. Version 2.3 of HL7 contains 120 different possible segment definitions that could be used in any given message, but the use of many of these is optional as they will not be relevant in all circumstances. Message length itself is not limited, but the maximum field length suggested is 64 k.

Segments are further structured to contain a number of predefined fields, which further define the contents of the data segment. Individual fields may repeat within a segment, for

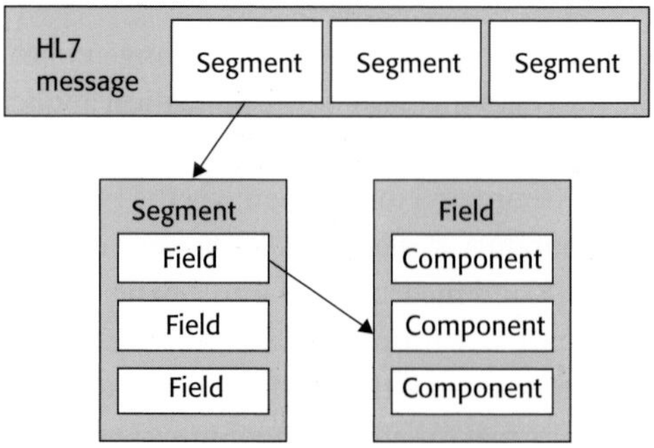
HL7 message
Segment
Segment
Segment
Segment
Field
Field
Field
Field
Component
Component
Component

Figure 20.9 HL7 messages have a hierarchically decomposed structure, and are assembled from a set of pre-defined composite components.

Table 20.3 HL7 defines several different types of messages, and the segments that each different message must contain. This ADT message has six separate segments describing the admission of a patient.

Message type: ADT (admission, discharge and transfer)
Event: Admit a patient

1	MSH	Message header	(R)
2	EVN	Event type	(R)
3	PID	Patient identification	(R)
4	PV1	Patient visit	(R)
5	NK1	Next of kin	(R)
6	DG1	Diagnosis information	

Required segments are labelled R.

example to carry a sequence of different values from a laboratory test. For example, the PID segment in HL7 version 2.3 consists of 2 mandatory fields, person name and person ID, as well as 28 others that are not mandatory (Table 20.4).

Fields may have their own internal structure, and these are known as composite data types. For example, **XPN** is one of the fields in the **PID** segment, and stands for 'extended person name'. **XPN** is composed of 7 data elements (Table 20.5).

The HL7 encoding rules translate the message structure into a string of characters that can be transmitted between applications. For example, encoding rules state that composites are delimited by | characters, and that the components of each composite are separated by ^ characters. For example, we could encode the name 'Mr. John M. Brown' into the **XPN** field as

|Brown^John^M^Mr|

and a whole **PID** segment could be encoded as

PID||05975^^^2^ID|54721||Brown^John^M^Mr|Brown^John^M^Mr|19591203|M||B|
54HIGHST^^KENSINGTON^NSW^2055^AUSTRALIA||(02)731–359|||M|NON|
8000034~29086|999|

Table 20.4 HL7 message segments may contain a number of pre-defined fields (after NHS IT Standards Handbook, 2001).

ST	String
TX	Text
FT	Formatted text
NM	Numeric
DT	Date
TM	Time
TS	Time stamp
PL	Person location
XPN	Person name
XAD	Address
XTN	Telephone number
ID	Coded value (HL7 table)
IS	Coded value (user defined)
CM	Composite
CN	ID and name
CQ	Quantity and units

Table 20.5 The HL7 XPN field is a composite structure: HL7 message fields may contain a number of pre-defined components.

#	Name
1	Family name
2	Given name
3	Middle initial or name
4	Suffix
5	Prefix
6	Degree
7	Name type code

In some ways we can liken the HL7 message structure to a compositional terminology, in that we build up messages from pre-defined components, according to encoding rules that control that composition in a limited way. However, since HL7 does no more than define data types, it is neutral to the meaning of any message's contents. There are no mechanisms in HL7, for example, to make sure the content of a message is clinically meaningful or correct, as this is considered to be in the domain of the applications that send or receive the messages.

HL7 is also developing standards for the representation of clinical documents such as discharge summaries and consultation notes (Dolin *et al.*, 2000). These document standards comprise the HL7 Clinical Document Architecture (CDA). CDA documents are encoded in Extensible Markup Language (XML), and derive their semantics from the HL7 Reference Information Model (RIM) and use RIM data types. The RIM is HL7's information model of the healthcare domain.

20.6 Computer and communication systems are merging

Despite technical difference, one abiding impression from the preceding discussion should be that computer and communication systems are in many ways similar. In fact, the separation of communication and computer systems is breaking down.

Although there are significant differences in the ways both types of system are optimized, they are being put to similar uses. Computer networks are increasingly being used for communication, and communication networks are becoming ever more reliant on computers to deliver complex communication services. Thus, the telephone network, originally designed for voice, is also used to ship data between computers, acting as an extension to local computer networks. Using the Internet, multitudes of local networks have been connected together to create a global computer network that rivals, and sometimes overlays, the existing telecommunications network.

Equally, computer networks such as the Internet, once designed to exchange data, are now being used to carry image and sound. Indeed, it is now possible to use packet-switched systems to deliver voice telephony. Recall that most voice traffic on a telecommunications network is already broken up into small packets and reassembled without the speakers being aware. Although the methods currently used are highly optimized to deliver voice, as computer packet networks grow in bandwidth and reliability they are being used to carry voice calls, independently of the telephone network. To say that this is a challenge to the existing shape of the telecommunications industry is an understatement.

All these signs point to a growing convergence between computer and communication networks. Both have had traditional strengths and weaknesses. Through the convergence of these two quite different systems, new architectures are emerging that try to capture the best aspects of both (Figure 20.10). Computer networks, for their part, are highly flexible. One can buy software and deploy it on to a personal computer, without any constraints from the network to which the computer is connected. The network itself is relatively simple in the way it provides connections between computers, since it traditionally has been designed around packet-based asynchronous data transfer. The net effect has been that it has been very easy to deploy new programs (or 'services' in telecommunication parlance), whereas connectivity has been expensive, with local organizations having to build their own networks.

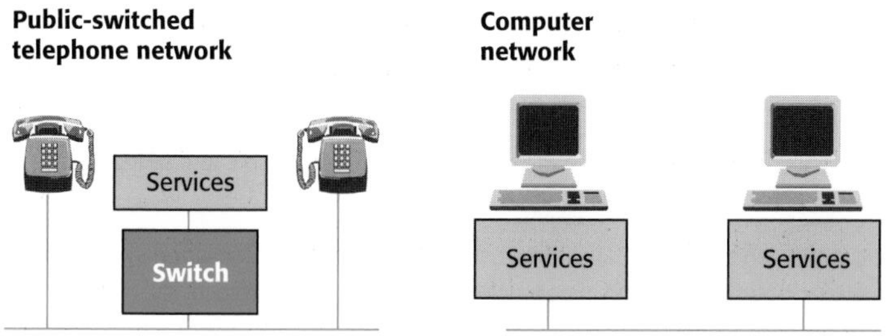
Public-switched telephone network
Services
Switch
Computer network
Services
Services

Figure 20.10 The architecture of telecommunication networks favours centralized control of services, whereas computer networks favour a distributed local ownership. As these architectures converge, emerging systems will begin to inherit characteristics from both.

In contrast, telecommunication networks traditionally provided an immediate and rich network of connections to subscribers. This was achieved through relatively complicated and sophisticated public-switching systems. All the communications services such as 0800 numbers resided in these centralized switching systems. The user's personal terminal (in this case the telephone) depends entirely on the network to provide any new services. Thus one could not go out and buy a new program to load into a private telephone. The consequence of this has been that telephone services are controlled by telecommunications companies, are expensive to develop and evolve very slowly in comparison to computer network services.

One can summarize the differences by noting that in a computer network the service 'intelligence' is distributed across the computers attached to the network, whereas in a telecommunications system it is centralized within the network.

One can immediately see the need for a system that offers high-speed reliable connections to a global network, with the flexibility of a service deployment of a computer network. Indeed, the telecommunications industry has struggled with these issues for several years, working on so-called **intelligent network** architectures that might one day supersede the existing one.

In the meantime, the computer industry has quietly sidestepped these issues by fashioning the Internet into a system that will soon have most of the desired characteristics of this hybrid network. Mobile Internet services using the wireless application protocol (WAP) use existing telecommunications infrastructure as well as computer networks to deliver hybrid systems that combine to provide previously unimagined possibilities (Box 22.5). As we shall see in Part 7, the implications of the Internet are thus as fundamental to the existing telecommunications and computing industries, as to those who use their services.

Discussion points

1 IP is the asynchronous networking protocol used on the Internet. How suited is IP to real-time services such as voice telephony (sometimes known as voice over IP), compared to ATM?

2 There are usually several competing standards or technological systems in the marketplace for any given application. What do you think determines whether a technology, protocol or standard is ultimately dominant?

3 The finer details of different technologies are probably not relevant or even of interest to most healthcare workers. They want to drive the car, not know what goes on under the bonnet. Do you agree with this sentiment?

Chapter summary

1 Rules governing how a conversation may proceed are called a communication protocol, and define how a message is to be constructed, how its receipt is to be acknowledged, how turn taking should occur, and errors might be repaired.

2 The International Organization for Standardization (ISO) has developed the **open system interconnection (OSI)** seven-layer model that is used almost universally to define the protocol layers for communicating between heterogeneous computers.

3 A communications channel can be either a dedicated circuit, or a shared resource. **Circuit-switched networks** provide a complete circuit between the communicating parties. **Packet-switched systems** transport separate packets of data that can come from a number of different sources on a common channel.

4 A channel's capacity to carry data is called its **bandwidth**, usually measured in bits per second.

5 The type of data transfer protocol used over a communications network contributes to the eventual bandwidth. The **Integrated Service Digital Network (ISDN)** and **Asynchronous Transfer Mode (ATM)** systems are currently the most important standard protocols for communicating with multimedia.

6 There are several competing standards for the provision of mobile telephony arising from Europe, Japan and the United States. All these systems deliver more or less the same basic set of services, including voice communications, data communications, and messaging or paging functions. Of these, for the present the **GSM** system is the most widely adopted on a global scale.

7 **Bluetooth** allows many personal devices to interact using short-range wireless communication to create a personal area network (PAN) or for individuals to use their devices to form a temporary *ad hoc* network to share information.

8 **HL7** is an international standard for electronic data exchange in healthcare, and defines the format and content of the messages that pass between medical applications.

9 There is a growing convergence between computer and communication networks, with merged networks such as the Internet now providing both communication and information services.

CHAPTER 21

Clinical communication and telemedicine

With such a long history of application of information technologies in healthcare, it is surprising that communication technologies have only recently become a focus for attention. It is difficult to explain this delay, but it may well reflect the perception that communication processes for the most part are considered human processes. Technology, when it has been used, has been relatively simple and disappeared into the background. The telephone, for example, is an unremarkable and commonplace item in most people's working day. The enthusiasm and novelty associated with its introduction a century ago have disappeared. In contrast, the development of information technologies dominated most of the second half of the twentieth century.

It was only in the last decade of the twentieth century that developments in communication technologies again accelerated. As the limitations of information technology have become apparent, and the potential for communication technologies has emerged, many have now returned to examine how communication technologies can be applied to healthcare. In this closing chapter of Part 6, various human and organizational problems with communication are explored. With the understanding of communication technologies developed in the previous chapters, an attempt is made to assess critically when these technologies are of benefit.

21.1 Telemedicine supports clinical care with communication technologies

Most of the effort in deploying communication technologies in healthcare is associated with the field of **telemedicine**. Definitions of telemedicine abound. For many, it has a particularly narrow technological definition. Specifically, it is seen by some to be the use of video-conferencing techniques to deliver consultation and care at a distance. Unfortunately, technology-driven definitions usually end up focusing more on the technologies than the problems that need to be solved. In particular, they miss the many opportunities for solving problems that do not encompass a given technology. So it is with telemedicine. Healthcare has many and varied communication needs, and video-based technologies are only one of many solutions that should be explored. Indeed, many solutions to communication problems are never technological, but require changes in human and organizational processes.

Others narrowly see telemedicine as discipline based, and restricted only to interactions between doctors and patients. They invoke terms such as **telehealth** or **telecare** to indicate a broader field that involves all health professionals. Within this text, telemedicine is understood to be an inclusive term, and covers all healthcare professionals, as well as the consumers of health services.

The essence of telemedicine is the exchange of information at a distance, whether that information is voice, an image, elements of a medical record or commands to a surgical robot. It seems reasonable to think of telemedicine as the **remote communication of information to facilitate clinical care.** And it is not a new enterprise – Einthoven experimented with telephone transmissions using his new invention, the electrocardiograph, at the beginning of the last century (Nymo, 1993).

At its inception, telemedicine was essentially about providing communication links between medical experts and remote locations. It is now clear that the healthcare system suffers enormous inefficiencies because of its poor communication infrastructure, and many see telemedicine as a critical way of reducing that cost. Consequently, telemedicine has now become a significant area both for research and development, as well as health service investment.

As one might expect, the renewed interest in telemedicine also has much to do with the excitement of new technologies. Telemedicine is often presented in the guise of sophisticated new communications technology for specialist activities like teleradiology and telepathology. These services are championed by telecommunication companies because they have the potential to become highly profitable businesses for them (Bowles and Teale, 1994). Perhaps influenced by these forces, much of the research in telemedicine is driven by the possibilities of technology rather than the needs of clinicians and patients.

Yet the communications infrastructure used by healthcare will not necessarily need to be special. The telecommunications market is competitive and the evolving options are numerous. Healthcare providers will be able to utilize the services of cable television, mobile cellular carriers and telecommunication companies. Further, communications technology does not need to be sophisticated to deliver benefit. For example, simple but appropriate use of today's telephone can make significant improvements to the delivery of care. Consequently, we will examine telemedicine from a problem-driven point of view, and only then examine the role that technologies have to play in their solution.

21.2 The evidence for the effectiveness of telemedicine remains weak

Telemedicine can be considered a health intervention designed to improve the care delivered to patients. We should therefore be able to identify the effects of the intervention and measure how large the effects are, just as we would for a new form of treatment like a medication. In the last few years, the body of literature describing the possible beneficial impacts of telemedical services has grown substantially. With the development of critical review methods and meta-analysis from evidence-based healthcare, many have turned to this large body of telemedicine literature to try and draw some general conclusions about the impact of telemedicine.

As with any class of intervention, including pharmaceuticals, success is not guaranteed, and it is likely that some specific telemedical interventions will be less successful than others. The big surprise in recent years is that almost all the independent and systematically conducted large-scale reviews of telemedicine have produced mixed to negative results (Table 21.1). The reviews typically fail to find evidence of benefit, rather than identifying evidence for lack of benefit, which is a critical distinction to make. In other words, despite the significant volume of literature on telemedicine, the content of the literature is as yet unable to answer basic questions about the value of telemedicine.

Summative evaluations of telemedicine can be made in three broad categories – a user's satisfaction with the service, the economic benefit of the service and any clinical outcome changes resulting from using the service (Taylor, 1998).

User satisfaction with telemedicine

User satisfaction studies seek to determine whether users are happy with a service, and thus do not necessarily attempt to compare a service with others. Satisfaction is necessarily a very subjective measure, and many variables may affect it. Consequently, simple assessments of satisfaction may not reveal much about the underlying reasons for attitudes to a service. Satisfaction surveys are also prone to positive biases. For example, patients may rate a telemedicine service positively simply because of the novelty factor associated with new technology, or because they wish to please those providing the service and asking them questions (Taylor, 1998).

Mair and Whitten (2000) reviewed 32 studies that reported on patient satisfaction with a telemedicine service. All the studies reported good levels of patient satisfaction, but most used simple survey instruments to measure satisfaction. Many studies had small sample sizes and low response rates, and most used volunteers or physician referrals and provided no information about refusal rates. The authors argue that the current research fails to provide satisfactory explanations for the reasons underlying patient satisfaction with telemedicine, and that generalizations about satisfaction are difficult because of the methodological deficiencies of the current evidence.

Williams *et al.* (2001) conducted a larger review of 93 studies and made similar findings. Reported levels of patient satisfaction with telemedicine are consistently greater than 80%, and frequently reported at 100%. However, the studies themselves had significant limitations. Only 20% included an independent control group. One-third of studies were based on samples of less than 20 patients, and only 21% had samples of over 100 patients. Only 33% of the studies included a measure of preference between telemedicine and face-to-face consultation.

Economic benefit of telemedicine

Economic analyses determine if there is a cost-benefit in using telemedicine to deliver health services. Economic analyses can look at savings that accrue from reduction in travel costs and time for patients or clinicians, as well as the freeing up of resources such as time to attend to

Table 21.1 Summary of key critical reviews examining the impact of telemedicine.

Review	Number of studies	Main conclusions
Broad reviews of telemedicine		
Roine *et al.* (2001)	50 of 1124 studies reviewed met review criteria	Most studies were pilot projects and of low quality. Some evidence for teleradiology, teleneurosurgery, telepsychiatry, echocardiogram transmission, electronic referrals enabling e-mail consultations, video-conferencing between primary and secondary care. Teleradiology can save costs
Hailey *et al.* (2002)	66 of 1323 studies reviewed met review criteria	As above. Few papers considered routine use. Evidence for benefit in home care and monitoring. Teledermatology has cost disadvantages to healthcare providers, but not patients
User satisfaction reviews		
Mair and Whitten (2000)	32 studies reviewed	Teleconsultation seems acceptable to patients in a variety of circumstances. Methodological deficiencies limit generalizability of findings
Williams *et al.* (2001)	93 studies reviewed	Reported levels of satisfaction consistently greater than 80%, and frequently 100%. However, many studies methodologically weak
Economic analysis reviews		
Whitten *et al.* (2002)	24 of 612 studies reviewed met quality criteria	There is no good evidence that telemedicine is a cost-effective means of delivering healthcare
Clinical outcome reviews		
Currell *et al.* (2000)	Seven trials met selection criteria	There is little evidence of clinical benefits
Hersh *et al.* (2001)	25 studies reviewed	Evidence of clinical benefit limited to a few areas: home-based telemedicine for chronic diseases; surgical and neonatal intensive care; patient transfer in neurosurgery
Hersh *et al.* (2002)	58 studies reviewed	Few high-quality studies. Strongest evidence for efficacy in diagnostic and management decisions in psychiatry and dermatology

other tasks. Utility analyses look at the outcome of using the intervention. For example, if patients have fewer complications, then a utility can be assigned to that quality of life outcome, and a price can be placed on these utilities, as we saw in Chapter 8. Importantly, one must not only factor in the technical costs of running the service, but also the set-up costs, costs of educating staff, and long-term replacement costs which help determine whether a service is sustainable in the long run. The rapid change in the cost of technology may make it difficult to predict future cost-benefit from the current price arrangements. However, the cost of technology, as with most information technology, is never the major component of total costs.

Often forgotten are opportunity costs, which arise from things that cannot be done because of the intervention. For example, a telemedicine session may make it unnecessary for a patient to travel to a city, but had they made the trip, they might have used the opportunity to see other health professionals. Equally, staying at home may mean more time is spent with family. Such missed benefits can be assigned utilities and hence a 'price', but may not be included in narrow analysis of the service.

Recently much criticism has been directed at the quality of economic analyses of telemedicine (Mair *et al.*, 2000). In a rigorous review of 612 studies, Whitten *et al.* (2002) were only able to identify 24 studies that met criteria for good economic analysis. Most of these 24 studies were small-scale, short-term and pragmatic evaluations that offered few generalizable conclusions. The authors concluded that there is little published evidence to confirm whether or not telemedicine is a cost-effective alternative to standard healthcare delivery. One of the major weaknesses of the evidence base was its inability to identify circumstances where telemedicine was and was not cost-effective. The authors did not conclude that telemedicine was not cost-effective, but that no case can yet be made to indicate that it is.

Clinical outcome changes resulting from telemedicine

Clinical outcome impact is possibly the most difficult area to evaluate, since it typically requires large randomized trials before any effect can be statistically demonstrated. Given that many telemedicine projects are pilots or prototypes, they rarely reach the level of maturity needed to consider such evaluation. Consequently, although some good evidence of positive improvement in clinical outcomes does exist in isolated clinical contexts, broad support for the value of telemedicine on clinical outcomes is still weak.

A Cochrane review conducted in 2000 by Currell *et al.* identified seven clinical trials of telemedicine that met stringent criteria for inclusion. All the technological aspects of the interventions appeared to have been reliable, and to have been well accepted by patients. Although none of the studies showed any detrimental effects, neither according to the authors did they show unequivocal clinical benefits. Further, the findings did not constitute evidence of the safety of telemedicine. The authors concluded somewhat negatively that policy-makers should be cautious about recommending increased use and investment in unevaluated technologies.

In a broader review of 25 studies, Hersch *et al.* (2001) focused on evaluating the efficacy of telemedicine for health outcomes in home-based and office or hospital-based applications. The strongest evidence for the efficacy of telemedicine in clinical outcomes came from home-based telemedicine in the areas of chronic disease management, hypertension and AIDS. The value of home glucose monitoring in diabetes mellitus was considered conflicting. There was also reasonable evidence that telemedicine is comparable to face-to-face care in emergency medicine and was beneficial in surgical and neonatal intensive care units as well as patient transfer in neurosurgery. Despite the widespread use of telemedicine in virtually all of the major areas of healthcare, the authors concluded that there is still only a small amount of evidence that telemedicine results in clinical outcomes that are comparable to or better than face-to-face care.

Hersh *et al.* (2002) also reported a systematic review to evaluate the efficacy of telemedicine for making diagnostic and management decisions. Again, there were very few high-quality studies. The strongest evidence for the efficacy of telemedicine for diagnostic and management decisions came from the specialties of psychiatry and dermatology. There was reasonable evidence that general medical history and physical examinations performed via telemedicine had relatively good sensitivity and specificity. Some evidence for efficacy existed in cardiology and ophthalmology. Despite the widespread use of telemedicine, the authors felt that there was strong evidence that diagnostic and management decisions provided by telemedicine are comparable to face-to-face care in only a few clinical specialties.

In perhaps the largest review to date, Hailey *et al.* (2002) identified 1323 studies. Only 5% of these studies reported a comparison of a telemedicine application with the conventional means of providing services, making any comparative assessment problematic. Of those studies that offered a comparison, telemedicine had advantages over the alternative approach in 37 studies and some disadvantages in 13 studies, and the alternative approach had advantages over telemedicine in 5. The overall findings of authors presented a somewhat sober picture of the current state of evidence on the benefits of telemedicine. Useful data are emerging on some telemedicine applications, but good-quality studies are still scarce and the generalizability of most findings is rather limited.

Problems with the current telemedicine literature

There are numerous reasons for the current failure to identify clear benefits for telemedicine. As we saw in Chapter 11, the process of system evaluation is a complex one. The implementation of systems is an iterative cycle of formative, and then summative reviews of performance, and the effects of the technology itself cannot be measured independently of the broader socio-technical context within which it is placed.

We can identify a number reasons that a telemedical project might not succeed, based on a failure to recognize the complexity of system development and implementation:

- **Studies may be methodologically weak or flawed:** It seems that much of the telemedicine literature has focused on reports of user satisfaction, often of small pilot studies, rather than attempting to measure system effects in a quantitative way. Very few randomized controlled trials of mature and widely deployed systems have been made, possibly because of the cost and complexity of such exercises. The failure to compare telemedicine to alternative services prevents most studies from demonstrating the superiority of this type of service. Some authors suggest this is as much a failure of the peer review process in the biomedical journals that publish reports, as it is of researchers who design the studies (Whitten et al., 2002).
- **Studies falsely assume interventions are discrete or homogenous:** Unlike a medication, which is a clearly defined intervention, we saw in Chapter 19 that a communication system is a bundle of different components and the utility of the overall system is determined by the appropriateness of all the components together. Communication systems comprise technical components such as channel, service and interaction mode, and non-technical components such as the individuals operating the technology. Failure to recognize the impact of even one of these variables may mean it is highly likely the system will not meet expectations. Equally, success in one clinical context will not necessarily guarantee success in another, as some of these variables will invariably have been altered between sites.
- **Studies may occur too early in the development cycle of the system:** It is important to use the appropriate methodology to assess rapidly evolving systems (Mowat *et al.*, 1997).

The iterative nature of system development means that early on, as systems are being developed from prototype to mature system, evaluation is necessarily formative, and it is reasonable to expect that modifications will need to be made before the system is 'bedded down'. Early emphasis on summative evaluation, such as a randomized controlled trial, is therefore not always appropriate. Pharmaceuticals typically spend 10 years in development before they are subjected to rigorous clinical trials, and we should equally expect communication systems to need 'laboratory time' to develop the system to an appropriate level of maturity.

- **Studies are technology-driven rather than problem- or task-driven:** If the motivating hypothesis behind a system is to demonstrate the value of a specific technology, then it is unlikely much thought has been given to understanding the specific tasks it is supporting, or defining their real requirements. A rational analysis of communication needs for many clinical problems may reveal that although an improved communication system is indeed needed, the need may actually be for improved organizational processes or policies rather than for the latest broadband technologies. Failure to recognize the underlying problem usually guarantees system failure.
- **Studies ignore the impact of socio-technical variables:** We know now that a communication system involves people, the messages they wish to convey, the technologies that mediate conversations, and the organizational structures that define and constrain the conversations that occur. Technology-driven research not only fails to understand the true needs of individuals, but also ignores the critical impact that other socio-technical variables have on success. Failure to address issues such as cultural responses to technology, educational needs, and the competing influence of other interactions on the new communication system is likely to result in project failure.

Although broad evidence in support of the value of telemedicine is still weak, there is much evidence for its value in specific clinical contexts. In the next section we look in more detail at the different roles that communication technology can play in supporting clinical processes.

21.3 Communication needs in healthcare vary widely

Communication tasks vary widely across the healthcare system. The needs of a doctor working as part of a close-knit team in a major hospital are very different from those of a nurse working in the community visiting patients in their homes. Consequently, the stresses on communication are equally varied.

It is helpful to separate communication needs into two groups. Firstly, specific **intra-organizational** needs exist within particular groups, such as hospitals or primary care centres. Secondly, there are significant **inter-organizational** needs that occur at the interfaces between significantly different organizations (Figure 21.1). The communication boundary between primary care givers in the community and hospital-based health services, for example, are characterized by the widely differing task styles and organizational structures of individuals within the two groups.

In the following sections, current work devoted to supporting communication within each of the areas of home, community, and hospitals is reviewed. Wherever possible, work that addresses communication at the interface between these sections of the healthcare system is also presented.

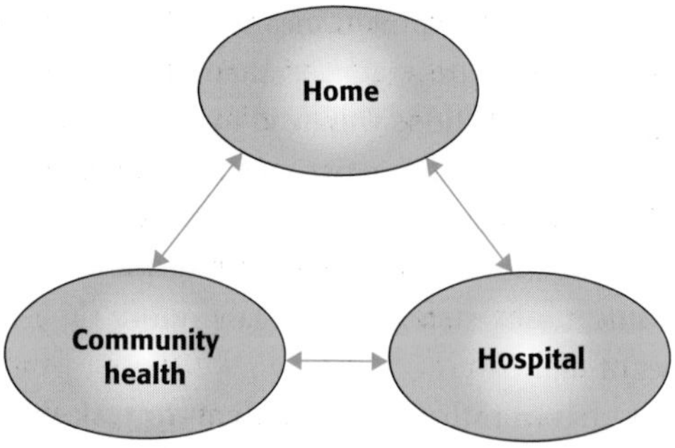
Home
Community health
Hospital

Figure 21.1
Major communication interfaces exist between primary care delivered in the community and tertiary institutions like hospitals, as well as between these and patients receiving care in the home.

21.4 Communication and home healthcare

The delivery of healthcare in the home continues to grow as a proportion of the total healthcare sector. With ever-increasing bed-costs, patients are being discharged from hospitals earlier, or having care once associated with inpatient stays delivered entirely as an outpatient. Equally, the benefits of being in a familiar environment, and away from risks such as hospital-acquired infection, means that home care carries many added therapeutic benefits.

Typically, long-term home care patients might be managing a chronic illness such as insulin-dependent diabetes, or undergoing home dialysis for renal failure. The delivery of chemotherapeutic agents in the home is also an option for some cancer patients. Short-term care at home might be appropriate after early discharge from hospital after an operation.

Consequently, for some patients, care in the home can span many years for a single condition, but for others it represents only a brief episode. In either case, communication can support both patient and carer. Patients have a need for information about their care, which is to a greater or lesser extent self-managed in the home. As well as requiring access to factual information about their therapy, patients may simply need to interact with healthcare workers to assure themselves that they are managing their own care well.

For their part, carers will need access to data about the patient's physical and mental state to ensure that they remain well managed. The ability of patients to communicate this information themselves depends on their condition, their understanding of the process of care and its complexity. One thus might expect a young adult insulin-dependent diabetic to be able to be deeply involved in the communication of information, whereas an elderly patient may need much more assistance and simpler interactions.

Remote monitoring of patients at home

The most obvious way for healthcare workers to monitor the progress of individuals at home is to visit them in person. Approximately 1.5 million such home visits take place in the United States each year. However, it is said that in many of these visits, hands-on care is not needed.

For this reason, some have advocated that such interactions can occur over communication links, rather than through physical visits. The proposed benefits are economic, as well as an improvement in the efficiency of staff who would spend less time travelling, and presumably more time communicating with patients.

The simplest way one can carry out such remote monitoring is to schedule a regular telephone call. Leirer *et al.* (1991) used a voicemail system to automatically telephone medication reminders to elderly people at home, and showed that it did reduce both tardiness and complete forgetting. Two-way messaging using pagers has also been shown to be an acceptable method of sending reminders to HIV-positive patients, with the goal of improving their adherence to antiretroviral medications (Dunbar *et al.*, 2003). In a review of 19 similar studies, Krishna *et al.* (2002) found that automated telephone messages in general have been repeatedly shown to improve clinical outcomes for patients with chronic illness, whether delivering reminders or educational messages.

Using more sophisticated technology, nursing staff in another study used interactive video to do things like verify compliance with medication regimens, assess mental and emotional status, or check measurements such as blood sugar levels. Despite a high acceptance with nursing staff, 40% of patients in this study felt a face-to-face visit would have been preferable because it might have altered the care that was delivered (Allen *et al.*, 1996).

Despite the uncertainties in even this simple form of remote care, others are advocating much more complicated monitoring systems. For example, it is technically possible to install monitoring equipment in the home. Measurements such as blood pressure and cardiogram data can then be transmitted to a remote monitoring station (Rodriguez *et al.*, 1995; Doughty *et al.*, 1996).

This type of monitoring service is seen as way of allowing hospital patients to be discharged early, for example after surgery or a myocardial infarct, or for the management of elderly or chronically ill patients at home. The arguments for and against such communication services to the home are still unresolved, and await further study. Much of the impetus behind many home communication proposals seems to be either economic or technological. Where resources and staff are limited, or patients are in remote locations, they may indeed prove to be useful alternatives to routine care. It is equally clear that these arguments omit the clear need of some patients in the community to occasionally interact face-to-face with healthcare workers.

Patient access to healthcare workers

In normal circumstances, a combination of routine home visits and access via channels like the telephone may be sufficient for most patients. In difficult circumstances this arrangement may break down. For example, elderly patients may need to communicate with carers in an emergency, but might be unable to reach a telephone once the emergency has occurred. Fractures of the hip, strokes and heart attacks are all common problems that can leave elderly people in a vulnerable position in their own home.

To combat this risk, many elderly people have a personal alarm system connected to the public telephone system. There are many variations of this type of system. Usually they involve an individual wearing a pendant-style personal transmitter that can be activated with a simple button push. This activates an alarm at a control centre, which is then relayed to healthcare workers who will respond. Personal alarm systems serve over 1 million people in the United Kingdom, and 2–3 million people elsewhere (Fisk, 1995).

Patient access to information

Until recently, apart from the near ubiquitous use of the telephone, communication technology has played only a small role in information provision for patients. This is rapidly changing. For example, in the previous chapter we saw how one could use an interactive telephone system to deliver specialized information services. For example, patients could ring up an automated information system, and request it to fax them back specific pages of information.

Communications can be a critical component of public health campaigns, where a clear message is targeted into the broad population. The combination of an anti-smoking telephone helpline and a mass media campaign in Scotland managed to encourage about 82 000 smokers (5.9% of the adult smoking population) to make contact via the helpline over 1 year (Platt *et al.*, 1997). At 1 year follow-up nearly 25% of smokers who called the helpline were still not smoking, which is a very positive result. At the end of the second year of the campaign, smoking prevalence had dropped 6% among adults.

Communication services have also been shown to be successful when used for more chronic illnesses. In France, for example, many diabetic patients have had access to specialized information for quite some time. The service is based on Minitel, which is a small videotext terminal supplied free in France to all telephone subscribers. Using Minitel, some diabetic patients have had access to e-mail and an expert system customized to give individualized dietary advice based on information supplied by the patient regarding diet and exercise. Patients also had access to libraries of information, for example recipes. In a randomized trial, patients with access to information through the system demonstrated improved diabetic knowledge, improved dietary habits, and improved metabolic markers of disease control (fructosamine and HbA_1c) (Turnin *et al.*, 1992). Similar services can be easily provided across the Internet, which has a much richer functionality than the older Minitel system.

Clearly, for patients to master such relatively complicated communication and information resources, they have to be well trained, motivated and physically able to use these resources. Thus, independently of whichever technology is being employed to deliver information to patients, the most critical factors affecting compliance and correct usage will probably be human rather than technical.

21.5 Communication and primary care

There are significant organizational and communication challenges facing those delivering healthcare in the community. The model of shared care often adopted means that many different healthcare professionals may be involved in the management of an individual patient. During the course of routine management, a diabetic patient may, for example, interact with a primary care physician, a diabetic specialist nurse, a podiatrist and a dietician. There is thus a clear need for communication between these team members.

Working against this is the decentralized manner in which community services are organized, quite unlike a large hospital. Team members are unlikely to work in the same building, and may not even work in the same local area. Further, many workers will on occasion be on the move outside their office, for example carrying out home visits. In general practice even apparently simple activities such as ordering a laboratory test and receiving the report can involve many individuals, and many opportunities for inefficiency and error (Figure 21.2).

Primary care in many countries is under pressure, with diminishing resources being applied to growing consumer demands for access to care. Telephone services can be used to both provide information to patients who believe they need to visit a general practitioner, as well as actively triage the patient. For example, it may be possible to counsel a patient that no visit is required, direct them instead to a more appropriate service such as a hospital emergency

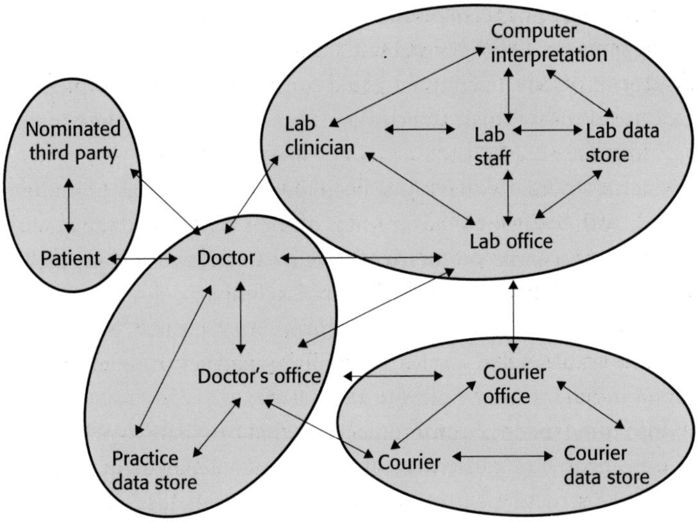
Computer interpretation
Nominated third party
Patient
Lab clinician
Lab staff
Lab data store
Lab office
Doctor
Doctor's office
Practice data store
Courier office
Courier
Courier data store

Figure 21.2
Possible communication pathways for a laboratory test ordered by a general practitioner.

department, or assist them by making an appointment with their general practitioner when this appears necessary.

Nurse-operated telephone triage has been shown to be both safe and effective as an out-of-hours service in primary care. One large-scale controlled study compared the impact of 7184 calls to a nurse triage point versus 7308 calls in the control group (Lattimer *et al.*, 1998). No increase in adverse events were noted during the trial, and the service resulted in a 69% reduction in telephone advice from the general practices, a 38% reduction in patient attendances to the practices and a 23% reduction in home visits.

In the UK, a service called NHS Direct has been set up to provide both information to consumers as well as acting as a triage point for the National Health Service (NHS). The system interacts with patients using multiple different channels and media, including a web presence, a call centre and information kiosks located in public areas. Even simple communication services are actually a complex bundle of components, often making evaluation difficult. With such a heterogeneous service as NHS Direct, one would expect no single metric to be available to determine effectiveness, nor would one expect benefits to be spread uniformly across the service.

Indeed, the evaluation of NHS Direct has proven to be difficult, given the complexity of the service (George, 2002). Some evidence suggests it has reduced the demand on emergency departments, which have received fewer telephone enquiries since the service came into operation (Jones and Playforth, 2001). However, little evidence exists that NHS Direct has significantly reduced demand on the NHS (Munro *et al.*, 2000) and therefore it is argued it is unlikely to be cheaper to run (Wootton, 2001). Lack of patient awareness of the service has confounded the analysis, as measures like cost-effectiveness for services with national reach are predicated on high levels of national awareness. Cost-effectiveness has proven to be an issue in other settings as well. A study of 32 paediatric call centres in the United States showed that all were losing on average $500 000 a year (Melzer and Poole, 1999).

Interface between primary care and specialist services

There has been a great emphasis in telemedicine on the interface between primary care and specialist services. There is a clear need for patient information to be exchanged between hospitals and primary care physicians at the time of admission to and discharge from hospital. The use of existing processes like the postal system to deliver such information is often criticized for tardiness and unreliability. In contrast, rapid communication of hospital discharge information using electronic data transfer mechanisms has been shown to be beneficial for general practitioners (Branger *et al.*, 1992).

Hospital discharge summaries have long been identified as a weak point between primary care and hospitals, both because of the tardiness of their arrival, and the quality of the information they contain. Discharge summaries arrive by a variety of means including the post, fax and e-mail. A randomized clinical trial in Canada compared discharge summaries created automatically from medical records against summaries created by voice dictation and demonstrated that the automated service can result in speedier completion of the summaries with no reduction in quality (van Walraven *et al.*, 1999).

Criticism is also often made of communications that originate in primary care, especially referral letters accompanying patients to the emergency department or specialists. Simple interventions such as structured forms may improve the quality of such communication (Harris *et al.*, 2002), but the wide variation in the types of message such letters might contain may require more complex, computer-assisted methods.

There has been significant recent effort in promoting methods that permit primary care practitioners to manage patients whom they would normally have referred to specialist centres, by supporting them with access to remote specialist advice. In one study, direct telephone access to a hospital-based cardiac monitoring centre was provided to primary care practitioners. They were able to consult with a cardiologist as needed, as well as transmit a 12-lead ECG (Shanit *et al.*, 1996). The centre in this study provided a 24-hour continuous service. Possible outcomes of the discussion were that the practitioner continued to manage the patient, that the patient was referred to a cardiology clinic, or in the case of suspected myocardial infarction, rapid hospital admission was arranged with pre-warning of hospital medical teams. A trial of 2563 patients over 18 months indicated that the service was perceived to be valuable, but no comparative cost-benefit analysis was performed.

In a pilot of video-based consultation for dermatological problems, the primary care practitioner was able to discuss patient cases interactively with a dermatologist, with the patient present. Over half of the patients could then be dealt with by the general practitioner immediately after consultation (Jones *et al.*, 1996). Common wisdom sees this type of service as a useful means of screening patients before they are seen by specialists, especially if travel is involved. However, in this study the patients suggested that they preferred an initial face-to-face consultation with the specialist dermatologist, and that the teleconsultation would have been better used for subsequent review of their progress.

Similar studies in Norway have identified other benefits to this type of remote telemedical consultation. The skill level of isolated practitioners was raised through repeated interactions with remote specialists and by having to manage cases that were previously referred (Akelsen and Lillehaug, 1993). This may arise through the dynamics of the relationship between remote practitioner and specialist. Unlike most educational settings, both are motivated to form a coach and apprentice relationship for the immediate management of a patient.

In Chapter 19 we saw that it is still unclear in what precise circumstances video-based consultations are most appropriate. Although there are some benefits in accessing remote expertise, there are limitations to the current technologies. It is well known for example, that during a clinical encounter a significant component of the information conveyed between practitioner and patient is non-verbal (Pendleton *et al.*, 1984). Tone of voice, facial expression and posture all convey subtle information cues that are interpreted by the patient. Technology can act either to distort these cues, or to filter them out. In some cases this might be beneficial. A patient may be less distressed if they are unable to pick up cues that the practitioner is worried about a situation. Equally, a patient's distress might increase if cues are misinterpreted because they are unfamiliar with the dynamics of the video-consultation. These effects will vary with the type of communication channel used, and the practitioner's skills at using the channel. Having a good 'video manner' may well soon be as important as having a good telephone manner.

21.6 Communication and hospitals

Telemedical systems, as we have seen, have been actively explored at the interface between hospital-based specialist services and primary care. Similar problems exist between small hospitals, which may not have access to the highly specialized personnel that can be found in larger institutions like teaching hospitals. Indeed, with the growing number of sub-specialities in clinical medicine, it is now unlikely that any one institution has a representative from every feasible medical sub-speciality within their institution. For this reason, there is a need to share highly specialized expertise across different hospitals, sometimes large distances apart.

Inter-hospital communication

There is now some evidence that remote consultation, using telemedical facilities such as video-conferencing, is able to assist with this problem of distribution of expertise (e.g. Doolittle and Allen, 1996). It has been shown, for example, that when a general radiologist is able to consult with a remote specialist, sharing views of radiographs using low-resolution video, then the general radiologist's diagnostic accuracy improved (Franken and Berbaum, 1996). It now seems accepted that, with appropriate technology, digitally transmitted images can in principle match existing imaging methods (e.g. Franken *et al.*, 1995; Martel *et al.*, 1995). The cost of achieving such results varies with the type of imaging task being attempted.

Triage models, similar to those explored in primary care, can limit the number of patients who need to be seen by limited sub-speciality resources. For example, in one study, general pathologists reviewed and reported on cases, and referred difficult cases to remote specialists by sending them high-resolution images (Bhattacharyya *et al.*, 1995).

In another study, patients were offered access to specialist medical practitioners in a different country. Patients were able to travel there or to have a consultation by video-link. Choosing the video-conferencing option changed patients' desires to travel overseas. Of those seeking consultation, 20% initially wished to travel for treatment, but after the teleconsultation only 6% chose this option (Richardson *et al.*, 1996).

Most of these studies throw up evidence that advanced communication systems and services are valuable. What remains unclear is whether there is any real cost-benefit from this approach. Indeed, it is becoming clear that the application of such technologies is beneficial only in particular sets of circumstances.

For example, comparing the costs of providing a rural population with radiology services from a small community-based unit, against a teleradiology system, the communication option fared poorly in one study (Halvorsen and Kristiansen, 1996). The study showed that the existing community-based system was the most cost-efficient, and the telemedical option the most expensive. The inconvenience caused when patients had to travel for specialist investigations was not factored into the study, nor was the possibility that some communities might not have access to local expertise.

Overall, the cost savings from installing any communication system must vary for different communities. The amount of resource saved, however measured, depends on many variables. These include:

- the size of population served
- the utilization rates of the services that are being augmented by the communication option
- the distances workers or patients might otherwise need to travel
- the effectiveness of local services in comparison to the telemedical options.

There is also evidence that some types of task are not entirely suited to the remote consultation model. Microbiologists, for example, probably need three-dimensional image information, as well as non-visual data like smell, before remote interpretation of microbiology specimens becomes feasible (Akelsen *et al.*, 1995).

As always, it is important to not overlook simpler solutions to communication problems, if they exist. It is not always appropriate or necessary, for example, to use video-based consultation. In many cases, the communication needs of a specialist consultation may be met by use of the telephone alone (McLaren, 1995). Rather than purchasing systems permitting real-time video-conferencing, images can be sent across computer networks. Standard e-mail systems are capable of transmitting text and image, and are more than able to manage the task of sending still images such as pathology slides or radiographs (Della Mea *et al.*, 1996). Once images have been received remotely, they can be viewed simultaneously and discussed over the telephone. Simple methods now exist to enhance this further, so that viewers can mark or point to sections of an image, and have these markings appear at the remote site.

Intra-hospital communication

Almost all of the current telemedical research is focused on the interfaces between hospitals and community services or the home. Very little work has been done to understand the internal communication dynamics and requirements of hospitals. Yet it should be apparent that any hospital is a complex organization, and that good communication processes must be fundamental to its operation.

Thus, although much effort has been devoted to developing the electronic patient record, there has been minimal exploration of what communication systems can be developed to support hospital operation. However, a critical examination of the characteristics of the hospital as a workplace can identify clear areas in which there is significant potential for improvement. Two areas in particular deserve discussion – the need to support mobility, and the need for asynchronous messaging.

Mobility

In contrast to other populations such as office workers or clinic-based healthcare workers, hospital workers are highly mobile during their working day. Nursing staff are perhaps least mobile, spending most of their day moving around their home ward. Medical staff may have to move widely across a hospital campus. Senior medical staff may also have to move off campus, to attend other hospitals or clinics. Nevertheless, it is important that staff remain within reach during the working day.

At present the commonest solution to this problem of contacting mobile staff is provided by radio-paging. Pagers are almost ubiquitous in modern hospitals, and staff may carry several of these. For example, a pager might be issued to each individual. Other pagers are issued to members of teams, for example a 'crash' team that needs to respond to critical emergencies such as cardiac arrests within the hospital. Pagers thus serve to permit communication both with named individuals, and individuals occupying labelled roles such as 'surgeon on call' (Smith *et al.*, 1991; Coiera, 1996b).

Pagers have several drawbacks. Invariably, in a busy work environment people move about and telephones are a pooled resource that quickly become engaged. As someone is paged, they answer the call to find either that the number given is now engaged, or that the caller has moved on to another ward location. The end result is often a game of 'telephone tag'.

The provision of mobile telephones bypasses many of these problems. The call set-up delays inherent in paging are eliminated, and the number of communication access points is multiplied through personal handsets. The value of mobile communications in a clinical environment is starting to be appreciated, but at present it remains an underutilized option (e.g. Fitzpatrick and Vineski, 1993). As with any technology, there are some drawbacks. At a practical level, some healthcare workers can choose to hide behind a paging system, effectively choosing which calls to answer on the basis of their current state. This form of call screening may no longer be possible if individuals have personal mobile telephones. The reduced costs of contacting colleagues and increased benefits of being contactable may be at the cost of decreased control of communication and increased interruption. At present it appears that the benefits significantly outweigh the costs, but formal studies are needed to confirm this.

Asynchronous communications

Hospitals are highly interrupt-driven environments (Coiera, 1996b). Interruptions to the normal flow of work are caused by the paging and telephone systems, as well as the result of impromptu face-to-face meeting by colleagues (e.g. being stopped in the corridor). The team-based nature of work also demands that clinicians communicate frequently with team members throughout the working day.

For example, nearly a third of communication events in a study of emergency department practice were classified as interruptions, meaning that they were not initiated by the observed subject, and occurred using a synchronous communication channel such as face-to-face conversation. This gave a rate of 11.15 interruptions per hour for all subjects (Coiera *et al.*, 2002). Even higher interruption rates were identified for individual clinical roles. Medical registrars and nurse coordinators experienced rates of 23.5 and 24.9 interruptions per hour (Spencer and Logan, 2002). In contrast, nurses and junior doctors had rates of 9.2 and 8.3 interruptions per hour.

The consequence of such frequent interruptions is that hospital workers have to repeatedly suspend active tasks to deal with the interruption, and then return to the previous task. Suspending tasks and then returning to them imposes a cognitive load (Box 8.2), and may result in tasks being forgotten, or left incomplete (Parker and Coiera, 2000). There thus is a cost in time and efficiency arising out of the interrupt-driven nature of the hospital work environment.

In part, the interruptive nature of hospitals is a result of the communication practices and systems in place in these organizations. For example, external telephone calls are one major source of interruption in emergency departments, especially if clinical staff are expected to suspend their current tasks to handle the calls. A simple organizational change, such as the introduction of a dedicated communications clerk who fields all incoming calls, has the potential to significantly reduce the communication load on clinical staff.

More generally, many hospitals do not at present routinely offer asynchronous channels such as voicemail or e-mail. It is likely that some of the interruptions delivered through synchronous systems like the telephone and pager system could be handled by asynchronous channels. For example, updates on patient results or non-urgent requests to complete tasks could be sent by voicemail or e-mail. As long as it is felt by those sending such messages that they definitely will be attended to, then some of the cause of interruption can be shifted on to these asynchronous systems. There thus seems to be a need for a concomitant change in communication process as well as the technology for such changes to be effective. The evidence that such asynchronous systems are of genuine benefit is slowly accumulating (e.g. Withers, 1988).

One of the limitations to the introduction of e-mail systems is the lack of access points around a campus, for many of the same reasons that access to telephony is limited. The mobility of workers is perhaps one of the main issues. This is why mobile computers are being introduced into the hospital environment (Forman and Zahorjan, 1994). Connected by wireless links, these small devices provide access to the hospital computer network.

The main driver for introducing such systems is to provide an easy way to capture clinical data and enter it into the hospital record system, or to retrieve data from it (e.g. Labkoff *et al.*, 1995; MacNeill and Huang, 1996). One additional benefit of mobile computing will be mobile access to e-mail. However, more advanced systems will be able to provide even richer services. Integrating mobile telephony, paging and access to the hospital network through lightweight portable devices, newer systems can combine the functionality of the telephone with that of the computer (e.g. Coiera, 1996b).

21.7 Researching clinical communication

The potential for the clinical application of communication technologies is indeed great, but there is still much to learn and several key research questions are apparent. Perhaps most crucially, it is still unclear which scientific principles should be applied in matching the needs of particular tasks with communication and information technology. Inevitably, any design theory will centre around good interaction design, and consequently include a socio-technical foundation. Communication systems include people, technologies and physical settings, and all these elements need to be considered in the design process. The notion of common ground between communicating agents (Figure 4.4) offers one way of conceiving of communication requirements (Coiera, 2000). Box 21.1 explores in detail how the notion of common ground can be used to choose between different technology options.

Secondly, our understanding of the effects of technology on communication is also in its infancy. Researchers in the field of human–computer interaction feel that before these technologies can be successfully introduced, the way in which individuals communicate needs to be understood (McCarthy and Monk, 1994). In one recent study, the presence of a computer during doctor–patient consultations had detectable negative effects on the way doctors communicated (Greatbatch *et al.*, 1993). While they were at the computer, doctors confined themselves to short responses to patient questions, delayed responding, glanced at the screen in preference to the patient, or structured the interview around the computer rather than the patient.

Box 21.1
When is conversation better than computation?

One of the great informatics challenges is to develop a set of principles that will guide the design and implementation of information and communication systems, based on the characteristics of the people using the system, their specific needs and constraints, and the attributes of different technological components (Coiera, 2000).

From an informatics viewpoint, we can take a 'first principles' approach that regards all informatics tasks as model construction and application. In simple terms, we can say that information technologies require explicit formalizations of information processes for them to operate, whereas communication systems remain relatively informal to process models. A telephone, for example, needs no model of the conversation that occurs across it for it to operate. In contrast, a computer system would need to explicitly model any dialogue that occurs across it. From this point of view, we can say that there is a continuum of possible model formalization available to us. For a given task, system designers make an explicit choice to model some or all of a process, based on their perception of costs and benefits. When the choice is to formalize the process substantially, we will sometimes find computational solutions are used. When the task is left informal, we should instead find that communication solutions are required.

Searching for a similar characterization of the continuum, one can turn to the literature in psychology and linguistics. In particular, the psychological notion of *common ground* is a strong match with the notion of relative formality of model construction. Common ground refers to the knowledge shared by two communicating agents. For a conversation to occur, agents have to share knowledge about language as well as knowledge about the subject under discussion (Figure 4.4). We know intuitively, for example, that discussing a medical problem with a clinical colleague or with a patient results in very different conversations. Messages can be concise and much mutual knowledge assumed between colleagues, but explaining an issue to a non-expert requires the main message to be sent along with the background knowledge needed to make the message understandable.

Human agents therefore communicate more easily with others of similar occupation and educational background, since they have similar experiences, beliefs and knowledge. Further, the more individuals communicate, the more similar they become (Rogers, 1995). We can recognize sharing of common ground as a key reason that similar agents find it easy to converse with each other. Further, during the process of any given conversation, there are actually two separate streams of dialogue. The first is concerned with the specifics of the conversation, whilst the second is devoted to checking that messages have been understood, and may result in sharing of common ground when it is clear assumptions about shared knowledge do not hold. Thus building common ground requires mutual effort and consent between participating agents.

The notion of common ground holds whether we are discussing a conversational interaction between humans, or a human–computer interaction. For a computationally rendered information system, the system designer must create a model of what the user will want to do with the application. For their part, users will have to learn a model of how to operate the computer application. Where both computer and user share this common ground, the interaction should be succinct and effective. Where the user or system do not share mutual knowledge we run into difficulty. If the user lacks knowledge of the system's operation, the human–computer dialogue will be ineffective. Where the system does not model its context of use, it will be regarded as an inappropriate intrusion into the workplace.

Building common ground incurs costs for the participating agents. For example, a computer user spends some time up front learning the functions of a system in anticipation of having to use them for future interactions. Inevitably, not everything that can be 'said' to the computer is learnt in this way, and users also typically learn new features of a system as they interact with it for particular tasks. This means that agents have two broad classes of grounding choice:

Pre-emptive grounding

Agents can share knowledge in advance of a specific conversational task, assuming it will be needed in the future. They elect to bear the grounding cost ahead of time and risk the effort being wasted if it is never used. This is a good strategy when task time is limited. For example, training a medical emergency team on how to interact with each other makes sense because at the time of a real clinical emergency, there is no time for individuals to question each other to understand the meaning of any specific orders or requests. However, pre-emptive grounding is a bad strategy when the shared knowledge is never used and the time and effort in grounding becomes wasted. For example, training students with knowledge that is unlikely to be used when they face a task in the workplace is usually a poor allocation of resources. From first principles, the cost of pre-emptive grounding is proportionate to the amount of common ground an agent has to learn. For example, the length of

(*Contd.*)

Box 21.1
(*Contd.*)

messages increases, as does the cost of checking and maintaining the currency of the knowledge once received (Figure 21.3).

Just-in-time grounding

Agents can choose to share specific task knowledge only at the time they have a discussion. This is a good strategy when there are no other reasons to talk to an agent. For example, if the task or encounter is rare it probably does not make sense to expend resources in the anticipation of an unlikely event. Conversely, it is a bad strategy when there is limited task time for grounding at the time of the conversation. For example, if a rare event is nonetheless an urgent one, preparation is essential. Thus pilots, nuclear power plant operators and clinicians all train rigorously for rare but mission-critical events, since failure to prepare has potentially catastrophic consequences. Just-in-time is also a poor strategy if one of the agents involved in the dialogue is reluctant to expend energy learning. Thus computer system designers might face difficulties if they assume users are willing to spend time during the routine course of their day learning new features of their system, when the users are already overcommitted with other tasks. The cost of just-in-time grounding is inversely proportional to the amount of prior shared knowledge between agents. For example, a message between agents with a high degree of common ground will be very terse, but the length (and thus cost) of transmitting a message to an agent with little common ground will be greater (Figure 21.4).

Any given interaction between two agents usually involves costs borne at the time of the conversation, as well as costs borne previously in pre-emptive grounding (Figure 21.5). For information system designers we thus have a space of choices in regard to the amount of grounding we expect of the agents who will participate in organizational interactions. At the 'solid ground' end of the spectrum, tasks will require agents to share knowledge ahead of time for the task to be effectively or efficiently completed. At the other end of the spectrum there is 'shifting ground', where it is hard or uneconomic to decide what ground should be pre-emptively shared.

Thus, with 'solid ground' interactions, a user is expected to have learnt most of the formalities of using an information system, or conversely the system is expected to have adapted to the needs of the users. With 'shifting ground', the information system is designed to handle interactions that require new knowledge to be exchanged at the time of interaction. This may be in the form of online help to the user, or acquiring data from the user.

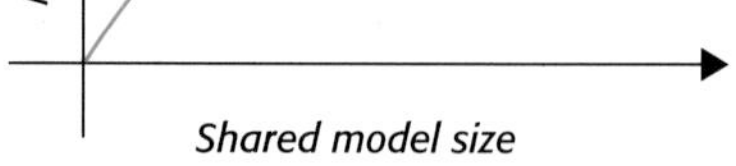
Model grounding cost
Shared model size

Figure 21.3
The cost of pre-emptive grounding increases with the amount of knowledge agents share – the more we share, the greater the cost of telling and maintaining.

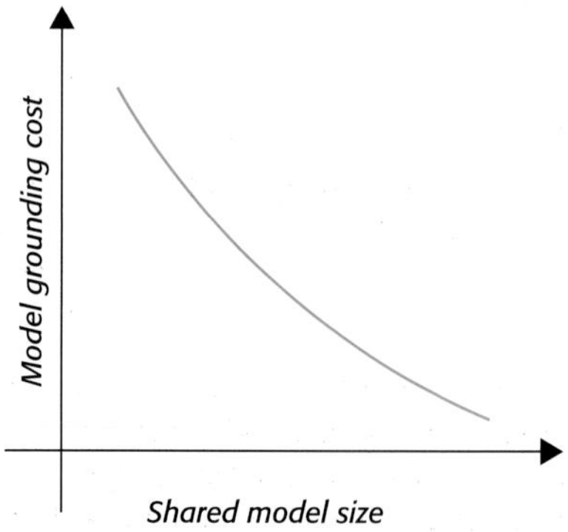
Model grounding cost
Shared model size

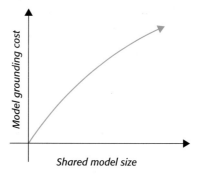

Figure 21.4
The cost of just-in-time grounding decreases with the amount of prior knowledge agents already share about a task – the less we share, the more I have to share now.

Common ground links the design of information and communication systems. It gives us the ability to explain why some communication systems work better than others, and may assist us in predicting whether or not new systems will work. It offers us an operational measurement that can be used to define the characteristics of specific interactions between agents, whether they are human or computational. Using it, we should be able to analyse the specifics of a particular set of interactions and make broad choices about whether they would be better served by communication or computational systems. It should also allow us to make finer grained distinctions about the dynamics of such interactions, for example with regard to the amount of grounding that needs to be supported within a specific human–machine conversation. With this in mind, we can now simply regard information models as part of the common ground of an organization and its members. We can choose to model any interaction across a spectrum from zero to a 'complete' formal description (Figures 9.3 and 21.6).

Further, the models we build of our organizational systems only have value when we interact with them through our information or communication systems. In other words, for computational tools to be of value, they have to share ground with humans. Users need to know how to use the system, and the system needs to be

(Contd.)

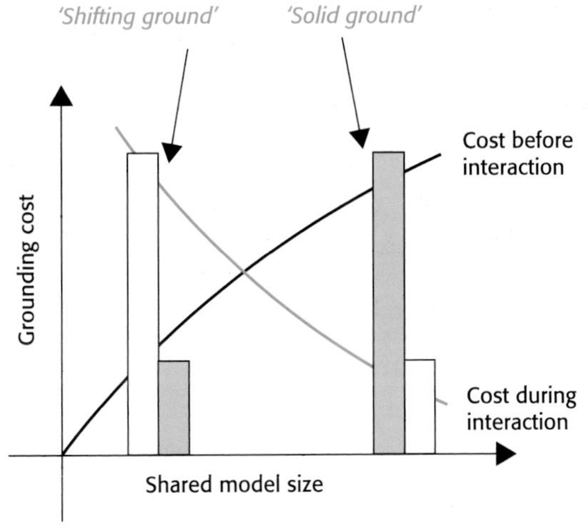
'Shifting ground'
'Solid ground'
Cost before interaction
Grounding cost
Cost during interaction
Shared model size

Figure 21.5
For any given interaction, some of the grounding costs are borne at the time of the interaction, and some have been taken earlier. For an information system designer, this means that there is a spectrum of options in designing the interaction between computer and user.

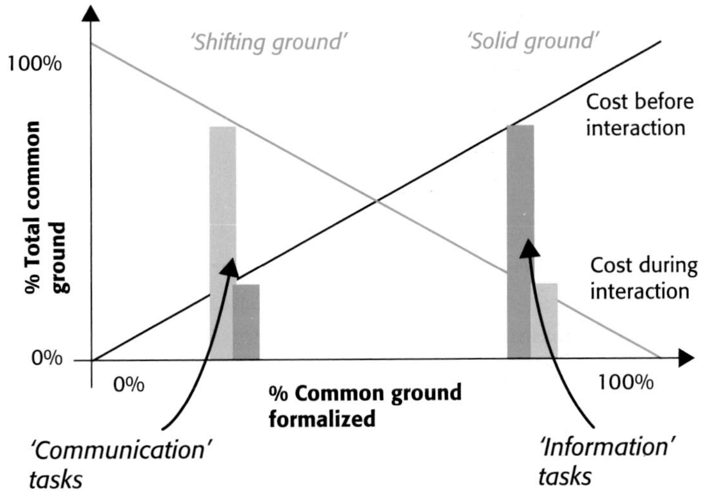
'Shifting ground'
'Solid ground'
100%
Cost before interaction
% Total common ground
Cost during interaction
0%
0%
% Common ground formalized
100%
'Communication' tasks
'Information' tasks

Figure 21.6 There is a continuum of common ground between agents that defines how much of the interaction can be modelled formally ahead of time, and how much needs to be left informal until the time of the interaction. Computational systems work well when substantial modelling can occur ahead of time; communication systems can be used when agents are unable to reliably model their interactions ahead of time.

Box 21.1 (*Contd.*)

fashioned to user's needs. If an information system is perfectly crafted to model the processes of an organization, but not the resource constraints of those who will need to learn to use it, then almost inevitably it will fail. Consequently we should no longer consider information models in isolation but rather include the models that users will need to carry with them. Simply building an information model without regard to how it will be shared with those who interact with it ignores the complex realities of the workplace, and does not factor in the costs and benefits of using the model for individuals.

'Pure' communication tools such as the telephone can now be seen to be neutral to any particular conversation that occurs over them, and need no common ground with the agents using them. As such they are well suited to supporting poorly grounded conversations, when it is hard to predict ahead of time what knowledge needs to be shared.

We thus favour the use of communication tools across 'shifting ground' with a high just-in-time grounding component. This may be because the interacting agents do not share sufficient ground or it may be that it simply is not worth the effort to do the modelling. The information transacted is thus often personal, local, informal, or rare. It is up to the agents having the discussion to share knowledge. The channel simply provides basic support to ensure the conversation takes place. Communication channels are thus used *de facto* when there are no computational tools to support the process.

Further, for highly grounded conversations, we know the agents will be able to have succinct conversations. One can predict that they will need lower bandwidth channels than would be the case if the message exchange were poorly grounded. Poorly grounded conversations in contrast will need higher bandwidth, since more information will have to be exchanged between the conversing agents. Building such common ground between agents may require the sharing of information objects such as images and designs.

In contrast, we favour computational tools when it is appropriate to formalize interactions ahead of time, and the users of the system are willing, able, and resourced to build common ground with the tool. Such interactions occur over 'solid ground', having a high pre-emptive grounding component. The information exchanged in such situations is worth formalizing, perhaps because it is stable, repetitive, archival, or mission critical. The computational system moves from being a passive channel to the interaction, to either modifying what is said, or becoming a conversational agent itself.

An information system designer also needs to take into account the common ground that is expected of the system users. For computational tools, there are also choices to be made between the traditional process of information modelling before system construction, and a more interactive approach to building models. Thus, a system designer may try to model all the user needs before the construction of a system, or engineer some flexibility into the architecture that allows personalization of the interaction for specific users. For example, a system may gather data about the frequency of different requests from a specific user, and customize its behaviour to optimize for the most frequent requests of the individual, rather than the population as a whole. Such computational systems build common ground with their users in a 'just-in-time' fashion, as well as having pre-emptive modelling to cover the commonest features users will need.

Clinical practice already revolves around communication, often by telephone, and important information exchanged in this way is often lost because it is not documented (Stoupa and Campbell, 1990). As we saw in Chapter 4, much of this information is informal. Capturing the informal information currently lost in healthcare's communication channels may soon become an important issue for those developing the formal electronic patient record. How one decides what information is important, and how that information is made available, are non-trivial questions involving issues of confidentiality and security, as well as the technology of storage and retrieval of voice recordings. The implications of this change in emphasis for the form and role of the electronic medical record are significant. Equally, the role of communications systems in supporting information retrieval should be reassessed. The telephone is an information system, albeit an informal one.

Probably the most immediate research challenges will be to focus the effect of introducing technologies that allow asynchronous communication. At present, devices like telephones and pagers interrupt individuals when communication is desired. The messages sent across asynchronous services like electronic mail and voicemail do not need to be answered immediately and so have the potential to significantly reduce the number of interruptions experienced by clinicians. Such messages may nevertheless carry important information. It will be critical to understand how such services can be designed to ensure that healthcare workers do not miss critical information, and equally are not inundated with a flood of irrelevant messages.

Finally, along with new communication possibilities, there come new medico-legal implications. The medico-legal position for teleconsultations is similar to that of telephone, fax, e-mail or letter. These all amount to the provision of advice from a distance, and the normal standards of care and skill will apply (Brahams, 1995). There thus may be circumstances when it is considered inappropriate **not** to use teleconsultation. For example, if moving a patient puts them at risk and teleconsultation is available, then the communication option may be most appropriate. Equally, in some circumstances it may be inappropriate to use it, perhaps because there is a likelihood that management will be sub-optimal compared to face-to-face care. Until the evidence accumulates to identify which situations are most suitable for teleconsultation, its appropriateness in any given circumstances will have to be argued on a case-by-case basis, quite probably in the courts.

In the United States the courts have already decided that radiologists are negligent if they fail to inform clinicians personally of a diagnosis. 'Communication of an unusual finding in an X-ray, so that it may be beneficially utilized, is as important as the finding itself.' Further, leaving a message with an intermediary is not enough – 'certain medical emergencies may require the most direct and immediate response involving personal consultation and exchange' (Kline and Kline, 1992). The fact that such communication requirements are beginning to be mandated reflects the community's changing perceptions of best clinical practice.

The next few years should see the research in telemedicine mature, as the number of high-quality well-designed trials of telemedicine systems grows. The main focus will become the application of communication technologies rather than their development. This represents the same shift in focus that was required of health informatics, which also initially spent much effort in developing technologies specifically for healthcare.

Discussion points

1. 'We should not invest in telemedical services until there is strong evidence to support their value.' Do you agree with this statement?
2. You are the project officer managing a new telemedicine project whose goal will be to improve communications between the emergency departments at your hospital and a small satellite hospital in a rural area. At the very first meeting you are informed by the CEO 'all of the video-conferencing equipment has now been ordered'. Do you think this project is going to succeed?
3. Are all interruptions necessarily bad? What would the consequence be of a 'no interruption' policy in a busy clinical setting?

Chapter summary

1 Telemedicine is the remote communication of information to facilitate clinical care.

2 Telemedicine can be evaluated in three broad categories – user satisfaction, economic benefit, and clinical outcome changes. Almost all independent and systematic large-scale reviews of telemedicine have failed to find evidence of benefit, rather than identifying evidence for lack of benefit.

3 Communication needs fall into two groups. Firstly, specific intra-organizational needs exist within particular groups, such as hospitals or primary care. Secondly, there are significant inter-organizational needs that occur at the interfaces between significantly different organizations.

4 Communications systems have a role in home healthcare, providing patients with access to information about their care and the ability to interact regularly with healthcare workers to assure themselves that they are managing their own care well.

5 In primary care there are communication needs at the interface between primary care and specialist services, and between primary care and patients. Video-based telemedical consultations are a possible solution to some of these needs, but their value still remains uncertain.

6 Very little work has been done to understand the internal communication dynamics and requirements of organizations like hospitals. There are clear needs, however, to have support for mobile and asynchronous communication.

PART 7

The Internet

CHAPTER 22

The Internet and World Wide Web

> Computers and automation have captured man's imagination. That is to say, like the psychiatrist's ink blot, they serve the imagination as symbols for all that is mysterious, potential, portentous. For when man is faced with ambiguity, with complex shadows he only partly understands, he rejects ambiguity and reads meaning into the shadows. And when he lacks the knowledge and technical means to find real meanings in the shadows, he reads into them the meanings in his own heart and mind … Computers are splendid ink blots.
> *H.A. Simon (1965), p. ix.*

The rise of the Internet presented us with a defining moment at the end of the last millennium. Some saw it as a technological revolution rivalling Gutenberg's invention of the printing press. Others saw it as just another tool that, like the telephone or television, would soon pass into common usage and leave our lives relatively unchanged. However, the Internet defies such simple analysis. It is not a single entity, but represents the conjunction of several quite different technological and social forces. Consequently, its implications for the way information is created, distributed and accessed are wide ranging. For healthcare in particular, the implications for the way healthcare is delivered are significant.

In previous sections of this book, the two fundamental informatics strands of information and communication systems were developed. In this section on the Internet, we will see how information and communication systems can combine, and the power that results from that combination. This chapter introduces the Internet and the Web, and explores the technical and social forces shaping it. The next chapter will look specifically at the way the Internet may be used in healthcare. The third chapter looks at the Internet as a social network, and shows how we can understand many of the features of Internet use through the principles of information economics.

22.1 The Internet has evolved through four stages

From a relatively humble beginning, the Internet has transformed completely in size, form and function. Historically, one can think of the Internet evolving through four relatively distinct stages, each one shaped in turn by its predecessors.

- It began in the United States in the late 1960s as a cold-war military research project, designed to ensure that communication lines remained open after nuclear strikes. This system slowly evolved in size and complexity until, in the mid-1980s, the Internet had become a global computer network.
- At that time it was used by many academic institutions, and a few commercial companies. During this second phase, its main use was for electronic messaging and the transfer of computer files. What followed next was a period of steady growth, as the population of users slowly expanded beyond industry and academia.
- It was not really until the third phase, with the introduction of the World Wide Web, that the massive growth today associated with the Internet occurred. The Web (WWW or W3) provides a simple and standard way to find and view documents on the Internet. Its ease of use, along with an ever-growing storehouse of publicly accessible information, combined to transform the Internet into a tool that the public at large was able to appreciate and wanted to use.
- The fourth phase, which we are now in, followed on relatively rapidly. It is characterized by the commercial and institutional exploitation of the Internet and its technologies. A constant stream of innovation in the way the Internet is being used,

Box 22.1
The end of the ice age

In the Victorian era, there was a global market in ice. The ice was harvested in cold countries like North America, and shipped around the world as far as the Indian sub-continent. The ice was transported in specially constructed ice-ships, then stored in huge warehouses upon arrival. Every good home had an ice chest in which they kept this precious commodity, and used it to keep food cool.

In the 1860s, competition in the form of artificial ice-making plants began to appear. Today the ice trade has disappeared. We no longer need to ship ice because technology has caused the nature of the market to change. Rather then shipping ice, we ship the stuff needed to make ice – energy. Energy is transported across great power grids that originate in huge power stations. The fundamental market need has not changed – we still want the ability to cool our food. What has changed is the way in which that need is met. The power industry and refrigerator manufacturers are the economic inheritors of the ice industries.

We can draw interesting economic parallels between the demise of the ice industry and the fate of printing. Books today are created in printing houses, and from there shipped around the globe, eventually to be stored in the huge warehouses we call libraries.

If the world of publishing is equivalent to the ice industry, then the Internet is equivalent to the power industry. The Internet does not ship documents printed on paper. It ships information down its data grid, which can be reconstituted into documents upon arrival. Just as a refrigerator sits at the edge of the power grid and takes in energy to produce cold, computers sit at the edge of the information grid, and take in information, converting it as needed into other forms. The parallel is striking.

The needs met by the 'information market' are the same before and after the arrival of the Internet, but the nature of that market has changed. The Internet thus heralds fundamental economic change. Old industries will disappear and new ones will emerge.

Although some changes will be rapid, others will undoubtedly be very slow. Libraries for example, will still be needed – at least until all their contents have been converted into electronic form. That process may be slow and expensive, and for some works the demand may be so small that it is easier to continue to warehouse them in libraries.

as well as in its underlying technologies, guarantees that change will be a feature for quite some time.

22.2 The Internet as a technological phenomenon

Essentially a network of networks, the Internet permits computers across the globe to communicate with each other. It evolved out of the Advanced Research Projects Network (ARPAnet) developed by the United States Department of Defence in the late 1960s (Lowe *et al.*, 1996). ARPAnet was built with the intention of developing computer networks that would be capable of surviving nuclear war. The challenge at that time was to develop methods for sharing information across diverse sites, and to keep these connections operational even if a disruption occurred at individual sites.

The result of this work was a standard internetworking protocol (IP), which regulates the way in which computers communicated with each other across the network. IP operates at layer 4 (network) of the OSI model (Table 20.1). Throughout the 1970s and early 1980s the Internet grew, as more and more small, mainly academic networks were joined on to it using the new IP.

Initially the information transmitted across the Internet consisted of text-based electronic mail, or computer files that were shipped from one site to another. These data files were often themselves complicated documents – for example, scientists commonly exchanged preliminary research papers in this way. There was no standard way that defined how these files should be created or viewed. Standard printer languages like Postscript gave some guarantee that a file generated on one computer system could be printed at another site, but it soon became clear that it would be desirable to send many different kinds of media, not just text, across the Internet. This **multimedia** added still and video images and voice to basic text.

Work that began at the European Particle Physics Laboratory (CERN) in 1989 resulted in a set of communication standards and software that provided Internet users with a simple way of creating and accessing such information. These standards allowed users to create and exchange text, image and video documents. The model for the way one could interact with these multimedia files also began to evolve.

In particular, the already well-understood notion of **hypertext** became particularly important. The notion of navigating around hypertext slowly evolved from the 1960s onwards, as computer scientists tried to find ways of managing complex and rapidly changing information that was distributed across many locations (Lowe *et al.*, 1996). A hypertext computer file includes links within it to other files, possibly located on a distant computer. Activating a hypertext link on a document permits a reader to view the document attached to the link. Hypertext document navigation is often characterized as being nonlinear. One can jump across documents, following references that appear of interest to a particular reader. Consequently different readers will follow different 'paths' through the space of hypertext documents, depending on their needs.

This work at CERN was successful in a way that was probably not foreseen by those who commenced the original research project. These standards were responsible for the appearance of a large number of interlinked multimedia files that were distributed across the Internet. This expanding global collection of interconnected information sources became known as the World Wide Web.

Today, these standards are in a state of constant evolution. It is unlikely that the Internet's creators could have foreseen, for example, that the Internet would be used for voice telephony, or that we could one day interact with virtual reality worlds across it. Equally, they could not have foreseen the size of the present Internet or its present rate of sustained growth. Perhaps of greater surprise is that the basic internetworking protocols developed out of the ARPAnet sustain a collection of networks far in excess of the number that was ever intended.

22.3 The Internet as a social phenomenon

The Internet has been around since the 1980s, but it was the advent of the World Wide Web that triggered its public growth. The Web permitted the general public to navigate easily across the global Internet and view a bewildering variety of information, from the bizarre and inaccurate, to the most up-to-date information available from scientific bodies, newspapers and academic journals.

By the end of the twentieth century, the Internet was in a phase of massive expansion, with monthly growth rates of well above 15%. For example, the OncoLink information resource provides oncologists with up-to-date clinical trial and treatment information, but also acts as an educational resource for cancer patients and their families. At its inception in March 1994, OncoLink was reportedly accessed 36 000 times that month (Buhle *et al.*, 1994). The figure for February 1999 was 5 957 448 accesses (Figure 22.1).

As more of these information services become available, even more people are persuaded to join. This 'network effect' is the same phenomenon of technology adoption reaching a critical mass that we have seen in the past with other technologies such as the telephone, the CD and the personal computer. When only a few people possessed them, there was insufficient market to develop the services and economies of scale that would make them mass market items. Once a certain threshold of ownership is exceeded, however, the market develops rapidly.

Associated with the growing public interest in the Internet is a brand of more extreme social futurism. Words like 'cyberspace' and 'virtual reality' combine with aspirations for social change to create visions of a future society based on a commerce of information

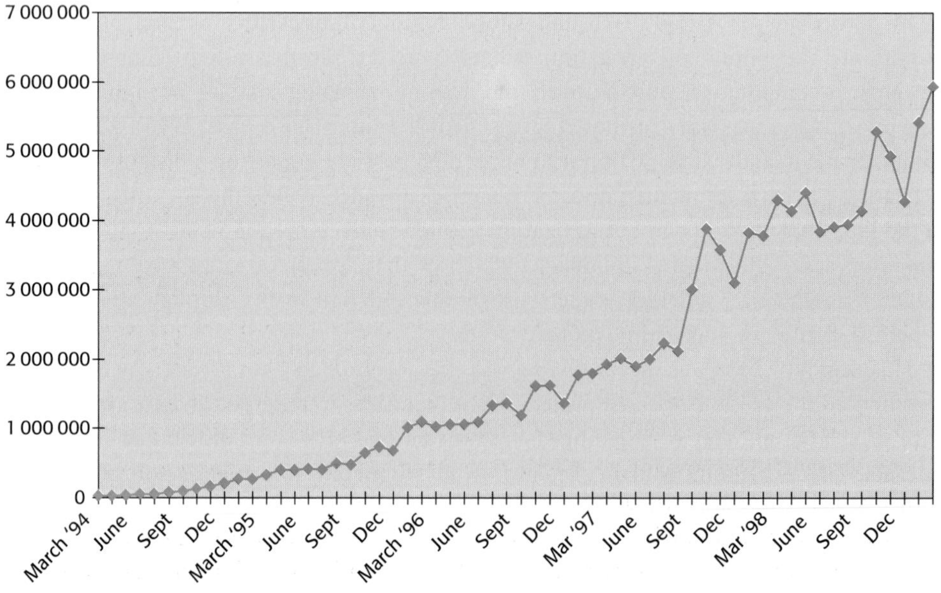

7 000 000
6 000 000
5 000 000
4 000 000
3 000 000
2 000 000
1 000 000
0
March '94
June
Sept
Dec
March '95
June
Sept
Dec
March '96
June
Sept
Dec
Mar '97
June
Sept
Dec
Mar '98
June
Sept
Dec

Figure 22.1 The rapid growth in Internet use is shown through the rise in total monthly accesses to the OncoLink World Wide Web site, which began service to the public in March 1994 (http://cancer.med.upenn.edu/).

(e.g. Negroponte, 1995). As unsurprising is the intellectual backlash of many who reject visions of a world in which people preferentially interact with others across computer networks rather than in more 'human' ways.

Perhaps more substantially, this brand of futurism has echoes of social reaction to many previous technologies. Everything from satellite communications, through to the Pill, radio, television, the telephone and the computer were all going to revolutionize society in the eyes of some commentators. In their own way, they often did, but never as fundamentally as was predicted.

A feature of the futurism associated with the Internet is the belief in a technology-enabled information society. Here, the freedom of creation, distribution and access to information is the mechanism through which many imagine the solution to a variety of social ills. As with any group of people engaged in radical thinking, there are elements both of truth and wishful thinking here. For example, much is now made of the 'digital divide', as the population of many resource-poor nations still have limited access to the Internet. Information is just one more global resource that is unequally shared between the peoples of the planet. No doubt faced with the end of the 'dot com' hysteria, the corporatization of the web, and the poor distribution of access to the Internet, many futurists have already dropped cyberspace in favour of a new liberation technology.

22.4 The Internet as a commercial phenomenon

The growth of the public's interest in the Internet initially caught most computer and telecommunications companies by surprise. Communication had traditionally been the preserve of the telecommunications industry, and the market for information provision on home computers was going to be dominated by CD-ROM technology. Today, a variety of industries are now capitalizing on the Internet, some more successfully than others. What initially made this particular market so ripe for exploitation was that it was fought over by so many separate industries, each a giant in its own right. Telecommunications carriers, cable television companies and personal computer companies, for example, believed that the Internet had the potential to either transform or wipe out their existing businesses.

The wealth and competitive aggression of such companies led to significant over-investment in Internet businesses, and fuelled the public equities bubble that resulted in the 'dot com' boom, and bust. It should be remembered that the Internet share market boom had little to do with the technologies being exploited, or their true potential. Rather, it was fuelled by greed and panic. So, despite the boom and bust, today the use of the Internet and Web continues to grow, and is becoming a commonplace element of everyday life for many people.

There are four basic Internet 'businesses' – transport, connection, services, and content.

- **Transport** refers to the industries that provide the physical networks upon which the Internet is built, and across which the basic bits of information are moved. This 'bit shipping' is the domain of telecommunication companies and the cable and wireless network operators, and is fiercely competitive. As it becomes increasingly cheap to ship bits, these industries are forced to look to other more profitable kinds of Internet business to maintain their profitability.
- Providing **connection** into the Internet is in itself a business. Increasingly, service providers offer network connections to the Internet for individuals or groups who do

not have the need, or cannot afford to build, their own networks. This is typically how most homes are presently connected to the Internet. Usually this involves signing a contract with a service provider who creates and maintains Internet accounts, and provides connection on some fee-for-service basis. Some of these service providers are well-established names such as CompuServe and America Online, but major computer companies have also moved into the service-provision business and are increasingly challenging them. This is seen by many as an attempt by these computer companies to establish a foothold in the potentially even more profitable businesses of service and content provision.

- For example, many diverse existing businesses can use the Internet to provide their **services** to a larger community of people. Customer information queries can now be satisfied by Web-based information sources, rather than needing to be handled by staff on the telephone. New means of advertising and marketing are also emerging. More fundamentally, the Internet provides businesses with new ways with which to interact with the public. These range from the ability to order pizza across the Internet through to browsing sales catalogues and placing orders, viewing homes with real estate agencies and to carrying out transactions with banks and other financial institutions.
- Finally, the Internet has created a new demand for information. So-called **content providers**, be they traditional publishers, or companies that control other forms of information (for example mailing lists) are able to sell their information on the Internet. Consider the difference in costs for a publisher of an encyclopaedia between its traditional business and an Internet-based one. Traditionally the public would be asked to buy a complete set of encyclopaedia volumes, representing a large personal investment by the family. Equally, the company has to invest considerably in sales staff to sell the books. The Internet business model is completely different. Here the public accesses an electronic version of the encyclopaedia on the Web. Every time a member of the public looks up information, the encyclopaedia company makes a small charge. So, a business that relied on making relatively few but large sales using a local sales force is transformed into a global company that makes a multitude of very small sales with no sales force. The implications of such business changes can be substantial.

22.5 The Internet as an enterprise phenomenon

Although initially a global phenomenon, the Internet provides a new model for the way organizations can organize their internal communication and information systems. Most major academic institutions and corporations manage their own internal computer networks, fulfilling similar communication and information functions to the wider Internet. The technological advances that have driven the growth of the Web on the external Internet are just as applicable to these internal networks. The use of Internet technologies on an internal computer network creates what is termed an internal Internet, or **intranet** (Figure 22.2).

There are numerous benefits of an intranet model for large organizations. Firstly, at a technological level, their existing networks may consist of a mixture of systems running different communication protocols. Managing such diversity is complex, expensive and time-consuming. Using IP allows a uniform protocol to be used across an enterprise's network. Just as attractively, the simplicity of the Web's multimedia and hypertext makes intranet systems much easier to use, and requires less specific training of staff.

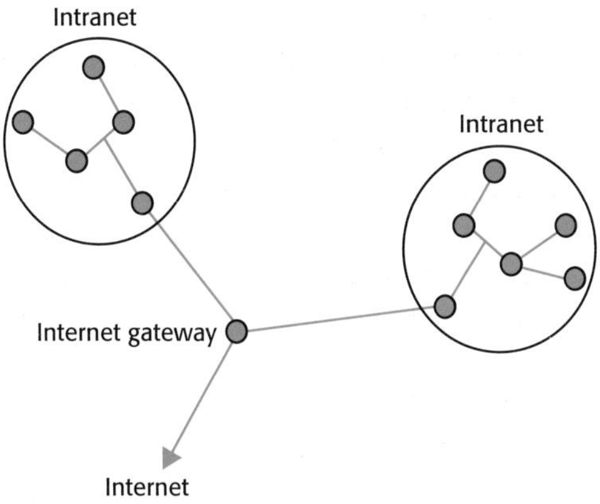
Intranet
Intranet
Internet gateway
Internet

Figure 22.2
Intranets are created from the computer networks within an organization like a hospital or a company, use Internet technologies and have the same benefits. They can also be connected by gateways to the open global Internet.

The model of information publication and access offered by the Web is also substantially different from the more traditional centralized corporate model. In the past, if an information service were to be made available, it would need to be created in conjunction with the organization's Information Systems (IS) department. If changes needed to be made to existing information resources, they also had to be funnelled through these same channels. The end result of this model for large organizations was that their computer systems tended to become large and complicated over time, and increasingly difficult and expensive to maintain. As the organization and its information requirements changed, the centrally managed systems become increasingly out of date, since they could not change at the same rate.

The Web model allows workers across an organization to create and locally maintain their own information services. For example, manuals and information packs can be placed online and updated without any central support being needed. In a hospital, the telephone directory, information packages for new patients and the daily report on bed occupancy could all be put on the hospital intranet.

22.6 Communication on the Internet

There are a variety of ways in which individuals and groups can communicate on the Internet, starting with basic services like e-mail, which can be combined to create more powerful services such as private mailing lists and newsgroups. We can broadly characterize such services as either being **information push**, in which messages are pushed out to targeted individuals, or **information pull**, in which access is based on individuals seeking or being pulled toward information sources. When messages are sent from one individual to another, this is called **peer-to-peer** communication. Sending a message to a select group of individuals is sometimes called **narrowcasting**, in contrast to widespread distribution, which we know as **broadcasting** (Table 22.1).

Mailing lists

An e-mail message is an example of a information push, peer-to-peer method that can also be used to narrowcast to multiple destinations. By drawing up pre-defined distribution lists

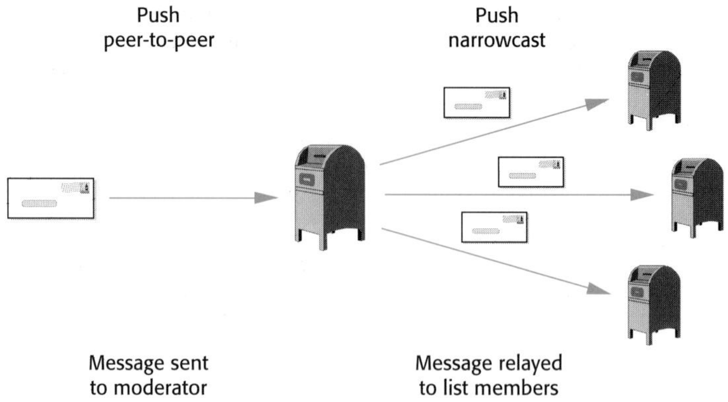
Push
peer-to-peer
Push
narrowcast
Message sent
to moderator
Message relayed
to list members

Figure 22.3
Mailing lists: before all the members of a mailing list receive a message, it is sent to the maintainer of the list, who acts as a gatekeeper, possesses the addresses of all list members and forwards messages to them.

Table 22.1 Types of communication modality, and some methods suited to these tasks.

Communication modality	Communication service
Peer-to-peer	E-mail, fax
Narrowcast	E-mail, fax lists
Broadcast	Web, newsgroups

of people, a mailing list can be created to allow a select group of people to carry out ongoing and private discussions by e-mail (Figure 22.3).

One or more individuals choose to maintain the list of names, and 'moderate' the group interactions. People wishing to join the list send requests to the moderator. People wishing to send a message to the group also send the message to the moderator. The moderator vets the message for appropriateness, and then sends it to the list. The speed of message distribution is thus dependent on the rapidity with which the moderator forwards messages. The moderator has significant and sometimes absolute control over the discussion that takes place in the group. For example, professional bodies may elect a moderator, draw up rules of conduct for message creation and distribution, or indeed have a panel of two or more individuals who collectively moderate messages.

Newsgroups and bulletin boards

Anyone with access to the Internet is able to access a wide variety of different discussion groups, read the messages placed in these groups and respond to messages by e-mail. Newsgroups are an example of the information pull communication method. Message responses can broadcast to the public, by posting back to the newsgroup, or be kept private by posting back only to the originator of the message (Figure 22.4).

Newsgroups are classified systematically, according to the type of discussion that takes place in each group (Figure 22.5). The organizational structure is usually taxonomic, resulting in a family tree of newsgroups. Thus the newsgroup *sci.med.informatics* belongs to the overall '*sci*' group devoted to scientific discussions, of which the '*med*' groups are in particular devoted to medical topics. Of the many medical newsgroups, this one is devoted to discussions about informatics.

Even if newsgroups may have a 'professional' topic, access to the group is universal. Thus it is just as likely to find a member of the public, perhaps currently under treatment, posting

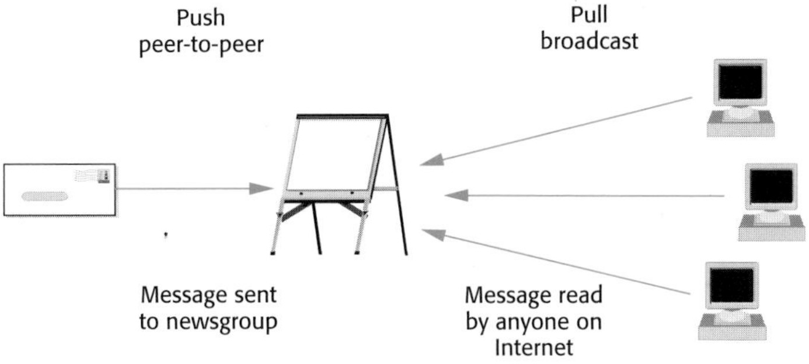
Push
peer-to-peer
Pull
broadcast
Message sent
to newsgroup
Message read
by anyone on
Internet

Figure 22.4
Newsgroups and bulletin boards are maintained by a moderator, who vets messages that are posted to the group. Once posted there, anyone with access to the group is able to read all current messages.

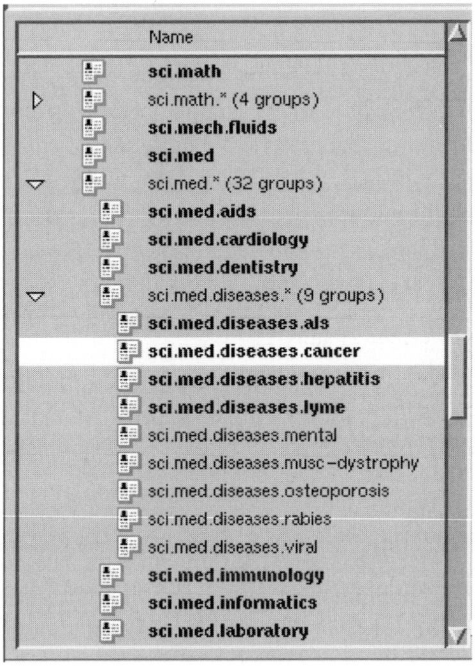
Name
sci.math
sci.math.* (4 groups)
sci.mech.fluids
sci.med
sci.med.* (32 groups)
sci.med.aids
sci.med.cardiology
sci.med.dentistry
sci.med.diseases.* (9 groups)
sci.med.diseases.als
sci.med.diseases.cancer
sci.med.diseases.hepatitis
sci.med.diseases.lyme
sci.med.diseases.mental
sci.med.diseases.musc-dystrophy
sci.med.diseases.osteoporosis
sci.med.diseases.rabies
sci.med.diseases.viral
sci.med.immunology
sci.med.informatics
sci.med.laboratory

Figure 22.5
Newsgroups are organized systematically, and classified according to subject. Messages appearing in a group are placed there by individuals who feel that their message will be appropriate to the group.

a question about their therapy, as it is to find clinicians discussing treatment options amongst themselves. This means some readers might consider particular messages posted to a group to be inappropriate.

Since one of the problems with newsgroups is the time and effort needed to read the many messages posted every day, the privacy and relative security of a mailing list can be very attractive. When it works well, however, this mix of readership can be very powerful. For example, patients in geographically isolated countries can post questions about their symptoms to a newsgroup, and receive a life-saving diagnosis from a specialist living in another country (M.F. Smith, 1996). Newsgroups have also proved to be a powerful medium for conveying information rapidly when other methods are inappropriate or restricted. For example, in areas of conflict or censorship, people have been able to send out information via the Internet, even when radio and television services in their own country have been shut down.

At its worst, people may post information that clinicians might consider ill-informed or dangerously incorrect. It is usually the nature of newsgroups that someone will quickly point out that information to the group, and explain why it is incorrect. Along with the Internet newsgroups, many larger service providers provide their own discussion forums and bulletin boards, available only to their subscribers. The content of the material that appears on these services is a current cause for concern, as some occasionally contravenes the laws of various countries, for reasons of either security or morality. Since by their very nature these systems are international, the legal implications of the material appearing on bulletin boards are still unclear. Some service providers chose to be very conservative in the discussion groups they supported. As a consequence, they close down groups that contain material breaking laws in any of the countries that their subscribers come from, even though the material may be acceptable in other countries.

22.7 The World Wide Web

In the same way that fax services overlay the telephone system, the Web sits on top of the Internet's transport system (Figure 22.6). Its originators developed it 'to be a pool of human knowledge, which would allow collaborators in remote sites to share ideas and all aspects of a common project' (Berners-Lee *et al.*, 1994). Conceptually the Web turns every computer on the Internet into a potential information source or library, and allows any other computer to look in on to these libraries and explore the information there. All these sources can further combine to create documents that exist on multiple computers and span the globe (Figure 22.7).

This expanding 'docuverse' is a new kind of library (Nelson, 1965), where information is created in one place and made immediately available everywhere. It is consequently almost infinitely flexible, allowing rapidly changing information to be both shared and updated quickly, in ways that traditional publishing is unable to achieve. Finally, because the Internet permits two-way transport, readers of documents can interact with and change them if the creators of the documents so desire. This kind of interaction of communication with information permits levels of collaboration that have previously not been possible.

What is perhaps surprising is that the establishment of the Web was achieved through the development and universal adoption of a relatively simple set of software and software standards for operation over the Internet. The CERN vision of a worldwide document pool meant that hypertext links permitted jumps to documents anywhere on the Internet. To make this happen, three technology standards had to be created:

- A standard way in which to create multimedia hypertext documents, called the **HyperText Markup Language (HTML)** (see Box 22.2).
- A standard way to give each document an address on the Internet so that it can be located, called its **Universal Resource Locator (URL)** (see Box 22.3).
- A standard way of transferring documents between computers, called the **HyperText Transfer Protocol (HTTP)** (see Box 22.4).

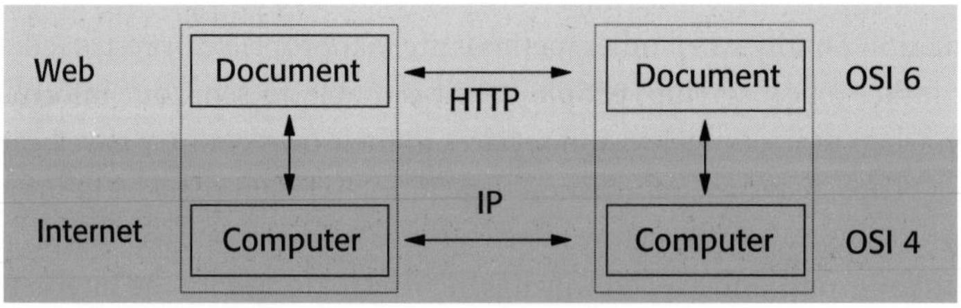
Web
Document
HTTP
Document
OSI 6
IP
Internet
Computer
Computer
OSI 4

Figure 22.6
The World Wide Web protocols are overlaid on top of the Internet, and provide a standard way for creating, finding and accessing documents.

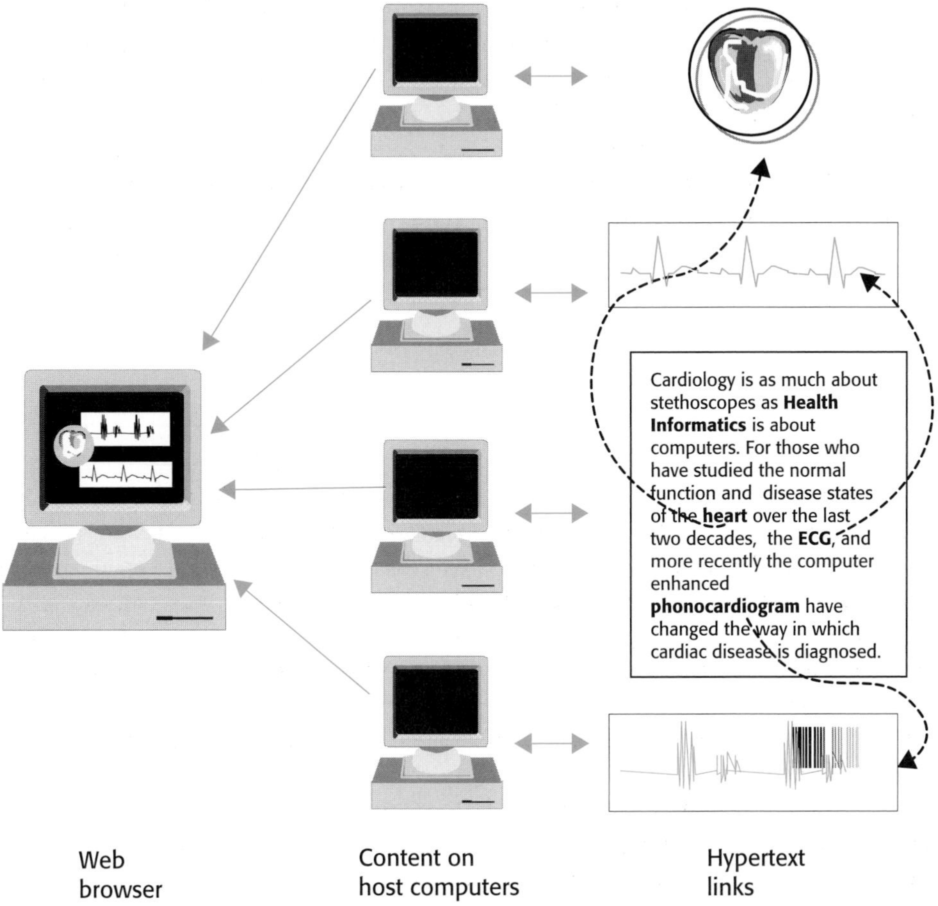
Cardiology is as much about stethoscopes as **Health Informatics** is about computers. For those who have studied the normal function and disease states of the **heart** over the last two decades, the **ECG**, and more recently the computer enhanced **phonocardiogram** have changed the way in which cardiac disease is diagnosed.
Web browser
Content on host computers
Hypertext links

Figure 22.7
Components of Web hypertext documents can be located on different computers. These multimedia documents may contain text, still or moving images and sound recordings.

Box 22.2
HTML: HyperText Markup Language

To allow hypertext documents to be created and read in a standard way, the researchers at CERN developed a language called HTML. This was a simplified subset of another standard called the Standard Generalized Markup Language (SGML). HTML defines the way in which a document should be structured so that it can be universally viewed on the Web. It defines a set of tags or codes that appear throughout a document. These tags define how the document's contents should be interpreted. For example, there are standard tags used when text has to appear in emphasized fonts, or for text to be centred or justified. These tags also define where images, sounds and hypertext links are to be found on the Web, and how they should appear in a document.

Browsers expect Web documents to be written in HTML. When they encounter the HTML codes in a document's text, they carry out its instructions to make the document appear as intended on the browser's system.

There is presently a tension between the desire to enhance the richness of Web documents and the need to maintain a common standard so that the concept of universal accessibility is maintained. The initial HTML standard was relatively simple, but language developers are keen to see it improve, permitting more sophisticated documents to be created. For example, programming languages like Java have been developed commercially to allow other programs to be attached to HTML documents. This means that arbitrarily complex behaviours can in principle be attached to hypertext documents.

However, as HTML evolves, the result is a proliferation of slightly different standards. Older Web browsers are already unable to interpret documents created according to more recent standards. Consequently the universality inherent in the original vision will gradually erode. For this problem to be solved, there needs to be a way for all Web users to have access to browsers incorporating the latest HTML standard. There also needs to be a guarantee that documents written in older versions of HTML remain readable as the standard evolves.

Box 22.3
URL: Universal Resource Locator

In the same way that there are Web standards for the way in which documents should be created, there are protocols that define how they should be accessed across the network. Just as HTTP insulates document creators from the specifics of an individual computer, an object's Web address is separate from the underlying protocols that are needed to find and transport it between computers. The address system is based around what is termed a Universal Resource Locator (URL).

There are several common ways in which files can be accessed. HTML documents are accessed according to HTTP. Files that are written in other formats could be retrieved using the older File Transfer Protocol (FTP).

The URL of an information object allows one to specify which protocol is to be used to access the object. So, for example, if one wanted to view an HTML document using HTTP, the URL would be of the form:

http://hostcomputername/objectname

If one wanted to copy the file across but not view it, the URL would be:

ftp://hostcomputername/objectname

Other protocols that are supported by the URL standard include Gopher, Telnet and Mailto. Mailto is used to indicate that an e-mail is to be sent to the address specified in the second part of the URL. Thus the URL *mailto:'bill@someplace.com'* will tell a browser that an e-mail is to be sent to the address specified in the section enclosed in quotes.

Box 22.4
HTTP: HyperText Transport Protocol

The Web is built around a client–server network architecture. This means that documents are placed on a computer that acts as a server. Other computers on the network are able to be clients of the server, sending requests to it for information. Upon receipt of a request, the server responds by delivering the requested information – which on the Web might be a document written in HTML. The exchange of requests and responses between client and server are made according to a network protocol that both client and server understand (Chapter 20). A protocol called the Hypertext Transport Protocol (HTTP) allows the exchange of HTML documents. HTTP is thus designed to transfer a variety of different data formats, including plain text, hypertext, plain image, audio and video.

Network protocols are generally of two types. Connection-oriented protocols set up a synchronous link between computers, requiring that the 'line' stay open for the duration of the connection. This is how a telephone connection is made, for example. Packet-oriented approaches like HTTP are asynchronous, and are more like sending a letter. Here a request is sent as a 'packet' to the server. This requires one connection, followed immediately upon delivery of the packet, by disconnection. Once it has processed the information contained in the requesting packet, the server responds by sending back information to the requesting client in a similar fashion. HTTP adopts this approach to make more efficient use of the network.

For most users, their window on to the Web is provided by a program called a **browser** (Figure 22.8). This program runs on their computer, and provides a means of interacting with the space of Web documents placed available on the Internet. Typically, a browser has the following basic functions:

- It acts as a navigation tool for moving around the Web.
- It provides mechanisms for retrieving and storing documents that have been found on the Web.
- It acts as a viewing tool for these multimedia hypertext documents.
- It acts as a communication port, connecting for example with e-mail systems.
- It may also incorporate methods for the creation of Web documents.

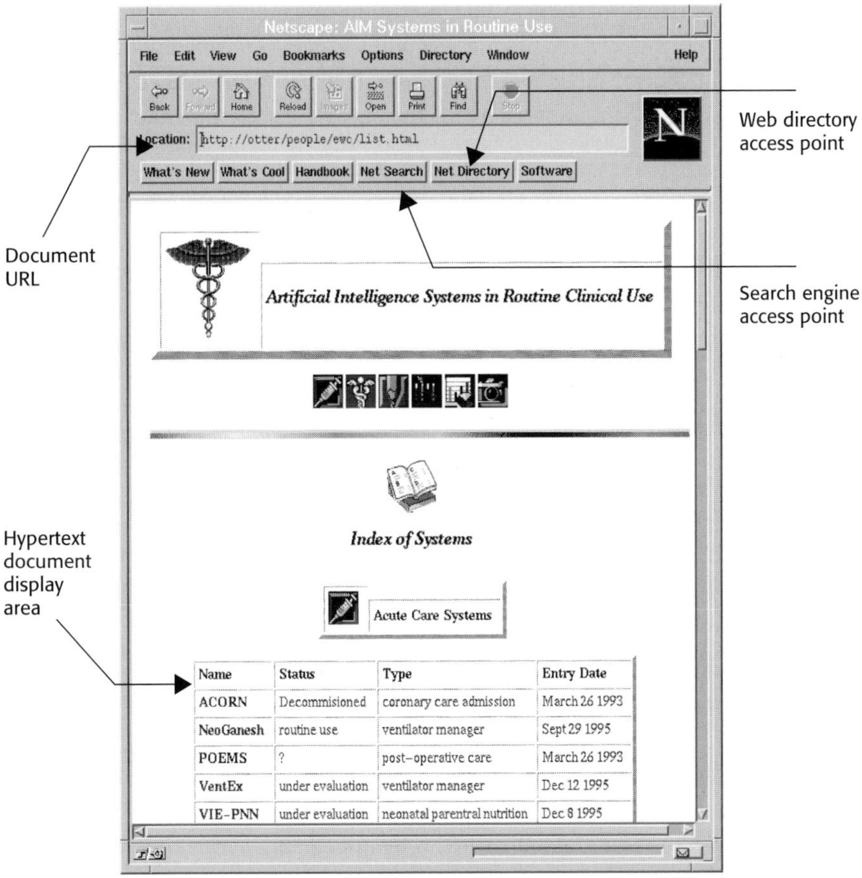
Netscape: AIM Systems in Routine Use
File Edit View Go Bookmarks Options Directory Window Help
Back Forward Home Reload Images Open Print Find Stop
Location: http://otter/people/ewc/list.html
What's New What's Cool Handbook Net Search Net Directory Software
Artificial Intelligence Systems in Routine Clinical Use
Index of Systems
Acute Care Systems
Name Status Type Entry Date
ACORN Decommisioned coronary care admission March 26 1993
NeoGanesh routine use ventilator manager Sept 29 1995
POEMS ? post-operative care March 26 1993
VentEx under evaluation ventilator manager Dec 12 1995
VIE-PNN under evaluation neonatal parentral nutrition Dec 8 1995
Web directory access point
Search engine access point
Document URL
Hypertext document display area

Figure 22.8
Web browsers provide mechanisms for accessing hypertext documents on the Web, as well as search and directory services.

Finding a document

Once connected into the Web, there are several different ways in which one can search the information space:

- **Specific address:** If the location of a document is explicitly known, then specifying its address (its URL) will permit a browser to directly request a document from the computer it is stored upon.
- **Directories:** Many directory services are offered on the Web, listing documents according to categories. These directories can be compiled in a number of ways. Initially it is usually possible in small subject areas for the creator of the directory to explore the Web manually, and list all sites that come within its scope. Once directories have become established, they attain a certain amount of popularity, and document creators themselves will inform the directory maintainers about their document.
- **Search engines:** Given the large number of documents that exist on the Web, and their constant state of flux, it is inevitable that much of the information on the Web is not indexed in the larger directories. One solution to this problem is to create keyword indexes of as many documents as possible. Using these indexes, a user specifies the words that are likely to be associated with the topic of interest, much as one would when specifying search criteria for articles at a library (see Chapter 6). Agent programs or

'Web crawlers' automatically traverse the Web, following links from one document to the next. They look for new documents, and store relevant information about these documents in the index. Some indexes just store document titles and addresses; others are far more ambitious and index all words that appear in a document, resulting in the creation of enormous databases.

Directories and search engines are powerful tools for exploring the information space of the Web. The problem of making the process of search tractable becomes ever harder as the number of documents on the Web grows. For example, using a search engine may result in many hundreds or even thousands of documents being identified with a set of keywords.

The whole area of search mechanisms attracts considerable attention at present, and new ways for filtering and ranking search results are being developed. Some of the larger search engines note which links people select after they have made a search, and use this information to give documents a ranking weight. The next time a similar search is performed, the documents selected by previous users are displayed higher up the search results. One potentially very promising avenue is for individuals to have a personal software agent. The agent might, for example, observe an individual's information search patterns, and see which type of documents tend to be retrieved. Using machine learning methods the program slowly builds up rules to identify documents that are likely to be appropriate in the future (see Chapter 26).

Publishing on the Web

The Web established HTML as a simple standard for the way in which multimedia and hypertext documents are written. The practical consequence of having all documents written in HTML is that they can be universally read by anyone on the Internet possessing a browser that can interpret HTML.

The information framework presented in Chapter 2 shows us how every information system can be understood to comprise data, a set of data models and data viewers. Web documents are all constructed according to a standard model that is specified by HTML. Browser software, resident on a client computer, incorporates the HTML model within it. HTML therefore provides a model that permits these document files to be interpreted when they are retrieved from the server by the browser (Figure 22.9).

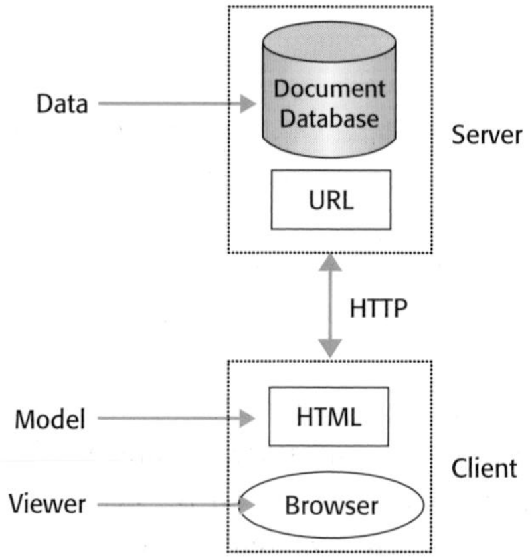
Data
Document Database
Server
URL
HTTP
Model
HTML
Client
Viewer
Browser

Figure 22.9
Data, models and views on the Web. A Web browser provides a view on to the data in a document, and interprets how to present it according the model described in HTML.

As a consequence, document creation is now decoupled from the needs of specific computer systems. This burden is now shifted on to those who create browser software, which must be developed specifically for different computer operating systems and architectures. By creating a document according to the HTML standard, document creators need know nothing about this underlying complexity. They are guaranteed that their document will appear approximately as intended, as long as a browser that understands HTML reads it. This has meant that it is much easier for information to be created and placed upon the Web. This has contributed substantially to the explosion of information made available on the Web, as the barrier to creating and distributing electronic documents has been significantly lowered.

The consequence of having such standard protocols for the retrieval of information, along with standard methods of creating documents, is a change in the way information is published. Normally the creator of a paper document is also responsible for its distribution. In an organization, for example, all the possible recipients of a document need to be identified, and the document copied and circulated to them (whether it be on paper or in electronic form). The Web model of publishing allows a document creator to put the burden of information access on to the reader. A document is placed in a known location, and is simply made available to all those who might be interested in it. This is the same model that is adopted when a document is placed on a notice board, and is available to anyone who cares to stop and read it.

There are several clear advantages to this model. Firstly, there is no need to specifically identify the name and location of all the people for whom a document is intended. As a corollary, the readership of a document can be widened considerably. Secondly, the costs of distribution are eliminated. Finally, since only one copy of the document is kept on the computer system of the individuals responsible for creating the document, it can be quickly updated. Consequently, readers of the document can always have access to the most up-to-date version of any document.

There are also clearly cases in which this particular model of publication would be inappropriate. For example, if urgent information needs to be communicated, then it may be more appropriate to send out a notice to all those who need to be informed. In this case, one might prefer to use e-mail for document distribution in preference, or in addition, to updating a Web document. It may be inappropriate for a hospital to place an urgent drug recall notice on its Intranet and not notify staff. Equally, it may be entirely appropriate for the minutes of a monthly meeting to be placed for viewing on a network without being announced.

22.8 Security on the Internet

The philosophy behind the Web is to provide open access to a global information space for everyone. It is this powerful vision, embodied in the open standards of Web technology, which has contributed so significantly to its growth. However, there is an increasing need to use mechanisms that permit restrictions to be placed on the shipment of information. In particular, security measures that either limit access to documents or prevent documents being read may be required.

Such security restrictions are essential, for example, with electronic commerce. When a financial transaction is made across the Internet, information like credit card or bank account numbers may need to be shipped across the network. Since it is often possible to covertly intercept traffic across the network, sending such information without any form of

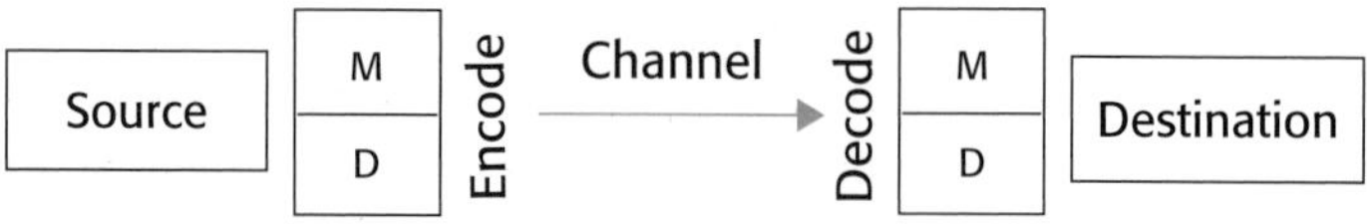
Source
M
D
Encode
Channel
Decode
M
D
Destination

Figure 22.10 Once data (D) have been encrypted according to a code, they can be securely transported across a communication channel like the Internet. To be able to decode the data, one must possess a key or code that is the model (M) used to encrypt the data.

protection is unsafe. Security is also of fundamental importance in healthcare, where confidential patient data are involved. Not only is there often a need to restrict who has the right to access electronic patient data files, it is also clearly important to prevent those data being intercepted when they are being transported across the Internet.

There are thus two complementary ways that a degree of security can be ensured for data placed upon the Web. The first involves setting up barriers to accessing data files. For example, an institution such as a hospital may set up an internal network or intranet. Access to the intranet is dependent on users knowing passwords to authenticate that they are privileged to use the system. By controlling which computers can access the network, which users have accounts, and the complexity of the password system, intranets can be relatively closed and secure systems. If a network is to be more open, for example using the Internet to allow access to documents, then the gateway between the Internet and the local system needs to be controlled. So-called **firewalls** are placed at the gateway to limit document access to appropriately authenticated users.

The second component of security is to prevent eavesdroppers outside a secure network from intercepting information traffic. To prevent access to such confidential information, these data need to be encrypted. Encryption basically scrambles data according to a predefined method, and only someone with access to the encryption code used is able to decode the data. In information model terms, a new model is introduced into the system, and only those in possession of the model are able to interpret the data (Figure 22.10).

Encrypted data are secure as long as the encryption code is itself secure. Just as powerful encryption schemes are created, there are those who seek to develop methods to crack these codes. As a consequence, when it is absolutely essential that data remain secure, there is a constant pressure to adopt ever more powerful encryption mechanisms. For situations in which total security is not necessary, it is still reasonable to use codes that are in principle decodable, accepting that it is unlikely that most people would have the knowledge or desire to do so.

22.9 Future Web advances

There is now a good deal of experimentation occurring with new methods of interaction on the Internet. Access to the Internet is broadening, as new devices and ways of connecting to the Web are developed. For example, wireless access to the Web from small mobile phones and palmtop devices is now possible (see Box 22.5). There is active research seeking to develop methods that allow interaction with others in virtual reality worlds across the Internet. In such worlds, people may be able to interact with each other through computer-rendered three-dimensional scenes (Raggett *et al.*, 1996). Such systems will no doubt produce newer interaction paradigms that will come into common use in the future.

Box 22.5
WAP and the wireless Internet

The technology for wireless access to Web-based services has evolved rapidly over the last few years, and several different options are now available. Using a wireless digital telephone system like GSM, mobile users have access to a data channel, which allows them to dial into a modem connected to a computer network, and access services on the network (Figure 20.7). If the phone is connected to a palmtop or laptop computer that runs a web browser, and the network being accessed connects to the Internet, then full access to the Web is available.

However, Internet standards such as HTML and HTTP are inefficient over mobile telephone networks, as they require large amounts of mainly text-based data to be sent. Standard HTML pages generally cannot be displayed effectively on the small screens of pocket-sized mobile devices, and navigation around and between screens is not easy using only one hand. Further, HTTP and TCP are not optimized for the intermittent coverage, long latencies and limited bandwidth associated with wireless networks. For example, HTTP sends its headers and commands in an inefficient text format instead of compressed binary. As a consequence, wireless web applications using these protocols are often slow, costly and difficult to use.

To meet these challenges, the Wireless Application Protocol (WAP) was developed to attempt to solve some of the technical problems of wireless Internet use. WAP is a new open, global communication protocol specification that allows mobile users with wireless devices to interact with information and services.

WAP takes a client–server approach. It incorporates a simple microbrowser into the mobile phone, requiring only limited resources on the mobile phone. The philosophy behind the WAP approach is to utilize as few resources as possible on the handheld device and put most of the network intelligence into a WAP gateway, which is a computer that sits between the Internet and mobile network and does most of the processing work to translate between WAP and Web documents.

WAP has been optimized to solve the problems of using standard Internet protocols over wireless networks, utilizing binary transmission for greater compression of data, and optimized for long latency and low to medium bandwidth. WAP sessions cope with intermittent coverage and can operate over a wide variety of wireless transports using IP where possible. WAP protocols are based on Internet standards such as HTTP. WAP documents are written in the Wireless Markup Language (WML), similar to HTML. WML makes better use of small screens and allows easy navigation with one hand without a full keyboard, and has built-in scalability from two-line text displays through to the full graphic screens on smart phones and communicators.

Like HTML, WML is derived from XML, the meta-language defined by the W3C. WML is thus like HTML in that both are XML applications, permitting XML specifications to be translated either into WML or HTML.

Most of the Web's content today is designed for humans to read, not for computer programs to manipulate meaningfully (Berners-Lee *et al.*, 2001). In particular, there is no easy way for a computer to understand any of the semantics of a web page. One page of text is as meaningful as another to a web browser, which is only interested in how to display the contents. Much effort is now being devoted to understand how web documents can be structured in a machine interpretable way that allows intelligent programs to make decisions based on the information they find as they traverse the Web. The task for the developers of this **Semantic Web** is to begin to add logic to the Web, to allow intelligent programs or agents to use rules and make inferences based on the information contained in Web sites. Since the meaning of particular words or terms varies from one context to another, the Semantic Web also envisions methods for allowing agents to use ontologies to help them understand the

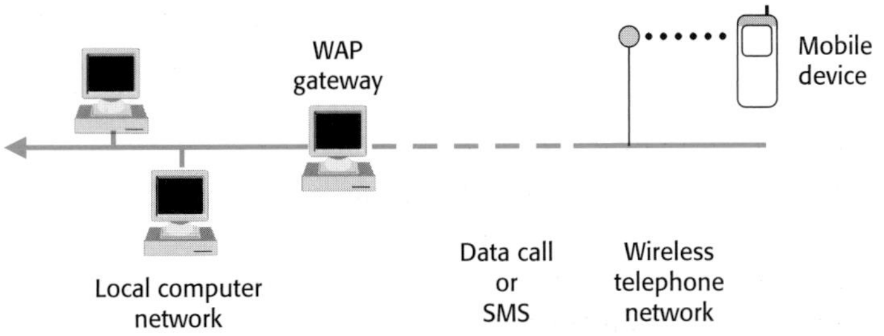
WAP
gateway
Mobile
device
Local computer
network
Data call
or
SMS
Wireless
telephone
network

Figure 22.11
WAP permits wirelesss telephone devices to connect to the Web.

specific type of information that different pages might contain. We shall return to the issue of building intelligent systems in more detail in Part 8 of this book.

Discussion points

1 Who controls the Internet?

2 Describe the search strategies you use to find information on the Web. How do they relate to the general strategy types presented in Chapter 7?

3 What is a chat room?

4 What was the 'dot com' boom all about?

5 What is spam, why is it possible, and what should be done about it?

Chapter summary

1 Essentially a network of networks, the Internet permits computers across the globe to communicate with each other. It evolved out of the Advanced Research Projects Agency Network (ARPAnet) developed by the United States Department of Defence in the late 1960s.

2 Shaped by technological, social and economic forces, the Internet represents a complex conjunction of phenomena.

3 In economic terms, there are four basic Internet 'businesses' – transport, connection, services, and content.

4 Internet technologies permit new means for the publication and distribution of information without, and within organizations. The use of Internet technologies on an internal computer network creates what is termed an internal Internet, or **intranet**.

5 We can characterize communication services as either being **information push**, in which messages are pushed at targeted individuals, or **information pull**, in which access is based on individuals seeking out or pulling information sources.

6 Messages sent from one individual to another are called **peer-to-peer** communication. Sending a message to a select group of individuals is called **narrowcasting**, and widespread distribution is known as **broadcasting.**

7 Several communication services are available on the Internet. With mailing lists, an e-mail message is sent to multiple destinations. Newsgroups are publicly accessible forums for discussion.

8 The Web has been created on top of the Internet's transport system. To make this happen, three technology standards had to be created:

- A standard way to create multimedia hypertext documents, called **HTML (HyperText Markup Language)**.
- A standard way to give each document an address called its **URL (Universal Resource Locator)**.
- A standard way of transferring documents between computers, called **HTTP (HyperText Transfer Protocol)**.

CHAPTER 23

Web health services

> Telegraphs are machines for conveying information over extensive lines with great rapidity. They have generally been established for the purpose of transmitting information during war, but the increasing wants of man will probably soon render them subservient to more peaceful objects. *Babbage (1833), p. 36.*

The Internet and the Web represent the most powerful instruments yet created for the creation and dissemination of information. Through the Internet, many of the assumptions about how information is created, distributed and communicated are gradually being broken down. The Internet is capable of providing a powerful distribution infrastructure over which healthcare organizations can move information. Further, the technical innovations associated with the Web provide tools for accessing and publishing that information. Indeed, it is because the Internet and Web are able to meet many of the information needs in healthcare that they have been adopted so rapidly. This contrasts starkly with earlier, and arguably more complex, information technology, which has generated far less enthusiasm within healthcare.

Consequently, the Web is often used as a vehicle for many of the telemedical services discussed in earlier chapters. However, the packet-based nature of current Internet technology means that the Web is still best suited to services which are transactional in nature, and do not have a strong synchronous requirement. The Web remains a poor vehicle for videoconferencing, for example, but is well suited to the transmission of large files such as clinical images, as long as there is not a need for them to be viewed in real time.

This chapter looks specifically at the ways in which healthcare can benefit from Web technologies. In particular, the way information can be published, distributed and accessed is examined in detail. The chapter concludes with an examination of the role of the Internet in evidence-based clinical practice, and looks ahead to some challenges that the growth of the Internet poses for healthcare.

23.1 The Web can support rapid publication and distribution of clinical information resources

In many ways, healthcare has always been information rich, but has been severely hampered by mechanisms for distribution and access to that information. As a consequence, one of the most tangible changes that comes from putting information on intranets, or the Internet, is a major improvement in information distribution and access. For consumers, clinical workers, researchers and students, access to health information can be improved in the following ways.

Amount of information

In the past, publishing information was associated with formal processes of manuscript preparation and physical publication by a publishing house or learned journal. As information technology has become more pervasive, the physical aspects of publication have shifted some of the act of publication closer to the creator of the original information. Anyone with word-processing and local printing facilities can create and distribute their own documents, either electronically or on paper. By using the Web, authors can also distribute their work.

With the cost of publication on the Internet being so low, and the ease of publication being so high, many people publish information that is clinically valuable, but that might not otherwise have an appropriate vehicle for publication. Much of this information is for local consumption but, by using the Internet, it becomes globally accessible. A large amount of material is available on the Web that is unavailable elsewhere. This extends from educational material created for local use, such as clinical guidelines, to specialized research data. For example, an enormous amount of information about the Human Genome project is available on the Internet that would in the past have been available to only those closely associated with the project (Hochstrasser *et al.*, 1995; Ouellette, 1999). For local intranets, the situation is much the same. The potential exists to make a large amount of information, from drug interaction data through to image libraries, available throughout an organization.

Speed of appearance

The rapidity with which changes in Web-based information can be made available to its readers cannot be matched by non-electronic distribution mechanisms.

Timeliness

A corollary of the speed of publication is the rapidity with which information is now able or permitted to change. Information is potentially always up to date, which is valuable for time-critical information needs. It is common for information sites on the Web to be updated regularly, often in response to feedback from those accessing the information. A negative consequence of the speed of Internet publication is that there is now a mismatch between the rapidity with which new scientific results can be disseminated, and the length of time required for careful peer review.

Version control

In contrast to other forms of publication, where multiple editions may exist (for example a clinical guideline), there is only one access point for a Web document, and it is always the current version. There are clear advantages here not just in timeliness, but in elimination of possible confusion between editions of an information source. Where older editions need to be kept, some Web sites maintain archives that can be accessed if needed.

Types of information

Many healthcare publications take full advantage of the multimedia and hypertext facilities offered on the Web, to create publications that could not have previously been possible. Indeed the quality of publicly available Web documents is now so high that many healthcare educational institutions use them. The University of Utah, for example, has an extensive library of anatomical pathology images called WebPath for its students. The Digital Anatomist is a Web-based anatomy atlas, used for teaching purposes (Brinkley *et al.*, 1997). At the University of Iowa a large set of teaching materials is assembled at their Virtual Hospital. The National Library of Medicine's Visible Human project is creating a complete, anatomically detailed, three-dimensional representation of the male and female human body and is making this available on the Internet. The project is collecting transverse CT, MRI and cryosection images of male and female cadavers at 1-millimetre intervals, and the data can be used for teaching and research purposes.

Permanence

Another important aspect on the Web is that our belief in the permanence of information begins to erode. Traditionally, with formal publication in an archival journal, the author of the work is making some commitment to the long-term stability of the work. Patient records fall into a similar category, since they too are created with the intent that they will enter a permanent archive. However, work that is incomplete or in its early stages can be just as easily distributed using the Internet, and the process of early distribution can allow widespread commentary and interaction with the work, to improve it before 'final' publication.

Manner of interaction

Web resources are not necessarily passive information repositories. They can be constructed to solicit input from the reader. From an educational point of view, the possibility for structured interaction with teaching materials on the Web is an exciting development. Web-based resources permit structured browsing, and problem exploration behaviours. One can now find Web sites that allow diagnostic problems to be posed for students, who are then able to search interactively for appropriate information amongst the patient data presented. Once the student submits answers to the problem set, they can then be assessed as necessary.

Searching

It has been commonplace to search for material published in journals, for example through a library, but other information has not been so accessible. One of the advantages of the Web is that, through the search engines and indexes that now exist, one can perform the same type of search on other kinds of information. For example, it is increasingly common for healthcare organizations to create their own sites on the Web. Here one can discover the activities of the group, their interests and their staff. It is often possible to e-mail individuals directly in this manner. As a consequence, one can now search globally for, find and communicate with individuals who have specialized expertise, in a manner that previously was not possible, even locally.

Remote collaboration

It is now common for healthcare to be delivered by teams whose members have differing skills, and who might be geographically quite distributed. This is also very much the case for healthcare research, where collaborations often extend across the world. A feature of collaboration is the need to create and exchange information amongst members of such teams. For some time, the notion of **groupware** has been explored within the information sciences. It emphasizes collaboration on common documents using shared information spaces on a network. The Web is more permissive than many early groupware offerings in this respect, since it allows individuals to create and distribute information with little regard to its structure. The Web intrinsically is a groupware platform, since it naturally facilitates common access to files in a distributed environment. Combining the Web's powerful information management tools with more basic Internet communication facilities like e-mail can thus contribute significantly to collaboration when individuals are separated by time or distance.

23.2 The electronic patient record can be built using Web technologies

In volume, the patient record must represent one of the largest components of published health knowledge. The need to publish and distribute portions of a patient record to all those involved in care, wherever they may be, is now an unavoidable consequence of the way in which healthcare is practised. As we saw in Chapter 10, the solution to this problem has been to move the patient record across to electronic systems.

Despite the promise of the EMR, several significant technical obstacles have hindered its widespread adoption:

- As organizations grow and obtain new information systems, there arises a need to integrate these with older or 'legacy' systems which continue to function in parts of the organization. Often the new and old systems are incompatible at many levels, and the integration is both technically challenging as well as expensive.
- One constant in the development of the EPR has been the running battle with obsolescence of the functional specification of these systems. Over time the needs of those using the system changes, as the practice of healthcare changes and the

organization develops. However, once a system has been implemented, it can prove very difficult to introduce new functionality without a major rewriting of the system software. For example, a system designed to carry out order-entry and result reporting is unlikely to be easily modified to allow viewing of clinical images, or browsing electronic documents from a library.

- There are as yet no internationally agreed standards on how a medical record should be structured, or the communication protocols that should be used to share medical records between institutions. As a consequence, it is very difficult to electronically exchange records between many institutions, as they are likely to be using different EMRs. It is possible to write translators between different systems. However, as we saw in Chapter 19, the number of possible communication links grows combinatorially with the number of agents. This means that for a given number of different EMRs, we will need a combinatorially larger number of translators between systems.

Many of these problems may be solved by using Web technologies to implement an EMR, since they provide open standards for developing medical information systems:

- Since the Web uses IP as its basic networking protocol, it is designed to interoperate with a variety of other networking standards, and should therefore support interaction both between different components of an organization's computer network including legacy systems, as well as interaction between different networks associated with disparate organizations. Rather than having to write many different communication protocol and information system translators, only one is needed per system, to the Web standards (Fraser *et al.*, 1997). The software components that translate between different information systems are sometimes called **interface engines**. Some other standards such as HL7 will also assist with messaging between institutions, and may in time also result in EMR document standards.
- The basic Web technology is designed specifically to handle multimedia, and imposes very few requirements for document display. Consequently, a Web browser is just as able to examine a document containing notes of a patient's progress, a form for ordering a laboratory test or a multimedia document from an electronic textbook. This flexibility in principle allows Web-based systems to introduce radically new functionality easily on to an existing system with only modest technical effort, and is a powerful argument for adopting Web technologies over existing methods for implementing the EMR.

Thus Web-based systems make little or no demands on the structure of knowledge, and emphasize ease of publication, distribution and access to information. As a consequence, many now consider that Web-based systems represent the ideal tool with which to build new EMRs as well as managing the problem of integrating existing or 'legacy' systems (Cimino *et al.*, 1995; Kohane *et al.*, 1996).

The Web is also seen as a mechanism to permit patients to access their medical records directly, from wherever they may be (Mandl *et al.*, 2001). Security and confidentiality remain critical barriers to the introduction of such free access. Since a Web-based electronic record can be built around a local Intranet, there is no inherent increase in security risk over traditional computer-based solutions. However, the security risks increase considerably when local information is distributed using the open and public Internet. Consequently, additional security features need to be incorporated into such systems. Recent experience has shown that such systems can be built to provide safe access to highly sensitive personal health information over the Internet. However, building systems that meet both patients' expectations for privacy and safety and their providers' expectations for convenience and usability remains a substantial challenge, as the security mechanisms may impose barriers to free access for clinicians, and require additional workload to authenticate their access (Masys *et al.*, 2002).

23.3 The dissemination of peer-reviewed scientific knowledge is enhanced through use of the Web

Tradition places biomedical journals at the pinnacle of healthcare publications. Their role is to solicit, scrutinize and then distribute the best scientific research. Yet the rigour of the review process places a significant delay between the submission of material and final publication. Once published, such material enters the archive, or long-term memory of healthcare knowledge.

Until recently, this was a successful process. Now, however, the delays in publication are leading to delays in the institution of appropriate treatments. Worse, the amount of information now being published weekly, in many thousands of journals, makes accessing that archive problematic.

As a result there has been a widespread shift to biomedical journals publishing on the Web. Major journals appear on the Web, sometimes in preference to or in advance of print. For example the *British Medical Journal*, the *New England Journal of Medicine*, the *Lancet* and the *Journal of the American Medical Association* are published in paper and Internet versions. For such journals, publication on the Internet has several advantages:

- **Speed of publication:** Eliminating the need to physically print journals, and then distribute them through a postal system, reduces the time between publication and appearance of a journal. Once published electronically on the Web, journals are immediately accessible. Increasingly, preprints of articles are available on web sites well ahead of the paper publication date. Sometimes papers in early draft form are also available, even before formal peer review.
- **Cost of publication, distribution and access:** The elimination of printing and distribution stages makes Web publishing cheaper than paper journals. Some newer journals from publishers like **Biomed Central** do not have a paper version at all, but exist only on the Web. For healthcare workers in some nations, particularly in the developing world, paper-based journals are not affordable, and the Internet may be their only means of keeping abreast of the latest research. However, the cost of access to academic journals is actually a global problem. The number of academic titles available grew by 84% in the UK in the mid-1990s, and by 45% in the US (Chittenden and Syal, 1995). As a consequence most major biomedical libraries are now unable to maintain broad paper collections of journals, and increasingly turn to Web versions of journals to manage costs.
- **Form of publication:** The multimedia and hypertext capacity for Web documents means that research appearing on the Web can appear in far richer forms than is possible on paper. For fields like clinical imaging, the Web adds an extra dimension to published research. One can create papers that contain text, graphics, sound, and moving images.
- **Content of publication:** The Internet's data capacity has significant implications for the way in which clinical research can be communicated. When clinical research is published

on paper, it is usually only possible to provide summaries of the study data because of page limits. Readers can examine the statistical methods used on the data, but not the raw data itself. When research is published on the Internet, such restrictions are minimal. A research paper can include all the data obtained during the investigation, and make them available to readers (Delamothe, 1996). This has an immediate benefit, allowing the validity of the study data to be reviewed. Many examples of scientific fraud are only detected when other researchers have eventually been permitted to examine the raw data. Secondly, and more positively, subsequent researchers can now use the published data. They may wish to reanalyse the data, either to check the conclusions reached, or to contribute to further research. This means that the life of a piece of healthcare research no longer needs to end upon publication. It can enter a living pool of data that contributes to ongoing research for many years to come.

- **Method of interaction:** The relationship of reader to text is changed on the Web, because of the potential for significant interaction between publisher and reader. Some journals have taken advantage of the two-way communication afforded by Internet publication to open up the peer-review process of articles to the journal's readership. By allowing rapid e-mail responses to articles to be posted on journal web sites, the opportunity for community feedback and discussion on new scientific papers is almost immediate.

These changes lead some to predict the 'death of biomedical journals' in their present form (LaPorte *et al.*, 1995). However, it is more likely that, freed from the limitations of paper, and taking advantage of the communication powers of the Internet, journals will change the role that they play. There will always be a need for an archival store of research, where important new ideas and experiences are recorded and, where necessary, priority of invention is established. It is just that the ways in which this archival store will be accessed will be vastly different.

23.4 Online systems can support continuing education and decision-making

All health professionals need to update their knowledge to keep up with changes in knowledge. This activity is often called **continuing professional education** (CPE) or **continuing medical education** (CME) when specifically addressing medical needs. Information technology is seen to have a role in the provision of clinical educational activities (Ward *et al.*, 2001). Virtual campuses can permit isolated or time-poor clinicians to participate in educational activities remotely. Educational packages can be developed around structured clinical problems, deliver multimedia content to students to interact with, and also connect online to allow rich interaction with academic staff by e-mail or chat room, and provide rapid assessment and feedback.

However, assessing the research about different educational activities, it is clear that in general traditional didactic measures such as lectures or formal exams to test understanding of educational materials do not change clinical performance or improve clinical care (Davis *et al.*, 1999). In contrast, interactive educational activities, structured around actual problems in the clinical workplace, are much more successful.

Consequently, an alternative idea to CPE as a distinct clinical activity has emerged. Recognizing that the body of biomedical knowledge has now grown to such an extent that it is no longer capable of mastery by individuals, even in sub-specialties, and also that learning works best when focused on issues in the clinical workplace, it has been proposed that in the future most CPE will consist of using online information technology to answer immediate clinical questions (Coiera and Dowton, 2000). The Internet is usually seen as the vehicle to support such online systems, since for professionals the sources of knowledge they will need are likely to be widely distributed and unlikely to come from a single source. Thus, the whole notion of CPE changes from one of periodic updates to a clinician's knowledge to a 'just-in-time' model where a clinician checks the medical knowledge base, potentially at every clinical encounter (Chueh and Barnett, 1997). In the just-in-time model, every time clinicians make a clinical decision, they consider whether they need to access the clinical evidence base.

The just-in-time model attempts to integrate information access into the routine activities of clinicians, and the mode of decision support can range from access to 'passive' knowledge sources on the Internet such as guidelines, manuals and textbooks, though to 'active' knowledge sources that interact with clinicians to assist in the formulation of diagnostic or treatment decisions.

Evaluation of the use and impact of online evidence systems has demonstrated significant use of evidence by clinical staff to support direct patient care, and examples of specific individual improvements in patient outcomes as a result of application of the evidence retrieved (Gosling *et al.*, 2003). In a survey of 5500 clinicians who used Web-based evidence resources, 88% reported that they thought this had the potential to improve patient care and 41% reported direct experience of this. Patterns of use of this system by 55 000 clinicians across the state of New South Wales demonstrated that evidence retrieval is principally related to direct patient care, but good use is also made of the system to support continuing education activities and research (Gosling *et al.*, 2003).

How likely are clinicians to use online systems to support CPE? As we saw in Chapter 14, there is at present widespread variation in the level of adoption of Internet-based evidence resources. Even amongst similar organizations, there can be wide variation in the level of access amongst seemingly similar clinical groups. Gosling *et al.* (2003) reported a web-log analysis of 181 499 bibliographic search sessions that were made over 7 months in the public hospitals of New South Wales, where Internet access to a broad range of evidence sources has been available to its 55 000 clinicians since 1997. The log analysis revealed a monthly rate of 48.5 sessions per 100 clinicians. There was considerable variation in rates of sessions (range 2.8–117.6/100 clinicians) for the 81 individual hospitals examined (Figure 23.1).

Studies investigating the barriers to the use of online evidence resources have identified a range of factors including insufficient training in both database searching and general IT skills. Organizational and social factors that promote discussion within the organization and the existence of 'champions' who enthusiastically support an innovation have also been shown to be important predictors of online literature searching and the use of point-of-care clinical information systems.

Problems with access to computers (Silverstein, 1995), and excessive amounts of information retrieved (Urquhart and Davies, 1997) have also been cited as barriers to online searching for evidence. Interestingly, the clinical perception of the adequacy of technical infrastructure and its objective performance may differ significantly. In a comparison between a hospital with high rates of online evidence use, and one with low use, there were similar speeds of information retrieval and similar numbers of computer terminals in both sites (Gosling *et al.*, 2003). Staff in the low-use institution complained about technical barriers, whereas those in the higher-use institution used the system despite frustrations with the speed. This indicates

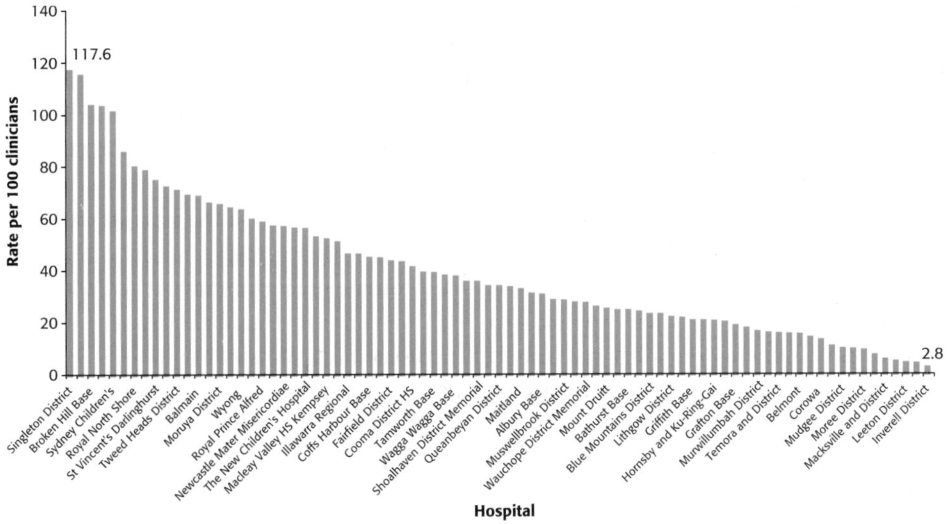
Rate per 100 clinicians
140
120
100
80
60
40
20
0
117.6
2.8
Singleton District
Broken Hill Base
Sydney Children's
Royal North Shore
St Vincent's Darlinghurst
Tweed Heads District
Balmain
Moruya District
Wyong
Royal Prince Alfred
Newcastle Mater Misericordiae
The New Children's Hospital
Macleay Valley HS Kempsey
Illawarra Regional
Coffs Harbour Base
Fairfield District
Cooma District HS
Tamworth Base
Wagga Wagga Base
Shoalhaven District Memorial
Queanbeyan District
Maitland
Albury Base
Muswellbrook District
Wauchope District Memorial
Mount Druitt
Bathurst Base
Blue Mountains District
Lithgow District
Griffith Base
Hornsby and Ku-Ring-Gai
Grafton Base
Murwillumbah District
Temora and District
Belmont
Corowa
Mudgee District
Moree District
Macksville and District
Leeton District
Inverell District
Hospital

Figure 23.1
There is a wide variation in monthly rates of access by hospital clinicians to Internet evidence resources, even in similar institutions. This graph shows the distribution of monthly rates of evidence usage per 100 clinicians amongst 81 public hospitals in New South Wales, Australia (© NSW Department of Health).

that other cultural and organizational factors were more important than technical barriers such as speed of searching time. This finding provides support for a socio-technical view of the integration of technology into organizations, which emphasizes the important role organizational culture has on uptake of technology (Kaplan, 2001).

This evidence does suggest that with appropriate education, support and effort to introducing systems that do not disrupt clinical workflow, online evidence systems will be used to support CPE and clinical problem-solving. However, the evidence also suggests that they may be used for only a small portion of clinician decision problems. This is because, as we saw in Chapter 19, it seems that the preferred mode of information access and decision-support for clinicians is face-to-face conversation with colleagues, even when online systems are available. Clinical work is complex, and is often rapidly moving and consensual, especially in hospital environments. One of the striking features of clinical work is that clinicians rely far more on informal interpersonal information exchange than on formal paper or computer records to satisfy their information requests. This is in part because information is not always easily available from formal sources, but more often is simply because on most occasions conversation is a more appropriate mechanism for information exchange.

23.5 Patients may access healthcare information on the Web

It is clear that access to healthcare information on the Internet will be of major benefit to patients. As we saw earlier, Web mechanisms make it possible for patients to access their electronic health records online. There are already numerous electronic discussion groups in which patients may ask questions and share experience. Some health-related Internet sites offer e-mail advice on a fee-for-service basis. Others provide free access to information. It is important to realize that information on the Internet is accessible from most parts of the globe, and that once made public, information access and dissemination are largely uncontrolled, and uncontrollable.

An information mass market is developing on the Internet, where the general public has access to a wide variety of health-related material, often of variable quality or relevance

(Bower, 1996). High-quality resources are now in existence, which offer clear and up-to-date information on diagnosis and treatment. However, poor-quality resources also continue to proliferate. The proportion of patients who have access to this information source will continue to grow over the years, as will the quantity of information placed on the Internet. It may still be the case that in some areas a higher percentage of patients than general practitioners have access to the Internet.

For healthcare systems in which patients are free to participate in their choice of treatment, the Internet provides a rich source of information on treatment options. Since such information may potentially vary from the most up-to-date practice guidelines from leading clinical centres, to out-of-date or inaccurate recommendations, managing patient expectations and requests may represent a greater challenge than it is at present. In countries in which healthcare provision is more centrally managed, even greater challenges exist. We must assume that patients have access to information on best practice from a variety of sources on the Internet and will demand it when it is known.

However, the health service is resource bound, and must attempt to ration treatment (Klein, 1995). Treatments that are the most cost-effective over a population may be favoured over treatments that are best in class. This will lead to a conflict between the informed desire of patients to obtain the best treatment for themselves as individuals, and the system's ability to deliver. Will individuals who have an almost unlimited access to information, but limited access to healthcare resource, tolerate sub-optimal care? Many conflicts may arise between a free market in information and a controlled market in healthcare.

Patients may be motivated to seek out the most recent literature for their condition, and can invest considerable effort in that search, but most practising clinicians are restricted in the time and effort they can devote to searching for information about individual patients. The Bolam principle, established in the UK in 1957, protects a doctor against a claim of negligence if other colleagues would have acted in the same manner (*Bolam v Friern Barnet, HMC* 1 WRL 582, 1957). The Bolam principle was overturned in an Australian court in 1995, and the same may happen in other countries where it applies, like the UK (Economist, 1995). Similarly in the US, some states have begun the move towards protecting healthcare workers against litigation if they treat a patient according to recognized guidelines. If the law were to judge a clinician negligent for failure to institute recognized best practice, then an informed patient population and an overworked clinical community provide a recipe for increasing litigation.

There is a risk that the Internet will spread poor-quality information to consumers

Along with the Internet's rapid growth has been an increasing concern about its potential to spread poor information to the public (Coiera, 1996a; Silberg *et al.*, 1997). There are also apparently anecdotes of patients coming to harm because of information obtained on the Internet (Weisbord *et al.*, 1997). Are we witnessing the beginning of an 'epidemic' of misinformation spread by the Internet, or are we seeing nothing more than a variation of what is endemic? Patients have always obtained information outside the formal healthcare system. Could it be that now there is simply a new 'carrier' called the Internet, and nothing else has changed?

The truth is that we know very little about epidemiology in health informatics. It is almost impossible to trace cause and effect as information moves through our human and technological systems. Their inherent complexity makes it hard to identify which information processes lead to unfavourable health outcomes. Although studies confirm the presence of poor-quality health information on the Internet (Culver *et al.*, 1997; Impiccatore *et al.*, 1997; McClung *et al.*, 1998), no work has clearly shown it has a positive or negative impact on public health outcomes (Wyatt, 1997).

Bessell *et al.* (2002) conducted a systematic review of 10 comparative studies of the effect of consumer use of online health information on decision-making, attitudes, knowledge, satisfaction, and health outcomes and utilization. The studies they examined evaluated the effectiveness of using the Internet to deliver a smoking cessation programme, cardiac and nutrition educational programmes, behavioural interventions for headache and weight loss, and pharmacy and augmentative services. All the studies showed some positive effects on health outcomes. However, the review concluded that the methodological quality of many studies was poor and there is still almost a complete lack of evidence of any effects consumer access to health information on the Internet may have on health outcomes.

Clearly more such studies are needed, but they may take time. Yet, with the exponential growth in the Internet, we may be in a situation where it is inappropriate to wait for complete results, and a 'precautionary principle' might have to be invoked. Acting while the problem is potentially controllable may be less risky than awaiting firm evidence of an out-of-control phenomenon.

As we shall explore in greater detail in the next chapter, compared to traditional media such as magazines and newspapers, electronic information can be infinitely duplicated at minimal cost, and is remarkably cheap to distribute. Given the effort required to generate high-quality information such as evidence-based guidelines, it becomes cheaper to produce poor-quality information that looks good, than high-quality information that is less well packaged. Consequently, producers of poor information may be at an advantage on the Internet, from where they could flood the entire information market with their product, and eventually diminish the market share of traditional media.

Official health information standards could be used to voluntarily label information and help the public make better choices. Indeed, sophisticated proposals along these lines are actively being explored (Eysenbach and Diepgen, 1999). However, a 1998 review of 47 different proposals for standards to label health information concluded that 'it is unclear whether they should exist in the first place, whether they measure what they claim to measure, or whether they lead to more harm than good' (Jadad and Gagliardi, 1998). By 2002 the same authors had found a further 51 new instruments designed to rate the quality of health information, none of which had been validated (Gagliardi and Jadad, 2002). Much of the problem lies in the inherent subjectivity of information. Quality can only be measured within the context of use, and public health information is used in many different ways. It is often designed to emphasize simplicity and intelligibility rather than scientific rigour, and needs to be understood by people with widely varying knowledge and abilities.

Assuming information standards are created, how would they be used? The television industry has come up with one mechanism. Using electronic labels embedded in the broadcast signal, the V-chip can block reception of material that is deemed unacceptable, for example screening violent material from children. The MedCERTAIN proposals (Eysenbach and Diepgen, 1999) suggest that we use similar Internet technologies to help the public sift good from bad. It is an approach that might work, with the public voluntarily using software filters to check Internet documents and only displaying those that have quality labels.

Effectively it is a proposal to create an immune system at information access points by placing recognition markers on documents. In a future where we might imagine new epidemics of misinformation spreading across the Internet, such immunity will never be perfect. The ability to mutate information pathogens and breach the immune defences will guarantee that the battle is never ending. Finding ways to attach labels is also a problem.

Eysenbach and Diepgen (1999) propose to distribute the load across the medical community. However, given the opportunity to review material on the Internet, participation rates amongst the medical population are reported to be very low (Bingham *et al.*, 1998). Consequently we may need an automated process for the scheme to succeed. Perhaps software agents will one day comb the Internet like cyber-immune cells. They could attach labels to all that they touch, or copy key fragments and bring these info-antigens back to enhance their host's immune memory. In a more hostile future, they might attack what they find.

23.6 Notification systems offer a rapid way of communicating with the clinical community

Although publishing using Web technologies is a powerful way to disseminate information, it is a passive or 'pull' broadcast medium. In many circumstances in healthcare, this model is inadequate. This is especially the case when it is necessary to make sure defined individuals receive critical information in a timely fashion. For example, a laboratory might wish to alert a clinician about a patient's test results. In this case, some form of 'push' peer-to-peer communication is more appropriate. If a government regulatory authority needs to issue an urgent bulletin informing healthcare workers about a public health warning, then a narrowcast push method may be more appropriate.

The Internet changes the way an organization is able to communicate through the distribution of information. It is often the case with publicly sensitive information that healthcare workers need to be notified in advance of the public, so that they can be prepared to deal with the consequences of such announcements. Much anxiety and confusion can result when this does not happen: a recent example in the UK arose when the public was informed of the withdrawal of certain forms of the oral contraceptive pill, but many general practitioners were not informed in advance of the announcement (Coiera, 1996a). In such cases, what is needed is a targeted narrowcast to healthcare workers, in advance of the broadcast to the general public.

Some rudimentary systems have already been put in place to communicate urgent public health information. Through a combination of fax, paging and e-mail technologies, it is possible to contact most people in developed countries. To solve the problem posed by the sheer number of individuals that need to be contacted, some authorities (e.g. in the UK) use a cascade communication system. Here, a message is passed on to a small group, who in turn relay it to their own regions according to locally maintained lists of names. Several cascade steps may be needed to get the multiplication effect needed to ensure that everyone is contacted within an appropriate time.

Contrast the complexity of this cascade system with one based on e-mail and computer-generated faxes, where a message can be sent once without any necessary intermediate steps. Lists of names can be maintained locally, to ensure accuracy, but can be made available on the Web to the organizations that need to access them. These lists can contain e-mail addresses, telephone or fax numbers, or whatever contact medium is most appropriate for different individuals. Once sent, the communication system is able to generate the message in the form appropriate to the facilities available for different individuals. Certainly, as more healthcare workers obtain routine Internet access, even this technical complexity can be sidestepped in favour of pure e-mail-based messaging.

Governmental bodies usually have well-developed systems for reporting adverse drug reactions, permitting the performance of newly licensed substances to be monitored. The type of incident reported need not be limited to drug reactions. For example, critical incidents during anaesthesia might relate to human error or device malfunction. Adverse or critical incidents during other types of procedure can also be submitted, possibly anonymously, to enhance the likelihood of obtaining reports (Staender *et al.*, 1996), and such reporting can also be done over an Internet service. For example, Web-based critical incident reporting systems have been set up for the anonymous capture of events, for example to collect a set of descriptions of critical incidents in anaesthesiology.

Computerized anonymous critical incident reporting has also been attempted in the emergency department as a tool in the quality assurance process (Pointer and Osur, 1987), primarily as a means of automating the process of acquiring, storing and analysing such reports. This computerized incident report system has been reported to be receiving approximately 100 reports per month, suggesting that when a system is well set up, clinical staff will be sufficiently motivated to report a fair number of critical incidents.

Globally, the World Health Organization (WHO) has developed FluNet, an Internet application linking the WHO network of influenza centres. This early-alert system for the global monitoring of influenza provides international and national authorities, the public and the media with full access to real-time epidemiological and virological information and is designed to improve management and enhance standardization of reporting (Flahault *et al.*, 1998). As we will see in Chapter 28, the Web also has a critical role to play in other forms of surveillance for infectious diseases, including intentional release as a form of bioterrorism.

23.7 The Internet has given rise to new types of healthcare service

The type of Internet uses that have been described so far represent extensions of existing processes. Although the technology is still relatively immature, there is a clear desire by many to see entirely new ways of delivering care created. This is in part due to a much bigger market that exists on the Web. From a commercial point of view this means that highly specialized services that would not be sustainable in a local region may now be able to survive on the Internet. Examples of some new healthcare services that have appeared on the Internet include:

Consultation by e-mail

E-mail is being used as a means for consumers and clinicians to obtain information from selected medical consultants in a timely manner. Using e-mail, clinicians encounter a wider pool of patients than in their physical practice, potentially of international scope. Patients for their part at best have rapid access to experts of international stature, if they should be willing to interact in this way. During one 33-month study covering of 1239 e-mail requests to a children's medical centre, 81% of e-mail requests were initiated by parents, relatives or guardians, 10% by physicians and 9% by other healthcare professionals (Borowitz and Wyatt, 1998). Consultation requests were received from 39 states and 37 other countries and on average, reading and responding to each e-mail took slightly less than 4 minutes. In 69%, there was a specific question about a particular child; in 9%, the requester sought a second opinion about a particular child; 22% requested general information concerning a disorder, treatment or medication. The study's authors concluded that e-mail correspondence with an unfamiliar consultant cannot substitute for examination and care by a physician. However, e-mail consultants can begin a dialogue with a person seeking information, ask clarifying questions, perhaps of information uncovered on the Internet, or direct people towards appropriate educational materials or other resources.

Such consultations may be carried out entirely by e-mail, or may in the future be a prelude to consultation taking place across a video-link. Some groups see many of these services as potentially powerful ways of generating revenue. For example, some internationally renowned centres of healthcare excellence now sell their expertise via telemedical video-links. As the need for specialized links for video-consultation diminish over the next decade, these services could potentially be provided by anyone with access to standard communication systems.

There remain many difficulties with e-mail as a consulting medium. Patients may not get the immediate response they would like, and clinicians may be swamped by more e-mail than they would care for. Advice given by e-mail is no doubt legally binding, but clinicians may not have had access to a physical exam, test results or the medical record. Consumers expect their personal details to be treated with privacy and confidentiality, but there are no safeguards that this will be the case with standard e-mail, especially when there is no established level of trust with the clinician apparently on the other side of the technology. E-mail is well suited to short messages between individuals who already share much common ground, and although the concept of e-mail consultation attracts most attention, it is likely that in the long run e-mail will be a routine communication tool between patients and their clinicians, discussing matters that arise between other more extensive interactions.

Brokering

Healthcare specialists offering to give advice to patients can register with a brokering service, which creates a list of specialists in different categories. Patients approach the brokering service and are put in contact with the specialist who is most suitable, perhaps because of experience, interests or geographical location. Such brokering services transcend state and national boundaries, and their implications are yet to be fully examined.

Third party medical record providers

The near universal accessibility of electronic files on the Internet, as we saw above, makes it an attractive technology for electronic medical records. An unexpected consequence of the technology has been that several companies now offer consumers Web sites where they can enter their own medical history, with a view to making their **personal health records** available to the many different clinicians who consumers may see over their lifetime. This model expects that eventually clinicians will be willing to access such records, which are not under their own control like traditional patient records, and enter in new data about the current encounter. Apart from the difficulties about ownership and control of the record associated with this model, there are also risks that the record structures chosen may not suit all clinicians, and it is unclear how complex data like images would be managed. There is also concern that, when the records are stored on computers either in different local jurisdictions, or even internationally, patients may lose their rights to control the uses their records are put to. For example, the laws in one country might prevent the secondary use of a patient's record, such as selling aggregate data to drug companies. However, if the record is stored in another country with different laws, patients may not realize they have forfeited their legal controls over the record's use.

Consequently, the delivery of healthcare services across the Internet is associated with legal uncertainty, since it allows clinicians to deliver care beyond state and national boundaries. Unfortunately most of the legal machinery developed to protect both patients and practitioners is based on the assumption that care takes place within tight geographic bounds, where particular laws have jurisdiction. It is difficult at present to know how one would take legal action for care delivered across national boundaries. Further, it is not clear how one would obtain reimbursement for such services, given that many patients would seek to recover costs from state funds or private health insurance schemes.

Discussion points

1 Should clinicians have unrestricted access to the Web in the workplace?

2 Biomedical librarians have championed the use of Internet technologies to improve clinician use of high-quality evidence. Early on, however, some strongly resisted clinicians using the Web to answer clinical questions. Can you imagine why?

3 Your organization runs separate information systems for the medical record, clinical laboratories and prescribing. Describe how Web technologies can be used to 'integrate' these systems.

4 What characteristics define a poor-quality document on the Web?

5 You are training consumers to use the Internet to obtain health information. What informatics skills will you teach them? Which resources would you recommend they use, and why?

6 A friend of yours has used e-mail to get a second opinion on a very difficult health problem they have from an 'expert' overseas, and the opinion is different from that of their current treating physician. What are you going to advise them to do?

Chapter summary

1 The Web can support rapid publication and distribution of clinical information by: increasing the amount of information available and the speed with which it can be published and kept up to date, minimizing problems of multiple versions of documents, allowing the use of multimedia and novel interactions and improving searchability.

2 The electronic patient record can be built using Web technologies, which support integration of multiple legacy systems through a single common set of standards for electronic communication and document presentation.

3 The dissemination of peer-reviewed scientific knowledge is enhanced through use of the Web. Peer-reviewed healthcare journals appearing on the Internet are able to publish more quickly and cheaply than paper editions, can utilize multimedia, allow readers to interact directly and deliver feedback, and make supporting data available when research papers are published.

4 Online systems can support continuing education and decision-making. CPE will increasingly consist of using online information technology to answer immediate clinical questions, but substantial socio-technical barriers remain at present.

5 Patients may access healthcare information on the Web but there is a risk that it will spread poor-quality information to consumers. However, there is still almost a complete lack of evidence of any effects consumer access to health information on the Internet may have on health outcomes.

6 Notification systems offer a rapid way of communicating with the clinical community, and can be used to alert clinicians to public health issues or get clinical feedback on critical incidents such as adverse drug reactions.

7 The Internet has given rise to new types of healthcare service including service brokering, e-mail consultation, third-party electronic medical records, and remote collaboration.

CHAPTER 24

Information economics and the Internet

> The idea that information can be stored in a changing world without an overwhelming depreciation in its value is false. *Weiner (1954), p. 120.*

The information space on the Internet we call the World Wide Web continues to grow, offering seemingly unlimited potential for the creation, storage and dissemination of information. Within healthcare, the Web is seen as offering us an answer to everything from the integration of our fragmented information systems, the delivery of accurate information to consumers, evidence-based medicine and the electronic medical record (EMR).

Yet, although it is beguiling to focus on the advantages of specific technical innovations on the Internet, it is much harder to predict their ultimate utility or impact. We have already seen, for example, that the diffusion, acceptance and ultimate success of any technology depends at least as much on the social system within which it is placed, as on the nature of the technology itself. Yet we still lack clear models of what it means to deliver information using a network technology like the Internet within a complex social system like health, and often struggle to explain what is so different about information systems built around traditional information technology, and Web-based implementations.

Surprisingly, economics may offer insights into the dynamics of information across networked systems. Its models invoke not just the specific technical advantages of one product over another, but the preferences and decisions of individuals who choose to use a product. In the specialist field known as information economics, we find theoretical and practical models for creating, diffusing and using information. Information economics also focuses on understanding how networks of individuals interact to exchange information, and the emergent properties of those interactions. As such, it provides informatics with a core set of theoretical results with wider application beyond the specifics of the Internet.

In this chapter, the basic properties of information as an economic good are introduced. Beginning with information production, the economic properties of information have substantial import for those publishing information on the Web, independently of whether their intent is commercial. Secondly, a basic economic analysis of the current growth of information on the Internet will be shown to have substantial implications for information retrieval by consumers.

24.1 Information has a value

Economic commentators regard any information that can be given a market value such as music, literature or a product design as an **information good**. Consequently the economic laws of supply and demand can be applied to the trading of information and assist us in understanding how much individuals might be wiling to pay for it, or under what circumstances it will or will not be profitable to produce it (Box 24.1) Indeed, any information that can be digitized is potentially a capital good (Varian, 1998). Within healthcare, we see many examples of the capital value of information. Consumers are willing to pay for health-related information that comes directly from clinical professionals or from mass media such as magazines. Clinicians pay for subscriptions to journals or purchase texts to maintain their skills, knowledge and professional standing. Pharmaceutical companies are happy to pay physicians for data about their prescribing behaviours so that they can be aggregated to reveal prescribing patterns for their products.

However, the characteristics of information goods deviate from those of a traditional traded good in a number of ways, with interesting consequences for producers and consumers (Davis and Stack, 1997; Morris-Suzuki, 1997; Kelly, 1998; Varian, 1998):

- You must experience information before you know what it is. Without reading a book or listening to music you will not know whether it is really worth buying. In contrast, there

Box 24.1
Information supply and demand

When costs and benefits are invoked for a particular product, be it physical or information, economics can assist in modelling its uptake into a community. The supply and demand for information can be modelled by graphing the quantity of product 'sold' – in this case the uptake of an information product such as a guideline – against the cost of the information for the producer and consumer (Figure 24.1). In traditional economics, price is expressed in monetary units, but in this case the price of creating and retrieving health information is a more complex blending of individual and societal costs and benefits.

The down-sloping demand curve shows that when information is cheap, consumers are more likely to seek it. Conversely, when the cost of information is high, demand is low. For information producers, the up-sloping supply curve shows the greater the return in creating a product, the more producers appear, increasing supply. However, electronic reproduction of information now means the cost of duplication is tending towards zero, flattening this curve.

The point at which supply and demand curves intersect represents the point of market equilibrium, where both equations are simultaneously satisfied. Any transactions occurring at prices away from the equilibrium result in unhappy consumers or producers, who then drive the market back to equilibrium as they try and minimize their dissatisfaction with the outcome (Frank, 1998). Thus, market equilibrium theoretically represents the optimum outcome for the system given the underlying cost and benefit structures. Changing costs or benefits will alter the shape of the supply and demand curves, resulting in a new equilibrium. If we want to increase the uptake of an information product we can alter either the supply or demand side (Figures 24.2 and 24.3).

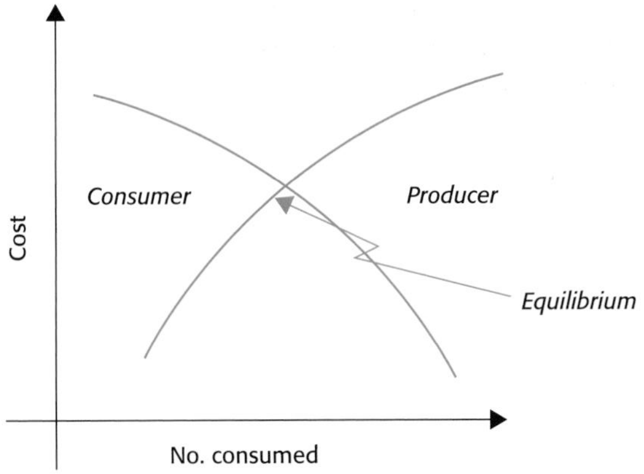
Consumer
Producer
Equilibrium
Cost
No. consumed

Figure 24.1
Supply and demand curves for information items. Demand is generated by a population of potential information consumers, and supply provided by a population of information creators.

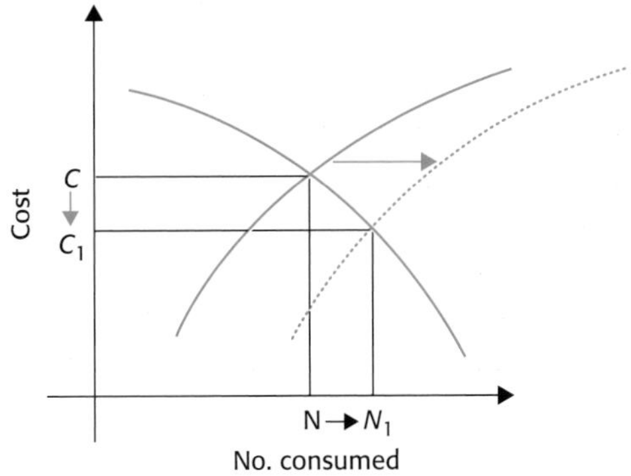
Cost
C
C1
N → N1
No. consumed

Figure 24.2
By reducing the cost of 'ownership' of an information product from C to C_1, the supply curve is shifted, resulting in a new equilibrium point and greater amounts of information being taken up.

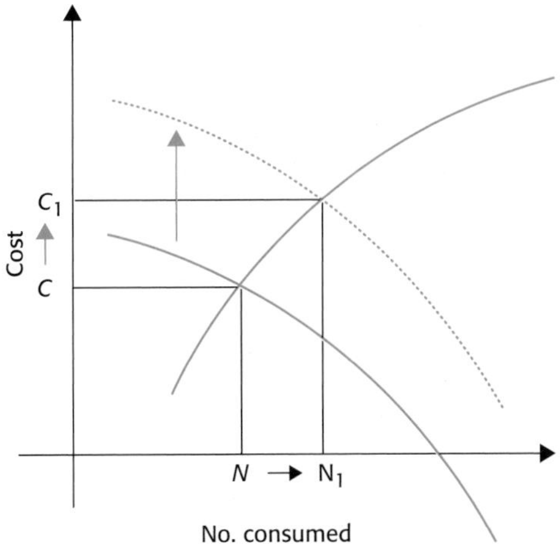
Cost
C1
C
N → N1
No. consumed

Figure 24.3
By increasing the perceived value of information, consumers are more willing to spend resources on it for a given cost, shifting the demand curve, and increasing the overall uptake of the information item into the community.

is no need to pre-use normal goods such as batteries or oranges since we can assume that these goods will deliver what is expected of them.

- Although production costs are typically high and fixed for information products, they can be copied cheaply (and indefinitely if in digital form). The master copy of a book, movie or soundtrack is expensive to produce, but copying it is cheap. On the Web, creating and maintaining the information content of a site is expensive, but making copies of it when consumers visit a site is almost zero in cost. In economic terms, the marginal costs of reproduction for information goods are low. Worse, initial production costs are 'sunk', in that they are incurred before mass reproduction and are not recoverable in the case of failure.

- Since digital information can be copied exactly, it is never consumed. Further, a possessor of information can transfer it to others without losing the information (unless we demand that they forget what they know!). Normal goods like apples, oranges or houses do not behave in this way. Consequently, the laws of supply and demand that depend on scarcity of a product do not easily apply to many information goods.
- Digital information can be transported at low cost (perhaps approaching free transmission across bulk communication networks).

When distribution costs are low, and the good itself is cheap to reproduce, producers can be drawn into ruinous price wars, driving the consumer price towards zero (Fishburn *et al.*, 1998). Consequently information can only acquire a proper market price when some form of monopoly protects it, for example through the protection of a patent or copyright, and this is the usual recourse for creating value and protecting investment.

However, pirates are well able to exploit irregularities in copyright laws to their advantage, and the information good in question need not even be digital for the enterprise to be worthwhile. In the nineteenth century, US copyright laws did not extend to foreign works, so publishers were able to rush popular works to the US for reproduction where they had an almost guaranteed market. Competition was intense, as the first to publish might only have had a matter of days before they too were copied. As a consequence, in 1843 pirated copies of Dickens' *Christmas Carol* sold for 6c in the US while the authorized version sold for $2.50 in England (Varian, 1998). Modern-day software and music pirates operate in a similar fashion.

When free distribution of information is the goal, then this behaviour of information to replicate and distribute at minimal cost is to be welcomed. When the owner of information seeks to generate revenue from the information, it is potentially disastrous. Any document placed on the Web is subject to similar pressures, as it can potentially be copied and subsequently be made available on another site. Unfortunately, copyright is weakened as a form of protection for Web documents, because information pirates can place duplicate documents on web servers residing in foreign countries that do not recognize or enforce the copyright. Further, the nature of the Web allows consumers living within a country with well-policed copyright laws to access these foreign pirated documents. Catching Web users accessing pirated information is non-trivial and perhaps more trouble than it is worth.

This leads to an obvious question. How does an information producer make money publishing on the Web? If consumers expect information to be virtually free, if producing information is expensive, and if once produced your competitors can steal your product, it may seem a forlorn proposition.

The answer is to avoid as much as possible creating information goods that must be traded in such openly competitive environments, and instead recreate the characteristics of a monopoly. These avoidance tactics may not ultimately prevent information leaking out from the owner and into a pirate market, but they all have the effect of delaying the inevitable. With sufficient delay, the information may no longer have commercial value, or the producer may have adequately recovered enough costs and generated revenue. Several tactics are commonly employed:

- Unlike most commodity items, most information goods are highly differentiated (Varian, 1998). Each article in a journal is different, and we would not necessarily consider one a direct substitute for another. However, there is enough similarity amongst information goods for there to be competition between them. Indeed, even though there may be differences present, consumers may not be able to discriminate. For example, a trained clinician may easily detect the difference between two self-help articles written for the general public, but a member of the public may not. In such cases, the reputation of the provider may be the only vehicle available for the general public to discriminate between information sources. Attaching the brand identity of a professional organization to an information site, for example, may ensure that consumers come there in preference to purely commercial information sources.

- It is often suggested that the Internet will herald a competitive pay-per-view model where consumers pay only for the information they read. For example, clinicians might only pay for the journal articles they download, rather than paying an annual subscription for the whole journal. Indeed, one of the big attractions of Web technologies is the potential to charge customers according to their usage of a product. However, in such an environment, items of information need to compete with each other, which would drive prices down towards zero. One way to avoid this is to charge a flat fee for entry into a Web site, and allow consumers to then take what they need. Comfortingly for information providers, there is theoretical and anecdotal evidence that customers may actually prefer paying a fixed fee for entry to a Web site rather than paying on a per-view basis (Fishburn *et al.*, 1998). For example, many pay-per-view TV schemes have flopped. Three main reasons probably lead to a preference for simple and predictable flat fees for access to information. Firstly, flat fees provide insurance against sudden large bills. Secondly, customers typically overestimate their potential usage, so they are happy to pay more. Thirdly, flat fees remove the worry of deciding whether downloading a specific information item is worth the money.
- It is also argued that producers will obtain more revenue for individual information items if they **bundle** them with other disparate items, and then sell access to the whole package. For example, software is most profitably sold bundled into a suite at cheaper cost than buying each of the individual items. Even though consumers may not need the whole bundle, they are happy to pay a higher price than for a single piece of software. Since the cost of manufacture for software is marginal, bundling returns greater revenue from individual consumers. So, selling access to a web site or a whole issue of an electronic journal not only may be favoured by consumers, but also may be more profitable for producers (Fishburn *et al.*, 1998).
- Information producers can also recover their fixed costs through creative pricing and marketing. It is common for different groups of consumers to pay different prices for different versions of the same information. Some consumers are happy to pay for an expensive hardback copy of a book because they will read it earlier. Others are happy to wait, and read the cheaper paperback. Some investors are happy to pay a high price for real-time stock quotes and complex financial analyses; others are happy to read free but delayed stock prices with little or no additional analysis. There are many dimensions along which one can 'version' information, including delay, user interface, convenience, image resolution, format, capability, features, comprehensiveness, annoyance and support (Shapiro and Varian, 1998). So, although an electronic journal may make its contents available for free to the general public, it may provide extra services to its fee-paying subscribers. For example, it may offer the ability to see articles before general release, advanced search and current awareness notification services, higher resolution images and access to links to related materials (Varian, 1996).

24.2 Consuming information on the Web is associated with search costs

As we have seen, information can never be consumed. However, as Herbert Simon has famously noted: 'What information consumes is rather obvious. It consumes the attention of its recipients. Hence a wealth of information creates a poverty of attention' (Kelly, 1998).

By all accounts, the store of information available on the Web is growing exponentially. However, the amount of information being accessed, or 'consumed', grows at best linearly. As Varian (1998) has pointed out, this leads to a variant of Malthus' law which showed that while the amount of food seemed to grow linearly, the number of stomachs grew exponentially (Box 24.2).

The uncomfortable consequence of this 'Malthusian law of information' is that **the fraction of information produced that is actually consumed will with time asymptotically approach zero.** In this case, the limiting factor is our ability to spend time consuming information. Our attention is the scarce resource.

The consequence of this ever-expanding information marketplace for information producers is that their success is increasingly dependent upon their ability to compete for the attention of information consumers. The consequences for consumers of information are equally problematic. Firstly and obviously, the demands on our attention are increasing. At the limit, information consumption has the potential to dominate all other tasks for our attention, unless individual limits to consumption are introduced.

As worryingly, theoretically it should become ever more expensive to find information. In particular, the costs of searching for and evaluating information have the potential to become increasingly expensive over time. If the amount of information is growing exponentially, then by implication, on average so too should the number of documents that match any particular search. Another way of restating this is to say that, for a given amount of search effort, the probability a finding a document on the Web will decrease with time. In other words, the seemingly inevitable consequence of a global growth in information supply is actually an 'information famine' where we cannot find what we need. The haystack just keeps growing, making it ever harder to find the needle.

The costs of searching for, evaluating and then purchasing any good are all **transaction costs.** Although they may not be factored into the final price paid for an item, they are

Box 24.2
Malthus' law

In nineteenth-century England, Thomas Malthus argued that a law of diminishing returns applied to the production of food, and he predicted that famine was the inevitable consequence for the human race (Frank, 1998). The problem was that while the amount of agricultural land was fixed, the human population continued to grow. Even with improved agriculture, beyond some point, the increased yield in food production per unit of land becomes ever smaller.

Malthus' logic was impeccable, but the human race has survived through the twentieth century and into the twenty-first. What Malthus did not foresee was that agricultural technology would increase food yields at the rate it did. Food production per capita in 1985 was 20 times as great as it was a century earlier, and outstripped the effects of a fixed supply in land and a growing population.

Some will argue that Malthus misunderstood the capacity for technology to improve food production, and that as long as we develop new technologies, we will always be able to feed ourselves. Yet Malthus' logic remains valid, and if the global population continues to grow, a time will come (perhaps long into the future) when the land cannot keep up with what is demanded of it. We only evade the law if we evade the rate-limiting step: the supply of land upon the earth, or our dependence upon it.

nonetheless a real part of the cost of doing business. So, while information on the Internet may ultimately become virtually free to obtain, the transaction costs in obtaining that information will not disappear. We can summarize by noting that the cost of an information transaction on the Internet is related to the amount of information placed on the Internet. Such costs are an example of a **negative network effect** or **negative externality** (see Box 24.3).

In this way, searching for information on the Web is subject to the same economic constraints that apply to searching for goods in a physical marketplace (Box 24.4). A traditional

Box 24.3
Externalities

An **externality** is a cost or benefit that falls on people who are not directly involved in an activity.

The Internet exhibits what are known as **positive externalities** or **network effects**, where the value of a good depends on the number of other people who use it. Thus, the more people that join the Internet, the more valuable an individual connection to the Internet becomes (Kelly, 1998). Other networks exhibit similar positive externalities. The value of the telephone or fax changed enormously once the network of individuals owning one grew, resulting in a sustaining positive feedback cycle of network growth. So, with positive network externalities, the actions of others enhance the value of joining the network.

In contrast, pollution arising out of the production of a commodity is an example of a **negative externality**. It affects not just those who manufacture or consume the product, but society as a whole (Frank, 1998). Since externalities are by definition not factored into prices, there is no economic incentive for producers to deal with them. The problem then is that negative externalities impose additional costs on others, but can be ignored by the producer. If one could somehow internalize the externality, for example by factoring the cost of pollution into taxation, then an incentive to minimize the negative effect is introduced. So, a tax based on the amount of pollution a producer generates has the effect of providing an incentive to minimize pollution.

The Internet also exhibits negative externalities. For example, when the number of users on the network exceeds its transmission capacity, they cause congestion. The resulting delay in transmission of e-mail, or long delays in document retrieval on the Web, imposes a cost on individual users. As long as the cost remains external to the system, there is no incentive to deal with the problem by individual users. However, if Internet usage became expensive at times of congestion, then the negative externality becomes internalized into the calculations of consumers, and there is an incentive to use the system at less congested times (Varian, 1998).

Box 24.4
Shopping with perfect information

We know that prices for similar items vary across different sellers. This price dispersion is a manifestation of lack of knowledge, or ignorance, in the marketplace (Stigler, 1961). If we always knew where the best buy was, then everyone would shop there. Alternatively, all the sellers would have to drop their price to match the lowest price. The reason people do not search exhaustively for the best deal is that search is expensive. It consumes time and effort, which are limited resources for us all. It is also the case that on average, prolonged searches show diminishing returns over time.

In the world of online commerce, things can be very different. For example, a consumer could use a software agent or 'shop-bot' to seek the best price for a particular item (Kephart and Greenwald, 1999). Searching with the agent incurs no real cost, since Internet transactions are virtually costless, as indeed is most information on the Internet. As a result, online sellers would be forced to price-match the lowest price to remain competitive in the shop-bot driven marketplace.

This is indeed what has happened. In one now infamous story, an online CD shopping agent offered to help customers find the cheapest CD from the online stores. As we would expect, prices started to come down among the online retailers to maintain sales. However, realizing the dilemma posed by perfect consumer information, most of the online sellers decided to block access to the shopping agent. In a single stroke they eliminated the potential for competing in a marketplace, which had the potential to drive their returns down close to zero.

Internet commerce also has the potential to drive prices up. If consumers can detect changes in prices more quickly than retailers, then a price drop favours the first price cutter. However, if retailers could detect price changes faster than consumers could, things change. So, if one firm drops its price, and is immediately matched by another firm before customers can act upon the change, then the first price cutter gets much less from the deal. So, the incentive to price-cut is diminished. In contrast, matching prices upwards is beneficial. Some evidence of a general upward drift in online prices through such price matching now exists (Varian, 1999).

way consumers minimize the search costs for goods is to seek out a trusted supplier that on average delivers a high-quality product at a good price. A department store, for example, can be seen as an organization whose main value is to search for superior goods for its customers, and then guarantee that they are of good quality. A store's good reputation results in a degree of consumer loyalty. Such reputation is a valuable item in itself, since it economizes on search for customers (Stigler, 1961) and therefore can be translated into a price added to the base cost of a good.

On the Web, information consumers can similarly minimize search costs by constraining their search to known areas that produce high-quality information which usually suits their needs. Such information **portals** thus act like traditional department stores. Unsurprisingly, there has already been fierce competition amongst Web portals for consumer attention and the consequent opportunity to attract what is most economically valuable to them – consumer loyalty maintained through reputation.

A related issue to the growth of information is that of information quality. If the main cost in creating and selling information online occurs at the time of production, then those producers with low production costs are in a position to swamp high-quality producers. For healthcare there are particular implications. For example, producing high-quality evidence-based guidelines for clinicians, or clear and accurate information for consumers is resource intensive. Consequently the rate at which good-quality health information is produced cannot match that at which poor information can be produced. Thus, producers of poor information may be at an advantage on the Internet, from where they could flood the entire information market with their product.

Solutions to this problem of information quantity include the use of legislation to limit the ability of producers of poor-quality content to publish on the Web, but the international reach of the Internet limits the effectiveness of any single nation's efforts. Alternatively, one could try to use quality labels that identify information of good standard, as discussed in the previous chapter. Many consumers solve the quality problem in the same way they solve the search problem. They seek information from portals that they judge to deliver good-quality information. Consequently, one of the Internet's challenges to healthcare is for us to find economic ways to provide trusted sources of information on the Web for consumers. Failure to do so leaves the health information market open to opportunists who may not share the same standards for information production, or the same goals in its dissemination.

However, despite all our best efforts, over time the rigid logic of the Malthusian law of information should theoretically swamp all the benefits of creating high-quality sites by information producers. And for consumers, it should swamp out the benefits of 'contracting out' information search costs to a trusted portal, labelling information or using search agents. Information will continue to increase exponentially, but our capacity to find what we need will not.

However, as with Malthus' prediction about the production of food, in the short term advances in technology might help avoid catastrophe. If we can increase the accuracy of information search technology at a rate greater than the rate at which information grows, then we can avoid our 'information famine'. At present, there is a large research effort focusing on Internet search technologies. For example, personalized search agents can help not just find information, but filter it according to the likelihood that it matches a consumer's needs. An agent could do this by learning from past experience. By building a computational model of what documents satisfied previous search criteria, the agent over time builds up knowledge about its user's needs. Since the rate-limiting step we have identified is a human's attention, and specifically the time it takes to sift through the results of a particular search, anything that reduces a human's need to specify exactly what is needed will improve the situation.

In a sense, we are entering a period of an escalating technological arms race between the production of information and our capacity to find information, and the ultimate outcome is not at all clear. However, even if improved search technology cannot change underlying economic principles, it can confer a relative advantage to individuals. When the possession of the best information is critical to an endeavour's success, then possessing a superior search technology confers relative advantage over one's competitors.

Conclusions

Information economics provides us with a challenging analysis of the future for information publication on the Internet. It shows that the grinding growth in information has profound consequences for both information producers as well as consumers. It will be harder for producers to push the information they create to the audience they want to see it. Consumers, on the other hand, are faced with parallel problems arising out of information oversupply and the limits of human attention. Technological innovation can be cast as our saviour, but in truth we still know very little about its power to help. At present, it is still very hard to know if we are heading for an information feast, or famine.

Discussion points

1. Should consumer health information be available free of charge?
2. Is it possible for a biomedical journal to publish only on the Web and not charge for access?
3. Why might people access poorer-quality information on the Web, when better-quality evidence-based resources are also available?
4. Is health information a public good, and if so, what is the role of government in its provision?

Chapter summary

1. Any information that can be given a market value, such as music, literature or a product design, is an **information good**. Consequently the economic laws of supply and demand can be applied to the trading of information and assist us in understanding how much individuals might be willing to pay for it, or under what circumstances it will or will not be profitable to produce it.
2. The characteristics of information goods deviate from those of traditional traded goods in a number of ways:
   - You must experience information before you know what it is.
   - Production costs are typically high and fixed for information products, but they can be copied cheaply and indefinitely if in digital form.
   - Since digital information can be copied exactly, it is never consumed. Further, a possessor of information can transfer it to others without losing the information.
   - Digital information can be transported at low cost, approaching free transmission across bulk communication networks.
3. Consuming information on the Web is associated with search costs, partly driven by the continuing growth in the amount of information available. The **Malthusian law of information** states that the fraction of information produced that is actually consumed will with time asymptote toward zero. In this case, the limiting factor is our ability to spend time consuming information. Our attention is the scarce resource.
4. The costs of searching for, evaluating and then purchasing any good are all transaction costs. Although information on the Internet may ultimately become virtually free to obtain, the transaction costs in obtaining that information will not disappear. The cost of an information transaction on the Internet is related to the amount of information placed on the Internet and is an example of a negative network effect or negative externality.

PART 8

Decision support systems

CHAPTER 25

Clinical decision support systems

From the very earliest moments in the modern history of the computer, scientists have dreamed of creating an 'electronic brain'. Of all the modern technological quests, this search to create artificially intelligent (AI) computer systems has been one of the most ambitious and, not surprisingly, controversial.

It also seems that very early on, scientists and clinicians alike were captivated by the potential such a technology might have in healthcare (e.g. Ledley and Lusted, 1959). With intelligent computers able to store and process vast stores of knowledge, the hope was that they would become perfect 'doctors in a box', assisting or surpassing clinicians with tasks like diagnosis.

With such motivations, a small but talented community of computer scientists and healthcare professionals set about shaping a research program for a new discipline called Artificial Intelligence in Medicine (AIM). These researchers had a bold vision of the way AIM would revolutionize healthcare, and push forward the frontiers of technology.

AI in medicine at that time was a largely US-based research community. Work originated out of a number of campuses, including MIT-Tufts, Pittsburgh, Stanford and Rutgers (e.g. Szolovits, 1982; Clancey and Shortliffe, 1984; Miller, 1988). The field attracted many of the best computer scientists and by any measure their output in the first decade of the field remains a remarkable achievement.

In reviewing this new field in 1984, Clancey and Shortliffe provided the following definition:

> Medical artificial intelligence is primarily concerned with the construction of AI programs that perform diagnosis and make therapy recommendations. Unlike medical applications based on other programming methods, such as purely statistical and probabilistic methods, medical AI programs are based on symbolic models of disease entities and their relationship to patient factors and clinical manifestations.

Much has changed since then, and today the importance of diagnosis as a task requiring computer support in routine clinical situations receives much less emphasis (Durinck *et al.*, 1994). The strict focus on the medical setting has now broadened across the healthcare spectrum, and instead of AIM systems, it is more typical to describe them as **clinical decision support systems** (CDSS). Intelligent systems today are thus found supporting medication prescribing, in clinical laboratories and educational settings, for clinical surveillance, or in data-rich areas like the intensive care setting.

Although there certainly have been ongoing challenges in developing such systems, they actually have proven their reliability and accuracy on repeated occasions (Shortliffe, 1987). Much of the difficulty experienced in introducing them has been socio-technical, and associated with the poor way in which they have fitted into clinical practice, either solving problems that were not perceived to be an issue, or imposing changes in the way clinicians worked. What is now being realized is that when they fill an appropriate role, intelligent programs do indeed offer significant benefits. One of the most important tasks now facing developers of AI-based systems is to characterize accurately those aspects of clinical practice that are best suited to the introduction of artificial intelligence systems.

In the remainder of this chapter, the initial focus thus remains on the different roles CDSS can play in clinical practice, looking particularly to see where clear successes can be identified, as well as looking to the future. Much of the material presumes familiarity with Chapters 2 and 8. The next chapter takes a more technological focus, and looks at the way CDSS are built. A variety of technologies including expert systems and neural networks will be discussed. The final chapters in this section look at several specialized topics where intelligent decision support is an essential component. We will look at the way CDSS can support the interpretation of patient signals that come off clinical monitoring devices, how they can assist in the surveillance for infectious diseases and public health challenges such as bioterrorism and how genome science is supported through bioinformatics.

25.1 AI can support both the creation and the use of clinical knowledge

Proponents of so-called 'strong' AI are interested in creating computer systems whose behaviour is at some level indistinguishable from that of humans (see Box 25.1). Success in strong AI would result in computer minds that might reside in autonomous physical beings like robots, or perhaps live in 'virtual' worlds such as the information space created by something like the Internet.

An alternative approach to strong AI is to look at human cognition and decide how it can be supported in complex or difficult situations. For example, fighter pilots may need the help of intelligent systems to assist in flying aircraft that are too complex for humans to operate on their own. These 'weak' AI systems are not intended to have an independent existence, but are a form of 'cognitive prosthesis' that supports a human in a variety of tasks.

CDSS are by and large intended to support healthcare workers in the normal course of their duties, assisting with tasks that rely on the manipulation of data and knowledge. An AI system could be running within an electronic medical record system, for example, and alert a clinician when it detects a contraindication to a planned treatment. It could also alert the clinician when it detected patterns in clinical data that suggested significant changes in a patient's condition.

Box 25.1
The Turing test

How will we know when a computer program has achieved an equivalent intelligence to a human? Is there some set of objective measures that can be assembled against which a computer program can be tested? Alan Turing was one of the founders of modern computer science and AI, whose intellectual achievements to this day remain astonishing in their breadth and importance. When he came to ponder this question, he brilliantly side-stepped the problem almost entirely.

In his opinion, there were no ultimately useful measures of intelligence. It was sufficient that an observer could not tell the difference in conversation between a human and a computer for us to conclude that the computer was intelligent. To cancel out any potential observer biases, Turing's test put the observer in a room, equipped with a computer keyboard and screen, and made the observer talk to the test subjects only using these. The observer would engage in a discussion with the test subjects using the printed word, much as one would today by exchanging e-mail with a remote colleague. If a set of observers could not distinguish the computer from another human in over 50% of cases, then Turing felt that one had to accept that the computer was intelligent.

Another consequence of the Turing test is that it says nothing about how one builds an intelligent artefact, thus neatly avoiding discussions about whether the artefact needed to in anyway mimic the structure of the human brain or our cognitive processes. In Turing's mind, it really didn't matter how the system was built. Its intelligence should only be assessed on the basis of its overt behaviour.

There have been attempts to build systems that can pass Turing's test in recent years. Some have managed to convince at least some humans in a panel of judges that they too are human, but none has yet passed the mark set by Turing.

Along with tasks that require reasoning with clinical knowledge, AI systems also have a very different role to play in the process of scientific research. In particular, AI systems have the capacity to learn, leading to the discovery of new phenomena and the creation of clinical knowledge. For example, a computer system can be used to analyse large amounts of data, looking for complex patterns within it that suggest previously unexpected associations. Equally, with enough of a model of existing knowledge, an AI system can be used to show how a new set of experimental observations conflicts with the existing theories. We now examine such capabilities in more detail.

25.2 Reasoning with clinical knowledge

Knowledge-based systems are the commonest type of CDSS technology in routine clinical use. Also known as **expert systems**, they contain clinical knowledge, usually about a very specifically defined task, and are able to reason with data from individual patients to come up with reasoned conclusions. Although there are many variations, the knowledge within an expert system is typically represented in the form of a set of rules.

There are numerous reasons why more CDSS are not in routine use (Coiera, 1994a, b). Some require the existence of an electronic patient record system to supply their data, and most institutions and practices do not yet have all their working data available electronically. Others suffer from poor human interface design and so do not get used even if they are of benefit.

Much of the initial reluctance to use CDSS arose simply because they did not fit naturally into the process of care, and as a result using them required additional effort from already busy individuals. It is also true, but perhaps dangerous, to ascribe some of the reluctance to use early systems to the technophobia or computer illiteracy of healthcare workers. If a system is perceived by those using it to be beneficial, then it will be used. If not, independent of its true value, it will probably be rejected.

Happily, there are today very many systems that have made it into clinical use (Table 25.1). Many of these are small, but nevertheless make positive contributions to care. Others, like prescribing decision support systems, are in widespread use and for many clinicians form a routine part of their everyday practice.

There are many different types of clinical task to which CDSS can be applied.

Alerts and reminders

In real-time situations, an expert system attached to a patient monitoring device like an ECG or pulse oximeter can warn of changes in a patient's condition. In less acute circumstances, it might scan laboratory test results, drug or test order, or the EMR and then send reminders or warnings, either via immediate on-screen feedback or through a messaging system such as e-mail. Reminder systems are used to notify clinicians of important tasks that need to be done before an event occurs. For example, an outpatient clinic reminder system may generate a list of immunizations that each patient on the daily schedule requires (Randolph *et al.*, 1999).

Diagnostic assistance

When a patient's case is complex, rare or the person making the diagnosis is simply inexperienced, an expert system can help in the formulation of likely diagnoses based on patient data presented to it, and the system's understanding of illness, stored in its knowledge base. Diagnostic assistance is often needed with complex data, such as the ECG, where most clinicians can make straightforward diagnoses, but may miss rare presentations of common illnesses like myocardial infarction, or may struggle with formulating diagnoses that typically require specialized expertise.

Therapy critiquing and planning

Critiquing systems can look for inconsistencies, errors and omissions in an existing treatment plan, but do not assist in the generation of the plan. Critiquing systems can be applied to physician order-entry. For example, on entering an order for a blood transfusion a clinician may receive a message stating that the patient's haemoglobin level is above the transfusion threshold, and the clinician must justify the order by stating an indication, such as active bleeding (Randolph *et al.*, 1999). Planning systems, on the other hand, have more knowledge about the structure of treatment protocols and can be used to formulate a treatment on the basis of data about a patient's specific condition from the EMR and accepted treatment guidelines.

Prescribing decision support systems

One of the commonest clinical tasks is the prescription of medications, and PDSS can assist by checking for drug–drug interactions, dosage errors, and if connected to an EMR, for other prescribing contraindications such as allergy. PDSS are usually well received because they support a pre-existing routine task, and as well as improving the quality of the clinical decision, usually offer other benefits like automated script generation and sometimes electronic transmission of the script to a pharmacy.

Information retrieval

Finding evidence in support of clinical decisions is still difficult on the Web, and intelligent information retrieval systems can assist in formulating appropriately specific and accurate clinical questions; they can act as information filters, by reducing the number of documents found in response to a query to a Web search engine; and they can assist in identifying the most appropriate sources of evidence appropriate to a clinical question. More complex software 'agents' can be sent to search for and retrieve information to answer clinical questions, for example on the Internet. The agent may contain knowledge about its user's preferences and needs, and may also have some clinical knowledge to assist it in assessing the importance and utility of what it finds.

Image recognition and interpretation

Many clinical images can now be automatically interpreted, from plane radiographs to more complex images such as angiograms, CT and MRI scans. This is of value in mass screenings, for example, when the system can flag potentially abnormal images for detailed human attention.

Diagnostic and educational systems

In the first decade of AIM, most research systems were developed to assist clinicians in the process of diagnosis, typically with the intention that it would be used during a clinical

Table 25.1 A wide variety of CDSS have been placed into routine clinical use. These systems are typical examples.

System	Description
Acute care systems	
(Dugas *et al.*, 2002)	Decision support in hepatic surgery
POEMS (Sawar *et al.*, 1992)	Postoperative care decision support
VIE-PNN (Miksch *et al.*, 1993)	Parenteral nutrition planning for neonatal ICU
NéoGanesh (Dojat *et al.*, 1996)	ICU ventilator management
SETH (Darmoni *et al.*, 1993)	Clinical toxicology advisor
Laboratory systems	
GERMWATCHER (Kahn *et al.*,1993)	Analysis of nosocomial infections
HEPAXPERT I, II (Adlassnig *et al.*, 1991)	Interprets tests for hepatitis A and B
Acid–base expert system (Pince *et al.*, 1990)	Interpretation of acid–base disorders
MICROBIOLOGY/PHARMACY (Morrell *et al.*, 1993)	Monitors renal active antibiotic dosing
PEIRS (Edwards *et al.*, 1993)	Chemical pathology expert system
PUFF (Snow *et al.*, 1988)	Interprets pulmonary function tests
Pro.M.D.- CSF Diagnostics (Trendelenburg, 1994)	Interpretation of CSF findings
Educational systems	
DXPLAIN (Barnett *et al.*, 1987)	Internal medicine expert system
ILLIAD (Warner *et al.*, 1988)	Internal medicine expert system
HELP (Kuperman *et al.*, 1991)	Knowledge-based hospital information system
Quality assurance and administration	
Colorado Medicaid Utilization Review System	Quality review of drug prescribing practices
Managed Second Surgical Opinion System	Aetna Life and Casualty assessor system
Medical imaging	
PERFEX (Ezquerra *et al.*, 1993)	Interprets cardiac SPECT data
(Lindahl *et al.* 1999).	Classification of scintigrams

encounter with a patient. Most of these early systems did not develop further than the research laboratory, partly because they did not gain sufficient support from clinicians to permit their routine introduction.

DXplain is an example of one of these clinical decision support systems, developed at the Massachusetts General Hospital (Barnett *et al.*, 1987). It is used to assist in the process of diagnosis, taking a set of clinical findings including signs, symptoms, laboratory data and then producing a ranked list of diagnoses. It provides justification for each differential diagnosis, and suggests further investigations. The system contains a database of crude probabilities for over 4500 clinical manifestations that are associated with over 2000 different diseases.

DXplain is in routine use at a number of hospitals and medical schools, mostly for clinical education purposes, but is also available for clinical consultation. It also has a role as an electronic medical textbook. It is able to provide a description of over 2000 different diseases, emphasizing the signs and symptoms that occur in each disease and providing recent references appropriate for each specific disease.

Decision support systems need not be 'stand alone' but can be deeply integrated into an electronic medical record system. Indeed, such integration reduces the barriers to using such a system, by crafting them more closely into clinical working processes, rather than expecting workers to create new processes to use them.

The HELP system is an example of this type of knowledge-based hospital information system, which began operation in 1980 (Kuperman and Gardner, 1990; Kuperman *et al.*, 1991). It not only supports the routine applications of a hospital information system (HIS) including management of admissions and discharges and order-entry, but also provides a decision support function. The decision support system has been actively incorporated into the functions of the routine HIS applications. Decision support provides clinicians with alerts and reminders, data interpretation and patient diagnosis facilities, patient management suggestions and clinical protocols. Activation of the decision support is provided within the applications but can also be triggered automatically as clinical data are entered into the patient's computerized record.

Expert laboratory information systems

One of the most successful areas in which expert systems are applied is in the clinical laboratory. Practitioners may be unaware that although a pathologist has checked the printed report they receive from a laboratory, the whole report may now have been generated by a computer system that has automatically interpreted the test results. Examples of such systems include the following:

- The PUFF system for automatic interpretation of pulmonary function tests has been sold in its commercial form to hundreds of sites worldwide (Snow *et al.*, 1988). PUFF went into production at Pacific Presbyterian Medical Centre in San Francisco in 1977, making it one of the very earliest medical expert systems in use. Many thousands of cases later, it is still in routine use.
- A more general example of this type of system is PEIRS (Pathology Expert Interpretative Reporting System) (Edwards *et al.*, 1993). During its period of operation, PEIRS interpreted about 80–100 laboratory reports a day with a diagnostic accuracy of about 95%. It accounted for about 20% of all the reports generated by the hospital's chemical pathology department. PEIRS reported on thyroid function tests, arterial blood gases,

urine and plasma catecholamines, hCG (human chorionic gonadotrophin) and AFP (alfafetoprotein), glucose tolerance tests, cortisol, gastrin, cholinesterase phenotypes and parathyroid hormone-related peptide (PTH-RP).

Laboratory expert systems usually do not intrude into clinical practice. Rather, they are embedded within the process of care, and with the exception of laboratory staff, clinicians working with patients do not need to interact with them. For the ordering clinician, the system prints a report with a diagnostic hypothesis for consideration, but does not remove responsibility for information gathering, examination, assessment and treatment. For the pathologist, the system cuts down the workload of generating reports, without removing the need to check and correct them.

25.3 Machine learning systems can create new clinical knowledge

Learning is seen to be the quintessential characteristic of an intelligent being. Consequently, one of the driving ambitions of AI has been to develop computers that can learn from experience. The resulting developments in the AI sub-field of **machine learning** have resulted in a set of techniques that have the potential to alter the way in which knowledge is created.

All scientists are familiar with the statistical approach to data analysis. Given a particular hypothesis, statistical tests are applied to data to see if any relationships can be found between different parameters. Machine learning systems can go much further. They look at raw data and then attempt to hypothesize relationships within the data, and newer learning systems are able to produce quite complex characterizations of those relationships. In other words, they attempt to discover humanly understandable concepts.

Learning techniques include neural networks, but encompass a large variety of other methods as well, each with their own particular characteristic benefits and difficulties. Some systems are able to learn decision trees from examples taken from data (Quinlan, 1986). These trees look much like the decision trees discussed in Chapter 8, and can be used to help in diagnosis.

Healthcare has formed a rich test-bed for machine learning experiments in the past, allowing scientists to develop complex and powerful learning systems. Although there has been much practical use of expert systems in routine clinical settings, at present machine learning systems still seem to be used in a more experimental way. There are, however, many situations in which they can make a significant contribution.

- Machine learning systems can be used to develop the knowledge bases used by expert systems. Given a set of clinical cases that act as examples, a machine learning system can produce a systematic description of those clinical features that uniquely characterize the clinical conditions. This knowledge can be expressed in the form of simple rules, or often as a decision tree. A classic example of this type of system is KARDIO, which was developed to interpret ECGs (Bratko *et al.*, 1989).
- This approach can be extended to explore poorly understood areas of healthcare, and people now talk of the process of 'data mining' and of 'knowledge discovery' systems. For example, it is possible, using patient data, to automatically construct pathophysiological models that describe the functional relationships between the various measurements.

For example, Hau and Coiera (1997) describe a learning system that takes real-time patient data obtained during cardiac bypass surgery, and then creates models of normal and abnormal cardiac physiology. These models might be used to look for changes in a patient's condition if used at the time they are created. Alternatively, if used in a research setting, these models can serve as initial hypotheses that can drive further experimentation.
- One particularly exciting development has been the use of learning systems to discover new drugs. The learning system is given examples of one or more drugs that weakly exhibit a particular activity, and from a description of the chemical structure of those compounds, the learning system suggests which of the chemical attributes are necessary for that pharmacological activity. On the basis of the new characterization of chemical structure produced by the learning system, drug designers can try to design a new compound that has those characteristics. Currently, drug designers synthesize a number of analogues of the drug they wish to improve upon, and experiment with these to determine which exhibits the desired activity. By boot-strapping the process using the machine learning approach, the development of new drugs can be speeded up, and the costs significantly reduced. At present statistical analyses of activity are used to assist with analogue development, and machine learning techniques have been shown to at least equal if not outperform them, as well as having the benefit of generating knowledge in a form that is more easily understood by chemists (King *et al.*, 1992). Since such learning experiments are still in their infancy, significant developments can be expected here in the next few years.
- Machine learning has a potential role to play in the development of clinical guidelines. It is often the case that there are several different treatments for a given condition, with slightly different outcomes. It may not be clear, however, what features of one particular treatment method are responsible for the better results. If databases are kept of the outcomes of competing treatments, then machine learning systems can be used to identify features that are responsible for different outcomes.

25.4 Clinical decision support systems have repeatedly demonstrated their worth when evaluated

Many potential benefits from CDSS have been widely reported in the literature (Johnson and Feldman, 1995; Evans, 1996). The claims made fall into three broad categories (Sintchenko *et al.*, 2003):

- **improved patient safety**, e.g. through reduced medication errors and adverse events and improved medication and test ordering.
- **improved quality of care**, e.g. by increasing clinicians' available time for direct patient care, increased application of clinical pathways and guidelines, facilitating the use of up-to-date clinical evidence, improved clinical documentation and patient satisfaction.
- **improved efficiency in healthcare delivery**, e.g. by reducing costs through faster order processing, reductions in test duplication, decreased adverse events, and changed patterns of drug prescribing favouring cheaper but equally effective generic brands.

The evaluation of CDSS are often poorly conceptualized and implemented (Cushman, 1997; Heathfield *et al.*, 1998). In a systematic review of 55 CDSS evaluations, Sintchenko *et al.* (2003) found that less than a quarter involved a randomized controlled trial (Table 25.2).

Table 25.2 Evaluation methodologies used in CDSS evaluation studies (*N* = 55) (Sintchenko *et al.*, 2003).

Evaluation methodology	%
Before/after sample	27.27
RCT	23.64
Case-control	21.82
Case study	16.36
Qualitative	5.45
Not done	3.64
Longitudinal study	1.82

Table 25.3 Limitations of evaluation components of CDSS studies (Sintchenko *et al.*, 2003).

A focus on post-system implementation evaluation of users' perceptions of systems
A reliance on retrospective designs which are limited in their ability to determine the extent to which improvements in outcome and process indicators may be causally linked to the CDSS.
Rare adoption of a comprehensive approach to evaluation where a multi-method design is used to capture the impact of CDSS on multiple dimensions.
Concentration on assessment of technical and functionality issues, which are estimated to explain less than 20% of IT failures. Such evaluations have also failed to determine why useful and useable systems are often unsuccessful.
Expectations that improvements will be immediate. In the short term there is likely to be a decrease in productivity. Implementing information systems takes time and measuring its impact is complex thus a long-term evaluation strategy is required but rarely implemented.
Almost none use naturalistic design in routine clinical settings with real patients and most studies involved doctors and excluded other clinical or managerial staff.

Table 25.4 Impact measures chosen in CDSS evaluation studies (*N* = 55) (Sintchenko *et al.*, 2003)

	Impact measured		**Impact not measured**
	Improvement demonstrated (no. of studies)	**No significant impact (no. of studies)**	**No. and % of studies**
Process variables			
Confidence in decision	12	3	40 (73%)
Patterns of care	15	4	36 (66%)
Adherence to protocol	10	4	41 (75%)
Efficiency/cost	10	2	43 (78%)
Adverse effects	12	3	40 (73%)
Clinical outcomes			
Morbidity	1	5	49 (89%)
Mortality	0	3	52 (95%)

Evaluation of CDSS is complex, and there are many challenges in appropriately structuring such studies (Randolph *et al.*, 1999). Consequently many studies fall into traps such as overemphasizing user satisfaction as a measure of system success. Some of the most frequent limitations of CDSS studies are listed in Table 25.3. While CDSS are often justified on the basis of clinical benefit, evaluation often focuses on technical issues or on clinical processes. Measurement of clinical outcomes is still sadly rare amongst evaluation studies, and most studies that do attempt to measure clinical impact do so through process variables (Table 25.4).

Nevertheless, the growing pool of evidence on the impact of CDSS in delivering improvements in the quality, safety and efficiency of health is promising, mainly in relation to alerts and reminders, and PDSSs. The following sections demonstrate not only the value of decision support systems in clinical practice, but also the complexity of the evaluation task, the ongoing gaps in our knowledge about their effectiveness, and the richness and variety of form of decision support.

Improvement in patient safety

Overall, there is now a body of research which provides good evidence of the effectiveness of CDSS, specifically computerized medication order-entry systems, in increasing the safety of patients by reducing errors and adverse events and increasing the proportion of appropriate and safe prescribing decisions.

Reduction in medication errors and adverse drug events

The interest in electronic prescribing systems has been generated by growing evidence of their effectiveness in reducing medication errors, which are one of the most significant causes of iatrogenic injury, death and costs in hospitals (Thomas *et al.*, 1999; Institute of Medicine, 2000). In the US it is estimated that over 770 000 people are injured or die each year in hospitals as a result of adverse drug events (ADEs) (Kaushal and Bates, 2001). The greatest proportion (56%) of preventable ADEs occur at the drug ordering stage, and only 4% at dispensing (Bates *et al.*, 1995). Errors occurring at the earlier stages are more likely to be intercepted (48%) compared to those occurring at the administration stage (0%).

Physician order-entry (POE) systems are used to automate the process of prescription, and assist in the generating and communicating of computerized scripts. POE typically include a prescribing decision support module to check the prescription produced.

Computer-assisted prescriptions have been shown in one study to contain more than three times fewer errors than handwritten prescriptions and to be five times less likely to require pharmacist clarification (Bizovi *et al.*, 2002). The first convincing evidence that such performance translates into a clinically significant reduction in medication errors and adverse drug events comes from two seminal studies undertaken at the Brigham and Women's Hospital in Boston, Massachusetts (Bates *et al.*, 1998, 1999a,b). The PDSS was developed specifically by the hospital and offered clinical decision support such as allergy alerts and suggested drug doses.

The first study (Bates *et al.*, 1998) demonstrated a 55% reduction in potential adverse drug events (i.e. errors which did not result in injury but had the potential to do so) after the system was implemented. The rate of adverse drug events fell from 10.7/1000 patient days to 4.9/1000 patient days. The second study (Bates *et al.*, 1999a) demonstrated an 86% reduction in potential adverse drug events 4 years after implementation. Unexpectedly, the number of life-threatening potential adverse drug events increased from 11% pre-implementation to 95% after 5 months. The majority of these related to orders regarding potassium chloride, because the PDSS system made it easy to order large doses of intravenous potassium without specifying that it be given in divided doses. Once changes were made to the order screen for this drug, the number of life-threatening intercepted potential adverse events fell to zero. If these systems were implemented nationwide in the US, it has been calculated that they would prevent approximately 522 000 adverse drug events each year and if only 0.1% of such errors were fatal, over 500 deaths would be avoided (Birkmeyer *et al.*, 2000).

In a broad systematic review of the impact of CDSS on the practice of doctors and patient outcomes, Hunt *et al.* (1998) identified 68 studies, 15 of which involved CDSS to assist dosing of potentially toxic drugs. Of these, 8 focused on dosing of intravenous drugs and 6 found improvements following the introduction of the CDSS. Four of the 8 studies examined the impact on patient outcomes, yet only 1 found a significant benefit (Mungall *et al.*, 1994). The authors stated that the consistent pattern of evidence suggests that intravenous medications can be titrated more effectively using a CDSS than without one, if the pharmacokinetics are well understood.

Clinicians are often unaware of the mistakes made when they prescribe. In one study, doctors stated that they were unaware of the potential clinical situation leading to 44% of the clinically significant ADEs that were identified by an alert system (Raschke *et al.*, 1998). However, alerting a clinician to an ADE may not result in changes to clinical behaviour, possibly because in many cases no change is necessary. A US study of prescriptions for 2.3 million people in an ambulatory setting identified 43 000 alerts for 23 697 people. In 15% of instances when the physician was contacted, the alerts resulted in an immediate change in drug management, and in a further 9% there was agreement to review management at the next patient visit (Monane *et al.*, 1998).

Enhancing prescribing behaviour

PDSS systems have the potential to change prescribing patterns resulting in more cost-effective drug selection. Teich *et al.* (2000) examined four specific drug decision support interventions:

- prompt to use a cheaper generic drug when a more expensive drug was initially ordered
- presentation of a list of suggested drug doses for each medication ordered
- a highlighted recommended frequency of dose for specific intravenous drugs
- prompt to suggest the order of a blood thinning drug for patients prescribed bed rest.

For all drug ordering interventions an immediate positive impact was found, with greater compliance with the recommended drug orders. Compliance with the generic drug choice changed from around 14% before system implementation to over 80% 2 months after implementation, and to 97% compliance at 1- and 2-year follow-up. The proportion of drug orders that exceeded the recommended maximum dose dropped from 2% in the pre-implementation period to less than 0.3% 2 years after implementation.

Change in the frequency of dose to reflect the recommended frequency occurred, with 6% compliance before implementation moving to 94% compliance at 1-, 2- and 3-year follow-up. Orders for anticoagulants for patients prescribed bed rest increased from 24% before implementation to 54% at 2-year follow-up.

Improved quality of care

Multiple measures have been used to attempt to assess the impact of CDSS on quality of care. Most have examined changes in work practices, with the expectation that improvements in patient outcomes will follow. Examples of process measures include increased compliance with practice guidelines or clinical pathways and increases in the proportion of time available for direct patient care.

Direct measurement of health outcomes is rare, and this is largely attributable to the difficulty of undertaking such studies. One of the few such studies undertaken was in a general medical clinic where clinicians were randomized to a reminder system over a 2-year period (McDonald *et al.*, 1984). Patients eligible for a flu or pneumococcal vaccine, and who attended one of the clinicians who received the reminder system, experienced significantly fewer winter hospitalizations and emergency department visits than patients in the control group.

Improved compliance with clinical pathways and guidelines

Order-entry and results-reporting systems with embedded decision support can increase compliance with recommended clinical pathways and guidelines and have been shown to reduce rates of inappropriate diagnostic tests (Harpole *et al.*, 1997).

In a randomized trial of antibiotic guidelines, a proportion of clinicians were shown vancomycin prescribing guidelines when they attempted to order this antibiotic using an electronic prescribing system (Shojania *et al.*, 1998). The use of vancomycin dropped by 30% with the guidelines, and when it was prescribed, the medication was given for a significantly shorter duration than in the control group. The paediatricians in the control group also increased their use of the recommended dose, but by a smaller proportion. This change was attributed to a diffusion of the evidence from the members of the control group who were working in the same clinic.

Alerts have been demonstrated to result in faster treatment by highlighting patients whose medication needed review. For example, Rind *et al.* (1994) assessed the impact of an alert system that notified doctors of patients experiencing rising creatinine levels and receiving nephrotoxic medications. They found that the use of the alerts was associated with a significantly faster average response to change patients' medications. Although the absolute risk of renal impairment in these patients was low, the alert system reduced this by 55%. However, other studies have found alerts to be of little effect in changing clinician behaviour. In one study, reminders printed on daily hospital ward round reports were found to have little impact on physicians' implementation of preventative care (Overhage *et al.*, 1996).

Time released for patient care

One potential benefit of the implementation of order-entry systems is that they may allow clinicians to spend more time in direct patient care. Shu *et al.* (2001) undertook a study of the impact of POE on time spent ordering, and available time for other tasks at Massachusetts General Hospital in the US. After implementation interns spent 3% more of their time with patients (from 13–16%), 6% spent more of their time alone (32% versus 38%) and less time with other physicians (47% versus 41%).

Tierney *et al.* (1993) conducted a time and motion study to determine time spent by clinicians in the order-entry process. Use of the POE actually resulted in increased time writing orders compared to paper orders (59 minutes versus 26 minutes), but 6 minutes less per day was spent on recording routine patient record data. Admitting medication orders were filled on average 63 minutes faster and daily drug orders 34 minutes faster. These results highlight that single indicators of improved efficiency may be of limited use, and that the extent to which such systems release clinicians from administrative tasks will vary depending upon multiple factors such as the type of system used, professional group, tasks to be undertaken and experience with the system.

Improved efficiency of healthcare delivery processes

Studies on the impact of CDSS on the efficiency of healthcare delivery have focused on reductions in costs due to fewer medication errors and adverse drug events; increased efficiency in the execution of patient care, particularly in relation to tests and drug orders; and increased use of generic drug brands.

Several estimates of the money saved as a result of computerized physician order-entry systems have been made. At Brigham and Women's Hospital, order-entry systems are estimated to save about $5–10 million per year, largely owing to the increased use of less expensive tests and drugs. In the US one adverse drug event is estimated to add an average of $2000–6000 to a patient admission, and thus they are estimated to cost over $2 billion in total each year in US hospitals alone (Raschke *et al.*, 1998).

In a randomized controlled trial, Tierney *et al.* (1993) demonstrated that patients treated by physicians who used a POE containing decision support, which included costs of specific drugs and diagnostic tests, had less expensive hospital stays. Extrapolation of the cost savings due to reduced costs per admission was of the order of $3 million for the teaching hospital. However, no adjustments were made to account for fixed or marginal costs.

The central economic evaluation question is, 'What is the cost of delivery of the IT system and how does this relate to the benefits or value that have resulted?' (Bannister *et al.*, 2001). One of the greatest challenges with economic evaluation is that in addition to cost data, benefits need to be measured and assigned a monetary value, yet most studies ignore benefits for which a dollar value may not be assignable. True costing of the CDSS investment side is also complex and there is great debate about what should be included or excluded from such calculations. One approach that has been advocated is the balanced score card (Kaplan and Norton, 1992) which measures performance indicators for four systems – financial, effectiveness and efficiency of internal processes, the customer perspective and organizational learning and innovation (Van Grembergen and Van Bruggen, 1997; Protti, 2002).

Conclusions

The available evidence on the impact of CDSS to deliver improvements in the quality, safety and efficiency of health is promising. Reductions in medication and adverse drug events alone appear impressive. To date the majority of studies have been undertaken in the United States and importantly, most have involved CDSS systems that have been internally developed and customized for individual healthcare organizations. The question as to whether the impressive results from systems that are custom built will be more widely reproducible is yet to be answered (Poikonen and Leventhal, 1999).

Discussion points

1 Which clinical tasks are worth automating?

2 Who is responsible if a CDSS makes a recommendation to a clinician that results in patient harm?

3 Should clinicians be able to use a CDSS without any specific training, or should we consider a CDSS as a specialized piece of clinical equipment that requires the user to first pass a certification course?

Chapter summary

1 Artificial intelligence (AI) systems are intended to support healthcare workers with tasks that rely on the manipulation of data and knowledge.

2 Expert systems are the commonest type of CDSS in routine clinical use. They contain medical knowledge about a very specifically defined task. Their uses include:
- alerts and reminders
- diagnostic assistance
- therapy critiquing and planning
- prescribing decision support
- information retrieval
- image recognition and interpretation.

3 Reasons for the failure of many expert systems to be used clinically include dependence on an electronic medical record system to supply their data, poor human interface design, failure to fit naturally into the routine process of care, and reluctance or computer illiteracy of some healthcare workers.

4 Many expert systems are now in routine use in acute care settings, clinical laboratories and educational institutions, and incorporated into electronic medical record systems.

5 Some CDSS systems have the capacity to learn, leading to the discovery of new phenomena and the creation of medical knowledge. These machine learning systems can be used to:
- develop the knowledge bases used by expert systems
- assist in the design of new drugs
- advance research in the development of pathophysiological models from experimental data.

6 Benefits from CDSS include improved patient safety, improved quality of care and improved efficiency in healthcare delivery.

CHAPTER 26

Intelligent systems

Workers in the field of artificial intelligence (AI) have over the years explored many different avenues in the quest to develop computational intelligence. Despite the many debates over whether one should build or 'evolve' intelligent behaviour, or whether we should replicate or merely simulate human cognitive processes, there has been much common ground among scientists. All probably agree for example, that for the behaviour we call 'intelligence' to be recreated in human-built artefacts, we need to develop methods that somehow capture knowledge about the world, and then manipulate that knowledge.

There is much ongoing discussion on just how explicit or detailed such knowledge needs to be. At one extreme we find a camp that feels that intelligence often emerges from the interaction of simple reasoning agents and their environment. These workers in the field of 'artificial life' are inspired by biology, citing for example the way a colony of ants can exhibit intelligent behaviour despite each ant being a relatively simple creature. As a consequence, they see little need to fill AI systems with detailed knowledge about the world (Steels and Brooks, 1995).

At the other extreme sit those researchers who believe an AI system needs to have its intelligence pre-programmed (e.g. Genesereth and Nilsson, 1988). These researchers feel that an AI should contain large amounts of knowledge about the world. This knowledge might need to cover everything from what most of us would call common sense through to complex technical knowledge that might come from a textbook.

From the point of CDSS, we are interested in these debates from a practical level, in so far as they can provide techniques that can be applied to healthcare. As we saw in the last chapter, AI offers methods for constructing computer systems that can carry out tasks that require some understanding of the world for their execution. In other words, intelligent systems have some capacity to capture, and then reason with, health knowledge.

Given the richness and technical complexity of AI, it would be impossible to cover the breadth of issues involved in constructing intelligent systems here. This chapter simply attempts to sketch the broad issues involved in developing the sort of AI system that is likely to be encountered in clinical practice over the next decade. More comprehensive and specialized texts deal with this subject in far greater depth (e.g. Russell and Norvig, 2002).

26.1 Before reasoning about the world, knowledge must be captured and represented

We saw in the previous chapter that AI systems can have two quite distinct capabilities. Some are able to take clinical knowledge and use it to reason from data. Other learning systems are able to take data, and help discover the relationships that might exist between different data elements to create new knowledge.

At a very abstract level, we can consider these AI systems either helping to generate models, or using these models to come up with some inference (Figure 26.1). It follows then that the designer of an AI program has several distinct problems to consider.

On what task will the AI system be used?

A recurring theme throughout this book has been that the characteristics of a task determines the characteristics of the technology applied to it. This is just as true with complex AI systems. In particular, different **reasoning tasks** such as diagnosis, planning or learning need

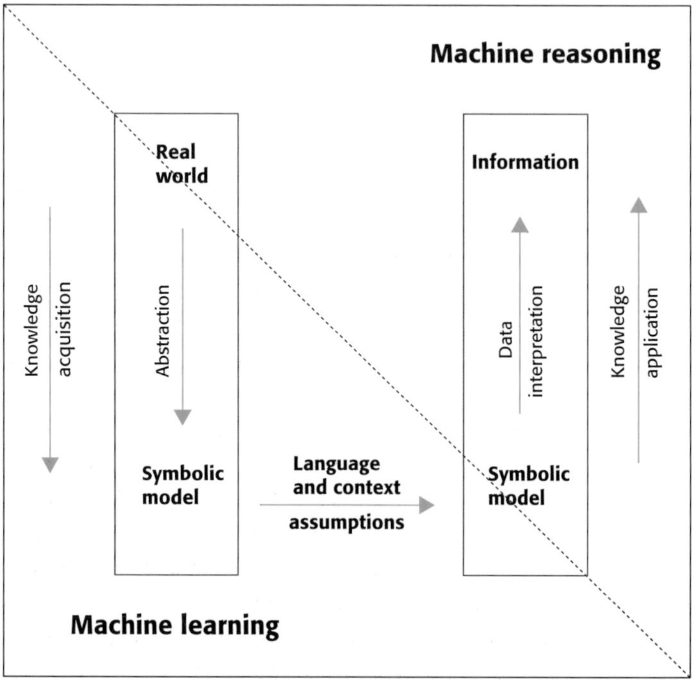

Machine reasoning
Real world
Information
Knowledge acquisition
Abstraction
Data interpretation
Knowledge application
Symbolic model
Language and context assumptions
Symbolic model
Machine learning

Figure 26.1
Machine learning programs can help acquire knowledge. AI programs like expert systems can apply that knowledge to reason about the world.

very different types of AI system. Consequently, a system designed to assist in the planning of chemotherapy is technically very different from one intended to detect malignant patterns in a mammogram.

In what circumstances will the task be executed?

The resources, skills and needs of individual workers, patients and institutions vary considerably. Consequently they will have very different requirements of a system, even if it apparently executes the same task. The amount of time available, the degree of accuracy expected of a decision, and the skill and training of the individual who might be using the system can all affect the way one designs a system. For example, a program designed to suggest diagnoses would need to perform very differently in different situations. If it is used to help with triage in a battlefield hospital, then it may need to focus on life-threatening conditions that can be actively managed. If it is used by a medical student in training, then it might suggest a long list of differential diagnoses and supply background reading and pathophysiological explanations.

What knowledge will the system have?

Human knowledge varies considerably in its level of detail and form. Some aspects of the world are very well defined, and could be expressed, for example, as a set of detailed mathematical equations. The designs of ventilator machines or the descriptions of some aspects of cardiovascular physiology fall into this group. When detailed models exist, they permit some form of explanation about why something occurs. In other areas, our knowledge is much slimmer. It might only be based on experience, and be captured as a set of aphorisms or rules of thumb. In this case, we are only able to say 'this is how it has been in my experience'. Thus, the quality of knowledge available has significant impact on how it can be use by an AI system. We would not expect an expert system, for example, to be able to generate explanations for a set of differential diagnoses if its knowledge only consisted of very simple rules of thumb.

How will that knowledge be presented to the computer?

Once it is clear just how much knowledge is available for a particular task, then a choice can be made about the best **knowledge representation** to use within the program. For example, we saw in Chapter 12 that computerized clinical guidelines could be represented in many different ways, and that the choice of representation depended on the way the guideline knowledge would be used. Similarly, for an expert system, it might be most appropriate to use a simple set of rules rather than a complex set of simultaneous differential equations to make a diagnosis, even though both are available. This might be because the equations take too long to solve or require too much data to be provided by the human user, or simply because the accuracy of the answer need only be approximate given the circumstances.

Once a task has been identified, the designer of the system needs to consider which reasoning method and which knowledge representation will be used. For example, the different reasoning methods one could use in arriving at a diagnosis might be to use statistics, rules of thumb, neural networks, comparison to past cases and so forth. The knowledge representation chosen is closely related to the reasoning method. For example, one would clearly need to use a model of disease based on probabilities to support a statistical reasoning method.

It is not possible here to cover the many different approaches to reasoning and representation devised by AI researchers. However, several of the most enduring and successful methodologies, including rule-based expert systems and neural networks, will be described. Since they represent quite different approaches to the problems of reasoning and representation, contrasting them will help to demonstrate the complex issues behind attempts to devise intelligent systems.

26.2 Rule-based expert systems

An expert system is a program that captures elements of human expertise and performs reasoning tasks that normally rely on specialist knowledge. Examples include programs that can diagnose the cause of abdominal or chest pain, based on clinical observations fed to the program. Expert systems perform best in straightforward tasks, which have a pre-defined and relatively narrow scope, and perform poorly on ill-defined tasks that rely on general or commonsense knowledge.

In an expert system, the knowledge is usually represented as a set of rules. The reasoning method is usually either logical or probabilistic. An expert system consists of three basic components (Figure 26.2):

- a knowledge base, which contains the rules necessary for the completion of its task
- a **working memory** in which data and conclusions can be stored
- an **inference engine** which matches rules to data to derive its conclusions.

For a task like interpreting an ECG, an example of a rule that could be used to detect asystole might be:

RuleASY1:
If heart rate = 0
then conclude asystole

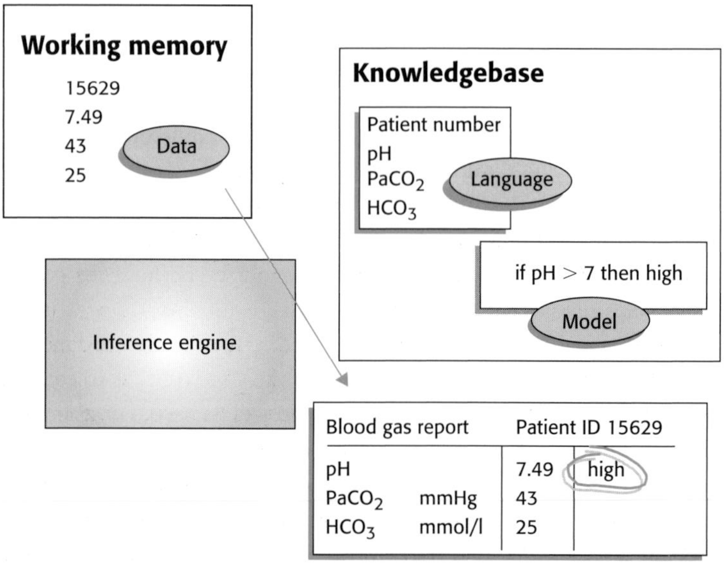
Working memory
15629
7.49
43
25
Data
Knowledgebase
Patient number
pH
$PaCO_2$
HCO_3
Language
if pH > 7 then high
Model
Inference engine
Blood gas report
Patient ID 15629
pH
7.49
high
$PaCO_2$
mmHg
43
HCO_3
mmol/l
25

Figure 26.2
An expert system has three components responsible for modelling knowledge, storing data and carrying out reasoning procedures.

If the expert system was attached to a patient monitor then a second rule whose role was to filter out false asystole alarms in the presence of a normal arterial waveform might be:

Rule ASY2:
If asystole
and (ABP is pulsatile **and** in the normal range)
then retract asystole

In the presence of a zero heart rate, the expert system would first match rule ASY1 and conclude that asystole was present. However, if it next succeeded in matching all the conditions in rule ASY2, then it would fire this second rule, which would effectively filter out the previous asystole alarm. If rule ASY2 could not be fired because the arterial pressure was abnormal, then the initial conclusion that asystole was present would remain.

Rules tend to become much more complicated than the simple examples presented here, and the process of manual knowledge acquisition from human experts can become a drawn-out affair. To counter this problem, much machine learning research has gone into developing techniques to automate the acquisition of knowledge in the form of rules or decision trees from databases of cases (e.g. Quinlan, 1986).

For the rules in the previous example, reasoning was based on the application of simple logical rules of inference like deduction or abduction (see Chapter 8). If the knowledge available to manage a problem was less certain, then the rules could use probabilities. For example:

RuleASY1:
If heart rate = 0
then conclude asystole with probability (0.8)

RuleASY2:
If heart rate = 0
then conclude 'ECG leads fallen off' with probability (0.2)

In this case, the inference engine would be designed to come up with the most probable conclusion, based on an assessment of the data and the known probabilities. One of the commonest probabilistic inference rules used in expert systems is the classic Bayes' theorem, which was also introduced in Chapter 8.

26.3 Belief networks

Although probabilities can be expressed in rules, it is more common for them to be captured in a **belief network**, which is a graphical way of representing the probability relationships between different events, similar to a finite state machine. Belief networks are also often called Bayesian networks, influence diagrams or causal probabilistic networks.

Finite state machines were introduced in Chapter 12 as a way of connecting related clinical events. A finite state machine represents processes as a series of different states, and connects them together with links that specify a transition condition that indicates how one traverses from one state to another (Figure 12.2). In a probabilistic network, the states represent clinical events such as the presence of a symptom, and diseases, and the links represent conditional probabilities between the events (Figure 26.3). Each node is assigned a probability that represents its likelihood of occurrence in the population in question. Next, connections between nodes record the conditional probability that if a parent node is true, then the child node will be true.

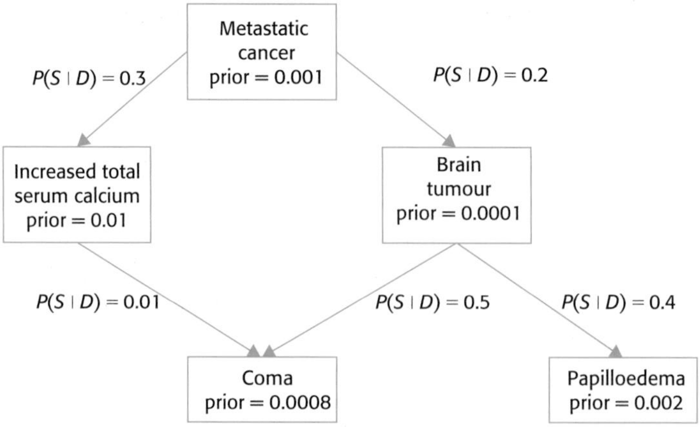
Metastatic
cancer
prior = 0.001
P(S | D) = 0.3
P(S | D) = 0.2
Increased total
serum calcium
prior = 0.01
Brain
tumour
prior = 0.0001
P(S | D) = 0.01
P(S | D) = 0.5
P(S | D) = 0.4
Coma
prior = 0.0008
Papilloedema
prior = 0.002

Figure 26.3
A simple Bayesian belief network for metastatic cancer. The prior probability of each event is recorded at the node representing it, and the conditional probability of one event giving rise to another is encoded in the links between the nodes (after Cooper, 1988).

Bayes' rule is typically the inference procedure used on belief networks. So, for example, if we are told certain clinical findings are true, then based upon the conditional probabilities recorded in the belief network, Bayes' rule is used to calculate the likelihood of different diseases. Often networks are many layers deep, and the inference procedure essentially percolates through the network calculating probabilities for events. Intermediate nodes between clinical findings and diseases might include intermediate pathophysiological states such as right-sided heart failure.

There are several potential restrictions with belief networks that may limit their usefulness in some clinical situations.:

- Bayes' rule in its traditional form only works for independent events, as we saw in Chapter 8. Belief networks may, however, need to record dependent states, and alternative formulations to Bayes' rule, designed for such dependencies, need to be used in such situations.
- Probability values may not always be available to build the network.

Interestingly, belief networks actually record two different types of knowledge. The first clearly are probabilities. The second is the causal structure of events. Although the formal power of Bayesian inference is attractive, the actual construction of the causal structures is not a formal science. The choice of states to include in the network, and the way they are or are not connected, strongly influences the behaviour of the network. Alternative probabilistic methods to represent clinical processes and determine likely outcomes include Markov models and Monte Carlo simulation methods.

26.4 Neural networks

Neural networks are computer programs whose internal function is based upon a simple model of the neurone (Kohonen, 1988). Networks are composed of layers of neurones (or nodes) with interconnections between the nodes in each layer (Figure 26.4).

For example, a network might be built to connect a set of observations with a set of diagnoses. Each input node would be assigned to a different datum. Each output node would similarly have a corresponding diagnosis assigned to it. The network is then told which

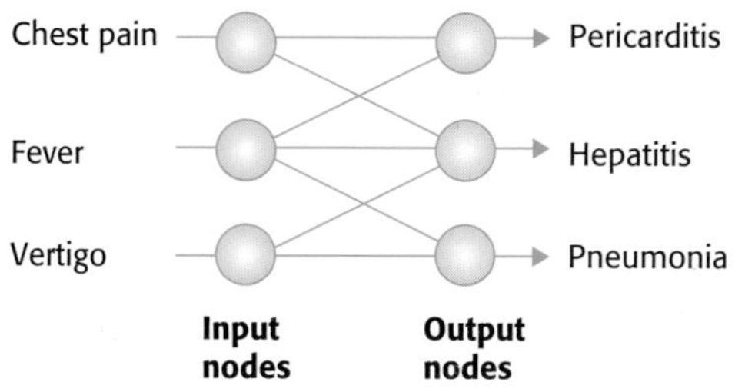
Chest pain
Fever
Vertigo
Pericarditis
Hepatitis
Pneumonia
Input nodes
Output nodes

Figure 26.4 A two-layer neural network. Input nodes on the left receive a pattern to be classified, and output nodes on the right are triggered to produce a classification. The sum of the signals received at an output node determine whether or not it will fire.

observations have been detected, and the output node that has been most 'stimulated' by the input data is then preferentially fired, thus producing a diagnosis.

The knowledge associating combinations of observations and diagnoses is stored within the connections of the network. The strength of the connections between different nodes is modelled as a weight on that connection. The stronger the connection between nodes, the greater the assigned weight. Thus, in contrast to an expert system, knowledge in a network is captured in a way that is not easily understood when inspected.

The reasoning procedure is similarly inspired by the way neurones fire once a certain level of activation has been reached. A node in the network fires when the sum of its inputs exceeds a predetermined threshold. These inputs are determined by the number of input connections that have been fired, and the weights upon those connections. Thus, when a net is presented with a pattern on its input nodes, it will output a recognition pattern determined by the weights on the connections between layers.

These weights in a network are obtained by a period of training. A raw network is presented with examples of the data patterns it is intended to recognize, and the weights in the net are slowly adjusted until it achieves the desired output. A neural network thus actually encodes within its weights a discriminating function that is optimized to distinguish the different classes present within its training set.

In theory, any such discriminant function can be approximated by a network (Stinchombe and White, 1989). Despite initial claims of uniqueness for the computational properties of neural nets, it is becoming clear that they have clear and important relationships with a number of more traditional discrimination methods including Markov models (Bourland and Wellekens, 1990), Bayesian networks and decision trees.

The properties of neural networks make them useful both for pattern recognition tasks and real-time signal interpretation. Neural networks have been used to recognize ECG patterns (Pietka, 1989), identify artefacts in arterial blood pressure signals (Sebald, 1989), in image recognition (e.g. ultrasound; Nikoonahad and Liu, 1990) and in the development of clinical diagnostic systems (Hart and Wyatt, 1989).

Although the interpretative facility of nets has found numerous applications, they are limited by their inability to explain their conclusions. The reasoning by which a net selects a class is hidden within the distributed weights, and is unintelligible as an explanation. Nets are thus limited to interpreting patterns where no explanation or justification for selecting a conclusion is necessary. Since the need to justify a clinical diagnosis is recognized as an important part of the process of decision support, this limits the application of nets in such tasks.

26.5 Model-based systems

One of the important contributions of AI has been a growing understanding of the ways in which knowledge can be represented and manipulated. Rule-based representations of knowledge, as we have seen, are only appropriate for narrowly defined problems like diagnosing chest pain. Humans deal with a broader class of problems by invoking other types of knowledge than the rules of thumb that are typically stored in an expert system.

Especially with difficult or rare problems, humans may attempt to reason from first principles, using models of pathophysiology or biochemistry to explain a set of clinical manifestations. For example, when several diseases are present at one time, it may only be possible to unravel the constellation of symptoms and signs by recourse to disease models. This contrasts with the simple structure of rules which record commonly seen patterns of disease, and which can only deal with interactions by explicitly enumerating them. The vast number of possible interactions makes such an enumeration of rules impractical (Coiera, 1990).

Model-based systems (sometimes called second-generation expert systems) are designed to utilize disease models in the hope that they will be able to cover a broader set of clinical problems than possible with rules (Uckun, 1992). These models might be constructed from a variety of different representations including mathematical models of physiological relationships, compartmental system models, or indeed statistical models.

As is often the case in healthcare, formal models of disease phenomena are often not available or are poorly formalized. In such cases, there is evidence that clinicians carry around looser models, expressible in non-numeric or qualitative terms (Kuipers and Kassirer, 1984). Such qualitative representations of knowledge have now been formalized, and can be used to capture useful portions of healthcare knowledge (Coiera, 1992a). These representations have actually proved to be useful in diagnosis (e.g. Ironi *et al.*, 1990), and patient monitoring (e.g. Coiera, 1990; Widman, 1992; Uckun *et al.*, 1993).

Model-based systems are perceived as being better at explanation than 'shallower' rule-based systems, and better at dealing with novel or complex problems. They are also, however, more computationally expensive to run. In other words, it takes longer to solve a problem using these systems (although for most common problems, the difference is probably not going to be appreciable). This is because it takes longer to reason a problem out from first principles than it does to simply recognize it from previous experience. Thus there is a move among researchers to build systems which combine the two sorts of system, having on the one hand the facility to invoke deep pathophysiological models should they be needed, but also being able to rely on efficient rules whenever they are applicable.

26.6 The choice of reasoning and representation methods should be based on the needs of the task

It is still not uncommon to find individuals advocating that one method of reasoning is generally superior to another. In the early days of AIM, there was an extended discussion over the comparative value of probabilistic reasoning and heuristic (or rule of thumb) expert systems. This was superseded by those who argued for the inherent superiority of brain-inspired neural networks. In their turn, proponents for fuzzy systems, evolutionary computing and genetic algorithms have all made similar claims.

In truth, there is now sufficient understanding of the strengths and weakness of each of these competing reasoning and representation schemes to permit some rational choices to be made. As a system designer, one can thus imagine a toolbox of different techniques being available. Depending on the particular problem to be solved, the most appropriate method can be selected.

26.7 Intelligent decision support systems have their limits

While expert systems and neural networks can perform at clinically acceptable levels, as with humans there are inherent difficulties in the reasoning process. These limitations need to be made explicit, and should be borne in mind by clinicians who use automated interpretation systems.

Data

Interpretative systems do not have eyes or ears, but are limited to accessing data provided to them electronically. This constitutes a potentially enormous amount of data to work with, but it means that critical pieces of contextual information may be unavailable. Thus computer interpretations need to be judged partly on the data available to the system when making its decision. This highlights the importance of designing an explanatory facility into expert systems, so that clinicians can understand the reasoning behind a particular recommendation by tracing the pieces of data that were used in its formulation.

The task of validating data may have to be one of the first tasks that an interpretative system undertakes. Many clues are available to suggest whether a datum represents a real measurement or is an error, but this is not always decidable solely on the basis of the electronic evidence. There may be no way for a machine to decide that a transducer is incorrectly positioned, or that blood specimens have been mixed up. Clinicians will always need to be wary of the quality of the data upon which interpretations have been made.

Knowledge

Knowledge is often incomplete, and this is an everyday reality in the practice of healthcare. Clinicians deal with physiological systems they only incompletely understand, and have evolved techniques for dealing with this uncertainty. Clinicians are able to acknowledge that they are performing at the edge of their expertise, and adjust their methods of handling a problem accordingly, but it is much harder to incorporate such a facility in a computer system.

Computers at present treat all knowledge equally. Although they are able to weigh up probabilities that a set of findings represent a particular condition, they do not take into account the likelihood that some pieces of knowledge are less reliable than others.

Further, most present-day systems are forced to utilize a static knowledge base. There are many techniques that can be used to update knowledge bases, but it is not necessarily the case that a system incorporates the latest knowledge on a subject.

The technical problems associated with the process of knowledge acquisition mean that there are always potential mistakes in the system. Just as a normal computer program can contain 'bugs', so a knowledge base can contain errors, since it is simply another form of program.

Wherever possible, the explanation offered by a system should be examined, to ensure that the logical flow of argument reflects current clinical understanding.

As we shall see at the end of the next chapter, the use of intelligent systems is also limited, not because of the flaws in the technical system, but because of the cognitive limitations of their human users.

Discussion points

1 Can machines think?

2 Which representational formalism is best suited to clinical decision support problems?

3 If a CDSS needs to provide explanations in support of its recommendations, which technology approach would you take and why?

4 What negative consequence do you imagine might arise from using a CDSS?

Chapter summary

1 Once a task has been identified, the designer of an AI system needs to consider which reasoning method and which knowledge representation will be used. For example, the different reasoning methods one could use in arriving at a diagnosis might be to use statistics, rules of thumb, neural networks and comparison with past cases. The knowledge representation chosen is closely related to the reasoning method.

2 An expert system is a program that captures elements of human expertise and performs reasoning tasks that normally rely on specialist knowledge. Expert systems perform best in straightforward tasks, which have a pre-defined and relatively narrow scope, and perform poorly on ill-defined tasks that rely on general or common sense knowledge.

3 An expert system consists of three basic components.
- a **knowledge base**, which contains the rules necessary for the completion of its task
- a **working memory** in which data and conclusions can be stored
- an **inference engine**, which matches rules to data to derive its conclusions.

4 Although probabilities can be expressed in rules, it is more common for them to be captured in a **belief network,** which is a graphical way of representing the probability relationships between different events, typically using Bayes' rule to draw inferences.

5 **Neural networks** are computer programs whose internal function is based on a simple model of the neurone. Networks are composed of layers of neurones (or nodes) with interconnections between the nodes in each layer.

6 **Model-based systems** (sometimes called second-generation expert systems) are designed to utilize disease models in the hope that they will be able to cover a broader set of clinical problems than possible with rules. These models might be constructed from a variety of different representations including mathematical models of physiological relationships, compartmental system models, or indeed statistical models.

7 AI systems are limited by the data they have access to, and the quality of the knowledge captured within their knowledge base.

CHAPTER 27

Intelligent monitoring and control

Patient monitoring systems are used to measure clinical parameters like the ECG or oxygen saturation. They are clinically commonplace devices and are found in many acute care settings. Through the introduction of advanced computer techniques, it is now possible to develop monitoring systems that automatically interpret patient signals. Rather than simply displaying measurements for clinicians to interpret, these intelligent monitoring devices can assist clinicians in the task of interpretation itself.

Similar techniques can be used to design intelligent therapeutic devices like patient ventilators or drug delivery systems. These devices are able to monitor patient status to control the delivery of therapy to a patient automatically. Such advances are made possible through developments in the fields of signal processing, pattern recognition and artificial intelligence.

This chapter will look at the role intelligent monitoring and control systems have to play in healthcare. The various levels of possible interpretation will be described, along with an introduction to the techniques that are used to create these interpretations.

27.1 Automated interpretation and control systems can assist in situations with high cognitive loads or varying expertise

The motivations for automating the interpretation of patient measurements and the control of patient systems are numerous. The most pressing arise from the difficulties clinicians face when they continuously monitor patient data, and are not unique to healthcare. They are also an issue, for example, in the design of systems used by airline pilots and nuclear power plant operators. These human factors include the problems of cognitive overload, varying expertise, and human error (Wickens and Hollands, 2000).

Cognitive overload

It should come as no surprise that clinicians may have difficulty in interpreting information presented to them on current patient monitoring systems (Weigner and Englund, 1990). There are finite limits to the cognitive resources, such as memory, that humans can devote to reasoning (Box 8.2). These resources can be overloaded by some activities at the cost of others. This cognitive overloading can result in the messages contained in critical patient information being missed or misinterpreted. There are several major mechanisms that contribute to this phenomenon in the clinical environment.

Firstly, the amount of information available on some monitoring systems may be greater than can be assimilated by an individual at one time. This **data overload** can result in the observer failing to notice significant events. Worse still, current monitors may flood clinicians with false alarms, providing further unnecessary distraction (Koski *et al.*, 1990).

This can be compounded by the clinical environment itself, which provides many distractions that compete with monitored data for the clinician's attention. These include tasks other than monitoring which might need to be carried out at the same time, especially in situations such as the emergency department, intensive care or the delivery of anaesthesia. All of these sources of distraction reduce the cognitive effort that can be devoted to signal interpretation, and increase the likelihood of an error of interpretation or a failure to notice data events.

Varying expertise

The level of expertise that individuals bring to a task like the interpretation of signals varies enormously, and it is not always possible for such deficits to be remedied by consultation with more skilled colleagues. Consequently, rare events may be missed or misinterpreted. Complexity is also introduced when more than one disease process is active in a patient. They may interact to alter the normal presentation of signals one expects. In the absence of previous experience, the only way such diagnoses can be made is to work back from first principles, often requiring a deep knowledge of the pathophysiological mechanisms involved.

Human error

Cognitive overload and inexperience are two of the major mechanisms that may lead to errors in diagnosis and selection of treatment. For example, most complications associated with anaesthesia, in which clinicians are highly dependent on the use of monitoring equipment to assess patient status, result from inadequate training or insufficient experience of the anaesthetist (Cooper *et al.*, 1984; Sykes, 1987).

There is, however, a wider literature on the causes and effects of human error (Reason, 1990). In particular, human reasoning is susceptible to certain biases that may result in incorrect conclusions being drawn, despite the evidence at hand (Box 8.3). The particular causes of error will vary significantly with the environment within which individuals are operating, as well as with the type of decision-making problems that face them.

There are several ways in which computer-based systems can assist in addressing such difficulties. Firstly, as we saw in Chapter 25, systems can be developed that issue alerts or alarms when clinically significant events are detected. There is now good evidence that such systems can have a positive effect on clinical outcomes, either by reducing the time between the event and its detection, or by preventing events being completely missed (Shea *et al.*, 1996).

Computer systems do not have value only as automated safety nets for busy clinicians. It is also possible to design computer systems capable of diagnosing clinical conditions, to assist with rare or complex cases (Patil, 1988). Much of the research in medical artificial intelligence over the last two decades has been devoted to this area, and impressive diagnostic performances have been demonstrated in many specialized medical domains (Clancey and Shortliffe, 1984).

At the other end of the scale, the process of data validation can be automated. At present it is up to the clinician to ascertain whether a measurement accurately reflects a patient's status, or is in error. In many situations, signal error is clear from the clinical context, but it can also manifest itself as subtle changes in the shape of a waveform. Without quite specialized expertise, clinicians may misinterpret measured data as being clinically significant, when in fact it reflects an error in the measurement system. For example, changes in the bedside height of a pressure transducer can significantly alter the measurements it produces.

27.2 Intelligent systems require access to additional data in the EMR before they can perform many complex functions

There are several basic requirements that must be met before a system for automatic interpretation or control can provide clinical benefit. Firstly, and most importantly, it is essential that any system developed actually fulfil a relevant clinical role. The long lag in the introduction of computerized decision support into healthcare is more probably due to failure on this point than because of technological limitations (Shortliffe, 1987). Systems must be developed to fit in with the work practices of clinicians, and to support decision-making processes that are clinically relevant. There is little advantage in developing a complex system that mimics interpretative skills already possessed by all clinicians. Rather, it should attempt to provide support for cognitive functions that clinicians perform poorly. Thus the development of intelligent systems is as dependent on developing an understanding of the cognitive patterns of the clinicians who will work with them as it is on advances in technology.

To ensure that monitored parameters are interpreted in clinical context, an intelligent system may also need access to clinical data other than the monitored signals themselves. This is because it may not be possible to come up with sufficiently useful interpretations without access to additional information about a patient. These data may include the medical record, current medications, and values from other devices such as the settings from an anaesthetic machine.

Pragmatic considerations suggest that, because of the slow and uneven way in which the electronic medical record (EMR) is coming into routine use, there needs to be a staged introduction of software capable of intelligent interpretation.

Current first-generation systems are relatively simple; they require minimal interaction with the clinician, and minimal or no interaction with the patient record system. Most of these are likely to be found embedded within normal clinical devices. For example, programs exist within current patient-monitoring devices that are capable of filtering out artefacts and suppressing false alarms.

The next level of system interpretation requires explicit interaction with clinicians, offering some form of active decision support. Such systems will come into their own as integrated EMRs become widespread and health professionals become more accustomed to computer assistance. They will be able to assist in the selection of tests and the formulation of diagnoses, as well as the selection of optimal therapies. Interaction will be necessary because, although such systems are capable of drawing conclusions from patient data, they will not have access to the complete clinical picture. The clinician must supply vital clinical context and therapeutic goals unavailable to the system.

The third stage of system introduction could consist of autonomous intelligent systems, capable of independent activity. These are at present almost entirely experimental, but could eventually form the heart of closed-loop systems. For example, drug delivery systems could automatically measure a drug's level and administer doses based on that measurement (Blom, 1991; Packer, 1990). The development of such closed-loop systems is at present hampered as much by legal and ethical issues as by technological considerations.

27.3 There are different levels of signal interpretation, each of which requires increasing amounts of clinical knowledge

Intelligent monitoring systems work by taking a raw data stream that comes from a measurement device attached in some way to a patient, like an ECG, and then apply a series of algorithms to transform that data stream into something that is clinically meaningful. This process of signal interpretation can occur at a number of levels, starting from a low-level assessment of the validity of a signal, through to a complex assessment of its clinical significance. The different levels of interpretation that a signal may pass through are illustrated in Figure 27.1.

A signal is first examined for evidence of artefact. Where possible, the signal is 'cleaned up' by removing the artefactual or noise components of the signal. Once it has been processed in this way, the modified signal is then presented to the next layer in the interpretative hierarchy.

Often a single measurement channel will contain sufficient information for a diagnosis to be made. In some circumstances, however, several alternative explanations might be possible, and a single channel does not contain enough information to disambiguate them. In such circumstances, an interpretative system can look for cross-signal correlations. In Figure 27.1, a flat portion of ECG trace is not diagnosed as an 'asystole' because examination of the corresponding arterial waveform reveals pulsatile behaviour consistent with normal cardiac function, and therefore there is more likely a problem with the ECG signal than with the patient.

A higher level of interpretation is also possible, taking into account relevant contextual patient information. This level is concerned with making decisions based on signal interpretations, and may include recommendations for further investigations or therapeutic actions. The tasks of artefact detection, single- and cross-channel interpretation and decision support will be examined in more detail below.

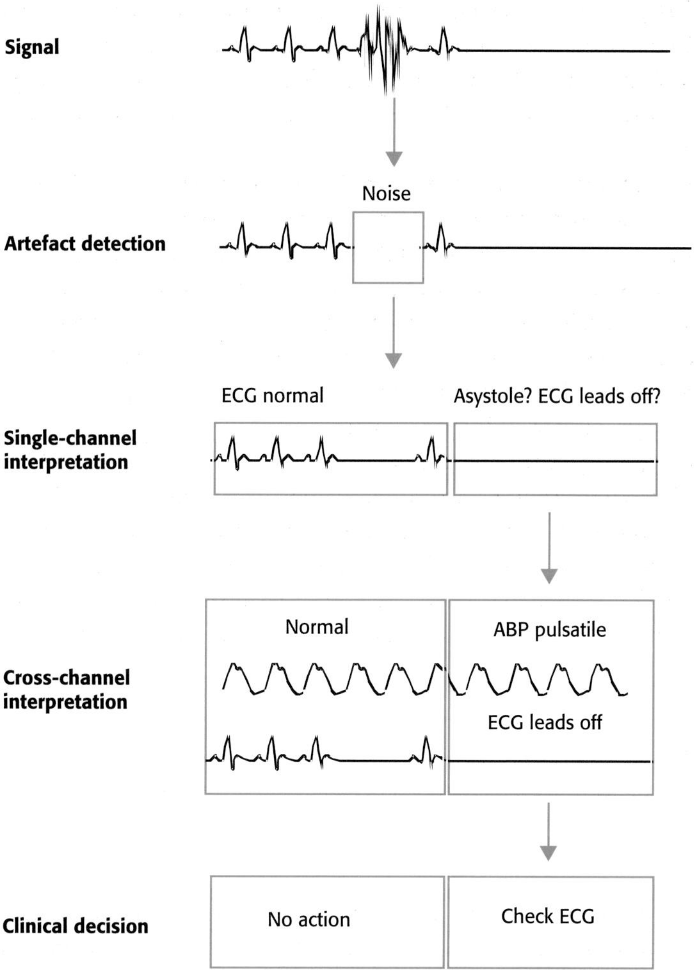
Signal
Noise
Artefact detection
ECG normal
Asystole? ECG leads off?
Single-channel interpretation
Normal
ABP pulsatile
ECG leads off
Cross-channel interpretation
Clinical decision
No action
Check ECG

Figure 27.1
Multiple levels of interpretation take a raw physiological signal and process it, with each level producing increasingly complex interpretations.

Artefact detection

The first task in signal interpretation is to decide whether the values that are measured are physiologically valid. In other words, is the signal genuine, is it distorted because of excessive noise resulting in a low signal to noise ratio, or is it distorted by a signal artefact from another source? A signal artefact is defined as any component of the measured signal that is unwanted. It may be caused by distortions introduced through the measurement apparatus. Indeed, an artefact may be due to another physiological process that is not of interest in the current context, such as a respiratory swing on an ECG trace. Thus 'one man's artefact is another's signal' (Rampil, 1987).

Artefact detection is important for several reasons:

- An artefact may be misinterpreted as a genuine clinical event and lead to an erroneous therapeutic intervention.
- Invalid but abnormal values that are not filtered can cause alarm systems to register false alarms.
- Artefact rejection improves the clarity of a signal when it is presented to a clinician for interpretation.

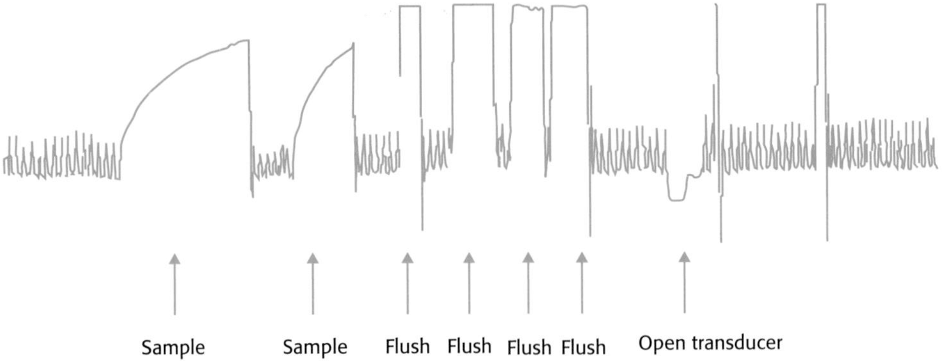
Sample
Sample
Flush
Flush
Flush
Flush
Open transducer

Figure 27.2
Examples of artefact on the arterial blood pressure channel.

There are many sources of artefact in the clinical environment. False heart rate values can be generated by diathermy noise during surgery or by patient movement. False high arterial blood pressure alarms are generated by flushing and sampling of arterial lines (Figure 27.2). These forms of artefact have contributed significantly to the generation of false alarms on patient monitoring equipment. Koski *et al.* (1990) found that only 10% of 1307 alarm events generated on cardiac postoperative patients were significant. Of these, 27% were due to artefacts, e.g. sampling of arterial blood. The net effect of the distraction caused by these high false alarm rates has been that clinicians have often turned off alarms intraoperatively, despite the concomitant increase in risk to the patient.

An artefact is best handled at its source through improvements in the design of the transducer system, or in low-level signal processing, but it is not always possible or practical to do so. The next best step is to filter out artefactual components of a signal or register their detection before using the signal for clinical interpretation. Many techniques have been developed to assist in this process, including Kalman filtering, rule-based expert systems, blackboard systems and neural networks. It is in the nature of artefacts that they cannot always be eliminated on the basis of a single signal, and cross-channel correlation may be needed, making artefact detection a feature at all levels of signal interpretation.

Single-channel interpretation

Having established that a signal is probably artefact free, the next stage in its interpretation is to decide whether it defines a clinically significant condition. This may be done simply by comparing the value to a pre-defined patient or population normal range, but in most cases such simple thresholding is of limited value.

- Firstly, clinically appropriate ranges cannot always be defined because the notion of the acceptable range for a patient may be highly context specific. One can in fact calculate statistically valid patient specific normal ranges (Harris, 1980; Nakano *et al.*, 1981) but these rely on an extended period of measurement stability, which may not be attainable in a clinical context.
- Further, the notion of an acceptable range is often tied up with expectations defined by the patient's expected outcome and current therapeutic interventions.
- Finally, even if one can decide upon an acceptable range for a specific parameter, the amount of information that a single out-of-range warning can convey is usually limited.

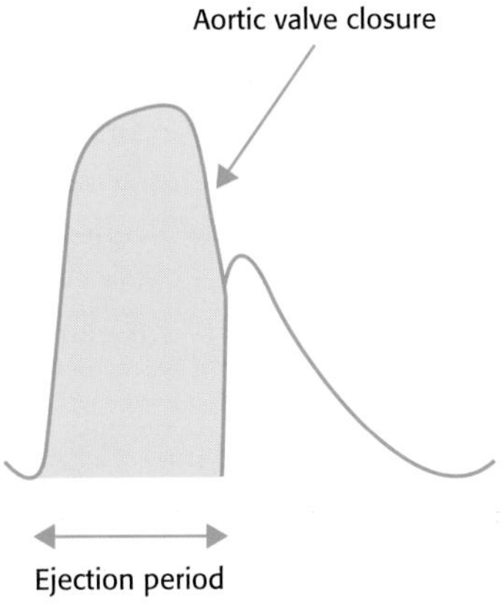
Aortic valve closure
Ejection period

Figure 27.3
Derivation of information from a waveform's shape. The systolic ejection area beneath the arterial pressure waveform gives an indirect measure of stroke volume. It is demarcated by the beginning of systole and the dicrotic notch caused by the closure of the aortic valve.

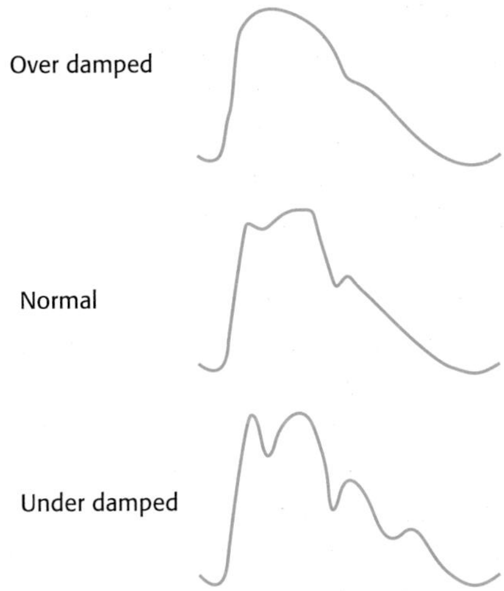
Over damped
Normal
Under damped

Figure 27.4
The shape of arterial pressure waves varies with the dynamic response of the catheter transducer. Analysis of the waveform frequency components following a fast flush can assist in detecting system damping and assist in optimizing pressure measurements (adapted from Gardner, 1981).

Even wildly abnormal values may have several possible interpretations. These limitations of simple threshold-based alarm techniques have spurred on the development of more complex techniques capable of delivering 'smart alarms' (Gravenstein *et al.*, 1987).

Much more information can be obtained from the analysis of a single channel if is a time varying, continuous waveform, like arterial pressure. Specific pressure artefacts such as sampling and flushing of the catheter line can be detected by their unique shape (Figure 27.2). Estimates of clinically useful measures such as cardiac stroke volume can be derived by analysing the area under the curve of the wave (Figure 27.3). It is even possible to analyse the frequency components of the pressure waveform to obtain information about the fidelity of the measurement system itself (Figure 27.4).

Alterations in the behaviour of a repetitive signal can also carry information. Changes in the ECG are a good example. Features such as the height of the QRS peak help to label individual components within beat complexes. The presence or absence of features like P waves, and the duration and regularity of intervals between waves and complexes, can carry diagnostic information about cardiac rhythm. However, it is not always possible to unambiguously label events in an ECG strip, and sometimes one needs to use additional contextual information to assist in the labelling process (e.g. Greenwald *et al.*, 1992).

Cross-channel interpretation

Often clinical conditions can only be identified by examining the signals on several different channels. Such cross-channel information is useful at several levels, starting with artefact detection and signal validation through to clinical diagnosis.

Cross-correlation for signal validation can be made with a number of sources depending on the signal being measured. The alternatives for correlating a signal include the following methods.

- **Same signal, different interpretation method:** If, for example, an error is suspected when the heart rate is derived by a simple peak detection algorithm, one could attempt to validate the value by comparing it to one derived using a different method on the same data.
- **Different physical source, but same signal:** Comparing different ECG leads is a common technique for validating changes seen on one lead. Patterns across leads also have diagnostic importance.
- **Different signal:** A flat ECG trace indicating asystole can be checked against the arterial pressure waveform or the plethysmograph, both of which should demonstrate pulsatile waves if the heart were contracting normally, and would lose their pulsatile characteristics if asystole was present.

Cross-channel information can also be used to identify conditions not detectable with single channels alone. Many clinical conditions can be distinguished by the time ordering of events in their natural history (Coiera, 1990). For example, the cause of a hypotensive episode may be deducible from the order in which changes occurred across heart rate, blood pressure and CVP (Figure 27.5). In the presence of a vasodilator, the arterial blood pressure drop would precede the reflex tachycardia and CVP fall. In the presence of hypovolaemia, the first parameter to shift would be the heart rate followed by CVP and blood pressure.

Making clinical decisions

Once a computer system is able to diagnose complex disease patterns from measured signals and data stored in electronic patient records, it is in a position to assist clinicians in making

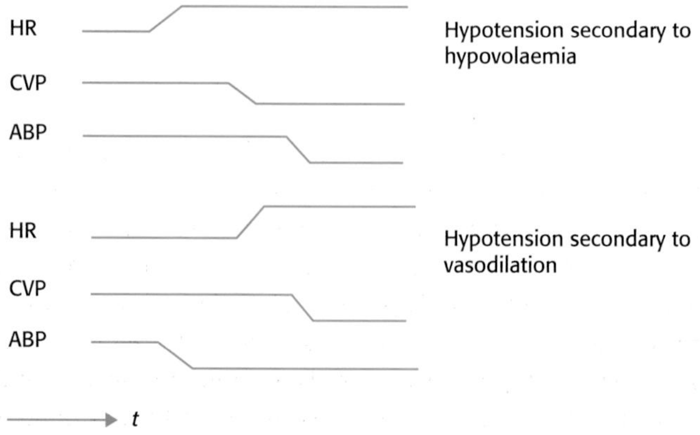
HR
CVP
ABP
Hypotension secondary to hypovolaemia
HR
CVP
ABP
Hypotension secondary to vasodilation
t

Figure 27.5 Time ordering of the onset of trends across different signals can help identify the onset of different clinical conditions. The cause of hypotension can be distinguished by the sequence of changes detected on heart rate (HR), central venous pressure (CVP) and arterial blood pressure (ABP).

therapeutic decisions. As noted earlier, intelligent interpretative systems can appear either as embedded systems hidden within instruments, or as explicit entities that can interact with a clinician.

The way in which an intelligent system is used affects its design. Systems that need to interact with humans may need to justify their decisions in a way that embedded systems do not. Equally, a system that acts as an advisor to a human is placed in a less critical position than one that acts independently to manage a patient's therapy. Although embedded interpretative systems are already starting to appear, those that require explicit interaction have yet to make a significant impact.

Decision support systems

The classic model of computer-based decision support requires a clinician to input details of a patient's clinical state, with the machine then suggesting one or more possible diagnoses. The MYCIN system is the archetype of this model, providing assistance with the selection of antibiotic therapy (Buchanan and Shortliffe, 1984). In practice, however, this model does not fit well with the realities of the clinical workplace.

Clinicians are often unable to spare the time required to use such systems. As a consequence, systems that offer different models of decision support have been developed. For example, to support the decision-making that is characteristic of anaesthetists in the operating room, work is currently underway to develop intelligent patient monitors and anaesthetic workstations (e.g. Loeb *et al.*, 1989).

Intelligent monitors will not only suppress spurious alarms generated by signal artefact, but will use cross-channel signal correlations to generate high-level diagnostic alarms. They have a role in assisting with clinical vigilance of slowly evolving conditions, and of conditions that have been missed because of distraction.

When integrated with an anaesthetic machine, a monitor system can also warn of faults within the gas delivery system, and possibly suggest corrective actions. Research is also under way exploring ways of integrating a predictive component into these systems. With such systems, a clinician could test changes to therapy before initiating them by simulating their effect on a mathematical model of the patient (Rutledge *et al.*, 1993).

Other modes of decision support include therapy planning systems, which develop a treatment protocol based on a patient's clinical status (Hickam *et al.*, 1985), and therapy critiquing systems that examine treatment plans generated by clinicians, and attempt to suggest improvements (Miller, 1983).

Autonomous therapeutic devices

In contrast to decision support systems, autonomous systems can operate independently of human interaction on complex tasks. Perhaps the most studied application area is ventilator management. Programs have been designed to adjust ventilator settings automatically in response to measurements of a patient's respiratory status. Early research into systems that could wean patients from ventilators (Fagan *et al.*, 1984) has led to more ambitious projects that seek to take control of most of the tasks associated with ventilator management (e.g. Hayes-Roth *et al.*, 1992). Such projects may in the long term provide new classes of therapeutic devices, although it is clear that their successful introduction will require continued advances in sensor design (e.g. implantable glucose sensors for insulin delivery systems), and in the technologies for signal interpretation.

27.4 Intelligent monitoring systems use a variety of methods for interpretation

Intelligent signal interpretation involves two broad tasks. Firstly, distinct events within a signal are identified using pattern recognition methods, e.g. detecting individual peaks in an ECG signal. Secondly, a meaningful label is assigned to the detected events using pattern interpretation methods, e.g. picking a QRS complex from a T wave, and interpreting its clinical significance. There have been significant advances with techniques for performing both these tasks, and new methodologies have emerged, several specifically from research in AI.

Pattern recognition techniques extract significant events from a clinical signal. For example, they detect edges and curves in pictures, or letters, letter groups and words from speech. Pattern detection techniques vary in the way they model events within signals. For example they may be based on statistical models, in which the frequency of certain patterns is used in the recognition process. Many classic recognition techniques have clinical application, such as blackboard systems (Nii, 1989) (initially developed for speech recognition) and Markov models. Neural networks are an alternative technique for pattern recognition, and they have become of increasing interest to the biomedical research community in recent years.

Once patterns have been identified within a signal, they need to be interpreted. It is with this task that techniques from AI have made major contributions over the last two decades, especially through the introduction of expert systems. Rule-based systems are more suited to cross-channel interpretation of signals than lower level signal processing.

Clinically deployed expert systems perform a variety of tasks from the interpretation of ECGs (Greenwald *et al.*, 1992) to analysis of laboratory results such as thyroid hormone assays (Horn *et al.*, 1985). Experimental expert systems have been developed with more ambitious goals in mind, including systems that can interpret respiratory parameters and automatically adjust ventilator settings during the process of weaning a patient off a ventilator (Fagan *et al.*, 1984).

27.5 Use of intelligent monitors can produce new types of error because of automation bias in the user

At the end of Chapter 26 a list of the limitations of intelligent decision support systems was presented, noting that their performance is bounded by the quality of the data that they have access to, and the quality of the knowledge captured within their knowledge base. One of the recurrent themes of this book is that one should never only evaluate the performance of a system in strictly technical terms, but rather consider it more broadly in socio-technical terms. When considering the limitations of intelligent monitoring systems, as with any form of CDSS, we should therefore think of the system as being composed of humans, the machines they use and the organizational context in which they come together to solve tasks.

One of the motivations for the development of intelligent monitoring systems and CDSS is a reduction in human error. However, studies show that, while they do indeed significantly reduce the errors they were designed to, their use introduces new unanticipated errors, associated with the cognitive limitations of humans. One of the error types associated with intelligent monitoring systems is known as **automation bias**, where people using an automated decision aid will act as the aid directs them to, irrespective of the correctness of the suggested action.

In a laboratory experiment by Skitka *et al.* (1999), users were given a simulated flight task, and some had the benefit of using a computer that monitored system states and made decision recommendations. When the aid worked perfectly, the users of the system outperformed those who did not use it. However, when the computer aid was very reliable, but not perfectly so, and occasionally failed to prompt the user when action was needed, or incorrectly made a prompt to carry out an action when none was needed, the situation changed. The participants in the study without the aid outperformed their counterparts who used the computer. Those using the aid made **errors of omission** (they missed events because the system did not prompt them to do so) as well as **errors of commission** (they did what the decision aid told them to do, even when it contradicted their training and other available indicators). In the study, those using an aid only had 59% accuracy on the omission error events, compared to 97% for the non-computer users, and performance was even worse on the commission error opportunities, with an accuracy of only 35%.

There are many possible explanations for these types of error. It has been suggested that humans who trust a computer system shed responsibility for tasks, and devolve them to the computer system. Computer users may as a result develop an 'out of loop unfamiliarity' with the system they are meant to be monitoring, because they have delegated the monitoring of data to the automated aid, and so they have effectively taken themselves out of the decision loop (Wickens and Hollands, 2000). If an urgent event were to occur, the consequence of this unfamiliarity may be that it takes much longer to develop situational awareness, because the human is unfamiliar with the current state of the data, and needs to develop a mental model that may take more time than is available to solve the problem. In contrast, without a decision aid, the human has no choice but to maintain an active mental model of the state of the system being monitored.

Recent evidence suggests that explicit training in automation bias has a short-term benefit only, but making individuals personally accountable for their decisions does seem to reduce automation bias. Specifically, if individuals are told that their actions are socially accountable, because the data of their performance are being recorded, and that they will be held accountable for the outcome of their performance, then individuals spend more time verifying the correctness of the decision aid's suggestions by checking data, and therefore make fewer errors (Skitka *et al.*, 2000).

Conclusions

It is already the case that much monitoring technology is poorly understood by the clinicians who use it, and that clinicians are often unaware of how to use or interpret their output correctly. As more intelligence is added to the devices that populate the clinical workplace, there is an even greater need to understand their advantages and limitations.

There is no doubt that advances in AI will gradually change many of the ways clinicians handle day-to-day problems and that they will greatly improve many aspects of the clinical process. Of necessity, the high level at which these systems will perform, assisting in both diagnosis and therapy, means that they have a direct impact on patient care.

It will often only be the clinician who will be in a position to assess the conclusions of these systems. Rather than accepting these as a given, however, the onus remains on those who use them to do so correctly. Although it will not always be necessary to understand the details of the technologies used, and indeed these will continue to evolve, it is necessary to understand their nature and in particular the types of mistake that they are prone to make.

Discussion points

1 What evaluation data would you require before being convinced to allow an intelligent system to take total control over a clinical function such as running an IV pump or managing a ventilator?

2 Is it possible to run a modern intensive care unit without intelligent monitoring devices?

3 In what circumstances is it permissible for a clinician to disable the alarms and warnings function on a monitoring device?

Chapter summary

1 The automated interpretation of patient measurements is needed because of the difficulties clinicians face when they continuously monitor patient data. These human factors include the problems of cognitive overload, varying expertise and human error.

2 Signal interpretation can occur at a number of levels, starting with artefact detection and removal, moving through to a complex assessment of its clinical significance.

3 Interpretations can be based on data within a single channel, such as arterial blood pressure, or look at multiple channels for cross-correlations and temporal patterns.

4 Once interpretations have been made, they can be presented for the consideration of a human, or can be used in closed-loop devices to autonomously control patient therapy, including ventilators and IV medication delivery.

5 Intelligent signal interpretation can be divided into two tasks:

- identification of distinct events within a signal using pattern recognition methods, e.g. detecting individual peaks in an ECG signal
- assigning a meaningful label to the detected events using pattern interpretation methods, e.g. picking a QRS complex from a T wave, and interpreting its clinical significance.

6 Neural networks are good at pattern recognition, but have limited ability to explain their conclusions. Expert systems are well suited to use in situations in which the system's user needs some form of explanation of reasoning.

7 Use of intelligent monitors can produce new types of error because of automation bias in the user, resulting in the generation of errors of commission or omission. Personal accountability for performance seems to reduce automation bias.

CHAPTER 28

Biosurveillance

Bioterrorism is the malicious introduction of biological agents such as viruses, bacteria and toxins into a civilian population. The most likely scenario for a bioterrorist attack would be a covert and unnoticed release of a biological agent into a major urban centre (Tucker, 1997; CDC, 2000). In such a situation it will be the civilian system, and in particular local hospitals, community physicians and the public health system that are the first detector and first responder (Franz *et al.*, 1997; CDC, 2000). An appropriate response by emergency departments and hospitals could significantly limit the morbidity and mortality of biological warfare agents (Richards *et al.*, 1999).

Given the potential for widespread and large-scale civilian casualties, much effort is currently focused on developing biosurveillance systems that rapidly detect and report suspected attacks, and result in the rapid mobilization of appropriate responses to the incident. One of the specific challenges faced by public authorities is the short window of opportunity that exists between the first cases being identified and a second wave of the population becoming ill through person-to-person transmission. During that window, public authorities will need to determine that an attack has occurred, identify the organism or agent, and commence prevention strategies such as mass vaccination or administration of prophylaxis (CDC, 2000).

The bioterrorist threat challenges the public health system to create biosurveillance systems that maximize the likelihood of the early detection of bioterrorist events, as well as ensuring the rapid and direct reporting of these events to appropriate bodies. Computer-based disease surveillance systems have been in place since at least the mid-1980s (Graitcer and Burton, 1987). However, it is only recently that the focus has shifted from improving internal reporting processes for public health authorities, to extending electronic reporting to the clinical workplace. This chapter examines the role that decision support and Internet technologies may play in assisting clinicians in the detection of biological terrorist attacks both as a means of rapid electronic reporting and through the provision of diagnostic decision support.

28.1 Event reporting = detection + recognition + communication

For a bioterrorist event to be identified rapidly and accurately, several critical events must occur:

- **The event needs to be detected.** Some potential bioagents may present themselves in dramatic ways that should attract clinician attention. For example, botulism results as progressive neuromuscular paralysis resulting in respiratory failure. However, non-specific symptoms like fever, chills, malaise and fatigue are unlikely to raise clinical suspicion as unusual events yet may herald infection by anthrax, brucellosis, plague, Q fever, viral encephalitis, tularaemia and the viral haemorrhagic fevers – all commonly discussed as potential bioterrorist agents (Franz *et al.*, 1997). If an event is indistinguishable from the 'background noise' of other normal clinical presentations, then it will not be recognized. Where the clinical presentation of a bioagent attack is ambiguous and easily confused with other presentations, one needs to consider mechanisms that somehow increase the signal to noise ratio so that clinicians recognize the clinical presentation as something worthy of attention. The probability of detection is higher if there is a pattern of rapid presentation of similar symptoms from many individuals, generating sufficient signal to be detectable. With most natural epidemics, the progressive exposure of people leads to a gradual rise in disease incidence. In contrast, a bioagent attack exposes a large number of people at the same time, producing a compressed epidemic curve with a peak in a matter of hours or days. For example, a staphylococcal enterotoxin B attack would cause patients to present in large numbers over a very short period of time, probably within 24 hours, in contrast to the naturally occurring pneumonias or influenza with patients presenting over a more prolonged interval (Franz *et al.*, 1997).
- **The event needs to be recognizable.** Where clinical recognition is a critical component in the surveillance process, then clinicians must have access to diagnostic knowledge to identify bioagent events and an awareness that they need actually to consult that knowledge. For an event to de diagnosed it must have a unique feature pattern. With many bioagents, the clinical pattern will be ambiguous, but the laboratory results will be pathognomonic. Even with an infection by a more recognizable disease like smallpox, it would require an astute clinician to distinguish the skin manifestations of this disease from other vesicular exanthems such as chickenpox, allergic contact dermatitis or erythema multiforme with bullae (Franz *et al.*, 1997). However, there is a risk that novel genetically engineered variants of organisms are used in bioterrorist attack, making rapid organism identification unlikely.
- **The existence of the event needs to be communicated rapidly.** Clinicians need to communicate to public health organizations capable of initiating a population

response. Further, such authorities need to communicate rapidly with clinicians working in the community, the public health system and the public, to raise the level of awareness to the point that clinicians and the public are able to commence responding in an appropriate manner. The execution of such a communication strategy requires both a communication infrastructure, as well as a well-organized plan for message sending.

We can deconstruct this process into a series of interconnecting communication flows, which evolve as a bioterrorist event unfolds and a biosurveillance system comes into action (Figure 28.1):

1 Sentinel presentation of patient(s) to clinician in absence of prior evidence of a bioterrorist event.
2 Clinician consults colleagues or evidence-resources such as online system of journals, texts and paper guidelines.
3 Clinician sends patient specimens to laboratory for testing.
4 Clinician (possibly) sends report to public health authority, before laboratory result.
5 Laboratory identifies bioagent in patient specimen.
6 Laboratory notifies referring clinician.
7 Laboratory notifies public health authority.
8 Public health authority sends out a communication to laboratories and clinicians in geographic region considered under threat, warning of potential bioterrorist event, and indicating clinical and laboratory signs to scan for, as well as commencing disaster management plan.
9 Patients present to clinician after public health authority warning.

At each step in this process, data and knowledge need to be brought to bear to make informed decisions under difficult time and resource constraints, and communication needs to be rapid and effective. We saw in Chapter 19 that a communication system involves people, the messages they wish to convey, the technologies that mediate conversations, and the organizational structures that define and constrain the conversations that are allowed to occur. Consequently, a biosurveillance system in the broadest sense is not just a piece of technology but a complex socio-technical system of people, processes, channels and tools. CDSS technology will probably be an indispensable tool in assisting clinicians make critical diagnoses, and that effective use of communication channels like the Internet may make the difference between local containment and wide spread of a bioagent amongst the population.

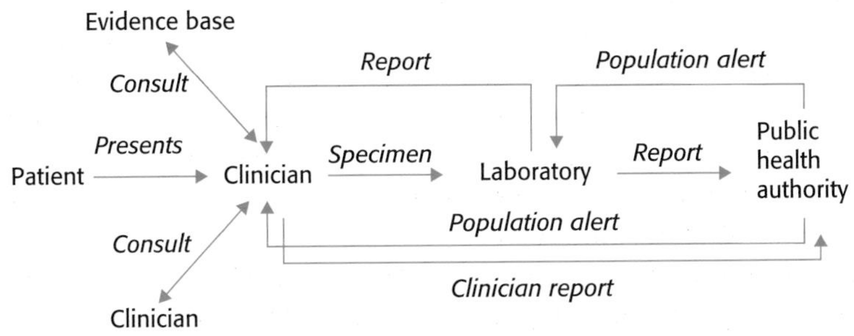
Evidence base
Consult
Report
Population alert
Presents
Patient
Clinician
Specimen
Laboratory
Report
Public health authority
Consult
Population alert
Clinician report
Clinician

Figure 28.1 Biosurveillance communication flows.

28.2 Infectious disease surveillance systems play a key role in bioagent detection

If they do detect a potential bioagent release, how likely are clinicians to report it to the appropriate authorities? Some data are available from existing infectious diseases surveillance programs. Many studies have shown that there is a substantial underreporting of notifiable infectious diseases by medical practitioners. Rushworth *et al.* (1991) reported that out of a series of 461 cases, clinicians reported 20.2%, whereas staff at diagnostic laboratories reported 75%. There was also a substantial time gap between the clinician and laboratory reports, with laboratories having a mean time of 8.1 days and clinicians of 13.2 days.

Many reasons have been advanced to explain the failure to comply with reporting requirements by clinicians, including medical practitioners being unaware of the need to notify, concerns about patient confidentiality, unclear communication channels, inadequate feedback by health departments to clinicians and practical difficulties including delays in delivery of notification forms.

In general, failure to comply with reporting by clinicians seems to be related to failures in communication between the managers of the surveillance system and the medical practitioners (Rushworth *et al.*, 1991). Healthcare providers are also often overworked, but are left to determine whether a patient meets public health surveillance case definitions and struggle with tracking down patient records and filling forms (CDC, 2000). This suggests that simplification of the notification process and timely feedback of surveillance information could be key to improving detection of infections diseases, and by analogy, bioterrorist agents.

Despite the superiority of manual laboratory reporting over clinician-initiated reporting, there is still a substantial delay associated with it. There are many reasons for the delay, including the use of batch testing of some specimens and the requirement to perform confirmatory testing before a final laboratory report is issued. Laboratory reporting of notifiable diseases can be speeded up by the introduction of automated data extraction and electronic communication to public health departments. Effler *et al.* (1999) showed that automated laboratory reporting doubled the number of reports received, detecting 91% of 357 illness reports, compared to 44% through the manual system. Further, electronic reports arrived an average of 3.8 days earlier than manual laboratory reports. The electronic reports in this study were also more likely to contain key information such as patient and physician telephone numbers. Effler *et al.* estimated that at least 80% of all notifiable laboratory reports, and probably more, could be detected and transmitted electronically.

Consequently, laboratories, and more specifically automated laboratory reporting systems, have a key role in the detection of attack by bioagents, since they will in all probability detect more infected patients and report them more quickly than the clinician-driven part of the 'detection apparatus'. Systems such as the CDC's National Electronic Disease Surveillance system (NEDSS) in the US should therefore be important at least as models, and perhaps as contributing infrastructure, to any bioagent detection system. There are a number of existing systems for infectious disease surveillance in the US, which are being turned to the biosurveillance task and they have been analysed for commonalities and differences (Lober *et al.*, 2002). Table 28.1 summarizes these technical systems and demonstrates a wide variation in system construction, including different communication, security and coding standards.

CDSSs also have a role to play in the automated detection of infections and have now been tested in a number of hospitals. The Infection Control Departments of Barnes and Jewish

Table 28.1 Comparison of existing biosurveillance systems (from Lober *et al.*, 2002).

System	Geography/population	Setting/data sources	Data transmission standards	Data update frequency	Data collection technique	Security protocol
Bergen County, New Jersey	County; 5 hospitals	ED	Text	Daily	Fax, e-mail, file transfer	–
Children's Hospital Boston	Metropolitan; 2 hospitals	ED	XML	Daily	Mining agent and reports	SSL
Denver Public Health	Metropolitan; 600 K, 25%	ED, EMS CAD, nurse advice line	ODBC	Daily (ED hourly)	Electronic from ED text and CAD, *ad hoc* queries	
Dept. of Defense/GEIS	14 countries, 395 installations (307 in USA, 88 other)	Military treatment facilities	Column-delineated	Daily	Data mining	Secure FTP vpn
EI Network	21 Pacific Rim countries	Disease alerts	Text, e-mail	2 weeks	Voluntary reporting	
Los Alamos/ University of New Mexico	2 counties, 2 EDs	ED	Http, XML	Voluntary	Reports	SSL
Regenstrief/Indiana University	Metropolitan; 11 hospitals, 5 health systems; 1.5 M, 95%	ED, hospital, physician groups	HL7	Real-time	HL7 over secure extranet	
Seattle–King County/ University of Washington	1 county, 3 hospital EDs, 9 PCC; 1.7 M, 20%	ED, primary care, EMS CAD	XML	Daily	Mining agent and reports	SSL
University of Pittsburgh	13 counties, 14 hospitals, 10 EDs; 3 M, 20%; 1.3 M, 37%	ED hospitals	HL7, ODBC	Real-time	HL7, free-text, processing physician case reporting	SSH

Abbreviations: CAD computer-assisted dispatching, ED emergency department, EMS emergency medical service, FTP file transfer protocol, GEIS US Department of Defense's Global Emerging Infectious Disease Surveillance, HL7 health level 7, ODBC open database connectivity, SSH secure shell, SSL secure sockets layer, VPN virtual private network, XML extensible mark-up language.

Hospitals St. Louis, Missouri has implemented an expert system called Reportable Diseases, which applies State public health department culture-based criteria for detecting 'significant' infections, which are required to be reported to the State. Reportable Diseases has been deployed at Barnes and Jewish Hospitals, which are tertiary-care teaching hospitals, since February 1995. Microbiology culture data from the hospital's laboratory system are monitored by two systems. One alerts clinical staff and one generates CDC reports. The first system, GermAlert, monitors microbiology culture data from the hospital's laboratory system. Using a rule base consisting of criteria developed by local infectious diseases experts, GermAlert scans the culture data and generates an alert to the infection control staff when a culture representing a 'significant' infection is detected. The second laboratory system, GermWatcher, uses a rule base consisting of a combination of the NNIS criteria and local hospital infection control policy to scan the culture data, and identify which cultures represent nosocomial infections. These infections are then reported to the CDC (Kahn *et al.*, 1993, 1995).

The advantage of expert systems is of course that they can look for patterns in data, and then correlate them with patient-specific data, to generate flags highlighting potentially suspicious cases. In a situation where the nature of the bioagent may be indeterminate, the combination of patient and laboratory data, perhaps also noting patterns in other similar cases, may generate the first signal of a bioterrorist event.

Although there are still substantial barriers to the introduction of clinical decision support technology to clinicians, laboratory-based systems such as GermWatcher are much more likely to be accepted. As we saw in Chapter 25, laboratory expert systems usually do not intrude into clinical practice. Rather, they are embedded within the process of care, and with the exception of laboratory staff, clinicians working with patients do not need to interact with them.

28.3 Clinical education alone is unlikely to enhance event detection and recognition

Since most bioterrorist disease presentations will be outside the experience of clinicians, it has been suggested that clinical personnel should be trained to recognize the symptoms of different bioagents (Simon, 1997; CDC, 2000). For example, it has been suggested that continuing professional education (CPE) courses should be arranged to familiarize clinicians with the signs and symptoms of anthrax infection, tularaemia, Q fever, brucellosis and other biological warfare agents that they would not normally encounter in their routine clinical practice (Tucker, 1997).

However, we know (see Chapter 23) that in general traditional didactic measures such as lectures or formal examinations do not change clinical performance or improve clinical care (Davis *et al.*, 1999). In contrast, interactive educational activities, structured around actual problems in the clinical workplace, are much more successful. This suggests that if educational programs are to be attempted, they would need to be somehow directly integrated into the routine clinical process, so that bioagents are routinely considered as a part of patient work-ups.

We can look to specific examples of atypical infectious diseases that pose substantial threats to the community to test the value of the direct educational approach. Legionnaire's disease, first detected in 1976, is probably the most important community-acquired atypical pneumonia. Yet after 25 years of clinical education, *Legionella* species are still underdiagnosed in patients with community-acquired pneumonia. When the diagnosis is made, it is usually made in the laboratory rather than on clinical suspicion (Waterer *et al.*, 2001).

Even with the current emphasis on evidence-based practice, and a profusion of clinical practice guidelines, there still seems to be a substantial barrier preventing the adoption of new clinical practices. Indeed, as we saw in Chapter 14, the uptake of evidence into clinical practice is low and this has been a cause of concern amongst proponents of evidence-based care. Practising clinicians, on the other hand, complain of being swamped by a growing tide of information. The consequence of this oversupply of evidence for information producers such as public health authorities is that their success in information dispersal is increasingly dependent upon their ability to compete for the attention of clinicians.

Consequently, it is unlikely that clinician awareness of bioterrorist risks will be substantially altered simply by the production of standard guidelines or CPE alone. For clinicians to be able to devote their scarce attention to bioagent risks, either it must become a routine part of their daily practice, or other means must be devised which reduce the costs of accessing such information.

28.4 Online evidence retrieval and CDSS can help support education and decision-making

We saw in Chapter 23 that in recent years an alternative idea to CPE as a distinct clinical activity has emerged. Recognizing that the body of biomedical knowledge has now grown to such an extent that it is no longer capable of being mastered by individuals, even in subspecialties, and also that learning works best when focused on issues in the clinical workplace, it has been proposed that in the future most CPE will consist of using online information technology to answer immediate clinical questions. Thus, the whole notion of CPE changes from one of periodic updates to a clinician's knowledge to a 'just-in-time' model where a clinician checks the medical knowledge base, potentially at every clinical encounter. In the just-in-time model, every time clinicians make a clinical decision, they consider whether they need to access the clinical evidence base.

The just-in-time model has echoes of earlier attempts to support clinical decision-making through the use of intelligent or expert computer systems. It differs in that it attempts to integrate the decision support system into the routine activities of clinicians, and that the mode of decision support can range from access to 'passive' knowledge sources like guidelines, manuals and textbooks, though to 'active' knowledge sources that interact with clinicians to assist in the formulation of diagnostic or treatment decisions.

How likely are clinicians to use online decision support? At present our detailed understanding of information transactions in the healthcare system is sadly limited, and the evidence is inconclusive. It suggests that with appropriate education, support and effort to introduce online systems that do not disrupt clinical workflow, they will be used. However, the evidence also suggests that these systems will only be used for a small portion of clinician decision problems. This is because it seems the preferred mode of information access and decision support for clinicians is face-to-face conversation with colleagues, even when online systems are available. Clinical work is complex, and is often rapidly moving and consensual, especially in hospital environments. One of the striking features of clinical work is that clinicians rely far more on informal interpersonal information exchange than formal paper or computer records to satisfy their information requests. This is in part because information is not always easily available from formal sources, but more often simply because conversation is a more appropriate mechanism for information exchange on most occasions.

Only sparse data are available to describe the volume of information transactions in healthcare, especially comparing formal information system transactions with informal interpersonal ones. The clinical communication space is large, as we saw in Chapter 19, and clearly varies from setting to setting. However, as the cumulative evidence suggests, the picture of heavy reliance on interpersonal exchanges for information transmission is repeated across most settings, varying from about 50% in clinics to about 90% in emergency departments.

These data suggest that any just-in-time decisions support for bioterrorist surveillance must recognize the importance of interpersonal communication, and provide assistance to clinicians in locating appropriate colleagues to discuss potential bioagent incidents, whether that be via phone, e-mail, or fax. An online just-in-time system can act as a knowledge portal, but sometimes that knowledge will be in the heads of other clinicians, and an online system needs to function as a communication tool, connecting clinicians with questions to those who have answers.

For those situations in which access to a guideline is appropriate, there are still confounding factors that need to be accounted for. Specifically, the context of care imposes widely different constraints on decision-making. Different user populations have different skill sets, education and resources and as a result their information needs may demand very different information presentations. One study estimates that up to 50% of the variation in compliance rate by clinicians with guidelines can be ascribed to the clinical setting (Grilli and Lomas, 1994). To combat this, context-specific versions of evidence can be created, perhaps using computerized user models that capture the specific needs of individual groups and permit some automatic tailoring of evidence before it is presented (Pratt and Sim, 1995).

28.5 The Web will need to be used in combination with other communication technologies to support biosurveillance

In this final section we re-examine the communication tasks associated with surveillance for bioterrorist events, and test whether the Web is capable of supporting the task, as well as examine what alternative channels or methods are available.

A clinician reports an event to a public health authority (clinician push narrowcast)

We can probably assume that the isolated presentation of a single patient with non-specific symptoms will not be detected as being different from the normal infectious disease case load. For clinicians to consider a patient to be affected by a bioagent, their threshold of suspicion needs to be raised by:

- multiple presentation of patients with similar symptoms
- symptoms that are unusual
- notification of a likely bioterrorist event by a public health authority.

In the absence of these, the sentinel patient is unlikely to be detected by clinicians, but may be detected by laboratory tests.

Notification is a clinician-initiated act and requires the clinician to have access to a communication channel, and to know which authority to contact and what message to tell the authority. The web is able to provide all these. It can provide a direct mechanism for sending electronic messages to designated addresses. It also supports structured reporting which permits a well-constructed message to be created and sent fairly rapidly.

However, the Web is not ubiquitous. It may be feasible to assume all major hospitals in many countries have (or could be made to have) Internet connections, but clinicians working in the community may not have ready access to the Web. Further, given the desire of clinicians to discuss issues, a structured report does not permit conversation. Clinicians would also require immediate feedback that their report had been received (Coiera and Tombs, 1998), given that they would have a degree of anxiety and concern surrounding the suspected bioagent event. This suggests that for reports with a high level of concern, a mixture of asynchronous (e.g. e-mail or Web forms) and synchronous (e.g. telephone) communication channels may be needed.

Consequently, any Web-based notification mechanism needs to be part of a larger reporting system which supports alternative channels for reporting, such as a telephone helpline, or rapid response to web reports with telephone calls to clinicians.

A clinician can request information to assist in deciding whether a patient has been exposed to a bioagent (clinician pull narrowcast)

In the situation in which clinicians are faced either with multiple presentation of patients with similar symptoms, or symptoms that are unusual, they may suspect that a bioagent is a possible cause, and wish to seek advice on whether their suspicions are well founded.

When clinicians have well-formed questions, have training to use online systems and have easy access to such systems, the web may be an appropriate delivery vehicle for decision support information, including both active and passive information services. Consequently, one can imagine that a web-based decision support system may be helpful to clinicians in such a situation.

However, when clinicians are unsure about a case before them, their questions may be ill formed, and traditionally discussion with colleagues seems to be the mode best suited to assist with decision-making. This suggests that for ill-formed clinical questions, face-to-face or telephone (synchronous) communication channels may be needed to augment to use of asynchronous channels that would deal with well-formed information seeking requests.

Further, the varying context of care may make it unacceptable to use computers as the interface into web systems. Providing access methods that are optimized to local needs can also enlarge the range of clinical contexts in which evidence is used. As we saw in Chapter 14, a clinician faced with an emergency that requires rapid decision-making is unlikely to browse at leisure through information on the Web, although that may be the perfect solution for less time-critical circumstances. The use of small mobile computing and communication devices, and voice-activated rather than text-based services, may help in circumstances where clinicians are mobile, hands are busy or time is limited.

This again suggests that a telephone helpline, similar to a poisons helpline, may be an essential part of any bioterrorist reporting system. The online tools and telephony can be brought together into a single sophisticated system design that incorporates voice and video communication over the Internet with the bioterrorist Web site. In cases in which clinicians are unsure of what they are dealing with, they may elect not to browse through information on the Web site or use interactive tools, but rather contact the helpline and use voice or video telephony which has been incorporated directly into the Web site design.

A stand-alone bioterrorist Web site is unlikely to be the best way of providing such support. The evidence cited earlier about the poor reporting behaviour of clinicians and the poor adoption of new practices suggests that it may be better in the near term to aim for a more general-purpose online system which supports many other clinical issues. For example, one could integrate bioterrorist support into an emergency department just-in-time decision support system. If the just-in-time model takes off in the near term, then it provides a natural entry point for educating clinicians about bioagents, prompting them to naturally consider specific bioagents at appropriate points in the diagnostic or treatment process, alongside other diagnostic alternatives.

From a theoretical point of view, this model is appealing since most informatics research now emphasizes that for new information systems to be successfully adopted after implementation, they need to blend naturally into the existing clinical workflow, rather than being a 'bolt-on' that imposes additional demands on clinicians. Embedding a new bioterrorist detection process on the top of existing work practices may substantially impede clinical work. Clinicians are often working to capacity and juggling multiple tasks. Imposing extra duties because of the introduction of an information system, without removing existing tasks, will limit the capacity of clinicians to perform their jobs in a time-critical way.

The successful integration of information relating to bioagents into just-in-time systems in the short term clearly is dependent to the extent to which any particular clinical institution has developed programs of culture change and developed information technology infrastructure to support this mode of work. It is equally appropriate to consider the benefit of using some bioterrorist surveillance resources to promote and support the national deployment of just-in-time systems, at least to critical nodes like emergency departments.

Public health authorities can contact a specific clinician in regard to a given patient (authority push synchronous narrowcast)

This form of communication task requires a point-to-point synchronous channel – from phone, pager and fax to face-to-face conversation. If telephony is integrated into a clinician's Web system, for example using a voice-over-IP service, then this may substitute for telephony. It may also add a degree of redundancy in the communication infrastructure if local telephony services are delivered via an independent telecommunication infrastructure, which could be a target for terrorist disruption. One advantage of Web-based communication is the capacity to view images, and a well-designed system that permitted the display of clinical images, radiological images and laboratory data would support a rich set of clinical interactions beyond the capability of traditional telephony.

Public health authorities can broadcast information to clinicians to raise their level of awareness and suspicion during a suspected bioagent exposure (authority push asynchronous broadcast)

If we consider clinicians to be an event detection system, then in normal circumstances their level of suspicion of bioterrorist attack is likely to be low. Even with repeated warnings to keep alert, in the absence of genuine threats, the information overload under which clinicians operate suggests that they will soon return to a low level of background awareness. Such a conclusion is supported by the poor performance of routine CPE in changing clinical practice. Consequently, it is the role of public health authorities to 'calibrate' physicians to a higher degree of suspicion during periods of suspected or confirmed bioterrorist attack, rather than to routinely remind clinicians to be alert in the absence of a genuine threat.

In such cases, the need is to maximize the reach of communication, aiming to maximize the audience reached. Given that clinicians are likely to be in a variety of locations, perhaps mobile, and have access to different communication channels at any given time, a clinical broadcast system relying solely on the Web will not act as a rapid emergency broadcast channel. Some form of public broadcast including radio, television and printed media might be considered. However, if the need is to reach clinicians without raising undue public concern, then an alternative broadcast system is required. An alternative strategy is to deliver highly specific messages to clinicians on pre-specified channels. For this to occur, a record needs to be kept of each clinician in an area, and the communication channels they have, e.g. telephone, mobile, pager, fax and mobile phone numbers, e-mail address.

The UK has an emergency 'cascade' system called Public Health Link, which operates in this way. Public Health Link is an electronic urgent communication system to health professionals that is initiated in the office of the Chief Medical Officer (similar to the Surgeon-General's office in the US). Messages cascade from the broadcasting health authority to a set of regions each with the responsibility of contacting the clinicians in their area, using the channels designated by clinicians ahead of time. Thus, urgent messages are sent to health authorities for onward cascade to nominated professionals, which may include general practitioners, practice nurses, community services pharmacists, medical directors in NHS Trusts, etc.

The system comprises a pager alert mechanism so that health authorities are aware when a message has been sent. Messages are classified as for cascade either within 6 hours (immediate) or 24 hours (urgent). The system aims to reach every clinician in the national health system in 24 hours. Urgent and immediate communications from the Chief Medical Officer on public health are transmitted on average 15 times a year and are most likely to be connected with issues about drugs, infections, vaccines or other public health matters. As well as being cascaded, the health link messages are archived at a Web site, where they can be viewed.

Conclusions

The problem of detection and reporting of suspected bioterrorist events by community clinicians is a complex one, and will not yield to simple strategies such as the introduction of stand-alone bioterrorist Web site accompanied by a clinician education programme.

A detailed analysis of the communication tasks associated with reporting does show many ways in which the Web and CDSSs, can play a significant part in the surveillance system.

However, the need for clinicians to interact with others to assist the decision process, as well as the demands of rapid notification in the event of a suspected bioterrorist event, demand a more integrated approach, using a mixture of communication channels and decision support systems.

Discussion points

1. What is the role of public education in biosurveillance?
2. Describe the socio-technical challenges to implementing a biosurveillance system.
3. How would you construct a biosurveillance system if the Web did not exist? What if CDSS did not exist?

Chapter summary

1. The bioterrorist threat challenges the public health system to create biosurveillance systems that maximize the likelihood of the early detection of bioterrorist events, as well as ensuring the rapid and direct reporting of these events.
2. For a bioterrorist event to be identified rapidly and accurately, several critical events must occur:
   - the event needs to be **detected**
   - the event needs to be **recognizable**
   - the existence of the event needs to be **communicated** rapidly.
3. A biosurveillance system in the broadest sense is not just a piece of technology but a complex socio-technical system of people, processes, channels and tools.
4. Infectious disease surveillance systems play a key role in bioagent detection. There is a substantial underreporting of notifiable infectious diseases by medical practitioners and consequently automated laboratory reporting systems have a key role in the detection of attack by bioagents, since they will in all probability detect more infected patients and report them more quickly.
5. CDSS can look for patterns in data, and correlate them with patient-specific data, to generate flags highlighting potentially suspicious or noting patterns in other similar cases, and may generate the first signal of a bioterrorist event.
6. Clinical education alone is unlikely to enhance event detection and recognition. Online evidence retrieval and CDSS can help support education and decision-making. However, an online just-in-time system needs to also function as a communication tool, connecting clinicians with questions to those who have answers.
7. The Web will need to be used in combination with other communication technologies such as fax, telephone and pagers to support biosurveillance.

CHAPTER 29

Bioinformatics

I. S. Kohane and E. Coiera

In the early 1980s, methods for DNA sequencing became widely available, and produced an exponential growth in molecular sequence data. Initially researchers had to painstakingly isolate individual genes and then attempt to associate them with specific functions or diseases. However, the arrival of bulk sequencing methods soon meant that for the first time, scientists could decode the genetic programmes for whole organisms.

From the mid-1990s onwards, genetic sequence data for the whole genome of organisms were amassed, including bacteria such as *Haemophilus influenza* and *Mycobacterium tuberculosis*, through to more complex multicellular organisms like the fruit fly *Drosophila melanogaster.* This frenetic activity culminated in the production of the draft sequence of the human genome. Completely sequenced genomes are now available for more than 100 organisms (Kanehisa and Bork, 2003).

Databases such as GenBank and EMBL (the European Molecular Biology Laboratory nucleotide sequence database) were developed to accommodate this growth in sequence data, and were made available to the research community through the Internet. In parallel, computational methods had to be developed to support retrieval and analysis of these large data sets. For example, scientists required algorithms to perform sequence similarity searches, so that they could find out whether the gene sequence data they were working with had already been identified or were similar to other documented genetic fragments.

Bioinformatics (or computational biology) is the name given to these computationally intense activities associated with the genome sciences. Bioinformatics is also concerned with the analysis of proteins and other elements of cell biology, and their exploitation to develop therapeutic agents (see Box 29.1).

Box 29.1
The bioinformatics family

Genomics: Determination of the DNA sequence of genes and, through the specialty of **functional genomics**, the identification of the functional role of these genes in cellular biology.
Proteomics: The study of all the proteins expressed within the cell. This includes determining the number, level, and turnover of all expressed proteins, their sequence, and protein interactions within the cell and across the cell membrane.
Transcriptomics: Study of mRNA molecules, which are involved in the transcription of DNA codes and their transport from the nucleus to the cell.
Glycomics: Study of cellular carbohydrates.
Metabolomics: Study of the small molecules generated in the synthetic and degradation pathways of cellular metabolism.
Pharmacogenomics: The identification of genetic markers that assist in predicting whether a patient will respond well to a therapy, or experience side effects.

In previous chapters we have examined decision support technologies from the point of view of the clinician who is faced with complex decisions in the workplace. In this final chapter on decision support technologies we explore bioinformatics and see how intelligent systems also have a critical role in supporting science and the development of therapeutic agents.

Indeed, the growth of bioinformatics has been driven as much by advances in informatics as by advances in basic biology. Although many see bioinformatics as a separate discipline to health informatics, in many ways it is a sub-discipline or speciality of the broader health informatics enterprise. We will thus also see how basic informatics technologies such as the EMR and the Internet are essential technologies if basic gene data are to be correlated with human health and disease.

This chapter is based on Kohane *et al.*'s (2003) text *Microarrays for an Integrative Genomics*, and the reader is directed to that text for a more detailed description of the field of bioinformatics, which has a particular emphasis on the use of microarray technologies. A brief primer on DNA biology is presented in Box 29.2, for those with limited biology training.

29.1 Genome science is rich in sequence data but poor in functional knowledge

Since DNA sequencing techniques were invented 25 years ago, the number of human gene sequences that have been identified has grown exponentially. In 2001 this rapid growth culminated in the entire human genome being sequenced as part of the **Human Genome Project**. In contrast, our knowledge of what these genes actually do has grown at a much slower rate.

In Figure 29.2, we can see that the number of entries in one of the major international public gene sequence repositories called GenBank (http://www.ncbi.nlm.nih.gov/Genbank/index.html) is rapidly outstripping the growth of Medline. As such, it demonstrates the large gap between our knowledge of the functioning of the genome and raw genomic data. Further, GenBank holds just a fraction of the available sequence data.

This volume of data must somehow be sifted and linked to human biology before it can have any meaning. Doing so exhaustively, reliably, and reproducibly is feasible only through the use of sophisticated algorithms and computer technology. However, the computational tools needed to extract knowledge from the gene data are still in their infancy, and novel tools are still needed to analyse the enormous databases.

Box 29.2
Gene biology

In almost all cells making up a living organism, there is an identical set of codes that regulate the function of the cell. This is encoded as one or more strands of the DNA molecule. The entire complement of DNA molecules of each organism is known as its **genome**. The overall function of the genome is to drive the generation of molecules, mostly proteins, which will regulate the metabolism of a cell and its response to the environment. The genome is the same in almost every cell in the human body. For instance, a liver cell and a brain cell have the same DNA content and code in their nucleus. What distinguishes cells in one organ or tissue from one another is that different portions of their DNA are active.

The structure of DNA

Each molecule of DNA may be viewed as a pair of chains of the nucleotide base molecules adenine (A), thymine (T), cytosine (C), and guanine (G). The two DNA strands join at each base-pairing, where A binds to T and C binds to G. DNA is able to undergo duplication, which occurs through the coordinated action of many molecules, including **DNA polymerases** (synthesizing new DNA), **DNA gyrases** (unwinding the molecule), and **DNA ligases** (concatenating segments together).

Transcription of DNA into RNA

In order for the genome to direct or effect changes in the cytoplasm of the cell, a transcriptional program needs to be activated to generate new proteins in the cell. DNA remains in the nucleus of the cell, but most proteins are needed in the cytoplasm of the cell where many of the cell's functions are performed. Thus, DNA must be copied into a transportable molecule called ribonucleic acid (RNA). A **gene** is a single segment of the coding region that is transcribed into RNA.

RNA is generated from the DNA template in the nucleus of the cell through a process called **transcription**. The RNA sequence of base pairs generated in transcription corresponds to that in the DNA molecules using the complementary *A-T, C-G,* with the principal distinction being that the nucleotide uracil (U) is substituted for the thymine (T) nucleotide. Thus, the RNA alphabet is *ACUG* instead of the DNA alphabet *ACTG*. The specific RNA that codes for proteins is called **messenger RNA (mRNA)**. A diagram of the genetic information flow, from DNA to RNA to protein, is illustrated in Figure 29.1.

(*Contd.*)

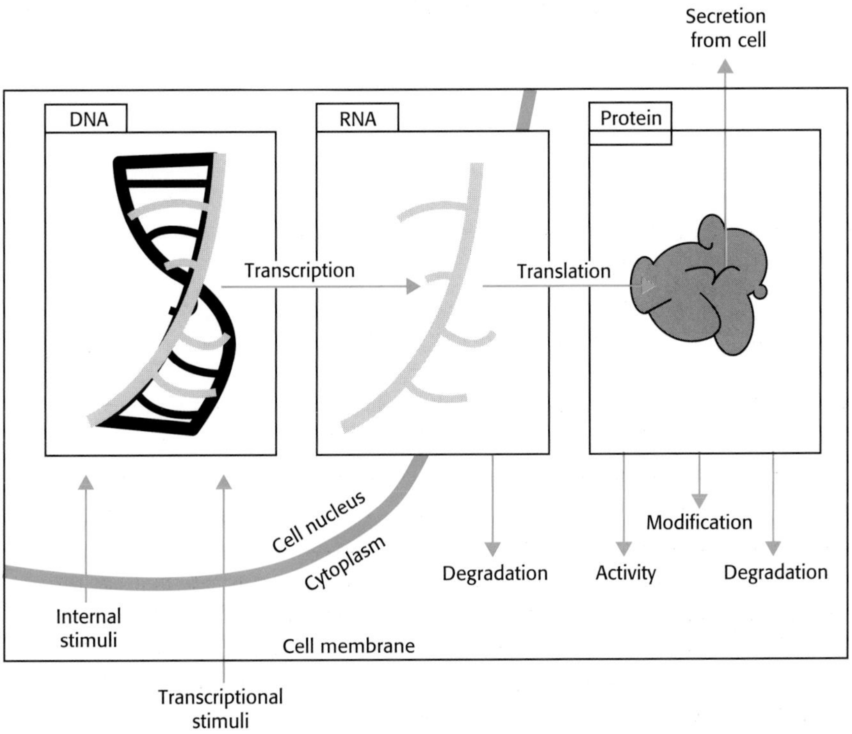
Secretion from cell
DNA
RNA
Protein
Transcription
Translation
Cell nucleus
Cytoplasm
Modification
Degradation
Activity
Degradation
Internal stimuli
Cell membrane
Transcriptional stimuli

Figure 29.1
Flow of genetic information, from DNA to RNA to protein. This simplified diagram shows how the production of specific proteins is governed by the DNA sequence through the production of RNA.

Box 29.2
(*Contd.*)

Structure and processing of RNA transcripts

Genes are not necessarily continuous. Instead, most genes contain **exons** (portions of the gene that will be placed into the mRNA) and **introns** (portions that will not appear in the mRNA but are 'spliced out' during transcription). Introns are not inert, however, and some functions have been recently discovered for them, such as promoter-like control of the transcription process. Further, introns are not always spliced consistently. If an intron is left in the mRNA, an **alternative splicing product** is created. Various tissue types can flexibly alter their gene products through alternative splicing. In fact, some cells can use the ratio of one alternative splicing to another to govern cellular behaviour.

After the splicing process, the mRNA molecule that has been generated is actively exported through nuclear pore complexes into the cell's cytoplasm. The cytoplasm is where the cellular machinery acts to generate the protein on the basis of the mRNA code. Specifically the ribosomal complex, which is a complex containing hundreds of proteins and special transfer RNA (tRNA) molecules, are directly involved in protein manufacture. A protein is built as a polymer or chain of amino acids, and the sequence of amino acids in a protein is determined by the mRNA template.

As an example, the DNA nucleotide sequence

GCT TGC AGA GCG

is transcribed into the mRNA sequence

GCU UGC AGA GCG

and is then transported into the cell cytoplasm, and translated into the amino acids

alanine cysteine arginine alanine

Note that both the initial GCU and the final GCG code for alanine because the code is degenerate (there is more than one way to code for some nucleotides); there are four codes for alanine in the standard genetic code.

Processing of amino acid chains

Once the protein is formed, it has to find the right place to perform its function, whether as a structural protein in the cytoskeleton, or as a cell membrane receptor, or as a hormone that is to be secreted by the cell. There is a complex cellular apparatus that determines this translocation process. One of the determinants of the location and handling of a polypeptide is a portion of the polypeptide called the **signal peptide**. This header of amino acids is recognized by the translocation machinery and directs the ribosome–mRNA complex to continue translation in a specific subcellular location, for example constructing and inserting a protein into the endoplasmic reticulum for further processing and secretion by the cell. Alternatively, particular proteins may be delivered after translation and chaperones can prevent proper folding until the protein reaches its correct destination.

Transcriptional programs

Initiation of the transcription process can be caused by external events or by a programmed event within the cell. For instance, the piezoelectric forces generated in bones through walking can gradually stimulate osteoblastic and osteoclastic transcriptional activity to cause bone remodelling. Similarly, heat shock or stress to the cell can cause rapid change or initiation of the transcriptional program. Additionally, changes in the microenvironment around the cell, such as the appearance of new micro- or macronutrients or the disappearance of these, will cause changes in the transcriptional program. Hormones secreted from distant organs bind to receptors that then directly or indirectly trigger a change in the transcriptional process. There are also fully autonomous, internally programmed sequences of transcriptional expression. A classic example of this is the internal pacemaker that governs our circadian rhythm. This is driven by the *clock* and *per* genes where, in the absence of any external stimuli, there is a recurring periodic pattern of transcriptional activity. Although this rhythmic pattern of transcription can be altered by external stimuli, it will continue initiating this pattern of transcription without any additional stimuli.

Finally, there are pathological internal derangements of the cell that can lead to transcriptional activity. Self-repair or damage-detection programs may be internal to the cell, and can trigger self-destruction (called **apoptosis**) under certain conditions, such as irreparable DNA damage. As another example, there may be a deletion mutation of a repressor gene causing the gene normally repressed to instead be highly active. There are many clinical instances of such disorders, such as familial male precocious puberty where puberty starts at infancy due to a mutation in the luteinizing hormone receptor. This receptor normally activates only when luteinizing hormone is bound, but with the mutation present, activation does not require binding.

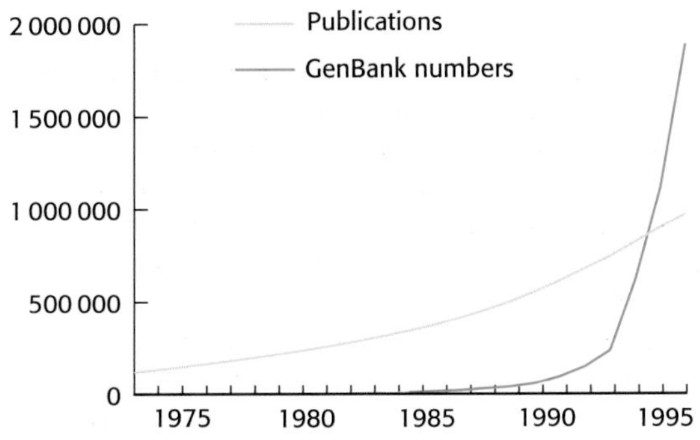
2 000 000
1 500 000
1 000 000
500 000
0
Publications
GenBank numbers
1975
1980
1985
1990
1995

Figure 29.2 Relative growth of Medline and GenBank. The cumulative growth of molecular biology and genetics literature (light grey) is compared here with DNA sequences (dark grey). Articles in the G5 (molecular biology and genetics) subset of Medline are plotted alongside DNA sequence records in GenBank over the same time period (after Ermolaeva *et al.*, 1998).

Bioinformatics tools are used in the quantitative and computational analysis of all forms of genomic data, including gene sequence, protein interactions and protein folding. The central hypothesis (or hope) of these methods is that, with improved techniques, one can analyse larger data sets and discover the 'true' biological functional pathways in gene regulation, and identify the characteristics of disease that most accurately predict the nature and course of disease.

29.2 Genome data can allow patient treatments to be highly tailored to the individual

The strong interest in decoding the human genome, and understanding the functional role that different genes play in health and disease, is driven by the hope that this will result in new ways of treating patients. Specifically, bioinformatics allows us to identify genes that indicate a patient's susceptibility to disease, assists in developing an understanding of the cellular pathways involved in generating the illness, and as a consequence provides an opportunity for the development of highly targeted therapies.

Consider the example of the analysis of large B-cell lymphoma conducted by Alizadeh *et al.* (2000). The researchers measured the expression level of thousands of genes in the lymphatic tissues of patients with this deadly malignancy of the lymphatic system, using DNA microarray technology. When a clustering analysis was performed to see which patients resembled one another the most on the basis of their gene expression pattern, two distinct clusters of patients were found. When the investigators examined the patients' histories it became apparent that the two clusters corresponded to two populations of patients with dramatically different mortality rates, as evidenced by a statistically significant difference in survival curves (Figure 29.3).

The implications of these two distinct mortality rates are profound:

- These investigators have discovered a new subcategory of large B-cell lymphoma, a new diagnosis with clinical significance.
- They have generated a tool that provides a new *prognosis*, so patients can be given much more precise estimates of their longevity.

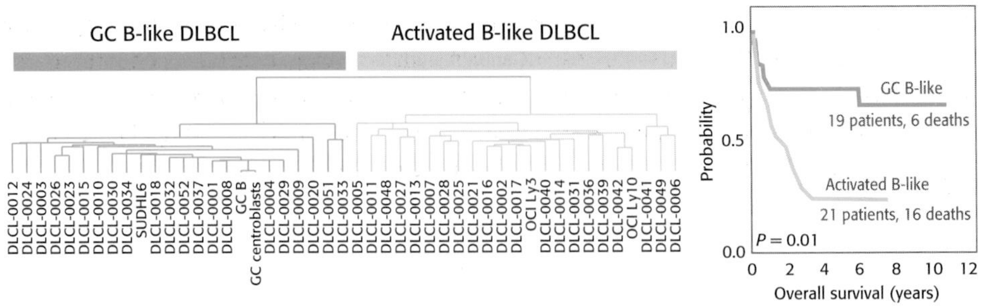
GC B-like DLBCL
Activated B-like DLBCL
Probability
1.0
0.5
0.0
GC B-like
19 patients, 6 deaths
Activated B-like
21 patients, 16 deaths
P = 0.01
0 2 4 6 8 10 12
Overall survival (years)

Figure 29.3 Subcategories of B-cell lymphoma determined by microarrays correspond clinically to duration of survival. On the left is a dendrogram (similar to a decision tree) that has been constructed across the samples of B-cell lymphoma, using an unsupervised learning technique. The top branch essentially defines an even split between the categories GC B-like DLBCL and Activated B-like DLBCL, but this distinction was never before made clinically. On the right are Kaplan–Meier survival curves of the patients from whom the samples were obtained. Patients whose cancer matched the Activated B-like DLBCL gene expression profile had a significantly worse prognosis (from Alizadeh *et al.*, 2000).

- A new *therapeutic* opportunity is provided, as the patients with an expression pattern predicting a poor response to standard therapy may be treated with different chemotherapy.
- There is a new *biomedical research* opportunity to uncover what it is about these two sub-populations that makes them so different in outcome and how that can be related to the differences in gene expression.

The range of potential bioinformatic approaches to the development of novel therapeutics is broad. Some are already having an impact on clinical practice, but others remain firmly experimental for the present.

Near patient testing

The identification of microorganisms has historically relied on culturing organisms or morphological identification in specialized laboratories. However, the ability to identify microorganisms genetically is enabling the detection, identification and characterization of infective pathogens to be done near the patient, whether at the hospital bedside, in general practice or at home (Borriello, 1999). Testing kits provide rapid analysis of a drop of blood, saliva or urine to detect if an infective pathogen is present and give an indication of its antimicrobial resistance potential. The technologies that make such test kits possible include microarrays or 'DNA chips'. Identifying genetic resistance markers allows a clinician to predict an organism's susceptibility to antimicrobial drugs, and select appropriate chemotherapy. The ability to identify how virulent an infection is likely to be, on the basis of genetic markers, should allow clinicians to make predictions of clinical outcome (Jenks, 1998). The detection of the flu virus or respiratory syncytial virus should reduce inappropriate antibiotic prescriptions. Near patient testing should also assist in controlling infectious disease in the community through rapid detection.

Pharmacogenomics

Bioinformatic analysis of genomic, pathological and clinical data from clinical trials can identify which sub-populations react well or poorly to a given drug. Simple genetic tests can then be used on prospective patients to determine whether they belong to a sub-population that is genetically predisposed to do well or poorly with that drug. Pharmacogenomics is thus likely to bring about a new age of personalized 'molecular' medicine, where a patient's unique genetic profile will be determined for certain drugs, with the aim of providing therapy that is targeted to their specific biological needs and is free from side effects.

Drug discovery

Genetic knowledge is enhancing our ability to design new drug therapies. For example, once the entire genome of an infective microorganism is available, it can be examined for potential molecular target sites for attack by specially designed drugs. Novel designer drugs such as *imatinib mesylate*, which interferes with the abnormal protein made in chronic myeloid leukaemia, have been produced using bioinformatics methods to identify and target specific human genetic markers (Bayat, 2002).

Gene therapies

For patients with genetically based chronic illnesses like cystic fibrosis, gene therapies are being pursued that should eventually offer the possibility of directly interacting with the defective genes to moderate, repress or disable the biochemical processes that result in the disease state.

29.3 Bioinformatics can answer many questions about the role of genes in human disease, but is limited by our ability to model biological processes

Now that the human genome has been sequenced (or, more accurately, now that a handful of human genomes have been sequenced), we are said to be in a postgenomic era. Knowing at least the draft outline for the human genome, we can begin to systematically deconstruct how the genetically programmed behaviour of human physiology is related to our genome. In this deconstruction, several kinds of biological information are available, including DNA sequences, physical maps, gene maps, gene polymorphism, protein structure, gene expression and protein interaction effects. By matching differences in phenotype (e.g. blood pressure, adult height) between individuals and their gene sequences, these phenotypic differences can be associated with a small span of the genome.

Functional genomics refers to the overall enterprise of deconstructing the genome and assigning biological function to genes. Functional genomics aims to use genome–phenotype associations to answer broad questions about the role of specific genes in health and disease. Examples of some of the broad questions that can be asked are:

- Given the effect of different drugs on cancer cell lines, which gene is the most predictive of the responsiveness of the cell line to the drugs?
- Given a known clinical distinction, such as between acute lymphocytic leukaemia (ALL) and acute myeloid leukaemia (AML), what is the minimal set of genes that can reliably distinguish these two diseases?

There is little doubt that one of the tremendous accomplishments of the Human Genome Project is that it has enabled a rigorous computational approach to identifying many questions of interest to the biological and clinical community at large. However, the danger of this success is a computational triumphalism, which believes that all the problems of disease will now rapidly be solved. Such a view relies on several dubious assumptions, most of them based on a misunderstanding of the nature of models, and in particular the complexity of biological models.

NP-computabilty
Some problems are harder to solve for computers than others. The time it takes for a computer to solve a problem can be characterized by the shape of the 'time it takes to solve it' function. Some problems can be solved in linear time, making them easy to solve. Harder problems are said to take polynomial time because the 'time to solve it' function is of polynomial form. A further class of potentially intractable problems have superpolynomial or exponential time solutions. These are known as non-deterministic polynomial time (NP) problems, as it cannot be said ahead of time how long it might take to solve them once you start, or even if an answer will be found (although by luck you might just solve them).

The first misunderstanding is that of **genetic reductionism**. Most bioinformaticians understand that physiology is the product of the genome and its interaction with the environment (see Box 2.1). In practice, however, a computationally oriented investigator often assumes that all regulation can be inferred from DNA sequences. They assume one can predict whether a change in nucleotide sequence will result in a different physiology. However, cellular metabolic pathways are substantially more complicated than this, and involve many levels of interaction between molecules (Figure 29.4).

The second dubious assumption is the computability of complex biochemical phenomena. One of the oldest branches of bioinformatics models molecular interactions such as the thermodynamics of protein folding. As yet, all the combined efforts and expertise of bioinformaticians have been unable to provide a thermodynamically sound folding pattern of a protein in a cell for as long as 1 microsecond. Furthermore, studies by computer scientists over the last 10 years (Lathrop, 1994; Berger and Leighton, 1998) suggest that the protein-folding problem is **NP-hard**. That is, the computational challenge belongs to a class of problems that is believed to be computationally unsolvable.

Therefore it seems unduly ambitious to imagine that within the next decade we will be able to generate robust models that can accurately predict the interactions of thousands of molecules from the transcription of RNA through to protein manufacture and function. We refer to this ambition as **interactional reductionism**.

The final questionable assumption is the **closed-world assumption** (Box 3.2). Both sequence level reductionism and interactional reductionism are based on the availability of a reliable and complete mechanistic model. That is, if a fertilized ovum can follow the genetic program to create a full human being after 9 months, then surely a computer program should be able to follow the same genetic code to infer all the physiological events determined by the genetic code. Indeed, there have been several efforts, such as the E-cell effort of Tomohita *et al.* (1999), which aimed to provide robust models of cellular function based on the known regulatory behaviour of cellular systems. Although such models are important, our knowledge of all the relevant parameters for these models is still grossly incomplete today.

These caricatured positions of traditional molecular biologists and computational biologists are, of course, overdrawn. When prompted, most investigators will acknowledge these complexities of functional genomics but may nonetheless often retreat to the simplifications and assumptions described above.

29.4 Bioinformatics is made possible by the development of new measurement and analysis technologies

Bioinformatics brings together all kinds of genomic and phenotypic data and then attempts to integrate them to extract new knowledge about organism function, all in an efficient,

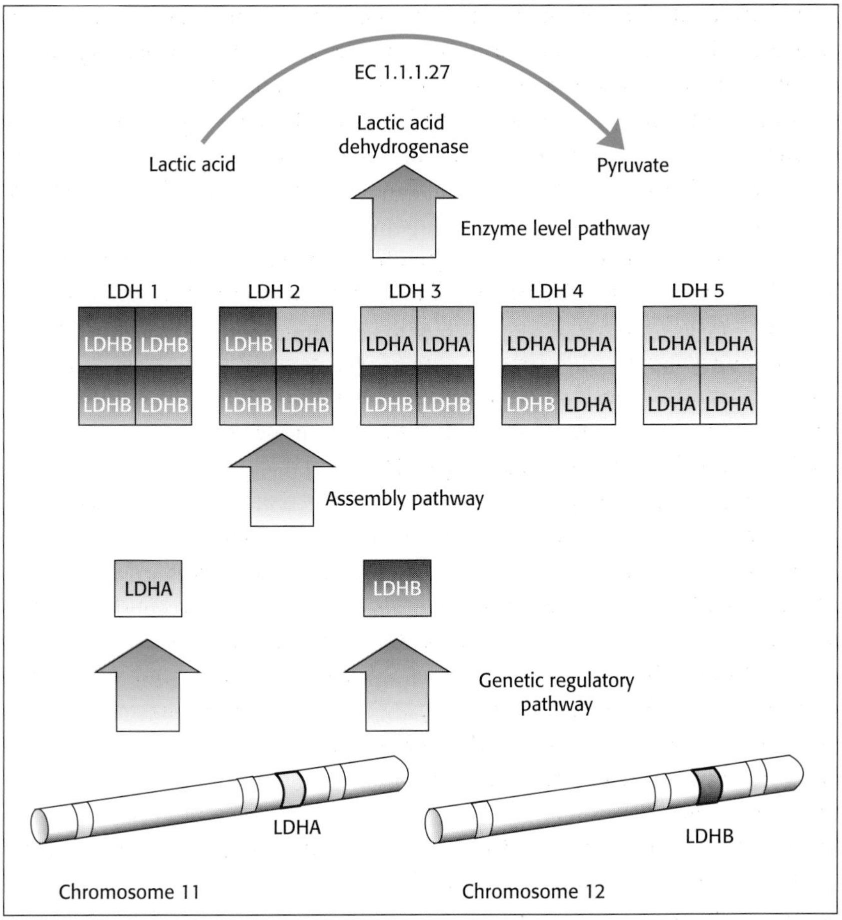
EC 1.1.1.27
Lactic acid
dehydrogenase
Lactic acid
Pyruvate
Enzyme level pathway
LDH 1
LDH 2
LDH 3
LDH 4
LDH 5
LDHB LDHB
LDHB LDHB
LDHB LDHA
LDHB LDHB
LDHA LDHA
LDHB LDHB
LDHA LDHA
LDHB LDHA
LDHA LDHA
LDHA LDHA
Assembly pathway
LDHA
LDHB
Genetic regulatory
pathway
LDHA
LDHB
Chromosome 11
Chromosome 12

Figure 29.4 An example of why discovery of pathways solely using gene expression measurements is difficult. At least three pathways are involved in the conversion of lactic acid to pyruvate. The highest enzyme level pathway involves the action of an enzyme called lactic acid dehydrogenase, designated EC 1.1.1.27. However, when one traverses to a lower-level pathway, one learns that the role of this enzyme is performed by five separate protein products, which appear in a binomial distribution. When one traverses lower, through the assembly pathway, one learns this distribution is present because of the various possible combinations of LDHA and LDHB, two individual protein subunits, of which four must be put together to make an active enzyme. Then, when one traverses even lower, through the genetic regulatory pathway, one learns that each of these subunits is regulated differently, and appears on different chromosomes. Not shown are the pathways involved in transcription, translation, movement of proteins to the appropriate locations, and movement of substrates into and out of the cells and organelles, and many other pathways.

large-scale, and timely fashion. For this functional genomic endeavour to succeed, bioinformatics has had to develop:

- methods to rapidly measure gene sequences and their expression in bulk
- methods to collect clinically relevant (phenotypic) data that measures human disease states
- methods that correlate the gene and phenotype data, and identify relevant associations
- methods for the storage and widespread dissemination of biological data.

The last few years have seen significant advances in each of these areas, although, as we have already seen, the production of gene data currently far outstrips our ability to carry out functional assessments of the meaning of genes.

Microarrays have enabled the large-scale measurement of gene activity

In the past, geneticists conducted clinical studies to identify the genes associated with a disease by obtaining DNA from a peripheral blood sample or a buccal smear from patients at risk. However, for some changes in genomic sequence, particularly with multigene regulation, the effects being studied can be so small that it would be hard to detect statistically significant correlations between genes and disease through population studies.

In contrast, functional genomic studies wish to directly measure the activity of the genes involved in a particular mechanism. There are many technologies that perform quantitative measurement of gene expression, but much of the current success in this field is centred on the development of **microarray technology**, where many genes can be measured simultaneously on a chip from a single tissue sample.

Microarrays, or 'DNA chips', are composed of a high-density array of DNA probes placed on a glass or nylon grid. Each probe is able to bind to and then recognize specified DNA segments in a sample. It is possible to manufacture single grids with many hundreds of thousands of different DNA probes. What distinguishes gene expression detection microarrays from earlier techniques is that they are able to measure tens of thousands of genes at a time and it is this quantitative change in the scale of gene measurement that has led to a qualitative change in our ability to understand regulatory processes occurring at the cellular level (Figure 29.5).

In microarray studies, mRNA is extracted from a sample of biological tissue and then a fluorescence-tagged complementary DNA (cDNA) copy of this mRNA is made. This tagged cDNA copy, called the **sample probe**, is then **hybridized** to a slide containing a grid of single-stranded cDNAs called **probes**. The probes are segments of DNA whose sequence is already known, and that have been built or placed in specific locations on this grid. A DNA sample probe will only hybridize with its complementary DNA probe. Since we know what DNA has been placed at each probe, we are therefore able to infer the type of DNA that has hybridized with it.

Hybridization is the interaction of complementary nucleic acid strands. Since DNA is a double-stranded structure held together by complementary interactions (in which C always binds to G, and A to T), complementary strands favourably bind or 'hybridize' to each other when separated.

Next, any unhybridized sample probes that are left are washed off and the microarray is lit by laser light and scanned. To determine the actual level of expression or concentration of DNA at a given probe, a digital image scanner records the brightness level at each grid location on the microarray. Studies have demonstrated that the brightness level is correlated with the absolute amount of RNA in the original sample, and by extension, the expression level of the gene associated with this RNA (Figure 29.6).

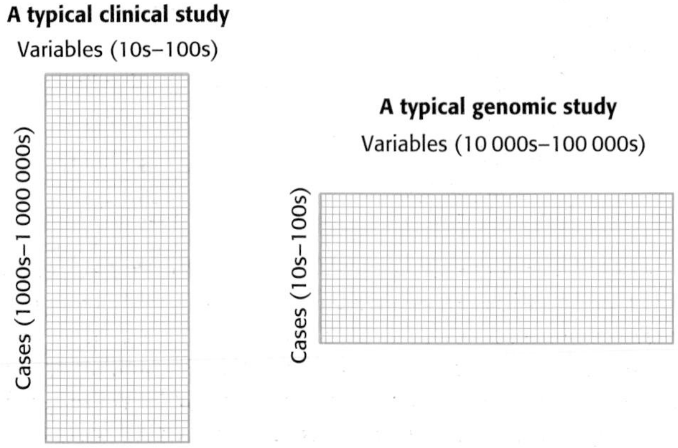
A typical clinical study
Variables (10s–100s)
Cases (1000s–1 000 000s)
A typical genomic study
Variables (10 000s–100 000s)
Cases (10s–100s)

Figure 29.5
Clinical studies typically measure few variables over many patients; gene studies typically measure many variables over few cases.

A characteristic of microarray technologies is that they enable the comprehensive measurement of the expression level of many genes simultaneously. Typical applications of microarrays include the quantification of RNA expression profiles of a sample under different experimental conditions, or the comparisons of two different samples.

The Internet has supported bioinformatics science by providing access to research and clinical databases

Some see the arrival of the Internet as the single most important computational advance in bioinformatics (Kanehisa and Bork, 2003), because it has transformed access to genetic sequence databases, software and the research literature. The Internet, with its ability to allow researchers to access databases irrespective of location, has facilitated the rapid sharing of new sequence data. Scientists not only publish their research results in biomedical journals, but add the new sequences to public databases, and make them immediately available for other researchers. There are two broad types of genetic database:

Databases of known genetic sequences can be used to identify unknown sequences obtained from patients

The introduction of the rapid sequence database search tool known as BLAST represented a major breakthrough for research scientists, as it allowed efficient search methods to examine the sequence data stored in genetic databases. A database search involves a comparison of the query DNA sequence against each sequence contained in the database. If a solid match is found for the query sequence, then the gene function may be predicted without the need for further laboratory experiments. BLAST looks for common patterns shared by two sequences and tries to extend these to obtain longer matches. BLAST (basic local alignment

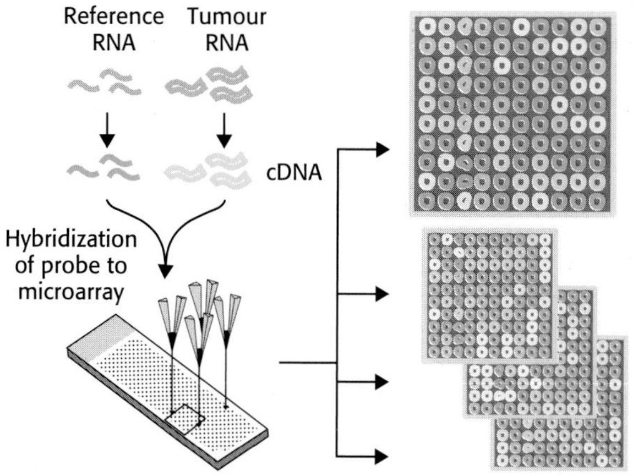
Reference RNA
Tumour RNA
cDNA
Hybridization of probe to microarray

Figure 29.6 An overview of procedures for preparing and analysing cDNA microarrays and tumour tissue, using robotically spotted microarray hybridized to two samples, each stained with two coloured dyes. Reference RNA and tumour RNA are labelled with different fluorescent dyes (dark orange for the reference and light orange for tumour) and hybridized to a microarray. The slides are scanned with a confocal laser-scanning microscope, and colour images are generated. Genes that have been upregulated in the tumour appear light orange, whereas those with decreased expression appear dark orange. Genes with similar levels of expression in the two samples appear grey.

search tool, www.ncbi.nlm.nih.gov/BLAST/) remains one of the best-known sites that provide this function.

Comprehensive descriptions of genetic disorders

A growing number of databases that contain genetic data of direct clinical relevance are now available for clinicians, including the Online Mendelian Inheritance in Man (OMIM) database (available at www3.ncbi.nlm.nih.gov/Omim/) which provides information on genetic disorders.

Phenotype data are stored in the patient medical record and require standard terminologies and ontologies to be meaningful

Functional genomics experiments can only have biological or clinical relevance if information external to the system being studied is also used. In experiments with the most obvious clinical relevance, such as finding genes that aid in the distinction between acute myeloid leukaemia (AML) and acute lymphoid leukaemia (ALL) (Golub *et al.*, 1999), the prognosis of large B-cell lymphoma (Alizadeh *et al.*, 2000) or pharmacogenomic prediction of gene targets for chemotherapy (Butte *et al.*, 2000), the correlation of external biological or clinical data with the gene expression data is central to the investigation.

If functional genomics is to lead to a change in the way in which clinical medicine is practised, then most studies will have to incorporate external data. That is, if we want to know how a gene expression pattern may predict mortality, a particular disease profile or drug responsiveness, we need to be at least as meticulous in characterizing the patients, their histories, and their tissues, as we are in obtaining the gene expression profile.

Electronic medical records

GenBank and the related genomic and protein databases are a central asset to functional genomics. In contrast, there are few, if any, shared clinical databases. Specifically, patient data in one information system can only rarely be transferred to another system in clinical practice. Yet, if properly constructed and maintained, electronic medical records (EMR) could provide an invaluable set of phenotypic data.

This contrast between the current state of genomic and clinical databases is somewhat deceptive. The Human Genome Project benefits from the elegant simplicity of the genetic code. There are relatively few items that GenBank requires for an entry to be a valid component to its database. The clinical care of human beings is more complex, requiring a detailed record of patient history and clinical measurements from serum chemistry to brain imaging.

It is therefore somewhat surprising that several efforts to develop clinical phenotype data models have been proposed, without much reference to existing efforts of the clinical informatics community. A more efficient mechanism might be for bioinformaticians to use existing clinical data models, such as the Health Level Seven (HL7) Reference Information Model (RIM).

Standardized vocabularies are needed for clinical phenotypes

Standardized clinical vocabularies are just as essential as standardized phenotypic data models. In the past, the lack of widely accepted standardized vocabularies for clinical care has greatly hampered the development of automated decision support tools and clinical research databases. Fortunately, as we saw in Chapter 17, many mature terminologies are now available. The US National Library of Medicine has invested large resources in the Unified Medical Language System (UMLS) to enable these different vocabularies to be interoperable, at least at a basic level. Nearly all of the most widely used vocabularies, such as Read codes, Medical Subject Headings, and Systematized Nomenclature of Medicine (SNOMED) are represented in the UMLS.

The same problems exist in bioinformatics. Many microarray technologies use their own system of accession numbers, which then have to be translated into a more widely used nomenclature such as LocusLink. When functional genomic investigations venture into the clinical domain, the lack of standardized clinical vocabularies will prevent the large-scale analysis of data. For example, if a set of genes is thought to be associated with a particular cardiac arrhythmia, this association will only be found if the nomenclature used to describe the arrhythmias in different clinical databases is drawn from the same standardized vocabulary.

Bio-ontologies

Individual biologists are usually expert in the specific area they are studying, and therefore are able to recognize the meaning of correlations found between genes, proteins or phenotypic features. However, the rapid growth in genetic and phenotypic data sets means that this process of assigning meaning to computer-identified associations will have to be automated. For a computer to be able to assign meaning, it will require access to a knowledge base that describes the domain of interest.

Ontologies are one form of domain knowledge that has attracted much interest in bioinformatics. The role of an ontology is to provide a conceptual map that allows automated reasoning to occur, and we have already encountered this concept several times in this book. For example, an ontology would allow a computer to recognize that 'penicillin is a kind of bone' is a nonsense association, even though an analysis of a data set found that many patients with osteomyelitis had been treated with penicillin. The ontology directs the identification of associations that are likely to be meaningful, so that a computer might decide that the most plausible of the associations it has found is that 'penicillin treats bone infections'.

In functional genomics, bio-ontologies refer to organized and formalized systems of concepts of biological relevance and the possible relationships between these concepts. For example, a bio-ontology would describe the kinds of relationships that exist between a gene and a protein, or a protein and a disease.

The Gene Ontology (GO) consortium is one of the more high-profile efforts that have developed in response to the pressing need for a unifying conceptual framework for genomics. The goal of the GO consortium is to provide a controlled vocabulary for the description of three independent ontologies (Ashburner *et al.*, 2000):

- **A description of molecular function:** This describes the biochemical activity of the entity such as whether it is a transcriptional factor, a transporter or an enzyme, without identifying where the functions occur or whether they are part of a larger biochemical process (Figure 29.7).
- **The cellular component within which gene products are located:** This provides localization of a gene product's molecular function, such as the ribosome or mitochondrion. Localization can help determine whether a function could occur through direct physical interaction between gene products or as a result of an indirect mechanism.

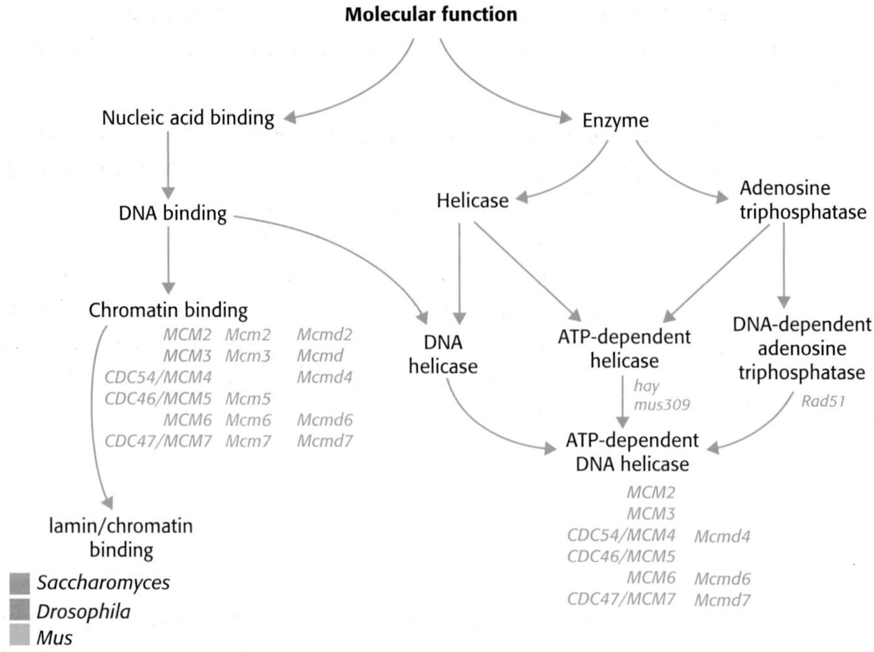

Molecular function
Nucleic acid binding
Enzyme
DNA binding
Helicase
Adenosine triphosphatase
Chromatin binding
MCM2 Mcm2 Mcmd2
MCM3 Mcm3 Mcmd
CDC54/MCM4 Mcmd4
CDC46/MCM5 Mcm5
MCM6 Mcm6 Mcmd6
CDC47/MCM7 Mcm7 Mcmd7
DNA helicase
ATP-dependent helicase
DNA-dependent adenosine triphosphatase
hay
mus309
Rad51
ATP-dependent DNA helicase
MCM2
MCM3
CDC54/MCM4 Mcmd4
CDC46/MCM5
MCM6 Mcmd6
CDC47/MCM7 Mcmd7
lamin/chromatin binding
Saccharomyces
Drosophila
Mus

Figure 29.7
The molecular function ontology of GO (from Ashburner *et al.*, 2000).

- **The biological process implemented by the gene products:** Biological process refers to a higher-order process, such as pyrimidime metabolism, protein translation or signal transduction.

The goal of such a set of ontologies is to allow queries to be made across a number of different databases, with the GO terms ensuring that the results from the different databases are biologically consistent.

Despite the limitations of the simple ontologies of GO, early efforts to annotate genomes using this infrastructure appear very promising, notably the GO annotations in the LocusLink site of the National Centre for Biotechnology Information (NCBI) (http://www.ncbi.nlm.nih.gov/LocusLink/).

Privacy of clinical data

As the fruits of the Human Genome Project are translated into clinical practice, personally identifiable genomic data will find their way into the EMR. Genomic information is likely to be much more predictive of current and future health status than most clinical measurements. Also, with very few exceptions, an individual's genome is uniquely identifying. In practice, however, the ease with which an individual can already be identified provides ample opportunity for breaches of privacy, even without genetic information.

Nonetheless, the architects of information systems storing genetic data can learn from the security architectures and privacy policies of conventional clinical information systems. The concerns voiced over the storage of personal genetic data will also probably generate new policies and security architectures that will enhance the confidentiality of all clinical information systems. When personal genetic data become incorporated into routine medical practice, it may also lead to an increase in the degree to which patients control their own medical record (Mandl *et al.*, 2001).

In theory, if privacy is to be protected, a database has to be truly anonymous, so that if it fell into the possession of an unscrupulous party, no harm could be done. There are two broad approaches to anonymizing a database:

- To delete or replace common identifying attributes, such as name, date of birth or address, which could be used very easily with external databases to identify the patient. The risk with this approach is that although it does indeed reduce the ease of identification, the records can still in principle be identifiable.
- To segregate those fields, including name and addresses, that would be the most revealing of the patient's identity and place them into a separate identification database controlled by a trusted third party who would only allow the patient data to be 'joined' to the non-identifying data with explicit permission of the patient or the institutional review board of a research institution.

Machine learning methods can assist in the discovery of associations between genetic and phenotypic data

We saw earlier that microarray data generate potentially many thousands of gene expression measurements from a few tissue samples, in contrast to typical clinical studies, which measure few variables over many cases. This high dimensionality of gene expression data poses problems for standard statistical analysis, since not enough data may be available to solve all the 'variables' in the data set, leaving it relatively undetermined. For example, to solve a linear equation of one variable, e.g. $4x = 5$, we only need one equation to find the value of the variable. To solve a linear equation of two variables, e.g. $y = 4x + b$, two equations are required. If we have tens of thousands of variables, but only hundreds of equations, then there will be thousands of potentially valid solutions. This is the essence of what constitutes an **underdetermined** system. High-dimensionality data sets are well known in machine learning, so it is not surprising that these techniques have found their way into functional genomics.

Machine learning techniques can be classified either as **supervised learning** or **unsupervised learning** techniques. These are also commonly known as classification techniques and clustering techniques, respectively. The two classes of techniques are distinguished by the presence of external labels on the data being examined:

- **Supervised learning:** Before applying a supervised learning technique, each datum needs to be assigned a label. For example, we would label a tissue as coming from a case of AML or ALL before learning which combinations of variables predicted those labels. This type of learning is used in neural network and decision tree construction, which can then be easily translated into diagnostic algorithms. The goal is typically to obtain a set of variables (e.g. expressed genes as measured on a microarray) that categorize a patient or tissue as part of a class of interest.
- **Unsupervised learning:** Here, data patterns are determined without labels. For example we may wish to find those genes that are co-regulated across all samples. The kinds of variables (also known as **features**) that characterize each case in a data set can be quite varied. Each case can include measures of clinical outcome, gene expression, gene sequence, drug exposure and proteomic measurements. Unsupervised techniques include relevance networks, dendrograms and self-organizing maps that analyse every

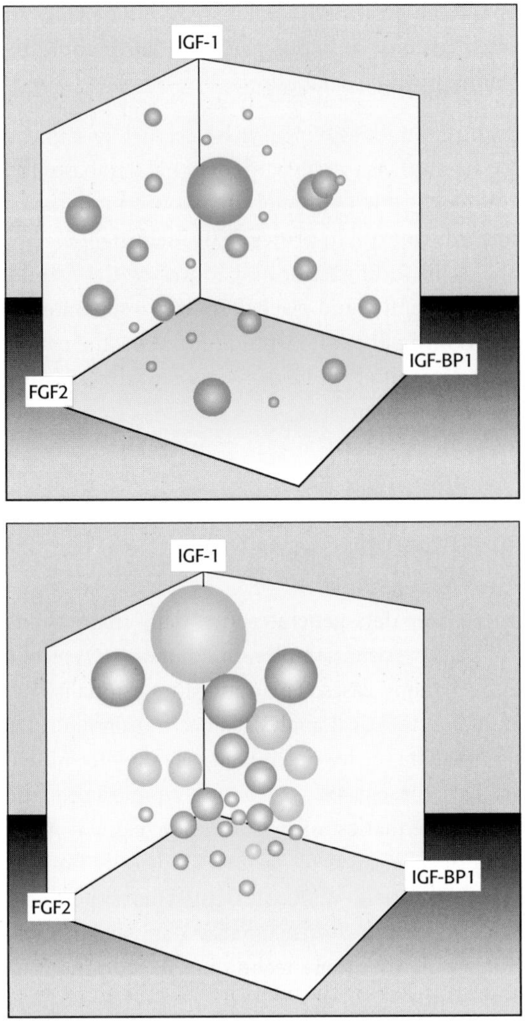
IGF-1
IGF-BP1
FGF2
IGF-1
IGF-BP1
FGF2

Figure 29.8
Expression space in which gene expression is loosely versus tightly coupled. If genes are tightly coupled in the expression space, they will tend to occupy a small subspace of expression space over any set of experiments. If, however, these genes are loosely coupled or even causally unrelated, then their expression levels will have little relation to one another and therefore tend to be scattered over a greater volume of the expression space.

possible pair of genes to determine whether a functional relationship exists between them. The end result of this analysis is a ranked list of hypotheses of pairs of genes that could work together. The typical application is to 'data mine' and either to find a completely novel cluster of genes with a hypothesized common function, or more commonly, to obtain a cluster of genes that appear to have patterns of expression that are similar to an already known gene (Figure 29.8).

The strengths of relationships found by clustering algorithms are not all necessarily novel or illuminating, however. For example, a case might include several thousand gene expression measurements and several hundred phenotypic measurements such as blood pressure (Figure 29.9). A clustering algorithm can be used to find those features that are most tightly coupled within the data set. However, the clustering algorithm may reveal more significant relationships between non-genomic variables than between genes. For example, if one looks at the effect of different drugs on a cancer cell line, then these drug effects might be tightly clustered around drugs that are derived from one another. Similarly, phenotypic features that are interdependent, such as height and weight, will also cluster together. The strength of these

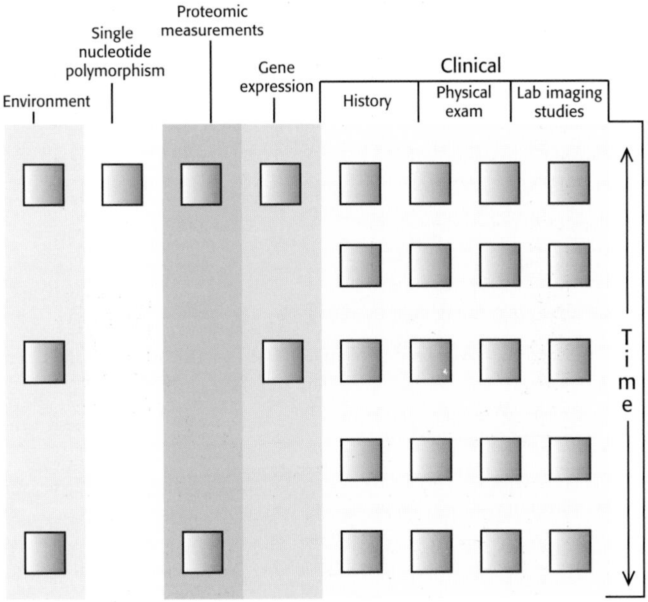
Proteomic measurements
Single nucleotide polymorphism
Environment
Gene expression
Clinical
History
Physical exam
Lab imaging studies
Time

Figure 29.9
Clustering more than only expression values. A full-fledged functional genomic study with clinical relevance will involve multiple and quite heterogeneous data types. The realities of clinical research and clinical care will ensure that there is a requirement for the handling of missing data.

obvious clusters will often dominate those of clusters that combine phenotypic and gene expression measurements.

Conclusions

Bioinformatics is a rapidly moving field, and although technically a subspecialty of health informatics, is in the short term likely to develop relatively independently of the broader health informatics agenda. However, as we have seen, the only way the functional genomic research programme can proceed is through the use of computational tools like machine learning, and through the use of phenotypic data, which is stored in the EMR. As such, it is inconceivable that clinically oriented bioinformatics will drift further away from health informatics in the longer term. Rather, the two will become more deeply entwined, as bioinformatics researchers become more dependent on health terminologies, ontologies and the EMR. Similarly, health informatics will start to change, as the influx of genetic data and knowledge changes the practice of medicine, and as a consequence alters the nature of the decision tasks in healthcare. In the future, clinical decision support systems, computer protocol systems, clinical vocabularies and the medical record will all have shifted in both design and function, as they incorporate the fruits of the bioinformatics revolution.

Discussion points

1 What is a gene chip?

2 In the future, clinicians will no longer need to carry out extensive examinations of patients. Rather, all we will need to treat patients is a map of their genome. Do you agree?

3 Are your genes your destiny?

4 What is data mining?

5 Describe how a clinician might use a gene chip in their office to deliver patient-specific care. Describe each of the major enabling technologies needed to make the whole system work.

6 Can you see any cultural or organizational barriers to the uptake of clinical bioinformatics technologies?

7 Decision theory incorporates probabilities and utilities into decision structures to capture both the likely biological outcomes of different treatments, as well as the values we assign to different outcomes. Will there be a place for values in genetic decisions?

8 Describe how you think bioinformatics will alter the path of health informatics.

9 Describe how you think health informatics will alter the path of bioinformatics.

10 Could the Human Genome Project have succeeded without computer technology?

11 Which attributes of the World Wide Web have been responsible for its pivotal role in the development of bioinformatics?

Chapter summary

1 **Bioinformatics** is the name given to the collection, organization and computational analysis of large biological data sets from genomics, proteomics, drug screening and medicinal chemistry sequences. Bioinformatics also includes the integration and 'mining' of the ever-expanding databases of information from these disciplines.

2 Since DNA sequencing techniques were invented 25 years ago, the number of human gene sequences that have been identified through experiments has grown exponentially. In contrast, our knowledge of what these genes actually do has grown at a much slower rate, demonstrating the large gap that has now opened up between our knowledge of the functioning of the genome and raw genomic data.

3 The strong interest in decoding the human genome, and understanding the functional role that different genes play in health and disease, is driven by the hope that such an understanding will result in new ways of treating patients, including new genetic therapies, but also the ability to genetically type individuals to determine which type of traditional therapy is most likely to be successful with them. New types of therapy are possible through the use of near patient testing systems, **pharmacogenomics**, genetically inspired drug discovery and gene therapies.

4 Although the Human Genome Project has been tremendously successful, there is danger of **computational triumphalism**, which believes that all the problems of disease will now rapidly be solved. However, such a view relies on several dubious assumptions, most based upon a misunderstanding of the nature of models, and in particular the complexity of biological models.

5 **Functional genomics** refers to the overall enterprise of deconstructing the genome and assigning biological function to genes, groups of genes, and particular gene interactions to answer broad questions about the role of specific genes in health and disease.

6 Functional genomics is made possible by the development of new measurement and analysis technologies:
- methods to rapidly measure gene sequences and their expression in bulk. in particular, **microarrays** have enabled the large-scale measurement of gene activity.
- methods to collect clinically relevant (phenotypic) data that measures human disease states. the EMR is an essential technology here, as are clinical vocabularies, **bio-ontologies** and methods to secure the privacy of medical records containing genetic information.
- methods that correlate the gene and phenotype data, and identify relevant associations. Machine learning methods can assist in the discovery of associations between genetic and phenotypic data, and can be classified either as supervised or unsupervised learning techniques. These are also commonly known as **classification techniques** and **clustering techniques** respectively.

Glossary

Abduction: A form of logical inference, commonly applied in the process of medical diagnosis. Given an observation, abduction generates all known causes. See also: Deduction, Induction, Inference.

Agent: Computer software constructed to operate with a degree of autonomy from its user, e.g. an agent may search the Internet for information based upon loose specifications provided by its user. Also, more generally, any human or computational entity capable of autonomous behaviour. See also: Artificial intelligence.

Algorithm: A set of instructions to programmatically carry out some task. In clinical practice algorithms usually, but not always, involve some form of numerical calculation. See also: Care pathway, Guideline, Protocol, Practice parameter.

Alphabet: The set of symbols that defines a particular language. See: Language.

Alternative splicing product: Variation in the way pre-mRNA is spliced together. Introns are typically spliced (removed) from pre-mRNA and the remaining exons are pieced together to form a contiguous transcript of mRNA (see Exon). However, the same set of introns may not always be spliced out, and the resultant mRNA may have a different combination of introns and exons. These alternative versions of the mRNA result in different downstream proteins being formed (alternative splicing products). Alternative splicing products are one reason why the number of gene products is much larger than the number of genes.

Application: Synonym for a computer program that carries out a specific type of task. Word-processors or spreadsheets are common applications available on personal computers.

Arden syntax: A language created to encode actions within a clinical protocol into a set of situation-action rules, for computer interpretation, and also to facilitate exchange between different institutions.

ARPAnet: Advanced Research Projects network. A computer network developed by the United States Department of Defence in the late 1960s, and the forerunner of today's Internet.

Artificial intelligence (AI): Any artefact, whether embodied solely in computer software, or a physical structure like a robot, that exhibits behaviours associated with human intelligence. Also the study of the science and methods for constructing such artefacts. See also: Turing test.

Artificial intelligence in medicine: The application of artificial intelligence methods to solve problems in medicine, e.g. developing expert systems to assist with diagnosis, or therapy planning. See also: Artificial intelligence, Expert system.

ASCII: American standard code for information interchange. Standard that defines a digital representation of alphabetic characters in text so that text files can be exchanged between computers.

Asynchronous communication: A mode of communication between two parties, when the exchange does not require both to be active participant in the conversation at the same time, e.g. sending a letter. See also: E-mail, Isochronous communication, Synchronous communication.

ATM (asynchronous transfer mode): A packet-based communication protocol that provides the high-bandwidth transmission rates required for multimedia communication. See also: Circuit-switched network, Packet-switched network.

Bandwidth: Amount of data that can be transmitted across a communication channel over a given period of time. See also: Bits per second, Channel capacity.

Base pair: The chemical structure that forms the units of DNA and RNA and that encode genetic information. The bases that make up the base pairs are adenine (A), guanine (G), thymine (T), cytosine (C), and uracil (U). See also: DNA.

Bayes' theorem: Theorem used to calculate the relative probability of an event given the probabilities of associated events. Used to calculate the probability of a disease given the frequencies of symptoms and signs within the disease and within the normal population. See also: Conditional probability, Posterior probability; Prior probability.

Bioinformatics: The collection, organization, and analysis of large amounts of biological data, using computers and databases. Historically, bioinformatics concerned itself with the analysis of the sequences of genes and their products (proteins), but the field has since expanded to the management, processing, analysis, and visualization of large quantities of data from genomics, proteomics, drug screening, and medicinal chemistry. Bioinformatics also includes the integration and 'mining' of the ever-expanding databases of information from these disciplines.

B-ISDN (broadband ISDN): A set of communication system standards for ATM systems. See: ATM, ISDN.

Bit: One binary digit, in base 2. The basic unit for electronically stored or transmitted data. See also: Byte.

Bits per second: A measure of data transmission rate. See also: Bit.

Bluetooth: Wireless communication system designed to allow many personal devices such as computers, mobile phones, and digital cameras to communicate with each other over a short range.

Boolean logic: A system of logic devised by Georges Boole that defined the meaning of linguistic notions like *and*, *or* and *not* to produce 'laws of thought' which had a clear syntax and semantics.

Broadband network: General term for a computer network capable of high-bandwidth transmission. See also: ATM.

Browser: A program used to view data, e.g. examining the contents of a database or knowledge base, or viewing documents on the World Wide Web. See also: Internet; Mosaic, World Wide Web.

Byte: Eight bits. Bytes are usually counted in kilobytes (1024 bytes), megabytes, and gigabytes. See also: Bit.

Care pathway: Describes the expected course of the patient's management and what actions need to be taken at every stage. See also: Algorithm, Guideline, Practice parameter, Protocol.

Case-based reasoning: An approach to computer reasoning that uses knowledge from a library of similar cases, rather than by accessing a knowledge base containing more generalized knowledge, such as a set of rules. See also: Artificial intelligence, Expert system.

Causal reasoning: A form of reasoning based on following from cause to effect, in contrast to other methods in which the connection is weaker, such as probabilistic association.

CERN (Conseil Européan pour la Recherche Nucléaire): The European Particle Physics Laboratory. It was here that the initial set of standards were developed to create the World Wide Web. See: HTML, HTTP, WWW.

Channel capacity: Amount of data that can be transmitted per unit time along a communication channel. Synonym: Bandwidth.

Channel: The connection between two parties that transports their messages, such as a telephone or e-mail.

Chromosome: One of the physically separate segments that together forms the genome, or total genetic material, of a cell. Chromosomes are long strands of genetic material, or DNA, that have been packaged and compressed by wrapping around proteins. The number and size of chromosomes varies from species to species. In humans, there are 23 pairs of chromosomes (a pair has one chromosome from each parent). One pair forms the sex chromosomes because they contain genes that determine sex. The chromosome carrying the male determining genes is designated Y and the corresponding female one is the X chromosome. The remaining pairs are called autosomes. Chromosome 1 is the largest and chromosome, 22 the smallest. Each chromosome has two 'arms' designated p and q.

Circuit-switched network: A communication network that connects parties by establishing a dedicated circuit between them. See also: Packet-switched network.

Client: A computer connected to a network that does not store all the data or software it uses, but retrieves it across the network from another computer that acts as a server. See also: Client–server architecture, Server.

Client–server architecture: A computer network architecture that places commonly used resources on centrally accessible server computers, which can be retrieved as they are needed across the network by client computers on the network. See also: Client, Server.

Closed-loop control: Completely automated system control method in which no part of the control system need be given over to humans. See also: Open-loop control.

Code: In medical terminological systems, the unique numerical identifier associated with a medical concept, which may be associated with a variety of terms, all with the same meaning. See also: Term.

Cognitive science: A multidisciplinary field studying human cognitive processes, including their relationship to technologically embodied models of cognition. See also: Artificial intelligence.

Communication protocol: The rules governing how a conversation may proceed between well-behaved agents. See also: OSI seven-layer model.

Complementary DNA (cDNA): DNA that is synthesized from a messenger RNA template; the single-stranded form is often used as a probe in physical mapping or for detecting RNA. Since cDNA is constructed from messenger RNA (after introns have been spliced out), it does not contain introns.

Computerized protocol: Clinical guideline or protocol stored on a computer system, so that it may be easily accessed or manipulated to support the delivery of care. See also: Clinical guideline.

Conditional probability: The probability that one event is true, given that another event is true. See: Bayes' theorem.

Connectionism: The study of the theory and application of neural networks. See: Neural network.

Control system: A system that utilizes measurement of its output and feedback to influence future behaviour based upon a measurement of past performance. See: Cybernetics, Feedback, System.

CPR (computer-based patient record): See: Electronic medical record.

CSCW (computer supported cooperative work): The study of computer systems developed to support groups of individuals work together. See also: Groupware.

Cybernetics: A name coined by Norbert Weiner in the 1950s to describe the study of feedback control systems and their application. Such systems were seen to exhibit properties associated with human intelligence and robotics, and so cybernetics was an early contributor to the theory of artificial intelligence.

Cyberspace: Popular term now associated with the Internet, which describes the notional information 'space' that is created across computer networks. See also: Virtual reality.

Database: A structured repository for data, consisting of a collection of data and their associated data model, and usually stored on a computer system. The existence of a regular and formal indexing structure permits rapid retrieval of individual elements of the database. See also: Knowledge base, Model.

Decision support system: General term for any computer application that enhances a human's ability to make decisions.

Decision tree: A method of representing knowledge which structures he elements of a decision into a tree-like fashion. Chance nodes in a decision tree represent alternative possibilities, and decision nodes represent alternative choices. The leaf nodes of the tree represent outcomes, which may be assigned a numerical utility. See also: Utility.

DECT: Digital European Cordless Telephony standard, which defines the architecture for wireless voice and data communication systems restricted to campus-size areas, rather than wide-area systems that would be publicly available.

Deduction: A method of logical inference. Given a cause, deduction infers all logical effects that might arise as a consequence. See also: Abduction, Induction, Inference.

Distributed computing: Term for computer systems in which data and programs are distributed across different computers on a network, and shared.

DNA (deoxyribonucleic acid): The chemical that forms the basis of the genetic material in virtually all living organisms. Structurally, DNA is composed of two strands that intertwine to form a springlike structure called the double helix. Attached to each backbone are chemical structures called bases (or nucleotides), which protrude away from the backbone toward the centre of the helix, and which come in four types: adenine, cytosine, guanine, and thymine (designated A, C, G, and T). In DNA, cytosine only forms optimal hydrogen bonding with guanine, and adenine only with thymine. These interactions across the many nucleotides in each strand hold the two strands together.

DTMF (dial tone multifrequency): The tones generated by punching in numbers on a telephone key-pad.

EDI (electronic data interchange): General term describing the need for healthcare applications to be able to exchange data, requiring the adoption of agreed common standards for the form and content of the messages passing between applications. See also: HL7.

Electronic mail: See E-mail.

Electronic medical record (EMR): A general term describing computer-based patient record systems. It is sometimes extended to include other functions such as order-entry for medications and tests, among others.

Electrophoresis: The use of electrical fields to separate charged biomolecules such as DNA, RNA, and proteins. DNA and RNA carry a net negative charge because of the numerous phosphate groups in their structure. In the process of gel electrophoresis, these biomolecules are put into wells of a solid matrix typically made of an inert substance such as agarose. When this gel is placed into a bath and an electrical charge applied across the gel, the biomolecules migrate and separate according to size in proportion to the amount of charge they carry. The biomolecules can be stained for viewing and isolated and purified from the gels for further analysis. Electrophoresis can be used to isolate pure biomolecules from a mixture or to analyse biomolecules (such as for DNA sequencing).

E-mail: Electronic mail. Messaging system available on computer networks, providing users with personal mail-boxes from which electronic messages can be sent and received.

EMR: See: Electronic medical record.

Enzyme: A protein that catalyses chemical reactions in a living cell. Enzymes are protein molecules whose function it is to speed the making and breaking of chemical bonds required for essential physiochemical reactions.

Epistemology: The philosophical study of knowledge.

EPR (electronic patient record): See: Electronic medical record.

Evidence-based medicine: A movement advocating the practice of medicine according to clinical guidelines, developed to reflect best-practice as captured from a meta-analysis of the clinical literature. See also: Clinical guideline, Meta-analysis, Protocol.

Exon: The protein-coding DNA sequences of a gene. See also: Intron.

Expected value: For a decision option, its expected value is the sum of the utilities of each different possible outcome of that option, each weighted by their own probability. See also: Decision tree, Utility.

Expert system: A computer program that contains expert knowledge about a particular problem, often in the form of a set of if-then rules that is able to solve problems at a level equivalent to or better than human experts. See also: Artificial intelligence.

FAQ (frequently asked questions): Common term for information lists available on the Internet, which has been compiled to newcomers to a particular subject, answering common questions that would otherwise often be asked by submitting e-mail requests to a newsgroup.

Feedback: Taking some or all of the output of a system and adding it to a system's own input. See also: System.

Finite state machine: A knowledge representation that makes different states in a process explicit, and connects them with links that specify some transition condition that specifies how one traverses from one state to another.

Firewall: A security barrier erected between a public computer network like the Internet and a local private computer network.

First principles, reasoning from: Use of a model of the mechanisms that control a system to predict or simulate the likely outcome if some of the inputs or internal structure of the system is altered. See also: System.

Formative assessment: Evaluation of the performance of an information system against user needs. See also: Summative assessment.

FTP (file transfer protocol): A computer protocol that allows electronic files to be sent and received in a uniform fashion across a computer network.

Functional genomics: The use of genetic technology to determine the function of newly discovered genes by determining their role in one or more model organisms. Functional genomics uses as its starting point the isolated gene whose function is to be determined, and then selects a model organism in which a homologue of that gene exists. This model organism can be as simple as a yeast cell or as complex as a nematode worm, a fruit fly or even a mouse.

Fuzzy logic: An artificial intelligence method for representing and reasoning with imprecisely specified knowledge, for example defining loose boundaries to distinguish 'low' from 'high' values. See also: Artificial intelligence, Qualitative reasoning.

Gene: The basic unit of heredity; the sequence of DNA that encodes all the information to make a protein. A gene may be activated or 'switched on' to make protein (referred to as gene expression) by these proteins that control when, where and how much protein is expressed from the gene. In the human genome, there are an estimated 30 000 genes (although recent studies suggest a larger number).

Gene product: The biochemical material, either RNA or protein, resulting from expression of a gene. The amount of gene product is used to measure how active a gene is; abnormal amounts can be correlated with disease-causing alleles. As gene products include all the alternative splicing products, there are estimated to be at least 100 000 distinct such products.

Gene therapy: The technology that uses genetic material for therapeutic purposes. This genetic material can be in the form of a gene, representative of a gene or cDNA, RNA, or even a small fragment of a gene. The introduced genetic material can be therapeutic in several ways: It can make a protein that is defective or missing in the patient's cells (as would be the case in a genetic disorder), or that will correct or modify a particular cellular function, or that elicits an immune response.

Grammar: The set of rules that together specify the allowed ways an alphabet can be put together to forms strings of symbols in a given language. See: Alphabet, Language, Syntax.

Group: A group collects together a number of different codes associated with medical events that are considered to be sufficiently similar for some purpose, e.g. the determination of an appropriate reimbursement for approximately similar clinical procedures or diseases. See also: Code, Term.

Groupware: A computer application that assists communication and shared working amongst groups of individuals with access to a common computer network, but who may be geographically or temporally separated. See also: CSCW.

GSM (global system of mobility): A widely adopted international standard for the architecture and operation of digital cellular telephony systems that can carry voice and data circuits, as well as short packet-data messages.

GUI (graphical user interface): That part of a computer application seen and interacted with by its user. Specifically, that part of the interface that is based upon visual structures like icons, which act as metaphors for the different functions supported by the application, e.g. deleting a file is enacted by dragging a visual symbol representing the file onto a trashcan icon.

Guideline: An agreed set of steps to be taken in the management of a clinical condition. See also: Algorithm, Care Pathway, Practice parameter, Protocol.

Hardware: For a computer system, all its physical components, as distinguished from the programs and data that are manipulated by the computer. See also: Software.

Heuristic: A rule of thumb that describes how things are commonly understood, without resorting to deeper or more formal knowledge. See also: Model-based reasoning.

HIS (hospital information system): Typically used to describe hospital computer systems with functions like patient admission and discharge, order entry for laboratory tests or medications, and billing functions. See also: Electronic medical record.

HL7 (Health Level 7): An international standard for electronic data exchange in healthcare, which defines the format and content of messages that pass between medical applications.

Home page: A document on the World Wide Web that acts as a front page or point of welcome to a collection of documents that may introduce an individual, organization, or point of interest.

Homeostasis: The use of feedback systems to keep a desired state. Often used to describe physiological steady-states. See also: Feedback.

HTML (hypertext markup language): The description language used to create hypertext documents that can be viewed on the World Wide Web. See also: HTTP, World Wide Web.

HTTP (hypertext transfer protocol): Communication protocol used on the Internet for the transfer of HTML documents. See also: HTML, World Wide Web.

Human–computer interaction: The study of the psychology and design principles associated with the way humans interact with computer systems.

Human–computer interface: The 'view' presented by a program to its user. Often literally a visual window that allows a program to be operated, an interface could just as easily be based on the recognition and synthesis of speech, or any other medium with which a human is able to sense or manipulate.

Hybridization: The interaction of complementary nucleic acid strands. Since DNA is a double-stranded structure held together by complementary interactions (in which C always binds to G, and A to T), complementary strands favourably re-anneal or 'hybridize' to each other when separated.

Hyperlink: A connection between hypertext documents, that allows a reader to trace concepts appearing in one document to related occurrence in other documents.

Hypertext: A method of presenting documents electronically that allows them to be read in a richly interconnected way. Rather than following a single document from beginning to end, sections of each document are connected to related occurrences in other documents via hyperlinks, permitting 'non-linear' reading following concepts of interest to the reader. See also: HTML, Hyperlink, World Wide Web.

ICD-9: The *International Classification of Diseases*, 9th edition. Published by the World Health Organization.

ICD-10: The *International Classification of Diseases*, 10th edition. Published by the World Health Organization.

Indifference probability: The probability at which a decision-maker is indifferent to the present outcome (*status quo*) or taking a gamble that might improve or worsen the situation. Used to determine utilities in the standard gamble method. See also: Standard gamble, Utility.

Induction: A method of logical inference used to suggest relationships from observations. This is the process of generalization we use to create models of the world. See also: Abduction, Deduction, Inference.

Inference: A logical conclusion drawn using one of several methods of reasoning, knowledge and data. See also: Abduction, Deduction, Induction.

Information superhighway: A popular term associated with the Internet, used to describe its role in the global mass transportation of information.

Information theory: Initially developed by Claude Shannon, describes the amount of data that can be transmitted across a channel given specific encoding techniques and noise in the signal. See: Channel.

Internet: Technically, a network of computer networks. Today, associated with a specific global computer network which is publicly accessible, and upon which the World Wide Web is based. See also: ARPAnet, World Wide Web.

Intranet: A computer network, based upon World Wide Web and Internet technologies, but whose scope is limited to an organization. An intranet may be connected to an Internet, so that there can be communication and flow of information between it and other intranets. See also: Internet, World Wide Web.

Intron: Non-coding portion of the gene that is spliced out from the nascent RNA transcript in the process of making an mRNA transcript. Frequently includes regulator elements (i.e. binding sites) in addition to those of the promoter.

IP (internetworking protocol): Communication protocol to allow different individual networks to communicate with each other. IP is the basis of the Internet's communication infrastructure.

IP address: The address of a computer on the Internet, which permits it to send and receive messages from other computers on the Internet.

ISDN (integrated services digital network): A digital telephone network that is designed to provide channels for voice and data services.

Isochronous communication: A communication process that operates at a regular interval to provide a certain minimum data rate, e.g. sending a communication with a guaranteed regularity in ATM. See also: Synchronous communication, Asynchronous communication, ATM.

Knowledge acquisition: Sub-speciality of artificial intelligence, usually associated with developing methods for capturing human knowledge and of converting it into a form that can be used by computer. See also: Machine learning, Expert system, Heuristic.

Knowledge base: A structured repository for knowledge, consisting of a collection of knowledge elements such as rules and their associated data model, or ontology. A knowledge base is a core component of an expert system. See also: Database, Expert system, Model, Ontology.

Knowledge-based system: See: Expert system.

LAN (local area network): A computer network limited to servicing computers in a small locality. See also: Intranet.

Language: A formal language specifies a way of constructing messages. A language is built from an alphabet of allowed symbols, which can be arranged according to rules that define the syntax of the language. See: Grammar.

Machine learning: Sub-speciality of artificial intelligence concerned with developing methods for software to learn from experience, or to extract knowledge from examples in a database. See also: Artificial intelligence, Knowledge acquisition.

Mailing list: A list of e-mail addresses for individuals. Used to distribute information to small groups of individuals, who may, for example, have shared interests. See also: E-mail.

Medline: Bibliographic database maintained by the National Library of Medicine in the US, which indexes articles published by most of the major biomedical journals.

Megabyte: 1 048 576 or 2^{20} bytes. See: Byte.

Messenger RNA (mRNA): The RNA that codes for proteins and is active in the cellular cytoplasm.

Meta-analysis: A statistical method that pools the results from multiple similar experiments, hoping that the improved power obtained from the combined data sets will identify statistically significant patterns that cannot be identified within the smaller sample sizes of individual studies.

Model: Any representation of a real object or phenomenon, or template for the creation of an object or phenomenon.

Model-based reasoning: Approach to the development of expert systems that uses formally defined models of systems, in contrast to more superficial rules of thumbs. See also Artificial intelligence, Heuristic.

Modem: Modulator–demodulator. Device used for converting a digital signal into tones that can be transmitted down a telephone wire.

Mosaic: The first commonly available World Wide Web browser for viewing hypertext documents, developed at CERN.

Multimedia: Computer systems or applications that are able to manipulate data in multiple forms, including still and video images, sound, and text.

Mutation: Any alteration to DNA that can potentially result in a change in the function of one or more genes. Mutations can be a change in a single base of DNA (point mutation) or a loss of base pairs (deletion) affecting a single gene, or a movement of chromosomal regions (translocation) affecting many genes. Some changes in DNA occur naturally and lead to no harmful effects; these changes in a population are called polymorphisms.

Network: Set of connected elements. For computers, any collection of computers connected together so that they are able to communicate, permitting the sharing of data or programs.

Neural computing: See: Connectionism.

Neural network: Computer program or system designed to mimic some aspects of neurone connections, including summation of action potentials, refractory periods and firing thresholds.

Newsgroup: A bulletin board service provided on a computer network like the Internet, where messages can be sent by e-mail and be viewed by those who have an interest in the contents of a particular newsgroup. See also: E-mail, Internet.

Noise: Unwanted signal that is added to a transmitted message while being carried along a channel, and distorts the message for the receiver. See: Channel.

Northern blot: RNA from a sample is spatially separated and distributed by mass on a gel. Radioactively labelled DNA or RNA strands with sequence complementary to the RNA segments from the sample are used to locate the position of those RNA segments.

Object-oriented programming: Computer languages and programming philosophy that emphasize modularity amongst the elements of a program and their sharing of properties and intercommunication.

Oligonucleotide: A short molecule consisting of several linked nucleotides (typically between 10 and 60) chained together and attached by covalent bonds.

Ontology: The set of concepts understood in a knowledge base. A formal ontology specifies a way of constructing a knowledge base about some part of the world. An ontology thus contains a set of allowed concepts, and rules which define the allowable relationships between concepts. See also: Knowledge base, Language.

Open reading frame: Regions in a nucleotide sequence that are bounded by start and stop codons and are therefore possible gene coding regions.

Open system: Computer industry term for computer hardware and software that is built to common public standards, allowing purchasers to select components from a variety of vendors and use them together.

Open-loop control: Partially automated control method in which a part of the control system is given over to humans.

OSI seven-layer model: International Organization for Standardization (ISO) model that defines the protocol layers for communicating between heterogeneous computers. See also: Communication protocol.

PABX (public area branch exchange): Telecommunication network switching station that connects telephones in an area with the wider telephone network.

Packet-switched network: Computer network which exchanges messages between different computers not by seizing a dedicated circuit, but by sending a message in a number of uniformly sized packets along common channels, shared with other computers. See also: Circuit-switched network.

Pharmacogenomics: The study of the pharmacological response to a drug by a population based on the genetic variation of that population. It has long been known that different individuals in a population respond to the same drug differently, and that these variations are due to variations in the molecular receptors being affected by the drug, or to differences in metabolic enzymes that clear the drug. Pharmacogenomics is the science of studying these variations at the molecular level. Applications of pharmacogenomics include reducing side effects, customizing drugs, improvement of clinical trials, and the rescue of some drugs that have been banned due to severe side effects in a small percentage of the eligible population.

Physician's workstation: A computer system designed to support the clinical tasks of doctors. See also: Electronic medical record.

Polymerase chain reaction (PCR): A technique used to amplify or generate large amounts of replica DNA or a segment of any DNA whose 'flanking' sequences are known. Oligonucleotide primers that bind these flanking sequences are used by an enzyme to copy the sequence in between the primers. Cycles of heat to break apart the DNA strands, cooling to allow the primers to bind, and heating again to allow the enzyme to copy the intervening sequence lead to doubling of the DNA present at each cycle.

Posterior probability: The probability that an event occurs with evidence both about the prior probability and also about the current case in question. See: Bayes' theorem, Prior probability.

PostScript: Commercial language that describes a common format for electronic documents that can be understood by printing devices and converted to paper documents or images on a screen.

Post-test probability: Posterior probability of an event, after a test to see if the event is true. See: Posterior probability, Pre-test probability.

Practice parameter: See: Care pathway.

Precision: The percentage of elements correctly matching a given attribute, out of all the elements identified as matching by a procedure.

Pre-test probability: Prior-probability of an event, ahead of a test. See: Post-test probability; Prior probability.

Prior probability: The probability that an event occurs in a population, with no evidence about the current case in question. See: Bayes' theorem.

Probe: Any biochemical agent that is labelled or tagged in some way so that it can be used to identify or isolate a gene, RNA or protein. Typically refers to the immobilized specified nucleic acid in a detection system.

Proteomics: The study of the entire protein complement or 'protein universe' of the cell. Mirroring genomics, proteomics aims to determine the entire suite of expressed proteins in a cell. This includes determining the number, level and turnover of all expressed proteins, their sequence and any post-translational modifications to the sequence, and protein–protein and protein–other molecule interactions within the cell, across the cell membrane and among (secreted) proteins.

Protocol: A set of instructions that describe the procedure to be followed when investigating a particular set of findings in a patient, or the method to be followed in the management of a given disease See also: Algorithm, Care pathway, Guideline, Practice parameter.

PSTN (public-switched telephone network): Providing ordinary voice-based telephone services.

Qualitative reasoning: A sub-speciality of artificial intelligence concerned with inference and knowledge representation when knowledge is not precisely defined, e.g. 'back of the envelope' calculations.

Randomized controlled trial (RCT): A form of scientific study that randomly allocates patients to either a group receiving a new treatment, or to a control group. If patients or scientists do not know which group patients are allocated to, the trial is a randomized blinded controlled trial. See also: Systematic review.

Read codes: Medical terminology system, developed initially for primary care medicine in the UK. Subsequently enlarged and developed to capture medical concepts in a wide variety of situations. See also: Terminology.

Reasoning: A method of thinking. See also: Inference.

Representation: The method chosen to model a process or object; for example, a building may be represented as a physical scale model, drawing or photograph. See also: Reasoning, Syntax.

RNA (ribonucleic acid): RNA is generated from the DNA template in the nucleus of the cell through a process called transcription, and is then exported into the cell cytoplasm from the nucleus where it begins the process of protein synthesis.

Rule-based expert system: See: Expert system.

Search engine: Computer program capable of seeking information on the World Wide Web (or indeed any large database) based upon search criteria specified by a user. See also: World Wide Web.

Semantics: The meaning associated with a set of symbols in a given language, which is determined by the syntactic structure of the symbols, as well as knowledge captured in an interpretative model. See also: Syntax.

Server: A computer on a network that stores commonly used resources such as data or programs, and makes these available on demand to clients on the network. See also: Client, Client–server architecture.

SGML (standard generalized markup language): Document definition language used in printing, and used as the basis for the creation of HTML. See also: HTML, XML.

Signal to noise ratio: Measure of the amount of noise that has been added to a message during transmission. See: Channel, Information theory.

SNOMED (systematized nomenclature of human and veterinary medicine): A commercially available general medical terminology, initially developed for the classification of pathological specimens. See also: Terminology.

Socio-technical system: The system created when people and technology together interact in an organization, emphasizing that both the human social, as well as technological, features contribute to the overall behaviour of the system.

Software: Synonym for computer program. See also: Application.

Southern blot: DNA from a sample is cut with restriction enzymes and the position of the fragments (e.g. on a gel) is determined by the fragment's molecular weight. Complementary strands of radioactively labelled DNA are used to identify the position of the DNA fragments on the gel.

Standard gamble: A method to get an individual to express a preference for an outcome where the value is unknown as a preference for a gamble where the value for the outcomes are known. See also. Indifference probability, Utility.

Summative assessment: Evaluation of an information system against formal functional metrics or organizational outcome measures. See also: Formative assessment.

Symbol: A representation that is used to signify a more complex concept. See: Model.

Synchronous communication: A mode of communication when two parties exchange messages across a communication channel at the same time, e.g. telephones. See also: Asynchronous communication, Isochronous communication.

Syntax: The rules of grammar that define the formal structure of a language. See also: Semantics.

System: A collection of component ideas, processes or objects which has an input and an output. See also: Feedback.

Systematic review: A formal process for searching for and then summarizing the evidence contained in scientific papers, to obtain an aggregate view. The review process uses statistical techniques to appropriately combine the individual statistical results of each paper, which ideally is a randomized trial. See also: Randomized controlled trial.

Telco: Abbreviation for telecommunication company.

Teleconsultation: Clinical consultation carried out using a telemedical service. See also: Telemedicine.

Telemedicine: The delivery of healthcare services between geographically separated individuals, using telecommunication systems, e.g. video-conferencing.

Term: In medical terminologies an agreed name for a medical condition or treatment. See also: Code, Terminology.

Terminal: A screen and keyboard system that provides access to a shared computer system, e.g. a mainframe or minicomputer. In contrast to computers on a modern network, terminals are not computers in their own right.

Terminology: A standard set of symbols or words used to describe the concepts, processes and objects of a given field of study. See also: Term.

Transcription factor: A molecule, typically a protein, which binds to DNA binding sites with some regulatory role in transcription. The binding (or unbinding) of a transcription factor from a promoter eventually leads to a change of transcription activity in the gene controlled by that promoter.

True negative rate (specificity)**:** The percentage of elements correctly detected as not matching a given attribute by a procedure, out of all the possible non-matching elements.

True positive rate (sensitivity)**:** The percentage of elements correctly detected as matching a given attribute by a procedure, out of all the possible correct elements.

Turing test: Proposed by Alan Turing, the test suggests that an artefact can be considered intelligent if its behaviour cannot be distinguished by humans from other humans in controlled circumstances. See also: Artificial intelligence.

URL (universal resource locator): The address for a document placed on the World Wide Web. See also: World Wide Web.

User interface: The view a user has of a computer program, usually understood to mean the visual look and feel of a program, but also extending to other modes of interaction, e.g. voice and touch.
Utility: A quantitative measure assigned to an outcome, expressing the preference for that outcome compared to others. See also: Decision tree.
Virtual reality: Computer-simulated environment within which humans are able to interact in some manner that approximates interactions in the physical world.
Vocabulary: See Terminology.
Voicemail: Computer-based telephone messaging system, capable of recording and storing messages, for later review or other processing, e.g. forwarding to other users. See also: E-mail.
W3: See: World Wide Web.
WAN (wide area network): Computer network extending beyond a local area such as a campus or office. See also: LAN.
World Wide Web: An easy-to-use hypertext document system developed for the Internet allowing users to access multimedia documents. See also: CERN, HTML, HTTP, Internet, URL.
WWW: See: World Wide Web.
XML (extensible markup language): A reduced version of SGML, designed for the Web, that allows customized tags to be embedded in documents. See: SGML.

References

Ackerman M, Ball M, Clayton PD, *et al.* (1994) Standards for medical identifiers, codes and messages needed to create an efficient computer-stored medical record. *Journal of the American Medical Informatics Association* **1**: 1–7.

Adlassnig KP, Horak W, Hepaxpert I (1991) Automatic interpretation of tests for hepatitis A and B. *MD Computing* **8**(2): 118–119.

Ahn W, Medin DL (1992) A two-stage model of category construction. *Cognitive Science* **16**: 81–121.

Akelsen S, Lillehaug S (1993) Teaching and learning aspects of remote medical consultation. *Telektronikk* **89**(1): 42–47.

Akelsen S, Hartviksen G, Vorland L (1995) Remote interpretation of microbiology specimens based on transmitted still images. *Journal of Telemedicine and Telecare* **1**: 229–233.

Alizadeh AA, Eisen MB, Davis RE, *et al.* (2000) Distinct types of diffuse large B-cell lymphoma identified by gene expression profiling. *Nature* **403**(6769): 503–511.

Allen A, Roman L, Cox R, Cardwell B (1996) Home health visits using a cable television network: user satisfaction. *Journal of Telemedicine and Telecare* **2** (Supplement 1): 92–94.

Anderson R (1995) NHS-wide networking and patient confidentiality. *British Medical Journal* **311**: 5–6.

Anonymous (2002) Implementing clinical practice guidelines: can guidelines be used to improve clinical practice? *Database of Abstracts of Reviews of Effectiveness* **1**(1).

Antman E, Lau J, Kupelnick B, Mosteller F, Chalmers T (1992) A comparison of the results of meta-analysis of randomised controlled trials and recommendations of clinical experts. *Journal of the American Medical Association* **268**: 240–248.

Arndt KA (1992) Information excess in medicine. *Archives of Dermatology* **128**: 1249–1256.

Ash J (1997) Organizational factors that influence information technology diffusion in academic health sciences centers. *Journal of the American Medical Informatics Association* **4**: 4102–4111.

Ashburner M, Ball CA, Blake JA, *et al.* (2000) Gene ontology: tool for the unification of biology. *Nature Genetics* **25**(1): 25–29.

Babbage C (1833) *On the Economy of Machinery and Manufactures*, 3rd edition. Charles Knight, London.

Baddeley AD (1982) *Your Memory, A User's Guide.* Macmillan, Basingstoke.

Bannister F, McCabe P, Remenyi D (2001) How much did we really pay for that? The awkward problem of information technology costs. *Electron Journal of Information Systems Evaluation* **5**(1).

Barnett GO, Sukenik HJ (1969) Hospital information systems. In: Dickson JF III, Brown JHU (eds) *Future Goals of Engineering in Biology and Medicine, Proceedings of an International Conference, September 1967, Washington DC*. Academic Press, New York.

Barnett GO, Cimino JJ, Huppa JA, *et al.* (1987) DXplain: an evolving diagnostic decision-support system. *Journal of the American Medical Association* **258**: 69–76.

Barrows RC, Clayton PD (1996) Privacy, confidentiality, and electronic medical records. *Journal of the American Medical Informatics Association* **3**: 139–148.

Bates D, Cullen D, Laird N, Peterson L, Small S, Servi D, *et al.* (1995) Incidence of adverse drug events and potential adverse drug events: implications for prevention. *Journal of the American Medical Association* **274**(1): 29–34.

Bates DW, Leape LL, Cullen DJ, *et al.* (1998) Effect of computerized physician order entry and a team intervention on prevention of serious medication errors. *Journal of the American Medical Association* **280**(15): 1311–1316.

Bates DW, Kuperman GJ, Rittenberg E, *et al.* (1999a) A randomized trial of a computer-based intervention to reduce utilization of redundant laboratory tests. *American Journal of Medicine* **106**(2): 144–150.

Bates DW, Teich JM, Lee J, Seger D, Kuperman GJ, *et al.* (1999b) The impact of computerized physician order entry on medication error prevention. *Journal of the American Medical Informatics Association* **6**(4): 313–321.

Bates D, Cohen M, Leape L, *et al.* (2001) Reducing the frequency of errors in medicine using information technology. *Journal of the American Medical Informatics Association* **8**: 301–308.

Bates M (1990) Where should the person stop and the information search interface start? *Information Processing and Management* **26**(5): 575–591.

Bayat A (2002) Bioinformatics. *British Medical Journal* **324**: 1018–1022.

Bean N (1996) Secrets of network success. *Physics World* (February): 30–34.

Berg M (1997) *Rationalizing Medical Work: Decision-support Techniques and Medical Practice.* MIT Press, Cambridge, MA.

Berger B, Leighton T (1998) Protein folding in the hydrophobic-hydrophilic (HP) model is NP-complete. *Journal of Computational Biology* **5**(1): 27–40.

Berners-Lee T, Calliau R, Luotonen A, Nielsen HF, Secret A (1994) The World Wide Web. *Communications of the ACM* **37**(8): 76–82.

Berners-Lee T, Hendler J, Lassila O (2001) The semantic web. *Scientific American* (May): 28–37.

Bero LA, Grilli R, Grimshaw JM, *et al.* (1998) Getting research findings into practice: closing the gap between research and practice: an overview of systematic reviews of interventions to promote the implementation of research findings. *British Medical Journal* **317**: 465–468.

Bessell TL, McDonald S, Silagy CA, *et al.* (2002) Do Internet interventions for consumers cause more harm than good? A systematic review. *Health Expectations* **5**: 28–37.

Bhagwat P (2001) Bluetooth: technology for short-range wireless apps. *IEEE Internet Computing* (May–June): 96–103.

Bhasale AL, Miller GC, Reid SE, *et al.* (1998) Analysing potential harm in Australian general practice: an incident-monitoring study. *Medical Journal of Australia* **169**: 73–76.

Bhattacharyya A, Davis JR, Halliday BE, *et al.* (1995) Case triage model for the practice of telepathology. *Telemedicine Journal* **1**(1): 9–17.

Bingham CM, Higgins G, Coleman R, Van der Weyden MB (1998) The *Medical Journal of Australia* internet peer-review study. *Lancet* **352**: 441–45.

Birkmeyer J, Birkmeyer C, Wennberg D, Young M (2000) *Leapfrog Patient Safety Standards: The Potential Benefits of Universal Adoption*. The Leapfrog Group, Washington, DC, pp. 1–32.

Bizovi KE, Beckley BE, McDade MC, *et al.* (2002) The effect of computer-assisted prescription writing on emergency department prescription errors. *Academic Emergency Medicine* **9**(11): 1168–1175.

Blom JA (1991) Expert control of the arterial blood pressure during surgery. *International Journal of Clinical Monitoring and Computing* **8**: 25–34.

Boden D (1994) *The Business of Talk – Organisations in Action*. Polity Press, London.

Borowitz SM, Wyatt JC (1998) The origin, content, and workload of e-mail consultations. *Journal of the American Medical Association* **280**: 1321–1324.

Borriello SP (1999) Near patient microbiological tests. *British Medical Journal* **319**: 298–301.

Bouhaddou O, Cofrin K, Larsen D, *et al.* (1993) Implementation of practice guidelines in a clinical setting using a computerized knowledge base (Iliad). *Proceedings of 17th Symposium on Computer Applications in Medical Care*, pp. 258–262.

Bourland H, Wellekens C (1990) Links between Markov models and multilayer perceptrons. *IEEE Transactions on Pattern Analysis and Machine Intelligence* **12**: 1167–1178.

Bower H (1996) Internet sees growth of unverified health claims. *British Medical Journal* **313**: 381.

Bowles RA, Teale R (1994) Communications services in support of collaborative health care. *BT Technology Journal* **12**(3): 29–44.

Brahams D (1995) The medicolegal implications of teleconsulting in the UK. *Journal of Telemedicine and Telecare* **1**: 196–201.

Branger PJ, van der Wouden JC, Schudel BR, *et al.* (1992) Electronic communication between providers of primary and secondary care. *British Medical Journal* **305**: 1068–1070.

Bratko I, Mozetic I, Lavrac N (1989) *KARDIO: A Study in Deep and Qualitative Knowledge for Expert Systems*. MIT Press, Cambridge, MA.

Brennan F (1994) On the relevance of discipline in informatics. *Journal of the American Medical Informatics Association* **1**: 200–201.

Brinkley JF, Bradley SW, Sundsten JW, Rosse C (1997) The digital anatomist information system and its use in the generation and delivery of web-based anatomy atlases. *Computers and Biomedical Research* **30**: 472–503.

Buchanan BG, Shortliffe EH (eds) (1984) *Rule-Based Expert Systems: the MYCIN Experiments of the Stanford Heuristic Programming Project*. Addison-Wesley, Reading, MA.

Buhle EL, Goldwein JW, Benjamin I (1994) OncoLink: a multimedia oncology information resource on the Internet. *Journal of the American Medical Informatics Association* (Symposium Supplement): 103–107.

Butte AJ, Tamayo P, Slonim D, *et al.* (2000) Discovering functional relationships between RNA expression and chemotherapeutic susceptibility using relevance networks. *Proceedings of the National Academy of Sciences of the USA* **97**(22): 12182–12186.

Cabral JE Jr, Kim Y (1996) Multimedia systems for telemedicine and their communication requirements. *IEEE Communications Magazine* (July): 20–27.

Caldwell BS, Uang S, Taha LH (1995) Appropriateness of communications media use in organizations: situation requirements and media characteristics. *Behaviour and Information Technology* **14**: 199–207.

Campbell JR, Payne TH (1994) A comparison of four schemes for codification of problem lists. *Proceedings of the Symposium on Computer Applications in Medicine. Journal of the American Medical Informatics Association* (Symposium Supplement): 201–204.

Campbell KE, Oliver DE, Spackman KA, Shortliffe EH (1998) Representing thoughts, words, and things in the UMLS. *Journal of the American Medical Informatics Association* **5**: 421–431.

CCC (1995) *A Guide to the Use of Tables of Equivalence between ICD-9 and ICD-10*. Report F6110, NHS Centre for Coding and Classification, Loughborough.

CDC (2000) Biological and chemical terrorism: strategic plan for preparedness and response. Recommendations of the Centres for Disease Control and Prevention Strategic Planning Workgroup. *Morbidity and Mortality Weekly Report* **4RR-4**: 49.

Chittenden M, Syal R (1995) Academic avalanche cripples libraries. *Sunday Times* (14 May).

Christakis D, Zimmerman F, Wright J, *et al.* (2001) A randomized controlled trial of point-of-care evidence to improve antibiotic prescribing practices for otitis media in children. *Pediatrics* **107**(2): 15–19.

Chueh H, Barnett GO (1997) 'Just-in-time' clinical information. *Academic Medicine* **72**: 512–517.

Cimino JJ (1994) Controlled medical vocabulary construction: methods from the CANON group. *Journal of the American Medical Informatics Association* **1**: 296–297.

Cimino JJ, Clayton PD (1994) Coping with changing controlled vocabularies. *Proceedings of the Symposium on Computer Applications in Medicine. Journal of the American Medical Informatics Association* (Symposium Supplement): 135–139.

Cimino JJ, Socratous SA, Clayton PD (1995) Internet as clinical information system: application development using the world wide web. *Journal of the American Medical Informatics Association* **2**: 273–84.

Clancey WJ (1993a) Notes on 'Epistemology of a rule-based expert system'. *Artificial Intelligence* **59**: 197–204.

Clancey WJ (1993b) Notes on 'Heuristic Classification'. *Artificial Intelligence* **59**: 191–196.

Clancey WJ, Shortliffe EH (eds) (1984) *Readings in Medical Artificial Intelligence – The First Decade*. Addison-Wesley, Reading, MA.

Clarke H, Brennan S (1991) Grounding in communication. In: Resnick LB, Levine J, Behreno SD (eds) *Perspectives on Socially Shared Cognition*. American Psychological Association, Washington, DC, pp. 127–149.

Cohen B (1986) *The Specification of Complex Systems*. Addison-Wesley, Reading, MA.

Coiera E (1990) Monitoring diseases with empirical and model-generated histories. *Artificial Intelligence in Medicine* **2**: 135–147.

Coiera E (1992a) The qualitative representation of physical systems. *Knowledge Engineering Review* **7**(1): 55–77.

Coiera E (1992b) Intermediate depth representations. *Artificial Intelligence in Medicine* **4**: 431–445.

Coiera E (1994a) Automated signal interpretation. In: Hutton P, Prys-Roberts C (eds) *Monitoring in Anaesthesia and Intensive Care*. Baillière Tindall, London, pp. 32–42.

Coiera E (1994b) Question the assumptions. In: Barahona P, Christensen JP (eds) *Knowledge and Decisions in Health Telematics – The Next Decade*. IOS Press, Amsterdam, pp. 61–66.

Coiera E (1996a) Editorial: The Internet's challenge to healthcare provision. *British Medical Journal* **311**: 2–4.

Coiera E (1996b) Clinical communication – a new informatics paradigm. *Proceedings of the 1996 AMIA Annual Fall Symposium. Journal of the American Medical Informatics Association* (Symposium Supplement): 17–21.

Coiera E (2000) When communication is better than computation. *Journal of the American Medical Informatics Association* **7**: 277–286.

Coiera E, Dowton SB (2000) Re-inventing ourselves – how innovations such as on-line 'just-in-time' CME may help bring about a genuinely evidence-based clinical practice. *Medical Journal of Australia* **173**: 343–344.

Coiera E, Lewis SCR (1994) Information Management System. European patent application 94302119.6, 24th March 1994. US patent application 08/409,444, 24 March 1995.

Coiera E, Tombs V (1998) Communication behaviours in a hospital setting – an observational study. *British Medical Journal* **316**: 673–677.

Coiera E, Jayasuriya R, Hardy J, Bannan A, Thorpe M (2002) Communication loads on clinicians in the emergency department. *Medical Journal of Australia* **176**: 415–418.

College of American Pathologists (2001) SNOMED® Clinical Terms TM Technical Specification – Core structure, Version 23 (2001-12-12). College of American Pathologists, Lakefield, IL.

Compton P, Jansen R (1990) A philosophical basis for knowledge acquisition. *Knowledge Acquisition* **2**: 241–257.

Compton P, Edwards G, Kang B, *et al.* (1992) Ripple down rules: turning knowledge acquisition into knowledge maintenance. *Artificial Intelligence in Medicine* **4**: 463–475.

Constable J (1994) Active voice. *British Journal of Healthcare Computing and Information Management* **11**: 30–31.

Cooper GF (1988) Computer-based medical diagnosis using belief networks and bounded probabilities. In: Miller PL (ed) *Selected Topics in Medical Artificial Intelligence.* Springer-Verlag, New York, pp. 85–98.

Cooper JB, Newbower RS, Kitz RJ (1984) An analysis of major errors and equipment failures in anaesthesia management: considerations for prevention and detection. *Anesthesiology* **60**(1): 34–42.

Côté RA, Rothwell DJ, Palotay JL, Beckett RS, Btochu L (1993) *The Systematized Nomenclature of Human and Veterinary Medicine – SNOMED International* (4 vols). College of American Pathologists, Lakefield, IL.

Covell DG, Uman GC, Manning PR (1985) Information needs in office practice: are they being met? *Annals of Internal Medicine* **103**: 596–599.

Cox DC (1995) Wireless personal communications: what is it? *IEEE Personal Communications* (April): 20–35.

Culver JD, Gerr F, Frumkin H (1997) Medical information on the Internet: a study of an electronic bulletin board. *Journal of General Internal Medicine* **12**: 466–470.

Currell R, Urquhart C, Wainwright P, Lewis R (2000) Telemedicine versus face to face patient care: effects on professional practice and health care outcomes (Cochrane Review). *Cochrane Library*, Issue 2. Oxford: Update Software.

Cushman R (1997) Serious technology assessment for health care information technology. *Journal of the American Medical Informatics Association* **4**(7): 259–265.

Cutler P (1979) *Problem Solving in Clinical Medicine – From Data to Diagnosis.* Williams & Wilkins, Baltimore, MD.

Darling G (2002) The impact of clinical practice guidelines and clinical trials on treatment decisions. *Surgical Oncology* **11**: 255–262.

Darmoni SJ, Massari P, Droy JM, Moirot E, Le Roy J (1993) SETH: an expert system for the management on acute drug poisoning in adults. *Computer Methods and Programs in Biomedicine* **43**: 171–176.

Davis D, O'Brien T, Freemantle N, *et al.* (1999) Impact of formal continuing medical education: do conferences, workshops, rounds, and other traditional continuing education activities change physician behaviours or health outcomes? *Journal of the American Medical Association* **282**: 867–874.

Davis J, Stack M (1997) The digital advantage. In: Davis J, Hirschl TA, Stack M (eds) *Cutting Edge – Technology, Information Capitalism and Social Revolution.* Verso, London, pp. 121–144.

Dawes MG (1996) On the need for evidence-based general and family practice. *Evidence Based Medicine* **1**: 68–69.

Dawkins R (1982) *The Extended Phenotype.* Oxford University Press, Oxford.

Degeling P, Kennedy J, Hill M, Carnegie M, Holt J (1998) Professional sub-cultures and hospital reform. Centre for Hospital Management and Information Systems Research, University of NSW, Sydney.

Delamothe T (1996) Whose data are they anyway? *British Medical Journal* **312**: 1241–1242.

Della Mea V, Forti S, Puglisi F, *et al.* (1996) Telepathology using Internet multimedia electronic mail: remote consultation on gastrointestinal pathology. *Journal of Telemedicine and Telecare* **2**: 28–34.

DeMarco T (1982) *Controlling Software Projects – Management, Measurement, Estimation.* Prentice Hall, Englewood Cliffs, NJ.

Devereaux P, Guyatt G (2002) Physicians' and patients' choices in evidence based practice. *British Medical Journal* **324**: 1350.

Dick RS, Steen EB (eds) (1991) *The Computer-based Patient Record – An Essential Technology for Health Care.* National Academy Press, Washington, DC.

Dick T (1833) *On the Improvement of Society by the Diffusion of Knowledge.* William Collins and Co., Glasgow.

Dickson JF III, Brown JHU (eds) (1969) *Future Goals of Engineering in Biology and Medicine, Proceedings of an International Conference, September 1967, Washington, DC.* Academic Press, New York.

Dojat M, Harf A, Touchard D, *et al.* (1996) Evaluation of a knowledge-based system providing ventilatory management and decision for extubation. *American Journal of Respiratory and Critical Care Medicine* **153**(3): 997–1004.

Dolin RH, Alschuler L, Boyer S, Beebe C (2000) An update on HL7's XML-based document representation standards. *Proceedings of the AMIA Annual Symposium*, pp. 190–194.

de Dombal FT, Dallos V, McAdam WAF (1991) Can computer aided teaching packages improve clinical care in patients with acute abdominal pain? *British Medical Journal* **302**: 1495–1497.

Doolittle GC, Allen A (1996) From acute leukaemia to multiple myeloma: clarification of a diagnosis using tele-oncology. *Journal of Telemedicine and Telecare* **2**: 119–121.

Doughty K, Cameron K, Garner P (1996) Three generations of telecare of the elderly. *Journal of Telemedicine and Telecare* **2**: 71–80.

Dugas M, Schauer R, Volk A, Rau H (2002) Interactive decision support in hepatic surgery. *BMC Medical Informatics and Decision Making* **2**(5).

Dunbar PJ, Madigan D, Grohskopf LA, *et al.* (2003) A two-way messaging system to enhance antiretroviral adherence. *Journal of the American Medical Informatics Association* **10**: 11–15.

Durinck J, Coiera E, Baud R, *et al.* (1994) The role of knowledge based systems in clinical practice. In: Barahona P, Christensen JP (eds) *Knowledge and Decisions in Health Telematics – The Next Decade*. IOS Press, Amsterdam, pp. 199–203.

East TD, Bohm SH, Wallace CJ, *et al.* (1992) A successful computerized protocol for clinical management of pressure control inverse ratio ventilation in ARDS patients. *Chest* **101**(3): 697–710.

EBMWG (1992) Evidence-Based Medicine Working Group. Evidence-based medicine. *Journal of the American Medical Association* **268**: 2420–2425.

Eccles M, McColl E, Steen N, *et al.* (2002) Effect of computerised evidence based guidelines on management of asthma and angina in adults in primary care: cluster randomised controlled trial. *British Medical Journal* **325**: 941.

Economist (1995) Doctors in the dock. *The Economist* (19 August): 23–24.

Edwards G, Compton P, Malor R, Srinivasan A, Lazarus L (1993) PEIRS: a pathologist maintained expert system for the interpretation of chemical pathology reports. *Pathology* **25**: 27–34.

Effler P, Ching-Lee M, Bogard A, *et al.* (1999) Statewide system of electronic notifiable disease reporting from clinical laboratories: comparing automated reporting with conventional methods. *Journal of the American Medical Association* **282**(19): 1845–1850.

Einstein A (1931) The world as I see it. In: *Living Philosophies*. Simon & Schuster, New York, pp. 3–7.

Elstein AS, Schwarz A (2002) Clinical problem solving and diagnostic decision making: selective review of the cognitive literature. *British Medical Journal* **324**: 729–732.

Elstein AS, Shulman LS, Sprafka SA (1978) *Medical Problem Solving – An Analysis of Clinical Reasoning*. Harvard University Press, Cambridge, MA.

Elting LS, Martin CG, Cantor SB, Rubenstein EB (1999) Influence of data display formats on physician investigators' decisions to stop clinical trials: prospective trial with repeated measures. *British Medical Journal* **318**: 1527–1531.

Ely JW, Oscheroff JA, Ebell MH, *et al.* (1999) Analysis of questions asked by family doctors regarding patient care. *British Medical Journal* **319**: 358–361.

Ermolaeva O, Rastogi M, Pruitt KD, *et al.* (1998) Data management and analysis for gene expression arrays. *Nature Genetics* **20**(1): 19–23.

Evans CE, Haynes RB, Gilbert JR, *et al.* (1984) Educational package on hypertension for primary care physicians. *Canadian Medical Association Journal* **130**: 719–722.

Evans D, Cimino JJ, Hersh WR, Huff SM, Bell DS (1994) Toward a medical-concept representational language. *Journal of the American Medical Informatics Association* **1**: 207–217.

Evans RW (1996) A critical perspective on the tools to support clinical decision making. *Transfusion* **36**: 671–673.

Eysenbach G, Diepgen TL (1999) Labeling and filtering of medical information on the Internet. *Methods of Information in Medicine* **38**: 80–88.

Ezquerra NF, Mullick R, Cooke CD, Krawczynska E, Garcia EV (1993) PERFEX: an expert system for interpreting perfusion images. Invited paper. *Expert Systems with Applications* **6**: 459–468.

Fafchamps D, Young CY, Tang PC (1991) Modeling work practices: Input to the design of a physician's workstation. *Proceedings of the 15th SCAMC*, 1991, pp. 788–792.

Fagan L, Shortliffe EH, Buchanan B (1984) Computer-based medical decision making: from MYCIN to VM. In: Clancey J, Shortliffe EH (eds) *Readings in Medical Artificial Intelligence – The First Decade*. Addison-Wesley, Reading, MA, pp. 241–255.

Feder G, Griffiths C, Highton C, *et al.* (1995) Do clinical guidelines introduced with practice based education improve care of asthmatic and diabetic patients? A randomised controlled trial in general practices in east London. *British Medical Journal* **311**: 1473–1478.

Feinstein AR (1967) *Clinical Judgement*. Williams & Wilkins, Baltimore, MD.

Feinstein AR (1973) The problems of the 'Problem Oriented Medical Record'. *Annals of Internal Medicine* **78**: 751.

Feinstein AR (1988) ICD, POR and DRG: unsolved scientific problems in the nosology of clinical medicine. *Archives of Internal Medicine* **148**: 2269–2274.

Fernow LC, Mackie C, McColl I, Rendall M (1978) The effect of problem-oriented medical records on clinical management controlled for patient risks. *Medical Care* **16**: 476–487.

Fishburn P, Odlyzko AM, Siders RC (1998) Fixed fee versus unit pricing for information goods: competition, equilibria and price wars. *First Monday* **2**: 7 (available at http:/www.firstmonday.dk/issues/issue2_7/odlyzko/).

Fisk MJ (1995) A comparison of personal response services in Canada and the UK. *Journal of Telemedicine and Telecare* **1**: 145–156.

Fitzpatrick K, Vineski E (1993) The role of cordless phones in improving patient care. *Physician Assistant* (June): 87–92.

Flahault A, Dias-Ferrao V, Chaberty P, *et al.* (1998) FluNet as a tool for global monitoring of influenza on the Web. *Journal of the American Medical Association* **280**: 1330–1332.

Fletcher RH (1974) Auditing problem-oriented records and traditional records. *New England Journal of Medicine* **290**: 829–833.

Forman GH, Zahorjan J (1994) The challenges of mobile computing. *IEEE Computer* (April): 38–47.

Fox J, Das S (2000) *Safe and Sound: Artificial Intelligence in Hazardous Applications*. AAAI and MIT Press, Cambridge, MA.

Fox J, Johns N, Rahmanzadeh A, Thomson R (1996) PROforma: a method and language for specifying clinical guidelines and protocols. *Proceedings of the Medical Informatics Europe – MIE*, pp. 516–520.

Frank RH (1998) *Microeconomics and Behavior*, 3rd edition. McGraw-Hill, New York.

Franken EA Jr, Berbaum KS (1996) Subspecialty radiology consultation by interactive telemedicine. *Journal of Telemedicine and Telecare* **2**: 35–41.

Franken EA, Berbaum KS, Smith WL, *et al.* (1995) Teleradiology for rural hospitals: analysis of a field study. *Journal of Telemedicine and Telecare* **1**: 202–208.

Franz DR, Jahrling PB, Friedlander AM, *et al.* (1997) Clinical recognition and management of patients exposed to biological warfare agents. *Journal of the American Medical Association* **278**: 399–411.

Fraser HS, Kohane IS, Long WJ (1997) Using the technology of the world wide web to manage clinical information. *British Medical Journal* **314**: 1600.

Fridsma DB, Ford P, Altman R (1994) A survey of patient access to electronic mail: attitudes, barriers and opportunities. *Proceedings of the Symposium on Computer*

Applications in Medicine. Journal of the American Medical Informatics Association (Symposium Supplement): 15–19.

Friedman CP, Wyatt JC (1997) *Evaluation Methods in Medical Informatics.* Springer, New York.

Friedman C, Huff SM, Hersh WR, Pattison-Gordon E, Cimino JJ (1995) The CANON Group's effort: working toward a merged model. *Journal of the American Medical Informatics Association* **2**: 4–18.

Gagliardi A, Jadad AR (2002) Examination of instruments used to rate quality of health information on the internet: chronicle of a voyage with an unclear destination. *British Medical Journal* **324**: 569–573.

Gall J (1986) *Systemantics – The Undergound Text of System's Lore. How Systems Really Work and How They Fail,* 2nd edition. The General Systemantic Press, Ann Arbor, MI.

Gardner RM (1981) Direct blood pressure measurements – dynamic response requirements. *Anesthesiology* **54**: 227–236.

Genesereth MR, Nilsson NJ (1988) *Logical Foundations of Artificial Intelligence.* Morgan Kauffman, Palo Alto, CA.

George S (2002) NHS Direct audited. *British Medical Journal* **324**: 558–559.

Gerrish K, Clayton J, Nolan M, Parker K, Morgan L (1999) Promoting evidence-based practice: managing change in the assessment of pressure damage risk. *Journal of Nursing Management* **7**(6): 355–362.

Gersenovic M (1995) The ICD family of classifications. *Methods of Information in Medicine* **34**: 172–175.

Gierl L, Feistle M, Muller H, *et al.* (1995) Task-specific authoring functions for end-users in a hospital information system. *Computer Methods and Programs in Biomedicine* **48**: 145–150.

Glance NS, Huberman BA (1994) The dynamics of social dilemmas. *Scientific American* (March): 58–63.

Glanville J, Haines M, Auston I (1998) Finding information on clinical effectiveness. *British Medical Journal* **317**: 200–203.

Glowinski AJ (1994) Integrating guidelines and the clinical record: the role of semantically constrained terminologies. In: Gordon C, Christensen JP (eds) *Health Telematics for Clinical Guidelines and Protocols.* IOS Press, Amsterdam.

Glowinski AJ, Coiera EW, O'Neil MJ (1991) The role of domain models in maintaining the consistency of large medical knowledge bases. *Proceedings of the Third AIME. Lecture Notes in Medical Informatics* **44**: 72–81.

Goble CA, Glowinski AJ, Jeffery KG (1993a) Semantic constraints in a medical information system. *Proceedings of the 11th BNCOD*, Worbuys B, Grundy AF (eds). *Lecture Notes in Computer Science* **696**: 40–57.

Goble CA, Glowinski AJ, Nowlan A, Rector A (1993b) A descriptive semantic formalism for medicine. *Proceedings of the 9th IEEE International Conference on Data Engineering.* IEEE Computer Society Press, Piscataway, NJ, pp. 624–632.

Golub TR, Slonim DK, *et al.* (1999) Molecular classification of cancer: class discovery and glass predication by gene expression monitoring. *Science* **286**(5439): 531–537.

Goodlee F (1994) The Cochrane Collaboration. *British Medical Journal* **309**: 969–970.

Gorman P (1993) Does the medical literature contain the evidence to answer the questions of primary care physicians? Preliminary findings of a study. *Proceedings of the 17th Annual Symposium on Computer Applications in Medical Care*, pp. 571–575.

Gorman PN (1995) Information needs of physicians. *Journal of the American Society for Information Sciences* **46**: 729–736.

Gosling AS, Westbrook JI, Coiera EW (2003) Variation in the use of online clinical evidence: a qualitative analysis. *International Journal of Medical Informatics* **69**(1): 1–16.

Graitcer PL, Burton AH (1987) The Epidemiological Surveillance Project: a computer-based system for disease surveillance. *American Journal of Preventive Medicine* **3**(3): 123–127.

Gravenstein J, Newbower R, Ream A, Smith N (eds) (1987) *The Automated Anaesthesia Record and Alarm Systems.* Butterworths, Boston.

Greatbatch D, Luff P, Heath C, Campion P (1993) Interpersonal communication and human-computer interaction: an examination of the use of computers in medical consultations. *Interacting with Computers* **5**(2): 193–216.

Greenes RA, Peleg M, Boxwala A, Tu S, Patel V, Shortliffe EH (2001) Sharable computer based clinical practice guidelines: rationale, obstacles, approaches, and prospects. *Proceedings of the Medinfo 2001*, pp. 201–206.

Greenhalgh T (1997) The Medline database. *British Medical Journal* **315**: 180–183.

Greenwald S, Patil R, Mark R (1992) Improved detection and classification of arrhythmias in noise-corrupted electrocardiograms using contextual information. *Biomedical Instrumentation and Technology* **26**(2):124–132.

Greenwood J, Sullivan J, Spence K, McDonald M (2000) Nursing scripts and the organizational influences on critical thinking: report of a study of neonatal nurses' clinical reasoning. *Journal of Advanced Nursing* **31**(5): 1106–1114.

Gregory J, Mattison JE, Linde C (1995) Naming notes: transitions from free text to structured entry. *Methods of Information in Medicine* **34**: 57–67.

Grice H (1975) Logic and conversation. In: Cole P, Morgan JL (eds) *Syntax and Semantics*, volume 3. Academic Press, New York, pp. 41–58.

Griffiths P, Riddington L (2001) Nurses' use of computer databases to identify evidence for practice – a cross-sectional questionnaire survey in a UK hospital. *Health Information and Libraries Journal* **18**(1): 2–9.

Grilli R, Lomas J (1994) Evaluating the message: the relationship between compliance rate and the subject of a practice guideline. *Medical Care* **32**(3): 202–213.

Grimshaw JM, Russell IT (1993) Effect of clinical guidelines on medical practice: a systematic review of rigorous evaluations. *Lancet* **342**(8883): 1317–1322.

Guyatt GH, Sinclair J, Cook DJ, Glasziou P (1999) Users' guides to the medical literature. *Journal of the American Medical Association* **281**: 1836–43.

Hailey D, Roine R, Ohinmaa A (2002) Systematic review of evidence for the benefits of telemedicine. *Journal of Telemedicine and Telecare* **8**(Suppl 1): 1–7.

Halvorsen PA, Kristiansen IS (1996) Radiology services for remote communities: cost minimisation study of telemedicine. *British Medical Journal* **312**: 1333–1336.

Harpole L, Khorasani R, Fiskio J, Kuperman G, Bates D (1997) Automated evidence based critiquing of orders for abdominal radiographics: impact on utilization and appropriateness. *Journal of the American Medical Informatics Association* **4**: 511–521.

Harris EK (1980) On the use of statistical models of within-person variation in long term studies of healthy individuals. *Clinical Chemistry* **26**: 383–391.

Harris MF, Giles A, O'Toole BI (2002) Communication across the divide. A trial of structured communication between general practice and emergency departments. *Australian Family Physician* **31**(2): 197–200.

Hart A, Wyatt J (1989) Connectionist models in medicine: an investigation of their potential. In: Hunter J, Vookson J, Wyatt J (eds) *Lecture Notes in Medical Informatics* **38**: 115–124.

Hau D, Coiera E (1997) Learning qualitative models of dynamic systems. *Machine Learning* **26**: 177–211.

Haycox A, Bagust A, Walley T (1999) Clinical guidelines – the hidden costs. *British Medical Journal* **318**: 391–393.

Hayes-Roth B, Washington R, Ash D, *et al.* (1992) Guardian: A prototype intelligent agent for intensive care monitoring. *Artificial Intelligence in Medicine* **4**: 165–185.

Haynes RB, McKibbon KA, Walker CJ (1990) Online access to MEDLINE in clinical settings. *Annals of Internal Medicine* **112**: 78–84.

Haynes RB, Wilczynski N, McKibbon KA, Walker CJ, Sinclair JC (1994) Developing optimal search strategies for detecting clinically sound studies in Medline. *Journal of the American Medical Informatics Association* **1**: 447–458.

Haynes RB, Sackett DL, Guyatt GH, Cook DJ, Muir Gray JA (1997) Transferring evidence from research into practice: 4. Overcoming barriers to application. *Evidence Based Medicine* **2**: 68–69.

Heathfield HA, Wyatt J (1993) Medical informatics: hiding our light under a bushel, or the emperor's new clothes? *Methods of Information in Medicine* **32**: 181–182.

Heathfield HA, Kirby J, Hardiker NR (1995) Data entry in computer-based care planning. *Computer Methods and Programs in Biomedicine* **48**: 103–107.

Heathfield H, Pitty D, Hanka R (1998) Evaluating information technology in health care: barriers and challenges. *British Medical Journal* **316**: 1959–1961.

Heinsohn J, Kudenko D, Nobel B, Profitlich H (1994) An empirical analysis of terminological representation systems. *Artificial Intelligence* **68**: 367–397.

Heitmann KU, Blobel B, Dudeck J (1999) *HL7 – Communication Standard in Medicine.* Verlag Alexander Mönch, Munich.

Henderson S, Crapo RO, Wallace CJ, East TD, Morris AH, Gardner RM (1992) Performance of computerised protocols for the management of arterial oxygenation in an intensive care unit. *International Journal of Clinical Monitoring and Computing* **8**: 271–280.

Henry S, Campbell K, Holzemer W (1993) Representation of nursing terms for the description of patient problems using SNOMED III. *Proceedings of the Symposium on Computer Applications in Medicine*, McGraw-Hill, New York, pp. 700–704.

Hersh WR (2002) *Information Retrieval: A Health and Biomedical Perspective*, 2nd edition. Springer, New York.

Hersh W, Hickam D (1998) How well do physicians use electronic information retrieval systems?: A framework for investigation and systematic review. *Journal of the American Medical Association* **280**(15): 1347–1352.

Hersh WR, Helfand M, Wallace J, *et al.* (2001) Clinical outcomes resulting from telemedicine interventions: a systematic review. *BMC Medical Informatics and Decision Making* **1**: 5.

Hersh W, Helfand M, Wallace J, *et al.* (2002) A systematic review of the efficacy of telemedicine for making diagnostic and management decisions. *Journal of Telemedicine and Telecare* **8**: 197–209.

Hickam DH, Shortliffe EH, Bischoff MB, Scott AC, Jacobs CD (1985) The treatment advice of a computer-based cancer chemotherapy protocol advisor. *Annals of Internal Medicine* **101**: 928–936.

Hochstrasser DF, Appel RD, Golaz O, Pasquali C, Sanchez JC, Bairoch A (1995) Sharing of worldwide spread knowledge using hypermedia facilities and fast communication protocols (Mosaic and World Wide Web): The example of ExPASy. *Methods of Information in Medicine* **34**: 75–78.

Hogarth RM (1986) Generalisation in decision research: the role of formal model. *IEEE Transactions on Systems, Man and Cybernetics* **16**(3): 439–449.

Hohnloser JH, Pürner F, Kadlec P (1995) Coding medical concepts: a controlled experiment with a computerised coding tool. *International Journal of Clinical Monitoring and Computing* **12**: 141–145.

Hohnloser JH, Pürner F, Soltanian H (1996) Improving coded data entry by an electronic patient record system. *Methods of Information in Medicine* **35**: 108–111.

Horn K, Compton P, Lazarus L, Quinlan JR (1985) An expert system for the interpretation of thyroid assays in a clinical laboratory. *Australian Computer Journal* **17**: 7–11.

Howell J, Higgins C (1990) Champions of change: identifying, understanding and supporting champions of technological innovations. *Organizational Dynamics* **40**: 40–55.

Humber M, Butterworth H, Fox J, Thomson R (2001) Medical decision support via the Internet: PROforma and Solo. *Proceedings of Medinfo 2001*, pp. 464–469.

Humphreys BL, Lindberg DA (1989) Building the Unified Medical Language System. *Proceedings of the Annual Symposium on Computer Applications in Medical Care*, pp. 475–480.

Hunink M, Glasziou P, Siegel J, *et al.* (2001) *Decision Making in Health and Medicine – Integrating Evidence and Values*. Cambridge University Press, Cambridge.

Hunt D, Haynes B, Hanna S, Smith K (1998) Effects of computer-based clinical decision support systems on physician performance and patient outcomes: a systematic review. *Journal of the American Medical Association* **280**(15): 1339–1346.

Hydo B (1995) *Designing an Effective Clinical Pathway for Stroke. American Journal of Nursing Continuing Education Series*; http://www.ajn.org/ajn/5.3/a503044e.1t.

Impiccatore P, Pandolfini C, Casella N, Bonati M (1997) Reliability of health information for the public on the World Wide Web: systematic survey of advice on managing fever in children at home. *British Medical Journal* **314**: 1875–1879.

Institute of Medicine (2000) *Crossing the Quality Chasm: A New Health System for the 21st Century*. National Academy of Sciences Press, Washington, DC.

Ironi L, Stefannelli M, Lanzola G (1990) Qualitative models in medical diagnosis. *Artificial Intelligence in Medicine* **2**: 85–101.

Jackson R, Feder G (1998) Guidelines for clinical guidelines. *British Medical Journal* **317**: 427–428.

Jadad AR, Gagliardi A (1998) Rating health information on the Internet. *Journal of the American Medical Association* **279**: 611–614.

Jenks PJ (1998) Microbial genome sequencing: beyond the double helix. *British Medical Journal* **317**: 1568–1571.

Johansen R, Sibbet D, Martin A, Mittman R, Saffo P (1991) *Leading Business Teams*. Addison-Wesley, Reading, MA.

Johnson KB, Feldman MJ (1995) Medical informatics and pediatrics. Decision-support systems. *Archives of Pediatric and Adolescent Medicine* **149**: 1371–1380.

Johnson PD, Tu SW, Booth N, Sugden B, Purves IN (2000) Using scenarios in chronic disease management guidelines for primary care. *Proceedings of the AMIA Annual Fall Symposium*, pp. 389–393.

Johnson P, Tu S, Jones N (2001) Achieving reuse of computable guideline systems. *Proceedings of Medinfo 2001*, pp. 99–103.

Jones DH, Crichton C, Macdonald A, Potts S, Sime D, *et al.* (1996) Teledermatology in the Highlands of Scotland. *Journal of Telemedicine and Telecare* **2**(Suppl 1): 7–9.

Jones J, Playforth MJ (2001) The effect of the introduction of NHS Direct on requests for telephone advice from an accident and emergency department. *Emergency Medicine Journal* **18**: 300–301.

Jousimaa J, Makela M, Kunnamo I, MacLennan G, Grimshaw JM (2002) Primary care guidelines on consultation practices: the effectiveness of computerized versus paper-based versions. A cluster randomized controlled trial among newly qualified primary care physicians. *International Journal of Technology Assessment in Health Care* **18**(3): 586–596.

Kafka F (1971) Investigations of a dog. In: *The Complete Stories*, Schocken Books, New York.

Kahn MG, Steib SA, Fraser VJ, Dunagan WC (1993) An expert system for culture-based infection control surveillance. *Proceedings of the Symposium on Computer Applications in Medical Care*. McGraw-Hill, New York, pp. 171–175.

Kahn MG, Steib SA, Spitznagel EL, Dunagan WC, Fraser VJ (1995) Improvement in user performance following development and routine use of an expert system. In: Greenes RA, Peterson HE, Protti DJ (eds) *MEDINFO '95, Edmonton, Alberta, Canada*. International Medical Informatics Association/Healthcare Computing and Communications Canada, pp. 1064–1067.

Kahneman D, Slovic P, Tversky A (eds) (1982) *Judgement Under Uncertainty: Heuristics and Biases*. Cambridge University Press, Cambridge.

Kanehisa M, Bork P (2003) Bioinformatics in the post-sequence era. *Nature Genetics* **33**(suppl.): 305–310.

Kaplan B (1997) Addressing organizational issues into the evaluation of medical systems. *Journal of the American Medical Informatics Association* **4**(2): 94–101.

Kaplan B (2001) Evaluating informatics applications – some alternative approaches: theory, social interactionism, and call for methodological pluralism. *International Journal of Medical Informatics* **64**: 39–56.

Kaplan R, Norton D (1992) The balanced scorecard – measures that drive performance. *Harvard Business Review* **70**(1): 71–79.

Kaushal R, Bates D (2001) Computerized physician order entry (CPOE) with clinical decision support systems (CDSSs). In: Shojania K, Duncan B, McDonald K, Wachter R (eds) *Making Health Care Safer: A Critical Analysis of Patient Safety Practices*. Evidence Report No. 43, Agency for Healthcare Research and Quality, San Francisco, pp. 59–70

Kay S, Purves IN (1996) Medical records and other stories: a narratological framework. *Methods of Information in Medicine* **35**: 72–87.

Kelly K (1998) *New Rules for the New Economy*. Fourth Estate, London.

Kent W (1978) *Data and Reality*. North-Holland, Amsterdam.

Kephart JO, Greenwald A (1999) Shopbot economics. *Proceedings of ECSQARU*, 5–9 July 1999, London, pp. 5–9; http://www.research.ibm.com/infoecon/researchpapers.html.

Kidd M, Mazza D (2000) Clinical practice guidelines and the computer on your desk. *Medical Journal of Australia* **173**: 373–375.

Kim JM, Frosdick P (2001) Description of a drug hierarchy in a concept-based reference terminology. *Proceedings of the AMIA Annual Symposium*, pp. 314–319.

King RD, Muggleton S, Lewis RA, Sternberg MJE (1992) Drug design by machine learning: the use of inductive logic programming to model the structure–activity relationship of trimethoprim analogues binding to dihydrofolate reductase. *Proceedings of the National Academy of Sciences of the USA* **89**: 11322–11326.

Klein GA, Calderwood R (1991) Decision models: some lessons from the field. *IEEE Transactions on Systems Man and Cybernetics* **21**(5): 1018–1026.

Klein MS, Ross FV, Adams DL, Gilbert CM (1994) Effect of online literature searching on length of stay and patient costs. *Academic Medicine* **69**(6): 489–495.

Klein R (1995) Priorities and rationing: pragmatism or principles? *British Medical Journal* **311**: 761–762.

Kline TJ, Kline TS (1992) Radiologists, communication and resolution **5**: a medicolegal issue. *Radiology* **184**: 131–134.

Kohane IS, Greenspun P, Fackler J, Cimino C, Szolovits P (1996) Building national electronic-medical record systems via the World Wide Web. *Journal of the American Medical Informatics Association* **3**: 191–207.

Kohane IS, Kho AT, Butte AJ (2003) *Microarrays for an Integrative Genomics*. MIT Press, Boston, MA.

Kohonen T (1988) An introduction to neural computing. *Neural Networks* **1**: 3–16.

Korzybski A (1958) *Science and Sanity: An Introduction to Non-Aristotelian Systems and General Semantics*, 4th edition. International Non-Aristotelian Library, Lakeville, CT.

Koski E, Makivirta A, Sukuvaara T, Kari A (1990) Frequency and reliability of alarms in the monitoring of cardiac postoperative patients. *International Journal of Clinical Monitoring and Computing* **7**: 129–133.

Krall LP, Beaser RS (1989) *Joslin Diabetes Manual*, 12th edition. Lea and Febiger, Philadelphia.

Krishna S, Balas EA, Boren SA, Maglaveras N (2002) Patient acceptance of educational voice messages: a review of controlled clinical studies. *Methods of Information in Medicine* **41**: 360–369.

Kuipers BJ, Kassirer JP (1984) Causal reasoning in medicine: analysis of a protocol. *Cognitive Science* **8**: 363–385.

Kuperman GJ, Gardner RM (1990) The impact of the HELP computer system on the LDS Hospital paper medical record. *Proceedings of the SCAMC*, 1990, pp. 673–637.

Kuperman GJ, Gardner RM, Pryor TA (1991) *The HELP System*. Springer-Verlag, New York.

Kuperman G, Sittig DF, Shabot M, Teich J (1999) Clinical decision support for hospital and critical care. *Journal of the Healthcare Information and Management Systems Society* **13**: 81–96.

Labkoff SE, Shah S, Greenes RA (1995) Patterns of information resource access in patient care: a study of the use of portable computers to support the clinical encounter. *Proceedings of the AMIA Spring Congress, Capturing the Clinical Encounter*, p. 33.

Lang GS, Dickie KJ (1978) *The Practice-Oriented Medical Record*. Aspen, Rockville, MA.

LaPorte RE (1995) Global public health and the information superhighway. *British Medical Journal* **308**: 1651–1652.

LaPorte RE, Marler E, Akazawa S, *et al.* (1995) The death of biomedical journals. *British Medical Journal* **310**: 1387–1389.

Lathrop RH (1994) The protein threading problem with sequence amino acid interaction preferences is NP-complete. *Protein Engineering* **7**(9): 1059.

Lattimer VL, George S, Thompson F, *et al.* (1998) Safety and effectiveness of nurse telephone consultation in out of hours primary care: randomised controlled trial. *British Medical Journal* **317**: 1054–1059.

Lawton LS (1993) *Integrated Digital Networks*. Sigma, Wilmslow, Cheshire.

Ledley RS, Lusted LB (1959) Reasoning foundations of medical diagnosis. *Science* **130**: 9–21.

Leirer VO, Morrow DG, Tanke ED, Pariante GM (1991) Elders' nonadherence: Its assessment and medication reminding by voice mail. *Gerontologist* **31**(4): 514–520.

Leveson NG, Turner CS (1993) An investigation of the Therac-25 accidents. *IEEE Computer* (July): 18–41.

Lewontin RC (1993) *The Doctrine of DNA – Biology as Ideology*. Penguin, London.

Lindahl D, Lanke J, Lundin A, Palmer J, Edenbrandt L (1999) Improved classifications of myocardial bull's-eye scintigrams with computer-based decision support system. *Journal of Nuclear Medicine* **40**(1): 96–101.

Lindberg DA, Humphreys BL, McCray AT (1993) The Unified Medical Language System. *Methods of Information in Medicine* **32**(4): 281–91.

Little AD (1992) *Telecommunications: Can It Help Solve America's Health Care Problems?* Little, Cambridge, MA.

Littlejohn SW (1996) *Theories of Human Communication*, 5th edition. Wadsworth, Belmont, CA.

Littlewood B (ed.) (1987) *Software Reliability – Achievement and Assessment*. Blackwell Scientific, Oxford.

Lobach DF, Hammond E (1997) Computerized decision support based on a clinical practice guideline improves compliance with care standards. *American Journal of Medicine* **102**: 89–98.

Lober WB, Karras BT, Wagner MM, *et al.* (2002) Roundtable on bioterrorism detection – information system-based surveillance. *Journal of the American Medical Informatics Association* **9**: 105–115.

Lock C (1996) What value do computers provide to NHS hospitals? *British Medical Journal* **312**: 1407–1410.

Loeb R, Brunner J, Westenskow D, *et al.* (1989) The Utah Anaesthesia Workstation. *Anesthesiology* **70**: 999–1007.

Lorenzi NM, Riley RT, Blyth JC, Southon G, Dixon BJ (1997) Antecedents of the people and organizational aspects of medical informatics: review of the literature. *Journal of the American Medical Informatics Association* **4**: 79–101.

Lowe HJ, Lomax EC, Polonkey SE (1996) The World Wide Web: a review of an emerging Internet-based technology for the distribution of biomedical information. *Journal of the American Medical Informatics Association* **3**: 1–14.

Ma H (1995) Mapping clause of Arden syntax with the HL7 and ASTM E 1238–88 standard. *International Journal of Bio-Medical Computing* **38**: 9–21.

MacNeill D, Huang V (1996) Pen computers in healthcare. *Pen Computing Magazine* (April): 18–25.

Mair F, Whitten P (2000) Systematic review of studies of patient satisfaction with telemedicine. *British Medical Journal* **320**: 1517–1520.

Mair FS, Haycox A, May C, Williams T (2000) A review of telemedicine cost-effectiveness studies. *Journal of Telemedicine and Telecare* **6**(Suppl 1): 38–40.

Majidi F, Enterline JP, Ashley MSB, *et al.* (1993) Chemotherapy and treatment scheduling: The Johns Hopkins Oncology Center Outpatient Department. *Proceedings of the 17th Annual Symposium on Computer Applications in Medical Care*, pp. 154–158.

Mandl KD, Szolovits P, Kohane IS (2001) Public standards and patients' control: how to keep electronic medical records accessible but private. *British Medical Journal* **322**(7281): 283–287.

Manias E, Street A (2000) Legitimation of nurses' knowledge through policies and protocols in clinical practice. *Journal of Advanced Nursing* **32**(6): 1467–1475.

Markus ML (1994) Electronic mail as the medium of managerial choice. *Organization Science* **5**(4): 502–527.

Martel J, Jimenez MD, Martin-Santos FJ, Lopez-Alonso A (1995) Accuracy of teleradiology in skeletal disorders: solitary bone lesions and fractures. *Journal of Telemedicine and Telecare* **1**: 13–18.

Martin J (1995) *The Great Transition – Using the Seven Disciplines of Enterprise Engineering to Align People, Technology, and Strategy*. AMACOM, American Management Association, New York.

Massaro T (1989) Introducing physician order entry at a major academic medical center: I. Impact on Organizational culture and behavior. *Academic Medicine* **64**(1): 20–25.

Masys D, Baker D, Butros A, Cowles KE (2002) Giving patients access to their medical records via the Internet: the PCASSO experience. *Journal of the American Medical Informatics Association* **9**: 181–191.

Mathews JJ (1983) The communication process in clinical settings. *Social Science and Medicine* **17**(18): 1371–1378.

Mays N, Pope C (1996) *Qualitative Research in Health Care*. British Medical Journal Publishing Group, London.

McCarthy JC, Monk AF (1994) Channels, conversation, co-operation and relevance: all you wanted to know about communication but were afraid to ask. *Collaborative Computing* **1**: 35–60.

McClung HJ, Murray RD, Heitlinger LA (1998) The Internet as a source for current patient information. *Pediatrics* **101**: E2.

McDonald C, Hui S, Smith D, *et al.* (1984) Reminders to physicians from an introspective computer medical record. *Annals of Internal Medicine* **100**: 130–138.

McLaren P (1995) Telepsychiatry in the USA. *Journal of Telemedicine and Telecare* **1**: 121.

McManus RJ, Wilson S, Delaney BC, *et al.* (1998) Review of the usefulness of contacting other experts when conducting a literature search for systematic reviews. *British Medical Journal* **317**: 1562–1563.

Medin D, Alton MW, Edelson SM, Freko D (1982) Correlated symptoms and simulated medical classifications. *Journal of Experimental Psychology* **9**: 607–625.

Melzer SM, Poole SR (1999) Computerized pediatric telephone triage and advice programs at children's hospitals: operating and financial characteristics. *Archives of Pediatric and Adolescent Medicine* **153**: 858–863.

Mikolanis S (1997) How to use the new E/M documentation guidelines, Part I: A step-by-step description of how to comply with HCFA's history-taking requirements. *ACP Observer* (November).

Miksch S, Dobner M, Horn W, Popow C (1993) VIE-PNN: an expert system for parenteral nutrition of neonates. *Proceedings of the 9th IEEE Conference on Artificial Intelligence for Applications (CAIA), Orlando, Florida*, pp. 285–291.

Miller PL (1983) Critiquing anesthetic management: the ATTENDING computer system. *Anesthesiology* **58**: 362–369.

Miller PL (1988) *Selected Topics in Medical Artificial Intelligence*. Springer, New York.

Monane M, Matthias D, Nagle BA, Kelly MA (1998) Improving prescribing patterns for the elderly through an online drug utilization review intervention: a system linking the physician, pharmacist and computer. *Journal of the American Medical Association* **280**: 1249–1252.

Monk R (1990) *Ludwig Wittgenstein – The Duty of Genius*. Jonathan Cape, London.

Morrell RM, Wasilauskas BL, Winslow RM (1993) Personal computer-based expert system for quality assurance of antimicrobial therapy. *American Journal of Hospital Pharmacy* **50**: 2067–2073.

Morris A, Wallace C, Menlove R, *et al.* (1994a) A randomized clinical trial of pressure-controlled inverse ratio ventilation and extracorporeal CO_2 removal from ARDS. *American Journal of Respiratory and Critical Care Medicine* **149**(2): 295–305.

Morris A, East T, Wallace C, *et al.* (1994b) Ethical implications of standardization of ICU care with computerized protocols. *Proceedings of the Symposium on Computer Applications in Medicine, Journal of the American Medical Informatics Association Symposium Supplement*, 501–505.

Morris-Suzuki T (1997) Capitalism in the computer age and afterward. In: Davis J, Hirschl TA, Stack M (eds) *Cutting Edge – Technology, Information Capitalism and Social Revolution*. Verso, London, pp. 57–72.

Mowat G, Bowner DJ, Brebner JA, *et al.* (1997) When and how to assess fast-changing technologies: a comparative study of four generic technologies. *Health Technology Assessment* **1**: 14.

Muir Gray JA, Haynes RB, Sackett DL, Cook DJ, Guyatt GH (1997) Transferring evidence from research into practice: 3. Developing evidence-based clinical policy. *Evidence Based Medicine* **2**: 36–38.

Mulrow CD (1994) Rationale for systematic reviews. *British Medical Journal* **309**: 597–599.

Mungall D, Anbe D, Forrester P (1994) Clinic trials and therapeutics: a prospective randomized comparison of the accuracy of computer-assisted versus GUSTO nomogram-directed heparin therapy. *Clinical Pharmacology and Therapeutics* **55**: 591–596.

Munro J, Nicholl J, O'Cathain A, Knowles E (2000) Impact of NHS Direct on demand for immediate care: observational study. *British Medical Journal* **321**: 150–153.

Murphy-Muth SM (1987) *Medical Records – Management in a Changing Environment*. Aspen, Rockville, MA.

Musen MA, Tu SW, Das AK, Shahar Y (1995) A component-based architecture for automation of protocol-directed care. *Proceedings of the 5th Conference on Artificial Intelligence in Medicine Europe (AIME), Lecture Notes in Artificial Intelligence* **934**: 1–13.

Nakano K, Atobe T, Hiraki Y, Yasaka T (1981) Estimation of subject-specific normal ranges based on some statistical models of an individual's physiological variations. *Medical Informatics* **6**(3): 195–205.

Negroponte N (1995) *Being Digital*. Knopf, New York.

Nelson TH (1965) A file structure for the complex, the changing and the indeterminate. *Proceedings of the 20th National ACM Conference*, pp. 84–100.

NHS Information Authority Standards Project group (2001) NHS IT Standards Handbook

Nii HP (1989) Blackboard systems. In: Barr A, Cohen P, Feigenbaum EA (eds) *The Handbook of Artificial Intelligence* Vol. IV. Addison-Wesley, Reading, MA, pp. 1–82.

Nikoonahad M, Liu DC (1990) Medical ultrasound imaging using neural networks. *Electronics Letters* **26**: 545–546.

Nisbett RE, Wilson TD (1977) Telling more than we can know: verbal reports on mental processes. *Psychological Review* **84**: 231–259.

Norman DA (1993) Cognition in the head and in the world: an introduction to the special issue on situated action. *Cognitive Science* **17**(1): 1–6.

Nygren E, Henriksson P (1992) Reading the medical record – 1. Analysis of physician's ways of reading the medical record. *Computer Methods and Programs in Biomedicine* **39**: 1–12.
Nymo J (1993) Telemedicine. *Telektronikk* **89**(1): 4–11.
Oesterlen F (1855) *Medical Logic* (English translation). Sydenham Society, London.
O'Neil M, Payne C, Read J (1995) Read Codes Version 3: A user led terminology. *Methods of Information in Medicine* **34**: 187–192.
Ouellette F (1999) Internet resources for the clinical geneticist. *Clinical Genetics* **56**: 179–185.
Overhage J, Tierney W, McDonald C (1996) Computer reminders to implement preventative care guidelines for hospitalised patients. *Archives of Internal Medicine* **156**(4): 1551–1556.
Packer JS (1990) Patient care using closed-loop computer control. *Computing and Control Engineering Journal* **1**(1): 23–28.
Padgett JE, Gunther CG, Hattori T (1995) Overview of wireless personal communications. *IEEE Communications Magazine* (January): 28–41.
Palmer S, Byford S, Raftery J (1999) Types of economic evaluation. *British Medical Journal* **318**: 1349.
Parker J, Coiera E (2000) Improving clinical communication: a view from psychology. *Journal of the American Medical Informatics Association* **7**: 453–461.
Paterson-Brown S, Wyatt J, Fisk N (1993) Are clinicians interested in up-to-date reviews of effective care? *British Medical Journal* **307**: 1464.
Paterson-Brown S, Fisk NM, Wyatt JC (1995) Uptake of meta-analytical overviews of effective care in English obstetric units. *British Journal of Obstetrics and Gynaecology* **102**: 297–301.
Patil RS (1988) Artificial intelligence techniques for diagnostic reasoning in medicine. In: Shrobe H (ed.) *Exploring Artificial Intelligence: Survey Talks from the National Conferences on Artificial Intelligence*. Morgan Kaufmann, San Mateo, CA, pp. 347–380.
Peleg M, Boxwala A, Ogunyemi O, *et al.* (2000) GLIF3: The evolution of a guideline representation format. *Proceedings of the AMIA Annual Fall Symposium*, pp. 645–649.
Peleg M, Tu S, Bury J, *et al.* (2003) Comparing computer-interpretable guideline models: a case-study approach. *Journal of the American Medical Informatics Association* **10**: 52–68.
Pendleton D, Schofield T, Tate P, Havelock P (1984) *The Consultation – An Approach to Learning and Teaching*. Oxford University Press, Oxford.
Phaal P (1994) *LAN Traffic Management*. Prentice Hall International, Hemel Hempstead.
Pietka E (1989) Neural nets for ECG classification. *Images of the 21st Century: IEEE Engineering in Medicine and Biology 11th Annual Conference*, pp. 2021–2022.
Pince H, Verberckmoes R, Willems JL (1990) Computer aided interpretation of acid-base disorders. *International Journal of Biomedical Computing* **25**: 177–192.
Platt S, Tannahill A, Watson J, Fraser E (1997) Effectiveness of antismoking telephone helpline: follow up survey. *British Medical Journal* **314**: 1371–1375.
Poikonen J, Leventhal J (1999) Medication-management issues at the point of care. *Journal of Healthcare Information Management* **13**(2): 43–51.
Pointer JE, Osur MA (1987) EMS Quality Assurance: a computerized incident reporting system. *Journal of Emergency Medicine* **5**: 513–517.
Popper K (1976) *Unended Quest*. Fontana, London.
Pratt W, Sim I (1995) Physician's information customizer (PIC): using a shareable user model to filter the medical literature. *Proceedings of the International Conference on Medical Informatics (MEDINFO '95)*, pp. 1447–1451.

Protti DJ (1995) The synergism of health/medical informatics revisited. *Methods of Information in Medicine*, **34**: 441–445.

Protti D (2002) A proposal to use a balanced scorecard to evaluate Information for Health: an information strategy for the modern NHS (1998–2005). *Computers in Biology and Medicine* **32**: 221–236.

Purves IN, Sugden B, Booth N, Sowerby M (1999) The PRODIGY project – the iterative development of the Release One model. *Proceedings of the AMIA Annual Symposium*, pp. 359–363.

Quinlan JR (1986) Induction of decision trees. *Machine Learning* **1**: 81–106.

Raggett D, Lam J, Alexander I (1996) *HTML 3: Electronic Publishing on the World Wide Web*. Addison-Wesley, Harlow.

Rampil IJ (1987) Intelligent detection of artifact. In: Gravenstein J, Newbower R, Ream A, Ty Smith N (eds) *The Automated Anaesthesia Record and Alarm Systems*. Butterworths, Boston, pp. 175–190.

Ramsay J, Barabesi A, Preece J (1996) Informal communication is about sharing objects and media. *Interacting with Computers* **8**(3): 277–283.

Randolph AG, Haynes RB, Wyatt JC, Cook DJ, Guyatt GH (1999) Users' guides to the medical literature: XVIII. How to use an article evaluating the clinical impact of a computer-based clinical decision support system. *Journal of the American Medical Association* **282**(1): 67–74.

Rao JN (1994) Follow up by telephone. *British Medical Journal* **309**: 1527–1528.

Raschke RA, Gollihare B, Wunderlich TA, *et al.* (1998) A computer alert system to prevent injury from adverse drug events: development and evaluation in a community teaching hospital. *Journal of the American Medical Association* **280**(15): 1317–1320.

Reason J (1990) *Human Error*. Cambridge University Press, Cambridge.

Rector AL, Nolan WA, Glowinski A (1993) Goals for concept representation in the GALEN project. *Proceedings of the 17th SCAMC*, pp. 414–418.

Rector AL, Solomon WD, Nolan WA, *et al.* (1995) A terminology server for medical language and medical information systems. *Methods of Information in Medicine* **34**: 147–157.

Reeves B, Nass C (1996) *The Media Equation*. Cambridge University Press, Cambridge.

Renaud-Salis JL (1994) Distributed clinical management-information systems: an enabling technology for future health care programmes. In: Barahona P, Christensen JP (eds) *Knowledge and Decisions in Health Telematics – The Next Decade*. IOS Press, Amsterdam, pp. 139–146.

Retsas A (2000) Barriers to using research evidence in nursing practice. *Journal of Advanced Nursing* **31**(3): 599–606.

Rice RE (1992) Task analyzability, use of new media, and effectiveness: a multi-site exploration of media richness. *Organization Science* **3**: 475–500.

Richards CF, Burstein JL, Waeckerle JF, Hutson HR (1999) Emergency physicians and biological terrorism. *Annals of Emergency Medicine* **34**(2): 183–190.

Richardson RJ, Goldberg MA, Sharif HS, Matthew D (1996) Implementing global telemedicine: experience with 1097 cases from the Middle East to the USA. *Journal of Telemedicine and Telecare* **2**(1): 79–82.

Rind D, Safran C, Phillips RS, *et al.* (1994) Effect of computer-based alerts on the treatment and outcomes of hospitalized patients. *Archives of Internal Medicine* **154**: 1511–1517.

Rodriguez MJ, Arredono MT, del Pozo F, *et al.* (1995) A home telecare management system. *Journal of Telemedicine and Telecare* **1**: 86–94.

Rogers EM (1995) *Diffusion of Innovations*, 4th edition. Free Press, New York.

Roine R, Ohinmaa A, Hailey D (2001) Assessing telemedicine: a systematic review of the literature. *Canadian Medical Association Journal* **165**(6): 765–771.

Roper WL, Winkenwerder W, Hackbarth GH, Krakauer H (1988) Effectiveness in health care – an initiative to evaluate and improve medical practice. *New England Journal of Medicine* **319**(18): 1197–1202.

Rosch E (1988) Principles of categorization. In: Rosch E, Lloyd BB (eds) *Readings in Cognitive Science*. Morgan Kaufmann, San Mateo, CA, pp. 312–322.

Rothwell DJ (1995) SNOMED-based knowledge representation. *Methods of Information in Medicine* **34**: 209–213.

Rushworth RL, Bell SM, Rubin GL, *et al.* (1991) Improving surveillance of infectious diseases in New South Wales. *Medical Journal of Australia* **154**: 828–831.

Russell S, Norvig P (2002) *Artificial Intelligence – A Modern Approach*. Prentice Hall, Englewood Cliffs, NJ.

Rutledge G, Thomsen G, Farr B, *et al.* (1993) The design and implementation of a ventilator-management advisor. *Artificial Intelligence in Medicine* **5**: 67–82.

Sable JH, Nash SK, Wang AY (2001) Culling a clinical terminology: a systematic approach to identifying problematic content. *Proceedings of the AMIA Annual Symposium*, pp. 578–583.

Sackett DL, Straus S (1998) Finding and applying evidence during clinical rounds: the 'Evidence Cart'. *Journal of the American Medical Association* **280**(15): 1336–1338.

Sackett DL, Straus SE, Richardson WS, Rosenberg W, Haynes RB (2000) *Evidence-Based Medicine – How to Practice and Teach EBM*. Churchill Livingstone, Edinburgh.

Safran C, Sands DZ, Rind DM (1998) Online medical records: a decade of experience. *Proceedings of EPRIMP*, pp. 67–74.

Sawar MJ, Brennan TG, Cole AJ, Stewart J (1992) An expert system for postoperative care (POEMS). *Proceedings of MEDINFO*, Geneva, Switzerland.

Schafer EA, Thane GD (1891) *Quain's Elements of Anatomy*, Vol. 1, Part III. Longmans, Green and Co., London.

Schulz EB, Barrett JW, Price C (1998) Read code quality assurance: from simple syntax to semantic stability. *Journal of the American Medical Informatics Association* **5**: 337–346.

Sebald A (1989) Use of neural networks for detection of artifacts in arterial pressure waveforms. *Images of the 21st Century – IEEE Engineering in Medicine and Biology 11th Annual Conference*, pp. 2034–2035.

Shaneyfelt TM, Mayo-Smith MF, Rothwangl J (1999) Are guidelines following guidelines? *Journal of the American Medical Association* **281**: 1900–1905.

Shanit D, Cheng A, Greenbaum RA (1996) Telecardiology: supporting the decision-making process in general practice. *Journal of Telemedicine and Telecare* **2**: 7–13.

Shapiro C, Varian HR (1998) *Information Rules: A Strategic Guide for the Network Economy*. Harvard Business School Press, Cambridge, MA.

Shea S, Sidell RV, DuMouchel W, *et al.* (1995) Computer-generated information messages directed to physicians: effect on length of hospital stay. *Journal of the American Medical Informatics Association* **2**: 58–64.

Shea S, DuMouchel RW, Bahamonde L (1996) A meta-analysis of 16 randomized controlled trials to evaluate computer-based clinical reminder systems for preventative care in the ambulatory setting. *Journal of the American Medical Informatics Association* **3**: 399–409.

Shiffman RN (1994) Towards effective implementation of a pediatric asthma guideline: Integration of decision support and clinical workflow support. *Proceedings of 18th Symposium on Computer Applications in Medical Care*, pp. 797–801.

Shiffman RN, Liaw Y, Brandt CA, Corb GJ (1999) Computer-based guideline implementation systems – a systematic review of functionality and effectiveness. *Journal of the American Medical Informatics Association* **6**: 104–114.

Shojania K, Yokoe D, Platt R, *et al.* (1998) Reducing vancomycin use utilizing a computer guideline. *Journal of American Medical Informatics Association* **5**(6): 554–562.

Shortliffe EH (1987) Computer programs to support clinical decision making. *Journal of the American Medical Association* **258**: 61–66.

Shu K, Boyle D, Spurr C, *et al.* (2001) Comparison of time spent writing orders on paper with computerized physician order entry. *Proceedings of Medinfo*, 2001, London. IOS Press, Amsterdam, pp. 1207–1211.

Silberg WM, Lundberg GD, Musacchio RA (1997) Editorial: Assessing, controlling, and assuring the quality of medical information on the Internet. *Journal of the American Medical Association* **276**: 1244–1245.

Silverstein J (1995) Strengthening the links between health sciences information users and providers. *Bulletin of the Medical Library Association* **83**(4): 407–417.

Sim I, Hlatky MA (1996) Growing pains of meta-analysis. *British Medical Journal* **313**: 702–703.

Simon HA (1965) *The Shape of Automation for Men and Management*. Harper & Row, New York.

Simon JD (1997) Biological terrorism – preparing to meet the threat. *Journal of the American Medical Association* **278**: 428–430.

Sintchenko V, Westbrook J, Tipper S, Mathie M, Coiera E (2003) *Electronic Decision Support Activities in Different Healthcare Settings in Australia*. Electronic Decision Support for Australia's Health Sector. National Electronic Decision Support Taskforce, Commonwealth of Australia; http://www.health.gov.au/healthonline/nedst.htm.

Skitka LJ, Mosier K, Burdick MD (1999) Does automation bias decision making? *International Journal of Human Computer Studies* **51**: 991–1006.

Skitka LJ, Mosier K, Burdick MD (2000) Accountability and automation bias. *International Journal of Human Computer Studies* **52**: 701–717.

Skolimowski H (1977) The twilight of physical descriptions and the ascent of normative models. In: Laszlo E (ed.) *The World System – Models, Norms, Variations*. G. Braziller, New York.

Slawson DC, Shaughnessy AF, Bennett JH (1994) Becoming a medical information master: feeling good about not knowing everything. *Journal of Family Practice* **38**: 505–513.

Smart S, Purves I (2001) The problems of large scale knowledge authoring and the PRODIGY solutions. *Proceedings of the AMIA Annual Symposium*, p. 835.

Smith BH, James NT, Sackett DL, *et al.* (1996) Correspondence: evidence based medicine. *British Medical Journal* **313**: 169–171.

Smith H, Gooding S, Brown R, Frew A (1998) Evaluation of readability and accuracy of information leaflets in general practice for patients with asthma. *British Medical Journal* **317**: 264–265.

Smith HT, Hennessy PA, Lunt GA (1991) An object-oriented framework for modelling organisational communication. In: Bowers JM, Benford SD (eds) *Studies in Computer Supported Cooperative Work*. Elsevier/North-Holland, Amsterdam, pp. 145–157.

Smith MF (1996) Telemedicine safety. *Journal of Telemedicine and Telecare* **2**(1): 33–36.

Smith R (1996a) The greatest breakthrough since fire or just more technology? *British Medical Journal* **312**: ii.

Smith R (1996b) What clinical information do doctors need? *British Medical Journal* **313**(7064): 1062–1067.

Snow MG, Fallat RJ, Tyler WR, Hsu SP (1988) Pulmonary consult: concept to application of an expert system. *Journal of Clinical Engineering* **13**(3): 201–205.

Sox H, Blatt M, Higgins M, Marton K (1988) *Medical Decision Making*. Butterworths, Stoneham, MA.

Spackman KA, Campbell KE, Cote RA (1997) SNOMED®: a reference terminology for health care. *Proceedings of the AMIA Annual Symposium*, pp. 640–644.

Spencer R, Logan P (2002) Role-based communication patterns within an emergency department setting. *Proceedings of the HIC.*

Staender S, Davies JM, Helmreich RL, Sexton B, Kaufmann M (1996) Anesthesia critical incident reporting system: an experience database. *Proceedings of Mednet '96 – European Congress of the Internet in Medicine*, pp. 44–45.

Steels L, Brooks R (eds) (1995) *The Artificial Life Route to Artificial Intelligence.* Lawrence Erlbaum Associates, New York.

Stigler GJ (1961) The economics of information. *Journal of Political Economy* **69**: 213–225; (reprinted in Lamberton DM, ed., *Economics of Information and Knowledge*, Penguin, Harmondsworth, 1971).

Stinchombe M, White H (1989) Multilayer feedforward networks are universal approximators. *Neural Networks* **2**: 359–366.

Stoupa R, Campbell J (1990) Documentation of ambulatory care rendered by telephone: Use of a computerized nursing module. *Proceedings of the Symposium on Computer Applications in Medicine.* IEEE Computer Society Press, Los Alamitos, CA, pp. 890–893.

Straus SE, Sackett DL (1998) Using research findings in clinical practice. *British Medical Journal* **317**: 339–342.

Sykes MK (1987) Essential monitoring. *British Journal of Anaesthesia* **59**: 901–912.

Szolovits P (1982) *Artificial Intelligence in Medicine.* AAAS Selected Symposia Series, Westview Press, CO.

Tanenbaum AS (2002) *Computer Networks*, 4th edition. Prentice Hall, Englewood Cliffs, NJ.

Tang PC, Fafchamps D, Shortliffe EH (1994) Traditional hospital records as a source of clinical data in the outpatient setting. *Proceedings of the SCAMC*, pp. 575–579.

Tang P, Jaworski MA, Fellencer CA, *et al.* (1996) Clinical information activities in diverse ambulatory care practices. *Proceedings of the American Medical Informatics Association Autumn Symposium*, pp. 12–16.

Tange HJ (1995) The paper-based patient record: is it really so bad? *Computer Methods and Programs in Biomedicine* **48**: 127–131.

Tange H (1996) How to approach the structuring of the medical record? Towards a model for flexible access to free text medical data. *International Journal of Biomedical computing* **42**: 27–34.

Tange HJ, Schouten HC, Kester ADM, Hasman A (1998) The granularity of medical narratives and its effect on the speed and completeness of information retrieval. *Journal of the American Medical Informatics Association* **5**: 571–582.

Taylor P (1998) A survey of research in telemedicine. **2**: Telemedicine services. *Journal of Telemedicine and Telecare* **4**: 63–71.

Teich J, Mercia PR, Schmiz J, Kuperman G, Spurr C, Bates D (2000) Effects of computerized physician order entry on prescribing practices. *Archives of Internal Medicine* **160**: 2741–2747.

Tenner E (1996) *Why Things Bite Back – Technology and the Revenge Effect.* London, Fourth Estate.

Thomas KW, Dayton CS, Peterson MW (1999) Evaluation of internet-based clinical decision support systems. *Journal of Medical Internet Research* **1**(2): E6.

Thompson LA, Ogden WC (1995) Visible speech improves human language understanding: implications for speech processing systems. *Artificial Intelligence Review* **9**: 347–358.

Thomsen GE, Pope D, East T, *et al.* (1993) Clinical performance of a rule-based decision support system for mechanical ventilation of ARDS patients. *Proceedings of the Symposium on Computer Applications in Medicine*. McGraw-Hill, New York, pp. 339–343.

Tierney W, Miller M, Overhage J, McDonald C (1993) Physician inpatient order writing on microcomputer workstations: effects on resource utilization. *Journal of the American Medical Association* **269**(3): 379–383.

Tomohita M, Hashimoto K, Takahashi K, *et al.* (1999) E-CELL: software environment for whole-cell simulation. *Bioinformatics* **15**(1): 72–84.

Trendelenburg C (1994) Interpretation of special findings in laboratory medicine and medical responsibility. *Laboratory Medicine* **18**: 545–582.

Trumbo CW (1998) Communication channels and risk information. *Science Communication* **20**(2): 190–203.

Tu SW, Kahn MG, Musen MA, *et al.* (1989) Episodic skeletal-plan refinement based upon temporal data. *Communications of the ACM* **32**(12): 1439–1455.

Tucker JB (1997) National health and medical services response to incidents of chemical and biological terrorism. *Journal of the American Medical Association* **276**(5): 362–368.

Tufo HM, Speidel JJ (1971) Problems with medical records. *Medical Care* **9**: 509–517.

Tura C, Ruiz L, Holtzer C, Schapiro J, Viciana P, González J, *et al.* (2002) Clinical utility of HIV-1 genotyping and expert advice: the Havana trial. *AIDS* **1**(16): 209–218.

Turnin MG, Beddok RH, Clottes JP, *et al.* (1992) Telematic expert system Diabeto. *Diabetes Care* **15**: 204–212.

Tuttle MS (1994) The position of the CANON group: A reality check. *Journal of the American Medical Informatics Association* **1**: 298–299.

Tuttle MS, Nelson SJ (1994) The role of the UMLS in 'storing' and 'sharing' across systems. *International Journal of Bio-Medical Computing* **34**: 207–237.

Tuttle MS, Cole WG, Sherertz DD, Nelson SJ (1995) Navigation to knowledge. *Methods of Information in Medicine* **34**: 214–231.

Tversky A, Kahneman D (1981) The framing of decisions and the psychology of choice. *Science* **211**: 453–458.

Uckun S (1992) Model-based reasoning in biomedicine. *Critical Reviews in Biomedical Engineering* **19**(4): 261–292.

Uckun S, Dawant B, Lindstrom D (1993) Model-based diagnosis in intensive care monitoring: the YAQ approach. *Artificial Intelligence in Medicine* **5**(1): 31–48.

University of Leeds (1994) Nuffield Institute for Health, University of Leeds; University of York Centre for Health Economics. NHS Centre for Reviews and Dissemination. Implementing clinical practice guidelines: can guidelines be used to improve clinical practice? *Effective Health Care* **8**: 1–12.

Urquhart C, Davies R (1997) EVINCE: The value of information in developing nursing knowledge and competence. *Health Libraries Review* **14**(2): 61–72.

Utterback JM (1994) *Mastering the Dynamics of Innovation*. Harvard Business School Press, Boston, MA.

van der Loo RP , Gennip EM van, Bakker AR, Hasman A, Rutten FF (1995) Evaluation of automated information systems in health care: an approach to classifying evaluative studies. *Computer Methods and Programs in Biomedicine* **48**: 45–52.

van der Lubbe JCA (1997) *Information Theory*. Cambridge University Press, Cambridge.

Van Grembergen W, Van Bruggen R (1997) Measuring and improving corporate information technology through the balanced scorecard. *Electronic Journal of Information Systems Evaluation* **1**: 1.

Van Leeuwin C (1998) *Perception*. In: Bechtel W, Graham G (eds) *A Companion to Cognitive Science*. Blackwell Science, Oxford, pp. 265–282.

van Walraven C , Laupacis A, Seth R, Wells G (1999) Dictated versus database-generated discharge summaries: a randomized clinical trial. *Canadian Medical Association Journal* **160**: 319–326.

Varian HR (1996) Pricing electronic journals. *D-Lib Magazine* (June); http://www.dlib.org/dlib/june96/06varian.html

Varian HR (1998) Markets for information goods. http://www.sims.berkeley.edu/~hal/people/hal/papers.html

Varian HR (1999) Market structure in the Network Age. http://www.sims.berkeley.edu/~hal/people/hal/papers.html

Vissers MC, Biert J, Linden CJ v d, Hasman A (1996) Effects of a supportive protocol processing system (protoVIEW) on clinical behaviour of residents in the accident and emergency department. *Computer Methods and Programs in Biomedicine* **49**: 177–184.

Wang D, Peleg M, Tu SW, *et al.* (2002) Representation primitives, process models and patient data in computer-interpretable clinical practice guidelines: a literature review of guideline representation models. *International Journal of Medical Informatics* **68**: 59–70.

Ward JPT, Gordon J, Field MJ, Lehmann HP (2001) Communication and information technology in medical education. *Lancet* **357**: 792–796.

Warner HR, Haug P, Bouhaddou O, *et al.* (1988) Iliad: an expert consultant to teach differential diagnosis. *Proceedings of the SCAMC*, p. 371.

Waterer GW, Baselski VS, Wunderink RG (2001) *Legionella* and community-acquired pneumonia: a review of current diagnostic tests from a clinician's viewpoint. *American Journal of Medicine* **110**: 41–48.

Weed LL (1968) Medical records that guide and teach. *New England Journal of Medicine* **278**: 593–599; 652–657.

Weigner MB, Englund CE (1990) Ergonomic and human factors affecting anesthetic vigilance and monitoring performance in the operating room environment. *Anesthesiology* **73**(5): 995–1021.

Weiner N (1954) *The Human Use of Human Beings*. Eyre and Spottiswood, London.

Weingarten SR, Henning JM, Badamgarav E, *et al.* (2002) Interventions used in disease management programmes for patients with chronic illness which ones work? Meta-analysis of published reports. *British Medical Journal* **325**: 925.

Weisbord SD, Soule JB, Kimmel PL (1997) Brief report: Poison on line – acute renal failure caused by oil of wormwood purchased through the Internet. *New England Journal of Medicine* **337**: 825.

Whittaker S (1995) Rethinking video as a technology for interpersonal communications: theory and design implications. *International Journal of Human Computer Studies* **42**: 501–529.

Whitten PS, Mair FS, Haycox A, *et al.* (2002) Systematic review of cost effectiveness studies of telemedicine interventions. *British Medical Journal* **324**: 1434–1437.

WHO (1977) *ICD-9, Manual of the International Statistical Classification of Diseases, Injuries and Causes of Death*. World Health Organization, Geneva.

WHO (1993) *ICD-10, International Statistical Classification of Diseases and Related Health Problems – 10th Revision*. World Health Organization, Geneva.

Wickens CD, Hollands JG (2000) *Engineering Psychology and Human Performance*, 3rd edition. Prentice Hall, Englewood Cliffs, NJ.

Wicker AW (1976) Attitudes v. actions: the relationship of verbal and overt responses to attitude objects. In: Warren N, Jahoda M (eds) *Attitudes*, 2nd edition. Penguin, London.

Widman LE (1992) A model-based approach to the diagnosis of cardiac arrhythmias. *Artificial Intelligence in Medicine* **4**: 1–19.

Williams E (1977) Experimental comparisons of face-to-face and mediated communication: a review. *Psychological Bulletin* **84**: 963–976.

Williams TL, May CR, Esmail A (2001) Limitations of patient satisfaction studies in telehealthcare: a systematic review of the literature. *Telemedicine Journal and e-Health* **7**(4): 293–316.

Wilson RM, Runciman WB, Gibberd RW, *et al.* (1995) The Quality in Australian Health Care Study. *Medical Journal of Australia* **163**: 458–471.

Winograd T (1997) The design of interaction. In: Denning PJ, Metcalfe RM (eds) *Beyond Calculation – The Next Fifty Years of Computing*. Springer, New York.

Wisniewski EJ, Medin DL (1994) On the interaction of theory and data in concept learning. *Cognitive Science* **18**: 221–281.

Withers CB (1988) Electronic voicemail: one hospital's experience. *Computers in Healthcare* **9**(1): 28–30.

Wittgenstein L (1953) *Philosophical Investigations*. Macmillan, New York.

Woolf S, Grol R, Hutchinson A, Eccles M, Grimshaw J (1999) Potential benefits, limitations, and harms of clinical guidelines. *British Medical Journal* **318**: 527–530.

Wootton R (2001) Recent advances: telemedicine. *British Medical Journal* **323**: 557–560.

Worrall G, Chaulk P, Freake D (1997) The effects of clinical practice guidelines on patient outcomes in primary care: a systematic review. *Canadian Medical Association Journal* **156**(12): 1705–1712.

Wright P, Jansen C, Wyatt J (1998) How to limit clinical errors in interpretation of data. *Lancet* **352**: 1539–1543.

Wyatt J (1987) The evaluation of clinical decision support systems: a discussion of the methodology used in the ACORN project. *Proceedings of AIME 87, Lecture Notes in Medical Informatics*, **33**: 15–24.

Wyatt J (1991) Use and sources of medical knowledge. *Lancet* **338**: 1368–1373.

Wyatt J (1995) Evidence-based decision support – Is it feasible? *Workshop on Decision Support in Primary and Secondary Care – Priorities for Implementation, NTRHA.*

Wyatt JC (1997) Commentary: measuring quality and impact of the World Wide Web. *British Medical Journal* **314**: 1879–1881.

Wyatt J, Wright P (1998) Design should help use of patients' data. *Lancet* **352**: 1375–1378.

Wyatt JC, Paterson-Brown S, Johanson R, *et al.* (1998) Randomised trial of educational visits to enhance use of systematic reviews in 25 obstetric units. *British Medical Journal* **317**: 1041–1046.

Young J, Ward J, Sladden M (1998) Do the beliefs of Australian general practitioners about the effectiveness of cancer screening accord with the evidence? *Journal of Medical Screening* **5**: 67–68.

Index

Abduction 83, **84**, 397
Abstraction 5, 8, 9, 180
Active protocol systems xxv, 154, 158–64
  alert-based reminding 160
  information technology and 158, **159**, 163, 164
    evaluation of 163, 164
  integrated into electronic medical records 168
  semi-automated record-keeping 159, 160
  task recommendations 160
  task reminders 160, 161
Admission, Discharge and Transfer 256
Advanced Research Projects Network 287
Adverse drug reactions
  CDSS and reductions in 340, 341
  reporting 315
Alerts
  early alert system 315
  electronic medical record reminders **120**, 121
  expert systems applied to xxvi, 334, 342
  protocol alert-based reminding 160
Algorithm 146, 397
  flowchart-like 168
  information systems 130
Aliasing 139
Ambulatory visit groups 206
America Online 290
Anchoring and adjustment heuristic 93
Answers, evaluating 77–9
Arden syntax 165, 397
ARNO 165
ARPAnet 287, 288, 397
Artefacts 8, 9, 358–60
Artificial heart **10**
Artificial intelligence xxvi, 331–3, 337, 345–8, 351, 352, 397
Artificial Intelligence in Medicine (AIM) 331, 332, 352, 397
Asynchronous channels 46
Asynchronous communication 237, 238, 275, 276, 280, 281, 397
Asynchronous transfer mode 249, **250**, 251, 252, 398
  transmission 250, **251**, *251*
Attitudinal bias 128
Australian Federal Government's Practice Incentives Program 176
Automation bias 364, 365
Autonomous therapeutic devices 363, 364
Availability heuristic 92, 93

Babbage, Charles 29
Bandwidth 248, 398
Basic level 195, 218, 219
Bayesian networks 349
Bayes' rule 350
Bayes' theorum 85, 86, **87,** 88, 89, 349, 350, 398
B-cell lymphoma 383, **384**
Belief networks 349, **350**
Biases
  attitudinal 128
  automation 365
  cognitive 41, 91
  presentation 93
  probability estimates 92–3
Bioinformatics xxii, xxvii, 379–96, 398
  Internet and 389, 390
Biological warfare, agents 368, 372
Biomedical equipment, control of 163
Bio-ontologies 391, **392**
Biosurveillance xxvii, 367–78
  clinical education 372, 373
  communication flows **369**
  communication technology in support of 374–7
  systems *371*
  Web in support of 372–7
Bioterrorism 367
  agents 368, 372
    infectious disease surveillance systems 370–2
  communication of events 368, 369
  detection of events 368
  recognition of events 368
Bit shipping 289
Blackboard systems 360, 364
BLAST 389, 390
Bluetooth **254**, 255, 398
Bolam principle 312
Boolean logic 60, **61**, 398
Braess' paradox **25**
Breadth-first search 70, **71**
Broadband 250, 398
Broadcasting 291, *292*, 314
Brokering services 316
Browser 296, 398
Bulletin boards 292, **293**, 294

Calculating machine 29
CAPSULE 165
Care pathways 146, *150*, 151, 159, 398
Cascade communication system 314, 377
Case-mix index 205, 206
Causal probabilistic networks 349
Causal structures 195, **196**
CDSS 332–5
  in biosurveillance 373, 374
  diagnostic 335, 336
  infectious disease surveillance systems 370, 372
  limits 353, 354
CERN 287, 294, 398
Chance nodes 89
Changing state 28
Circuit-switched systems 246, **247**, 399
Classification hierarchies 194, **195**, **196**, 203, 209
Classification systems 201–16
Classification techniques 393
Clinical audit 192
Clinical coding 197–200
  structured data-entry forms **199**
Clinical communication 261–82
  researching 276–81
Clinical data, privacy of 392, 393

Clinical databases 390
  anonymity 393
Clinical decision support systems 331–44
  benefits from 338, 340–3
  evaluation of 338, *339*
Clinical evidence 178
Clinical decision support systems, *see* CDSS
Clinical guidelines, *see* Guidelines
Clinical informatics xxii
Clinical knowledge, *see* Knowledge
Clinical practice xxii, xxiii
Clinical protocols 16, 18
Clinical studies **388**
Clinical Terms 206, 208, 212
Clinical Terms Project 207
Clinical vocabularies 390, 391
Closed-loop control of biomedical equipment 163, 358, 399
Closed-world assumption 26, 386
Clustering techniques 393, 394, **395**
Cochrane Collaboration 158, 171, 182
Coding xxvi, **193**, 194, 399
  problems with 217–28
  systems 196–200
    comparison *214*, 215, 216, 221, 222, 226
Cognitive biases 41, 91,
Cognitive overload 356
Cognitive prosthesis 332
Common ground 39, 277, 278, **279**, 280
Communicating 35–43
  attention limitations 41
  cognitive biases 41
  perceptual limitations 40, 41
Communication
  agents 235
  channels **37**, 38, 39, 47, 235, **236**
    dedicated 246
    shared 246–51
  devices 235
  failures 232
  home healthcare and 268–70
  hospitals and 273–6
  inter-hospital 273, 274
  intra-hospital 274–6
  policies 235
  primary care and 270–3
  protocol 244, **245**, 246, 399
    stack 245, 255
  requirements 236, *237*, 238, 239
    different time, different place 238
    different time, same place 237, 238
    in healthcare 267
    same time, different place 237
    same time, same place 236, 237
  services 235, *238*, 239–42
    media employed 238, 239
  space 232
  systems xxii, xxvi, 108, 109, 231–3, **234**, 235–43
    components 235
    interaction mode 235, 236
    merging with computer systems 258, 259
    wireless 252–5
    wireline 249–52
  technology 183, 244–60
Complex situation protocol 147
Compositional terminology 196, **197**
CompuServe 290
Computed tomography 19
Computer-based patient records, *see* Electronic patient records; Patient records
Computer-based protocols 156–68, **169**, 170, 181
Computer-generated reminders 121
Computer networks **259**
Computer-supported prescribing 120
Computer systems, merging with communication systems 258, 259
Concept creation 218, 219
Conditional probability 85, **86**, 399
Consensus review 183
Consultation by e-mail 315, 316
Content providers 290
Continuing medical education 309, 372
Continuing professional education 309, 310, 373
Cooperative principle 41, 42, 44
Copyright 322
Cordless Telephony 2 (CT2) 253
Critiquing systems 334
Cyber-immune cells 314
Cyberspace 288, 399

Data 13
  analysis 107
  capture 118
  condensation 122
  gathering 182
  genome 383–5
  interpretation 14, **15**, **18**, 19, 20
  mining 337, 394
  model 15
  overload 356
  stores 18
  structure **36**, 37
  views, generation by computers 18, 19
Databases 15, 18, 29, 60–5, 83, 181, 399
  clinical 390
  EMBL 379
  evidence-based healthcare 181
  GenBank 379, 380, **383**, 390
  keywords 64, 72
  limits 72
  OMIM 390
  query language 60
  query reformulation **73**
    semantic *74*
    syntactic 73, *74*
  questions
    performance *64*
  searching 66, 67, 73, 74, **75**
  search space 72
Data-oriented directory 45
Data-oriented messages 51
Decision control loop 102
Decision
  biases 41, 91, 92, 364, 365
  decision making 81–98
  node 93
  procedures 29, 30
  role of information technology in xxvii, 310, 331–44, 363
  support systems 331–44, 363, 373, 374, 399
    limits 353, 354
  trees 88, **89**, **94**, 93, 148, 153, 164, 399
Deduction 83, **84**, 400
DeMorgan's theorum **62**
Deoxyribonucleic acid, *see* DNA
Depth-first search 70, **71**, 76
  Design assumptions 9, 10, 180, **181**
  dominant 172
  information management cycle, designing a 136–9
  information system xxii, 22–9, **30**, 31, 32, 124–7, 130–9
  information system architecture 125
  for change 134–6
  human-computer interaction 131
  information 49
  interaction 132–4
  model 9
  protocol 180–188
  socio-technical 131,132
Designer drugs 385
Diagnosis related groups 205, 206
Diagnostic accuracy, information technology and 161
Diagnostic assistance, expert systems and 334–6
Dial tone multifrequency 242, 400
Digital Cellular system 1800 253
Digital divide 289
Digital European Cordless Telecommunications 253, 400
Disease-oriented evidence *58*, 59, 60, 79
DNA 7, 17, **381**, 400
  chips 384, 388, 389
Doctors, policies and procedures 178
Document complexity 47
Docuverse 294
Dominant design 172
Dot com boom 289
Drugs
  designer 385
  discovery 338, 385
  prescription, questions pursued *58*
DXplain 336

Early alert system 315
ECG
  faxing 108, 109
  intelligent monitoring and control **359**, 361, 362, 364
Economics
  information economics 172
  Internet and information economics 319–327
  analyses of information systems 130
  supply and demand 320, **321**
  system benefits 30, 263
  telemedicine 263–5
  view of guideline uptake 172
Education protocol 147
Electrocardiogram, *see* ECG
Electronic guidelines
  rate of uptake 163
  socio-technical system 163
Electronic journals 182
Electronic medical records xxvi, 52, 111–23, 357, 358, 390, 392, 400
  active protocol systems 168
  advantages 117–19
  alerts and reminders **120**, 121
  clinical audit 122
  clinical care 119, **120**, 121, 122
  computer-supported prescribing 120
  data
    capture 118
    condensation 122
    searching 119
  evaluation of the 117
  formal data models 118
  functions **114**
  outcomes assessment 122
  physical aspects 117–19
  protocol-guided care **120**, 121, 122, 145
  search engines 119
  security 119, 392, 393
  task-specific views of data **120**, 121, **122**
  Web technologies and 306–8, 311
  see also Patient record
Electronic prescribing 120
E-mail 238, **240**, 241, 253, 276, 400
  messages 291, 292, 314, 315
  consultation by 315, 316
EMBL 379
Encoding rules 256
Encryption **300**
EON 166, 167
Equilibrium state 137
Errors
  automation bias causing 364–5
  communication 232
  detection, costs of 224
  human 356, 357
  medication 35, 36, 120, 340–1
  memory 91
  modelling 4
  of commission 365
  of omission 365
  probability estimation as cause 92
  software, costs of error removal 126, **127**, 222
  Therac-25 4
Ethernet 251
Euclidean geometry **6**
European Particle Physics Laboratory (CERN) 287, 294
Evaluating answers
  complexity 78
  quality **78**, 79
  structure 78
  syntax 77
  terminology 77
  utility 79
Evaluation
  clinical decision support systems 338–43, *339*
  clinical outcomes 130, 265, 340–3
  computerized guidelines 163, 164
  economic 30, 263
  electronic medical records 117
  electronic prescribing 120, 341
  formative 127, 128–9
  guidelines 147, 173–4, 342
  guideline impact 173–4, 342
  information system 124–130
  online evidence systems 310–11
  protocol systems 147, 157, 159, 163–4
  summative 127, 129–30
  telemedicine 262–7
  user satisfaction 129, 263
Evidence
  clinical 178
  disease-oriented *58*, 59, 60, 79
  gathering 182
  online 310–11
  patient-oriented evidence that matters *58*, 59, 60, 79
  uptake 172–3
Evidence-based healthcare 143–55, 227, 400
  costs and benefits 175, 176
  databases 181
Evidence-based practice xxiii, 151
  costs and benefits 174, *175*, 176–8
  financial subsidies 176
  optimizing evidence 177
  organizational support 178
Expert systems 333, 334, *335*, **346**, 400
  alerts and reminders 334
  biosurveillance and 367–78
  diagnostic assistance 334
  image recognition and interpretation 335
  information retrieval 335
  laboratory information systems 336, 337
  rule-based **348**, 349
  therapy critiquing 334
  therapy planning 334
Expression space **394**
Externalities 325
Farr, William 202, 203
Fax 108–9, 253, 272, 314, 377
Faxing an ECG 108, 109
Feedback 26, **27**, **28**, 401
  control systems 137
Finite state machine 149, 349, 401
Firewalls 300, 401
Flowchart-like algorithms 168
Flowcharts 148, 149, 186
FluNet 315
Formal information systems xxv, 105–9
Functional genomics 385, 390, 401

GenBank 379, 380, **383**, 390
Gene
  biology **381**, 382, 401
  studies **388**
  therapy 385, 401
Gene Ontology consortium 391, 392
General Acknowledgement Originator 256
Genetic reductionism 386
Genome 381
  data, targeted therapies and 383–5
  sequenced 379
Genomics 380
GermAlert 372
GermWatcher 372
Global monitoring 315
Global system for mobile communications 252, **253**, 254, 401
  limitations 253, 254
  security 253
Glycomics 380
Grammar 14, 401
Grice's conversational maxims 41, 42, 44, 62, 245
Grounding, see Common Ground
Group **193**, 194, 401
Groupware 306, 401
Growth state 28
Guideline Interchange Format 167
Guideline representation languages 165–7
  Arden syntax 165
  Guideline Interchange Format 167
  Prodigy 166
  PRO*forma* 165, 167
  Protégé 166, 167
Guidelines 146–8, 401
  adherence to, information technology and 157, 159–61, 342
  clinical xxi, xxv, 79
    impact of 173, 174
    Internet and 158
    machine learning systems and 338
    presentation of 176
    uptake of 172, 173
  computer systems, developing 164
  distribution of 182, 183
  evaluation of 147
    computerized evidence-based 163, 164

Healthcare xxii, xxiii
capital value of information 320
classification systems 201–16
delivery processes, clinical decision support systems and efficiency of 343
international standard for electronic data exchange in, *see* HL7
terminologies xxvi, 201–16
see also Home healthcare
Healthcare Finance Administration 205
Health indexes 95
Health informatics xxi, xxii, xxv
Health Level Seven, *see* HL7
Helplines 270
HELP system 336
Heuristic 402
anchoring and adjustment 93
availability 92, 93
reasoning 89–93
search 70, *71*, 72
HIV infection 89, 93, 94
HL7 255–8, 402
Clinical Document Architecture 258
definitions *256*
message fields *257*
message structure **256**, 258
Reference Information Model 258, 390
Home healthcare
communication and 268–70
patient access to healthcare workers 269
patient access to information 269, 270
remote monitoring 268, 269
therapeutic benefit 268
Homeostasis 28, 402
Hospital discharge summaries 233, **234**, 272
Hospitals, communication and 273–6
HTML 294–6, 298, 299, 301, 402
HTTP 294, 296, 301, 402
Human error 356, 357
Human Genome Project 380, 386, 390, 392
Human mental models 4
Hybridization 388, 402
Hypertext 287, 294, **295**, 402
HyperText Markup Language, *see* HTML
HyperText Transport Protocol, *see* HTTP
Hypothesis generation 82, 90–2

Image recognition and interpretation, expert systems 335
Indifference probability 95, 96, 402
Induction 83, **84**, 402
Infectious disease surveillance systems 370–2
Inference engine 348
Inference procedure 15, 16
Influence diagrams 349
Info-antigens 314
Informal information systems 105–9
Informatics xxiii, xxiv, 124, 125
health xxi, xxii, xxv
tools xxi
see also Bioinformatics
Information 12–20
design *49*
marketplace 172
novelty 13
order 12
pull 291
push 291
retrieval, expert systems 335
supply and demand 320, **321**
transmission of **38**
value of 320–3
Information economics 172
Internet and 319–27
Information goods 320
characteristics 320–2
charges 322, 323
search costs 324–7
transaction costs 324, 325
Information management
cycle, designing a 136–9
loops 103–5, 111
systems 101–10, 137
Information systems xxii, 22–9, **30**, 31, 32
acceptance test 126
architecture design 125
designing 124–30, **131**, 132–40
algorithm 130
for change 134–6
computer program 130, 131
human–computer interaction 131
interaction space **132**, 133, 134
socio-technical system 131, 132
development 125, 126, **127**, 130
defining clinical needs 128, 129
evaluating 124–40
formal and informal 105–9, 111
formalization of 105, **106**, 107–9
functional specification 125
lifecycle of 125, 126
measuring impact of
clinical outcomes 130
economic analyses 130
user satisfaction studies 129
outcomes assessment 126
requirements analysis 125
software programming 125
system integration 126
time cycles 134, 135
unit test 126
user training 126
Information technology
active protocol systems 158, **159**, 163, 164
barriers to the use of 310, 311
decision making and 310
see also Decision support systems
diagnostic accuracy and 161
diagnostic assistance 334–6
education and 309, 310
Information theory 13, 402
Infrared links 252
Inputs 23, 24
Instantiation 7, 8, 180
Integrated record 49, **50**, 51
Integrated Service Digital Network 249, **250**
Intelligent monitoring and control xxvii, 355–66
artefact detection 358, 359, **360**
arterial pressure **361**
automation bias 364, 365
autonomous therapeutic devices 363, 364
cross-channel interpretation 362
decision support systems xxvi, 363
ECG **359**, 361, 362, 364
making clinical decisions 362, 363
methods used for interpretation 364
motivations for 355–7, 364
signal interpretation 358, **359**, 360–4
single-channel interpretation 360, 361
time ordering of trend onset **362**
Intelligent network architectures 259
Intelligent systems 345–54
Interaction design 132–4
Interactional reductionism 386
Interface engines 307
Inter-hospital communication 273, 274
International Classification of Diseases 122, 202–8, 210, 212, 217, 221, 222, 402
acceptance and use 203
classification structure *203*, **204**
history 202, 203
limitations 204, 205
purpose 202
International Classification of Functioning, Disability and Health 204
International Organization for Standardization 245, 404
Internet xxi, xxvi, 30, 182, 258, 259, 270, 285–94, 402
and bioinformatics 389, 390
'businesses' 289, 290
commercial phenomenon 289, 290
communication on the 291, *292*, 293, 294
bulletin boards 292, **293**, 294
mailing lists 291, **292**
newsgroups 292, **293**, 294
distribution of clinical practice guidelines 158
enterprise phenomenon 290, 291
evidence resources 309, 310, **311**
evolution of the 286, 287
expansion **288**
genome databases on the 379
information economics and the 319–27
internal, *see* Intranet
misinformation on the 312–14
poor-quality information on the 312–14, 326
publication of journals on the 308
publishing controls 158
security 299, 300, 307
social phenomenon 288, 289

technological phenomenon 287, 288
working protocol 287
Interruptive channels 46
Intra-hospital communication 274–6
Intranet 158, 290, **291**, 307, 402
IP 251, 307, 403
IrDA 255
Isochronous system 250, *251*, 403

Jargon 47
Java 295
Journals, publication on the Internet 308
Just-in-time grounding 278, 310, 372, 373, 376, **378**

Kalman filtering 360
KARDIO 337
Keywords *64*, 72
Kind-of hierarchy 195, **196**
Knowledge 13, **17**
background 59
base 15, 16, 29, 83, 183, 348, 403
clinical 55
gaps in 56–9
transfer of 56
discovery systems 337
foreground 59
model 15
representation 347
searching for 66, **67**
Knowledge-based systems 333, 403

Laboratory Observation Identifier Names and Codes, *see* LOINC
Language xxi, xxvi, 14, 191, 192, 403
Libraries 286
Linear accelerator 4
Literature
exponential growth 56, 144
searches 55, 58
Litigation 312
Lobachewsky–Bolyai geometry **6**
Local processes, protocol design including 185
Local resources, protocol design including 184
LocusLink 391
Logical deduction 16
LOINC 212
Long-term memory 90

Machine learning systems 337, 338, **346**, 403
associations between genetic and phenotypic data 393–5
clinical guideline development 338
drug discovery 338
knowledge-base development 337
Machine learning techniques 393, 394
MACRO 165
Magnetic resonance imaging 19
Mailing lists 291, 292, 403
Making decisions 81–98
Malthus' law of information 324, 326
Markov models 350, 364
MedCERTAIN proposals 313
Mediated interaction 132
Medical language 191, 192
Medical logic modules 165
Medical records
data, information design *49*
electronic 52, 111–23, 357, 358, 390, 392
see also Electronic medical records
functions of 112
paper based 112–17
Medical Subject Headings 391
Medical terminology 193
Medicare 205
Medication error 35, 36, 340–1
Medico-legal position of telecommunications 281
Medline 62, 63, *64*, 74, 380, **383**, 403
Memory 90, 91
Message
encoding rules 256
structure 235, 256
structuring 47, **48**, *49*, *53*
triggering events 256
Messages 44–9
channel choice 46, 47
data oriented *46*, 51, 235
public standard 49, 60
sending **39**
task oriented *46*, 51, 235
template oriented *46*, 51, 235
Meta-analysis 144, 183, 403
Metabolcomics 380
Metabolic pathways **387**
Microarrays 384, 388, **389**, 393
Microorganisms, identification 384
Minitel 270
Mnemonics 186
Mobile computers 276
Mobile telephones 239, 252, 253, 275
access to Web-based services 301
Model-based search 72
Model-based systems 352
Modelling error 4
Model, measure, manage cycle **102**, 103–5, 136, 151, 192
Models 3–11, 403
abstractions of the real world 4–7
data loss 5
distortion 5
purposes of 4–9
static 6
symbolic 13, **14**, 17
as templates 7, 8, **10**
Model theory 40
Monitor alarms, linked to protocol systems 162
Monitoring systems, *see* Intelligent monitoring and control
Monte Carlo simulation methods 350
Muller–Lyer illusion **40**
Multiaxial systems 196, 203, 209
Multimedia 237, 287, 403
Multiplexing **247**, 248, 249

Narrowcast communication 291, *292*, 314
Near patient testing 384
Needlestick injury 89, 93, 94
Negative externality 325
Network effect 288
negative 325
Networks 404
Advanced Research Projects Network 287
Bayesian 349
belief 349, **350**
causal probabilistic 349
computer networks **259**
Integrated Service Digital Network 249, **250**
neural 20, 350, **351**, 360, 364
personal area 254
Personal Communication Networks 253
telecommunication **259**
UMLS Semantic Network 214
Neural networks 20, 350, **351**, 360, 364, 404
Newsgroups 292, **293**, 294, 404
NHS Direct 271
Noise 38, 39, 235, 404
Non-deterministic polynomial time problems 386
Non-interruptive channels 46
Notification systems 314, 315
Nurse-operated telephone triage 271
Nurses, policies and procedures 178
nursing culture 178

OncoLink **288**
Online decision support, biosurveillance 373, 374
Online information technology 59
Online medical resources, barriers to use of 310, 311
Online Mendelian Inheritance in Man (OMIM) 390
Ontology 15, 16, 29, 165, 391, **392**, 404
Open-loop control of biomedical equipment 163, 404
Open system interconnection model 245
protocol layers *246*, 287
Optical illusions **40**
Order Message Originator 256
Order Response Originator 256
Outputs 23, 24

Pacemaker 19
Packet-switched systems 246, **247**, 404
Paging systems 239, 252, 253, 275
drawbacks 275

Paper-based medical record 112–17
advantages 114, 115, 117
disadvantages 115, 116
informational aspects 115, 116, 117
information entry 115, 116
information retrieval 116, 117
missing data 116
physical aspects 114, 115
Part–whole description 195, **196**
Passive protocol systems xxv, 154, 156–8
information technology and 156–8
Patent 322
Patient-oriented evidence that matters *58*, 59, 60, 79
Patient outcomes, protocols and 147
Patient records 49–53
computer-based 52
formal information system 111
functions of 112
integrated 49, **50**, 51
problem-oriented **50**, *51*, 52, 113
protocol-driven **50**, 51, 52
source-oriented **50**, 51, 52
structures 49–51
see also Electronic medical records; Paper-based medical record
Patients
access to information 269, 270, 311–14
history-taking 75, **76**, 77
physical examination 76, 77
protocol design including 184
Patient safety
clinical decision support systems and 340, 341
Patient specific knowledge 13
Pattern
matching 92
recognition techniques 364
Peer review 308
Peer-to-peer communication 291, *292*, 314
PEIRS system 336
Periodic table of elements 194
Permissive processes 154
Personal area network 254
Personal Communication Networks 253
Personal frequency estimates 93
Personal health records 316
see also Patient records
Pharmacogenomics 380, 384, 385, 404
Physiological monitors 19
Piconet 254
Pirates 322
Plain old telephony services 249, **250**
Portals 326
Posterior probability 86, 87, 405
Post-test probability 87, 405
Practice parameters 146, 405
Pre-emptive grounding 277, **278**
Prescribing
computer-supported 120
decision support systems 334, 340, 341
Prescriptive processes 154
Presentation bias 93
Pre-test probability 87, 405
Primary care
communication and 270–3
interface with specialist services 271–3
Prior probability 85, 87, 405
Privacy of clinical data 392, 393
Probability estimation 92, 93
Problem-oriented record **50**, *51*, 52
Problem-solving 81, **82**, 83
problem driven 124
technology driven 124
Process of care, protocols and 147
Prodigy 166
PRO*forma* 165, 167
Protégé 166, 167
Proteomics 380, 405
Protocol-based systems xxv
Protocol-driven
information systems **166**
order generation 161
record **50**, 51, 52
keeping 159, 160
Protocol-linked
device settings 163
monitor alarms 162
Protocol-modified data display 162
Protocols 143, 144, **145**, 146–55, 405
active use 154, 158–64
application of 153–4, 171
care pathways 150, 151
complex, chunking 149, **150**, 151
complexity 186
complex situations 147
computer-based 156–68, **169,** 170, 181, 399
constant review 187
construction 180–3
context of *185*, 186
definition 145
delegation of responsibility 146
demarcation of responsibility 147
departures from 152
design of 183–5
contextual factors 184, 185
designing 180, **181**, 182–8
disseminating 171, 173, 174
distribution of 182
education 147
entry criterion 148
form of 148
flowcharts 148, 149, 186
logical rules *149*
how to use 153, 154
languages 165–7
life cycle 151, 152
maintenance 180–3
ontology 165
passive use 154, 156–8
information technology and 156–8
patient outcomes and 147
process of care and 147
refinement 152
reflecting skill levels of users 186
representations 164–9
primitives, actions 167
primitives, decisions 167
primitives, intermediate states 167, 168
process model, nesting of guidelines 168
process model, scheduling constraints 168
research 145, 146
safety-critical 147
socio-technical barriers 171, 172, 178
specificity 186
stack **245**
structure of 148–50
terminology 146
uncommon conditions 147
usability 180
when to use 153
Public Health Link 377
Public health messages 47
Publishing on the Web 182, 183, 298, 299, 304, 305, 308, 309
PUFF system 336

Quality-adjusted life expectancy 96
Quality-adjusted life-year 96, 130
Quality labels 79
Quality of care, CDSS and 341, 342
Query language 19, 60
Questioning 55–65
Questions
general 62, **63**, 64
precise 62
pursued 57, *58*
specific 62, 63

Radiation overdose 4
Radio 252
RAGs 165
Randomized controlled trials 78, 405
Rare conditions, protocols 147
Rating scales 95
Read codes 206–8, 217, 391, 405
acceptance and use 207
classification structure *207*, 208
history 207
limitations 208
purpose 206
Read Codes Drug and Appliance Dictionary 208
Record-keeping, protocol-driven 159, 160
Reimann geometry **6**
Reminders
computer-generated 121
expert systems applied to 334
protocol driven 160–1
Remote monitoring 268, 269

Reportable Diseases 372
Representativeness heuristic 92
Research protocols 146
Resource utilization groups 206
Responsibility, delegation of 146
RetroGram 165
Ribonucleic acid, *see* RNA
Ripple-down systems 227, 228
RNA **381**, 405
Rule-based expert systems 348, 349, 360, 364, 405
Rules
Bayes' rule 350
encoding 256
of inference 16, 83
of logic 83, 84
of probability 84–6

Safety-critical protocol 147
Scatternet 255
Scientific hypothesis 6, 7
Search
accuracy *64*
engine 297, 298, 405
precision 63
space 68, **69**, **70**
analytic exploration 70, **71**, 72
database 72
systematic exploration of 70, **71**
specificity *64*
strategies 66–8, 70
analytic 70, 72
systematic 70, 72
structure **67**
terms *64*
tree **69**, 70
Searching 66–80
Second-generation expert systems 352
Security on the Internet 299, 300, 307
Semantic query reformulation *74*
Semantics 16, 405
Semantic Web 301
Service providers 289, 290
SGML 295, 405
Shannon, Claude 38
Short-message service 253
Signal to noise ratio 37, 406
Skeletal plan refinement 186
SNOMED 207–13, 217, 222, 391, 406
acceptance and use 209
classification structure 209, 210
codes **209**
history 208, 209
limitations 210
nomenclature and classification *209*
purpose 208
SNOMED Clinical Terms 210–13
acceptance and use 211
classification structure 211, *212*
core structure **211**
history 211
limitations 213
purpose 210, 211
SNOMED International 206, 208
classification structure *210*
modules *209*
SNOMED Reference Terminology *210*, 212
Social futurism 288, 289
Socio-technical system 131, 163, 406
Software development, costs of error removal 126, **127**, 222
Software pirates 322
Source-oriented record **50**, 51, 52
SPECIALIST Lexicon 214, 215
Staff, protocol design including 184, 185
Standard gamble 95, 406
Standard Generalized Markup Language, *see* SGML
State transitions 168
Steady state 28
Store-and-forward systems 238
Streptokinase 143
Structuring 44–54
Supervised learning 393
Synchronous channels 46
Synchronous communication 237, 406
Synchronous transfer mode transmission 250, **251**, *251*
Syntactic query reformulation 73, *74*
Syntax 16, 406
Systematized Nomenclature of Medicine, *see* SNOMED
Systems 22, 23, 406
arbitrary 28, 29
behaviour 24
closed 24
control 26
cybernetic 26
inputs 23, **24**
internal structure 25, 26
open 24
outputs 23, **24**
purposive 28, 29
state of 23, 24, 28

Task-oriented directory 45
Task-oriented messages 51
Task-specific data displays 162
Telecare 262
Telecommunication networks **259**
Teleconsultations 281, 406
medico-legal position 281
Telehealth 262
Telemedicine 261–82, 406
clinical outcome changes resulting from 265, 266
definition 261, 262
economic benefit of 263–5
effectiveness of 262, 263, *264*, 265–7
failure of studies of 266, 267
user satisfaction 263
Telephone 237, 268, 375, 376
Telephony, *see* Plain old telephony services
Television 237, 252
Template-directed directory 45
Template-directed messages 46, 51
Template-oriented structures 186
Term 193, 194, 406
Terminological systems
compositional 227
corresponding concepts 221, 222
universal 218–22
Terminology xxvi, 14, 191–17, 406
building 196, 197
compositional 196, **197**
costs of construction **224**
depth of knowledge 226
maintenance **223**, 224–6
mapping across **225**, 226
search costs 224, 225
enumerative
costs of construction **224**
depth of knowledge 226
maintenance **223**, 224
mapping across **225**, 226
search costs 224, 225
maintaining 222–8
Terms
context-dependence 219
evolution over time 221
purposive 220, 221
subjective 218, 219
Tests, independence of 88
Therac-25 linear accelerator 4
Therapy
individually tailored 383–5
planning, expert systems and 334
Third party medical record providers 316, 317
Three-loop model **103**, 104, 105, 111, 139, **151**, 152
Time trade-off 96
Token Ring 251
Transcription **381**, 382
Transcriptomics 380
Transmitting an ECG signal 109
Treatment
clinicians' beliefs about appropriate 56, 57
goals, protocol design including 184
Triage 273
Turing test 333, 406

UMLS 213–15, 391
acceptance and use 213
classification structure 213–15
history 213
limitations 215
purpose 213
UMLS Metathesaurus 214
UMLS Semantic Network 214
Unified Medical Language System, *see* UMLS

Universal Resource Locator *see* URL
Universal terminological systems 218–22
Unsupervised learning 393–5
URL 294, 296, 297, 406
US Guideline Clearinghouse 158
Utility 93, 94, 407
  estimation of 95, 96

Variance capture, semi-automated 163
Variances 152
Ventilator management xxvii, 363
Video-based consultations 272, 273
Video conferencing 237, 240, 251, 273, 274
Virtual reality 287, 288, 300, 407
Voicemail **241,** 242, 253, 268, 276, 407
Voice telephony 239, 287

WAP **301**
Web
  browsers **297**, **298**, 299, 307
  crawlers 298
  directories 297, 298
  see also World Wide Web
Web-based critical incident reporting systems 315
Web-based information sources 290, 310
Web Health Services 303–17
  information, patient access 311–14
  information distribution 304–6
Wireless Application Protocol, *see* WAP
Wireless communication systems 252–5
  bluetooth 254, 255
  global system for mobile communications 252–4
Wireless Markup Language, *see* WML
Wireline communication systems 249–52
  asynchronous transfer mode 249–52
  Integrated Service Digital Network 249, **250**
Wittgenstein, language games 220
WML 301
Word concepts **219**
Workflow management systems 161, 162
Working memory 90, 91, 348
World Health Organization 202, 203
World Wide Web xxvi, 286–8, 294–302, 407
  biosurveillance and the 374–7
  educational materials on the 305, 309
  electronic patient record on the 306–8
  future advances 300–2
  protocols **294**
  publishing on the 182, 183, 298, 299, 304, 305, 308, 309
  remote collaboration 306
  role in surveillance of infectious diseases 315
  search engine 297, 298
  wireless access 300, 301

Natural **highs**
for body & soul

70 instant energizers to banish everyday energy lows

Mary Lambert

hamlyn

First published in Great Britain in 2005 by
Hamlyn, a division of Octopus Publishing Group Ltd
2–4 Heron Quays, London E14 4JP

Distributed in the United States and Canada by
Sterling Publishing Co., Inc.
387 Park Avenue South, New York, NY 10016-8810

ISBN 0 600 61089 6
EAN 9780600610892

A CIP catalogue record for this book is available from the British Library

Printed and bound in China

10 9 8 7 6 5 4 3 2 1

Disclaimer

Yoga (see pages 50–51 and 124–125)
These postures can be practised quite safely; but to enjoy the full benefits of yoga, it is advisable to go to a yoga class with a trained teacher. If you are pregnant, are unfit or have a medical problem, consult your doctor before performing the postures.

Acupressure and reflexology (see pages 52–53, 64–65, 68–69 and 102–103)
Do not practise these routines if you have a heart condition, phlebitis, breast or lymphatic cancer, or in the first 16 weeks of pregnancy. Also do not use if your hands or feet have an infectious skin condition, are bruised or cut. If you have any other condition you are concerned about, such as diabetes, check with your doctor before treating yourself.

Chi kung (see pages 78–79)
These poses are quite safe to practise, but to learn chi kung fully it is advisable to attend a class. If you have a health problem, consult your doctor before practising chi kung.

6
Introduction

8
1 **What is energy?**

18
2 **Energy zappers**

24
3 **First steps**

27
4 **The energizer larder**

Instant energizers

38
5 **Wake up fresh**

54
6 **Mid-morning stress relief**

70
7 **Lunchtime revivers**

86
8 **Mid-afternoon boosters**

106
9 **Evening refreshers**

126
10 **Late-night cleansers**

142
Index

144
Acknowledgements

Introduction

In our lives today we often complain about a lack of energy. Our lives have become overcomplicated; we try to do too much, running ourselves ragged and ending up feeling tired and exhausted. Many of us are forced to work long hours, often while looking after a family as well, and there is precious little time left for us. Pollutants in the environment, daily commuting, a poor diet and a lack of sleep and exercise all take their toll on our energy levels. Added to this, as we get older our energy levels naturally decline, which makes it even more important to stay healthy and maintain energy throughout life.

Energy – Western and Eastern style

When we look at energy levels from the Western perspective, they are intrinsically linked to the life we lead. We obtain our energy from the food we eat, and the energetic ups and downs we suffer are caused by fluctuating blood-sugar levels if meals are missed or eaten late, or if we regularly ingest toxins by smoking or drinking alcohol, for example.

The Eastern view of energy is quite different: energy is seen from a holistic point of view, looking at the health of the mind, body and spirit of an individual. Eastern philosophers believe that they all need to be in balance for true wellbeing. Energy is a 'life force' in the body, which flows through invisible energy channels. When an Eastern health diagnosis is made, the energy flow is studied in detail and any blockage or stagnancy is treated. Overall, however, the philosophy is preventative, with the belief that if the energy flow is good, the body will stay healthy.

Re-energize your life

This book aims to show you how to keep your energy levels balanced holistically, because even if your diet and general lifestyle are good, you can be drained daily by stress, upsets at work or problems with friends and family. The Instant energizers' section (see pages 36–141) contains over 70 'mini' exercises or therapies to suit different times of the day. Each 'energizer' takes only a matter of minutes, so you can do it when you feel your energy levels dropping.

In time, you will discover how to listen to your all your body's energy needs and know when the time is right for an empowering mantra, a stimulating herbal tea or a relaxing neck and shoulder massage exercise to get you through another busy day.

Keeping your mind, body and spirit healthy will change your life, as you take time out to become more in tune with yourself and at peace with the world.

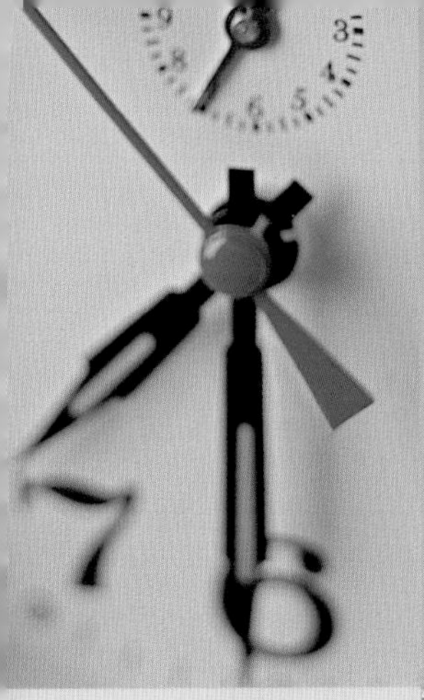

Energy is a 'life force' in the body, which flows through invisible energy channels.

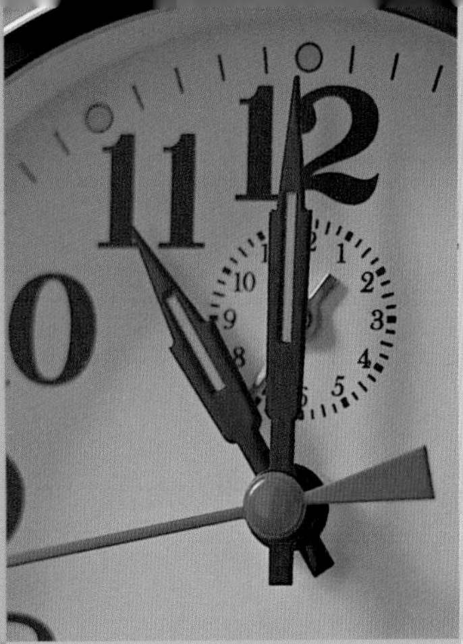

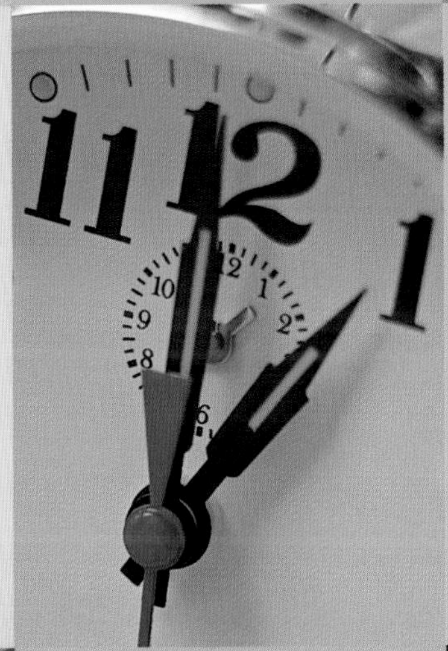

If energy flow is good, the body will stay healthy.

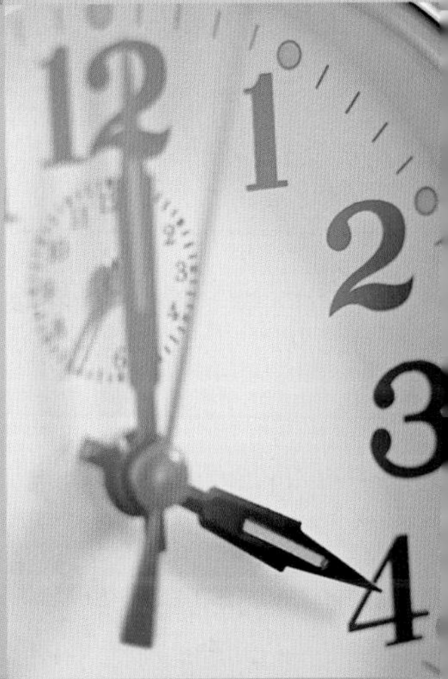

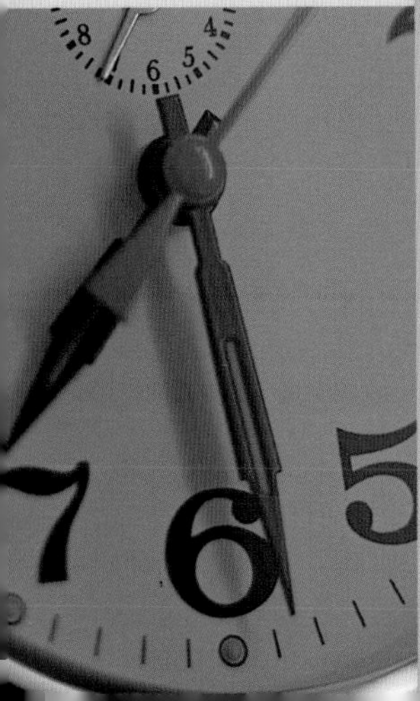

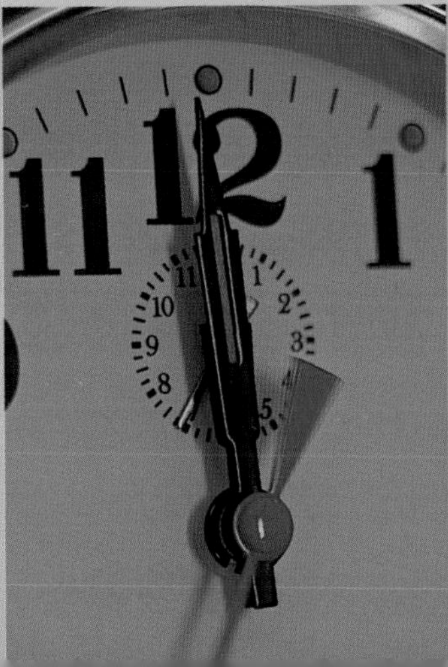

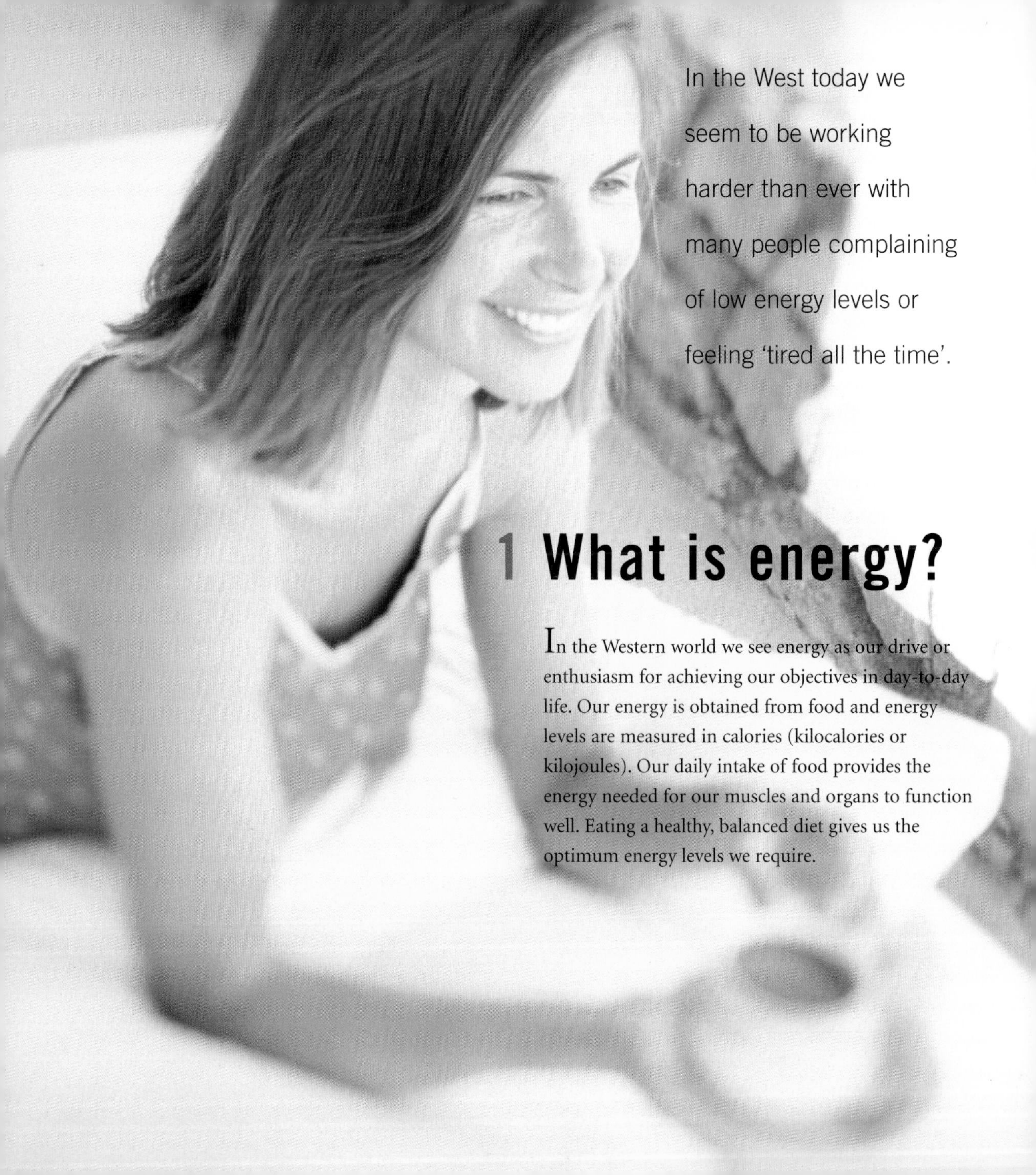

In the West today we seem to be working harder than ever with many people complaining of low energy levels or feeling 'tired all the time'.

1 What is energy?

In the Western world we see energy as our drive or enthusiasm for achieving our objectives in day-to-day life. Our energy is obtained from food and energy levels are measured in calories (kilocalories or kilojoules). Our daily intake of food provides the energy needed for our muscles and organs to function well. Eating a healthy, balanced diet gives us the optimum energy levels we require.

THE WESTERN CONCEPT OF **energy**

But in the West today we seem to be working harder than ever with many people complaining of low energy levels or feeling 'tired all the time', which basically results from neglecting normal physical, dietary and emotional needs. In today's busy world, people often eat on the go, indulging in a quick energy fix of sugary or processed foods when they need a pick-me-up. They regularly take limited exercise (if at all), have little time to relax and deprive themselves of sleep – no wonder, then, that energy levels often remain low.

The benefits of a good diet

Energy highs and lows relate to fluctuating blood-sugar levels – the more balanced and steady they are, the better we feel. Skipping meals or dieting disrupts these levels, lowering your energy. Blood-sugar levels start to drop within four hours of eating, so to counteract the inevitable dip eat three smaller meals (with some healthy snacks in between) at regular times throughout the day, rather than just eating two large meals a day.

Most of the energy from food comes in the form of carbohydrates (basically starches and sugars) and fats that 'fuel' the body. This food energy is released into the body with the help of micronutrients – vitamins and minerals that derive from the fruit and vegetables you eat. Protein provides some energy and keeps blood-sugar levels stable but it is mainly used for body maintenance and repair. Eating sugary or processed foods, which are often full of artificial additives, preservatives and flavourings, disrupts your energy levels. For example, if you snack on cakes or biscuits you get an instant burst of energy from the fast sugar release, but soon after your energy plummets again, leaving you tired and craving yet more sugar. Snacks such as fresh fruit and nuts, however, raise blood-sugar levels much more gradually, giving you a more sustained energy supply that keeps you going longer.

If you eat a healthy balanced diet but still complain of lethargy, it may be because you don't drink enough water. Being dehydrated can make you feel tired, so drink a glass of still water at room temperature every hour during the day, or keep a bottle of still mineral water by you. However, avoid drinking with meals as it hinders digestion.

The right balance of food

To keep you healthy and your energy levels stable, it is best to eat a varied and balanced diet with plenty of unrefined food and fresh produce, ideally organic. Include at least five portions of fruit and vegetables for essential vitamins and minerals; three or four portions of complex carbohydrates (unrefined) such as wholewheat bread, brown pasta and rice, potatoes and pulses; one or two portions of protein, such as fish (oily fish is ideal), meat, poultry, tofu, seeds or eggs plus a small amount of fat such as olive oil or butter.

HEALTHY SNACKS

Rebalance your blood-sugar levels throughout the day with these high-energy foods:

- dried fruit and nuts (salt-free)
- fresh fruit
- seeds (sunflower or pumpkin)
- raw vegetables with sour cream dip
- cereal bars (sugar-free)
- hummus and crispbread
- low-fat yogurt

The importance of sleep

Sleep is vital for a healthy body and mind. It allows the body to rest and restore itself. While we sleep, the healing and repair of cells, tissues, bones, muscles, nerves and organs takes place. When we are deprived of sleep, even for one night, our coping strategies weaken and we find it difficult to function properly. We feel fatigued and exhausted, lack concentration and have depleted energy levels. Worries and anxiety can cause disrupted sleep patterns, so any niggling issues need to be worked through before going to bed (see Late-night cleansers, pages 126–141). While some people can manage on a few hours, an average of 7–8 hours' sleep a night is normally enough to refresh, revitalize and re-energize our bodies.

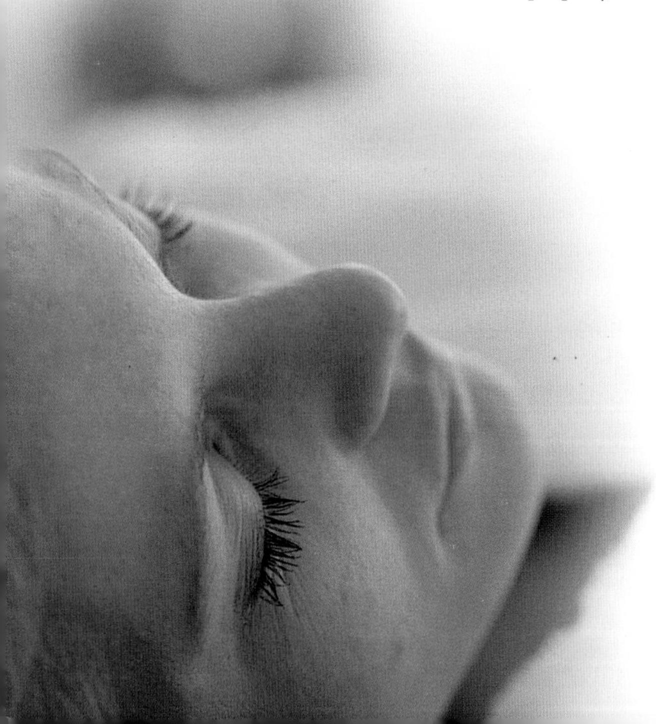

A regular exercise routine

Taking regular exercise tones your body muscles and improves how efficiently your organs work, particularly your heart and lungs. It makes you feel good about yourself, improves your sleep and boosts your overall energy so that you achieve more. You also benefit from the 'feel good factor' – the result of endorphins, the 'happy hormones' being released into the bloodstream.

The latest recommendation is for 30 minutes' exercise on most days of the week (you can even do it in 10-minute bouts if half an hour is hard to find). Ideally, combine some aerobic activity (where you work your lungs and heart hard until slightly breathless), such as fast walking, running, swimming or cycling, with stretching exercises to improve muscle suppleness; even some household chores, such as vacuuming, scrubbing floors or gardening, are aerobic activities. It is a good idea to also include some weight-bearing exercise such as tennis, dancing or skipping to strengthen your muscles and improve your bone density.

ENERGY, **Eastern-style**

Even when you have worked hard at balancing your energy levels by eating well, being more active, getting enough sleep and keeping your stress levels in check, you may still feel lethargic or listless and not really know why. According to the Eastern philosophy of energy you may be suffering from an energy blockage or stagnancy in one of your body's meridians (energy channels) that flow through your body or one of the chakras (spiritual energy centres). Eastern medicine aims to be preventative and works with the body's strengths and its natural inclination to heal itself. It looks at the body holistically and believes that either illness starts as an emotional upset or imbalance in one of the chakras that, if not dealt with, eventually manifests itself as a physical illness or illness in a part of the body that results from an emotional energy disturbance in energy points along one or more meridians.

Chi, prana or *ki*

In traditional Chinese medicine the body's energy or life force is known as *chi (qi)*. It is an invisible form of energy, similar to electromagnetic energy, that flows through a set of meridians or channels affecting the health of every cell in the body.

In Indian Ayurvedic medicine the body's energy force is known as *prana*. It moves through numerous meridians in the body, and needs to be balanced for good health in the same way as in traditional Chinese medicine.

In Japanese medicine the energy flow is called *ki*, and it works with the same meridians as in the Chinese system.

The meridians or *nadis*

Chi (qi) or the Japanese *ki* moves around the body through 12 main meridians and several minor ones. Six of the main meridians are yin and six are yang. Yin and yang are opposing forces that affect everything; one cannot act without the other: they are interdependent. Yin comes from the earth and is dark, passive and feminine, whereas yang comes from the sun and is light, active and male. To achieve optimum energy levels at all times, you need to keep a balance of both in the body.

Each main meridian connects to and is related to an organ or function. The yin meridians relate to the heart, liver, kidney, lung, pericardium (part of the heart) and spleen. The yang meridians relate to the triple-warmer (a metabolic zone), stomach, bladder, gall bladder, small intestines and large intestines. There are two extra meridians: the governor and conception. It is along these 14 meridians that 365 of the acupuncture points are found, all of which are named and numbered. When these are stimulated, stagnant or blocked energy can be shifted so that *chi* moves freely once again. When an imbalance is found in a person's body it can be related to an excessive emotional response such as rage, intense grief or sorrow or anxiety. For example, someone

THE BODY'S MERIDIANS

In Eastern medicine the body has 14 main meridians. Six are situated on each side of the body, one goes down the front and one goes down the back (see also page 11). Twelve of these are linked to internal organs and have an influence on them. The meridians are grouped in twos – one yin and one yang. Yin meridians are numbered from the lowest point, while yang meridians are numbered from the top. The acupressure points are situated all along these meridians, and stimulating them can help cure certain ailments (see pages 53 and 68–69). Massaging your skin along a meridian route can help balance the body.

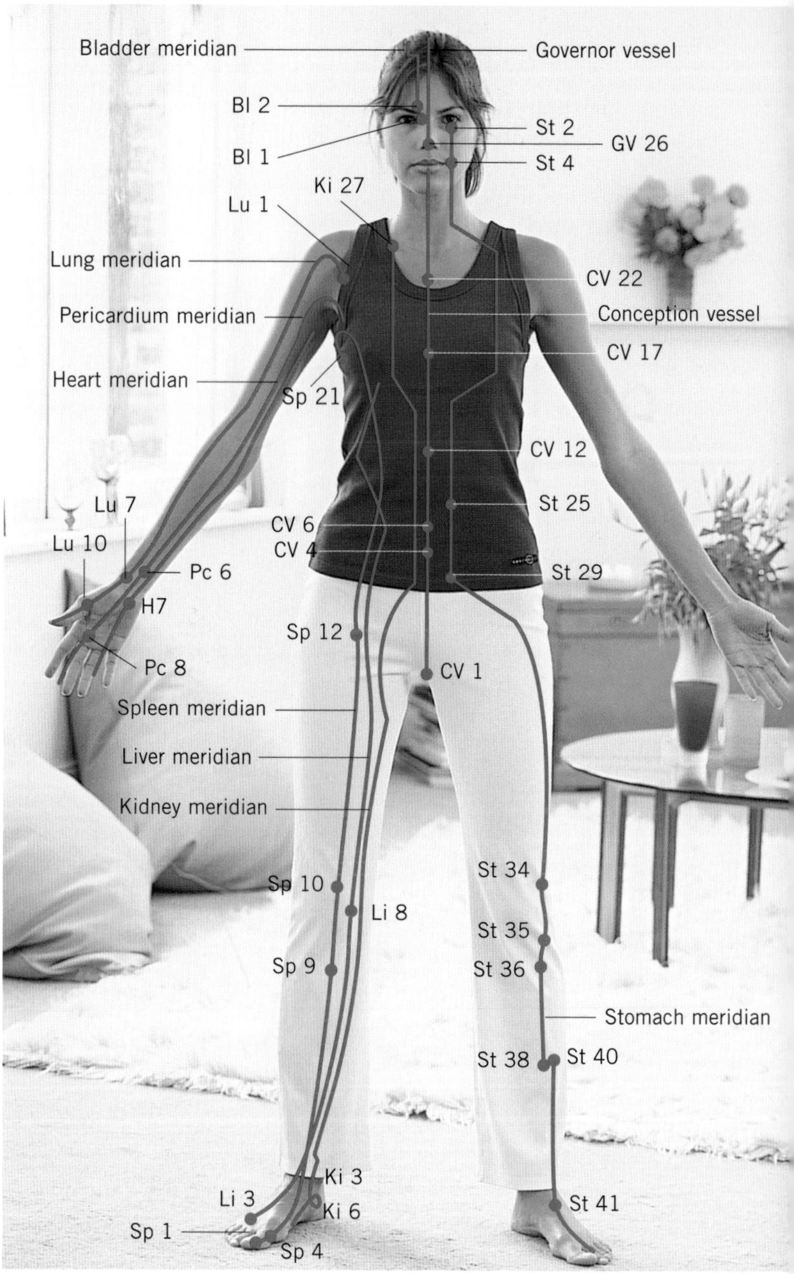
Bladder meridian
Governor vessel
Bl 2
St 2
GV 26
Bl 1
St 4
Ki 27
Lu 1
Lung meridian
CV 22
Pericardium meridian
Conception vessel
CV 17
Heart meridian
Sp 21
CV 12
Lu 7
St 25
CV 6
Lu 10
CV 4
Pc 6
St 29
H7
Sp 12
Pc 8
CV 1
Spleen meridian
Liver meridian
Kidney meridian
St 34
Sp 10
Li 8
St 35
Sp 9
St 36
Stomach meridian
St 38
St 40
Ki 3
Li 3
Ki 6
St 41
Sp 1
Sp 4

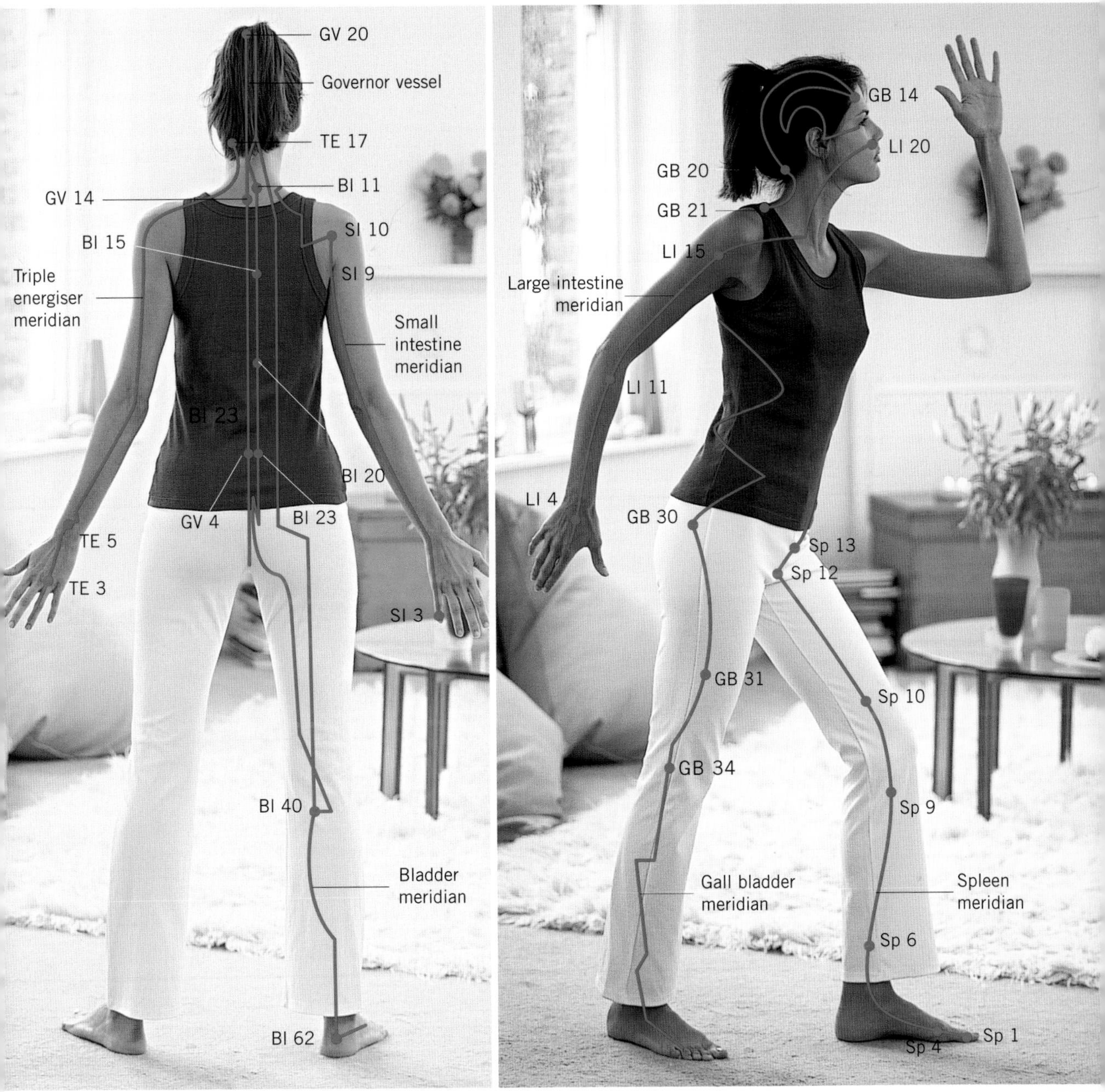
GV 20
Governor vessel
TE 17
Bl 11
GV 14
SI 10
Bl 15
SI 9
Triple energiser meridian
Small intestine meridian
Bl 23
Bl 20
GV 4
Bl 23
TE 5
TE 3
SI 3
Bl 40
Bladder meridian
Bl 62
GB 14
LI 20
GB 20
GB 21
LI 15
Large intestine meridian
LI 11
LI 4
GB 30
Sp 13
Sp 12
GB 31
Sp 10
GB 34
Sp 9
Gall bladder meridian
Spleen meridian
Sp 6
Sp 1
Sp 4

who suffers inappropriate anger can experience an imbalance in the liver.

The Indian energy, *prana*, moves through thousands of energy channels called *nadis* that form a network in the body. When energy flow is restricted, it is believed that toxins gather in that area causing physical stiffness and pain.

When hatha yoga (one of the main forms of yoga) is practised, three of the *nadis* are particularly important: the Sushumna nadi; the Pingala nadi (the sun channel); and the Idi nadi (the moon channel). Sushumna, the principal *nadi*, flows from the bottom of the spine to the top of the head. On its right-hand side flows the Pingala nadi, the active male channel that stimulates the physical body and transmits data from the left part of the brain, the rational side.

On the left-hand side flows the Idi nadi, the female channel that transmits consciousness to the body and sends messages from the right part of the brain, the creative side. Hatha yoga aims to balance these two life forces within the body.

The aura

To feel complete and function well, we all have a mind, body and spirit that need to be in harmony with one another. The philosophy of Indian and other Eastern therapies is to work towards achieving this harmony.

Many of us are good at worrying about the health of our physical bodies but we can too easily neglect our spiritual side. The aura is the subtle spiritual energy or electromagnetic field that surrounds a physical body. The more spiritually balanced we are, the wider our aura extends. An aura is oval in shape, with six coloured layers. The colours radiate from the

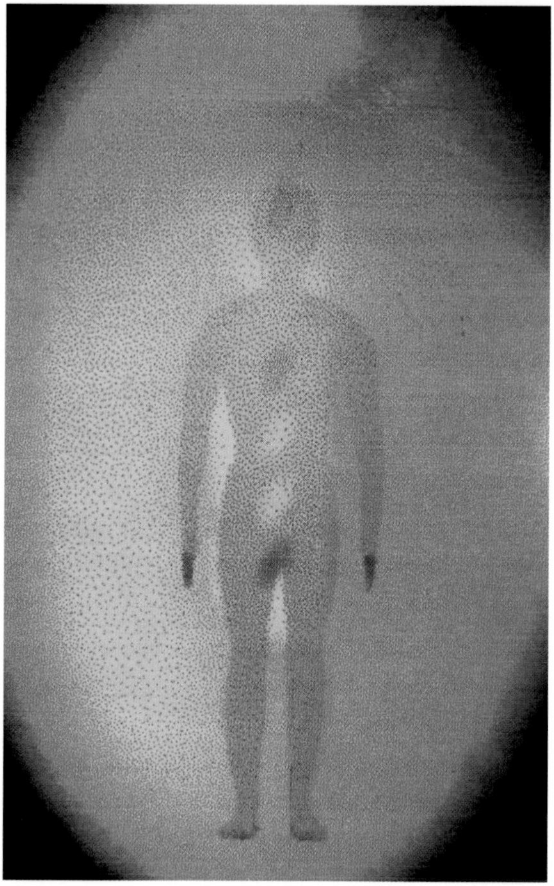

This healthy woman's aura has a lot of green, which indicates harmony, and yellow, which shows creativity.

major *chakras*: seven spiritual energy centres that penetrate all the layers. So the colours our aura projects change daily, showing the current state of our physical, emotional and spiritual health.

There are three main layers of the aura.

- The etheric body is the layer nearest to our physical body (and they are closely interwoven) but it vibrates at a higher level. The etheric level helps to transfer *prana* from the universe to our physical body.

- The second layer – the astra/emotional body – is wider and, because it is linked to the emotions, is often unbalanced. So, the colours of the aura change as we fluctuate from feeling wildly happy one day to being miserable or upset the next.
- The mental body, the third layer, harbours our thought patterns; this is where they turn from thoughts into actions. It is from here that unpleasant thoughts about someone are projected to that person, which can be emotionally damaging all round. If we think negative thoughts, we attract more in return; conversely, if we think positively, positive thoughts will abound.

The chakras

The word *chakra* is Sanskrit for 'wheel'; people who are psychic often see each *chakra* as a spinning wheel. Each chakra takes in energy from pulsating sunlight, and the Indians believe these spinning wheels are like lotus flowers, constantly opening and closing.

There are seven main *chakras* in the body:

- the red Root chakra at the base of the spine
- the orange Sacral chakra, below the navel
- the yellow Solar plexus chakra in the upper abdomen
- the green (or pink) Heart chakra in the centre of the chest
- the turquoise blue Throat chakra in the middle of the throat
- the indigo Third eye chakra in the middle of the forehead
- the violet Crown chakra on the top of the head.

Together the seven *chakra* colours make a rainbow, which in other cultures often represents the connection between our world and the gods.

Each *chakra* is associated with an emotional function and a body organ and is intrinsically linked to the endocrine system that controls the release of hormones in the body. So the *chakras* send energy to the endocrine system and vice versa.

When an imbalance occurs in a chakra, it either becomes smaller and spins more slowly, thereby affecting the health of the physical organs, or it spins faster and becomes larger, which can result in physical or emotional upset, such as an angry outburst or bursting into tears.

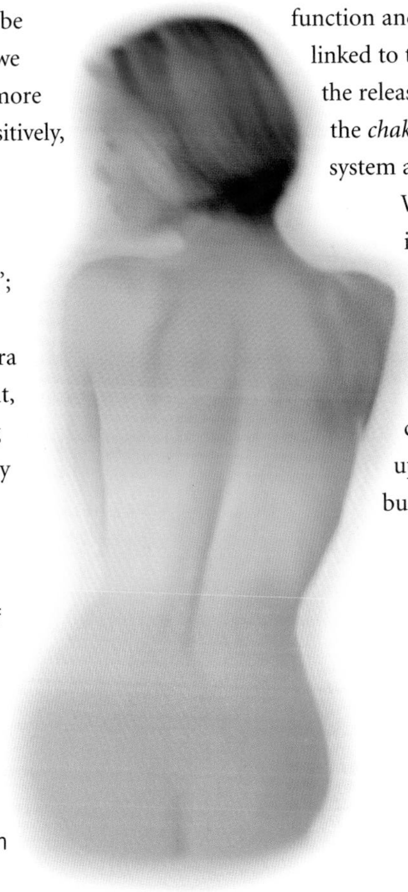

The seven *chakras* start at the base of the spine, with the Root chakra, and end with the Crown chakra, on top of the head.

jump-start YOUR ENERGY FLOW

There are many complementary therapies that can work alone or alongside conventional medicine to treat a general lethargy or lack of energy in the body. With some techniques or holistic exercise regimes you can do them yourself (see Instant energizers, pages 36–141) after learning the basics or following instructions; others, however, need to be performed by a qualified practitioner.

Energy-related therapies

Several therapies deal with correcting energy flow either through the body's meridians or *chakras*. With most therapies, a brief medical history is taken before diagnosis is made and any treatment begins.

Acupuncture

This powerful energy treatment is part of traditional Chinese medicine. A qualified acupuncturist performs the treatment. He or she makes a diagnosis by taking pulse readings and examining the face and tongue. For the treatment, fine sterilized needles are placed briefly in acupuncture points on the relevant organ meridian to remove a blockage or to stimulate sluggish *chi* flow.

Reflexology

This therapy is normally performed by a qualified reflexologist but you can do some simple treatments yourself (see pages 64–65 and 102–103). Although reflexology is linked to the Chinese meridian system, most therapists normally work with just ten vertical energy zones that start at the top of the head, branching out and stretching all the way to the fingers and toes; the main branches finish in the toes. In a treatment session, points are stimulated all over the feet or hands to boost energy circulation. Any blockages or imbalances can result in painful or slightly tender areas when pressed, and there may be some crystalline deposits that feel slightly 'crunchy' to the touch.

Feng shui

This Chinese art of furniture placement and *chi* flow in the home is performed by a feng shui consultant. He or she uses different techniques to achieve optimum energy circulation in the home and in work areas; consultants also advise people to clear out clutter, for example, as it causes debilitating energy blockages and stagnancy (see pages 94–97). Feng shui is often known as the 'acupuncture treatment of the home'.

Shiatsu

This Japanese therapy evolved alongside acupuncture and Chinese herbalism. Shiatsu literally means 'finger pressure', and practitioners use fingers, palms, elbows and other body parts to apply pressure to acupuncture points situated on the body's meridians to balance the energy systems.

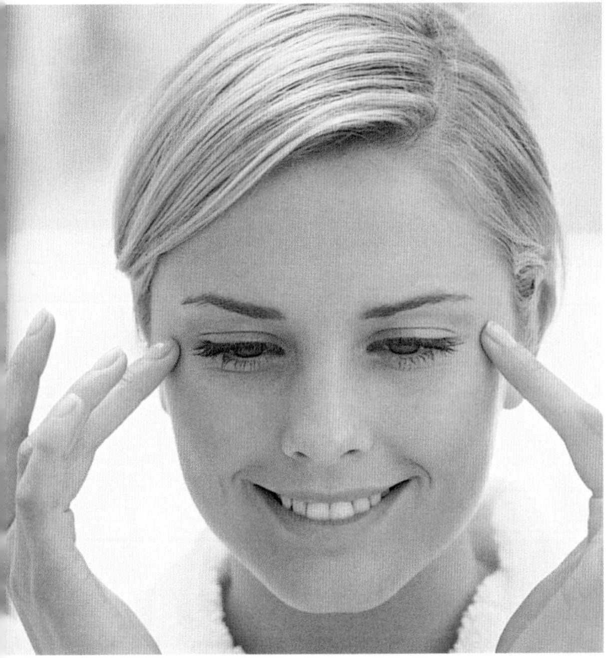

Acupressure

Similar to shiatsu, acupressure involves pressure being applied to acupuncture points along the body's meridians to increase *chi* flow and remove blockages. Unlike shiatsu, however, only thumbs and fingers are used to apply pressure to the points. Nowadays, it is a popular self-help technique that anybody can use (see pages 53 and 68–69).

Reiki

This Japanese hands-on healing therapy means 'universal life force energy'. A reiki therapist provides treatment, but training is available to all. It works with both the meridians and the *chakras*, and stimulates the body's innate healing system. This relaxing treatment shifts blockages, thereby promoting a better energy flow throughout the body.

Yoga

This Indian exercise discipline uses different postures, meditation and breathing techniques to allow a positive *prana* flow to purify the body, mind and spirit. The full practice of yoga is best learnt from a qualified teacher but you can enjoy its benefits by learning a few exercises (see pages 50–51 and 124–125).

Chi kung or qigong

This ancient Chinese exercise system, from which t'ai chi originates, is also part of traditional Chinese medicine. In chi kung, a qualified practitioner teaches stretching, breathing and visualization exercises to get *chi* moving through the meridians inside the body, but you can practise a few simple exercises yourself (see pages 78–79).

Self-help techniques

In addition to acupressure, yoga and chi kung, there are other simple self-help techniques you can learn to promote harmony and good energy flow. Visualization is one such technique; for example, focusing on the colour that is lacking in an underperforming *chakra* can help to rebalance body energy. Meditation, massage, muscle-releasing and breathing exercises can also alleviate stress and tension in the body, mind and emotions, helping to release toxins – the body's major energy drainers. You can pick and choose from over 70 energizers in the Instant energizers' section, see pages 36–141.

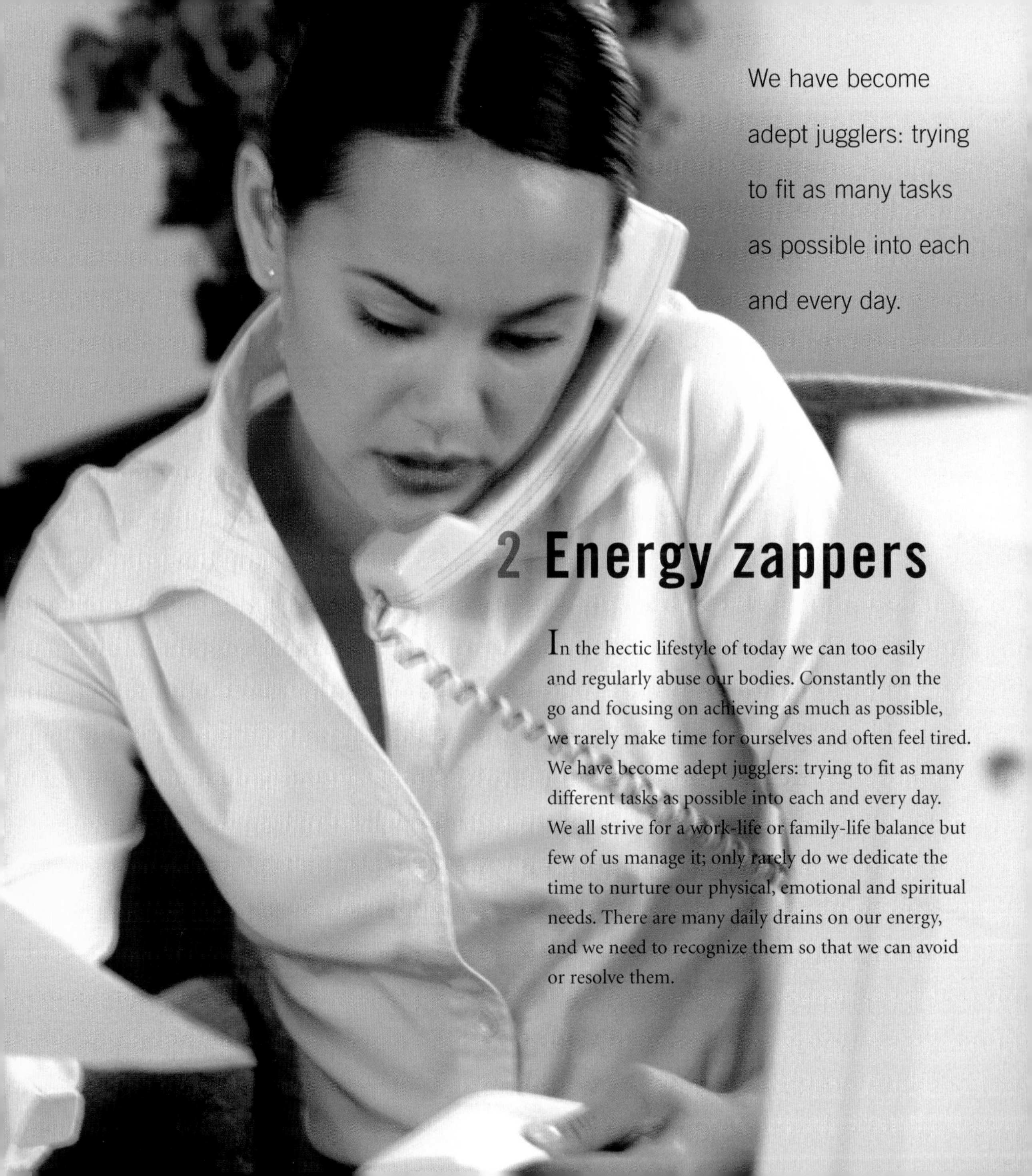

We have become adept jugglers: trying to fit as many tasks as possible into each and every day.

2 Energy zappers

In the hectic lifestyle of today we can too easily and regularly abuse our bodies. Constantly on the go and focusing on achieving as much as possible, we rarely make time for ourselves and often feel tired. We have become adept jugglers: trying to fit as many different tasks as possible into each and every day. We all strive for a work-life or family-life balance but few of us manage it; only rarely do we dedicate the time to nurture our physical, emotional and spiritual needs. There are many daily drains on our energy, and we need to recognize them so that we can avoid or resolve them.

WHAT IS ZAPPING YOUR **energy?**

Physical energy drains

As discussed earlier (see pages 8–9), to stay healthy with abundant energy, we need to eat a balanced and nutritious diet, get enough rest and sleep, and stay happy emotionally and spiritually. But when we are busy, or stressed, we can neglect our physical needs and our energy levels plummet.

Furthermore, we have the added problem of introducing toxins in the guise of alcohol, caffeine and nicotine into the body. Although we may rely on such stimulants, for example when we are trying to meet a deadline or entertain the kids on a rainy day, they actually work against us and upset the balance of our energy levels.

A sedentary lifestyle

Being inactive is an easy option when we are busy or overworked. Too many of us spend long hours every day working in one form or other without taking regular breaks, and we often drive everywhere (even short distances) rather than exercising by cycling or walking. But all our organs need a regular workout, particularly the heart, to thrive and make us feel good. A lack of physical activity reduces our energy levels, making us feel very lethargic and prone to mood swings.

Take action **Do some daily exercise – just a short, brisk walk will work your heart and lungs and make you feel much more energetic and generally better in yourself.**

Alcohol

This widely available stimulant is socially acceptable in many countries; many of us like to unwind from the day with a glass of wine or a beer. But alcohol is toxic to the body. Although enjoying a few glasses of red wine each week is thought to protect the heart, drinking to excess (more than 14 units for women, 21 units for men) strains the liver and reduces its ability to detoxify the body. Drinking too much alcohol also causes fatigue, dehydrates the body and brings on headaches. Furthermore, it disrupts sleep patterns and depletes the body of vital nutrients.

Take action **Keep your alcohol intake below recommended limits and drink plenty of water every day (see pages 9–10) to eliminate toxic wastes. It is a good idea to have at least one or two alcohol-free days each week, if possible.**

Caffeine

We mainly consume this powerful stimulant when we drink coffee or other caffeine-containing drinks, such as tea, cola drinks and hot chocolate. There is almost always enough time, it seems, to grab a coffee or tea to revive yourself. But drinking five to six cups of coffee on a daily basis is toxic to the body, wreaking havoc with the endocrine system. The stimulating effect induces the release of the hormone adrenaline, which promotes anxiety, restlessness, palpitations and insomnia. In addition, caffeine is addictive: you need

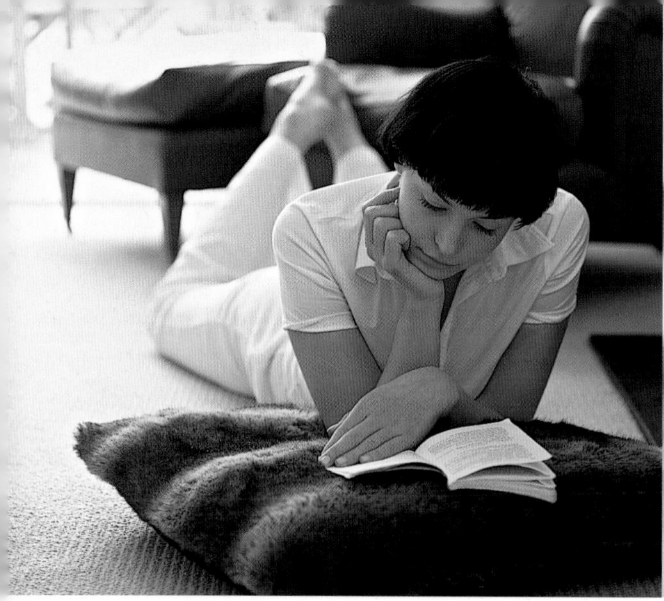
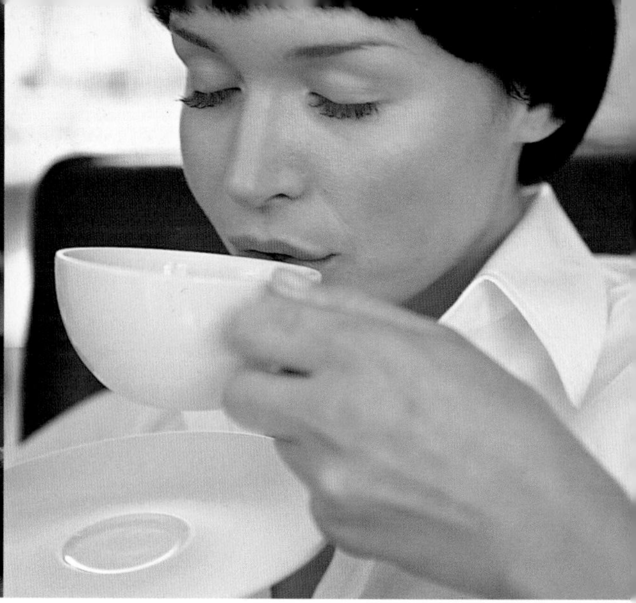

Try to limit your sedentary activities and drink more caffeine-free drinks and herbal teas.

to consume more over time to get the same buzz or lift and when you try to cut down the caffeine withdrawal brings on headaches.

Take action **Stay more balanced by drinking caffeine-free alternatives, such as dandelion coffee or herbal teas, or limit yourself to one to two cups of coffee or tea daily.**

Nicotine and other toxins

Cigarettes contain nicotine, which is another strong stimulant. Inhaling the smoke from a cigarette may ease muscular tension and stimulate the senses, but it also activates the nervous system, releasing stress hormones into the bloodstream. Smoking just one cigarette speeds your heart rate and raises your blood pressure, putting strain on your cardiovascular system as the flow of oxygen in the blood decreases. Smoking is a serious health hazard: it greatly increases the risks of lung cancer, heart disease and stroke. Thousands of other toxins are introduced into the body through smoking, including carbon monoxide (a by-product of the smoke), which decreases oxygen levels in the blood and damages body cells, reducing the natural detoxification process.

Take action **Stop smoking. You will have more energy within 24 hours as the carbon monoxide levels fall and oxygen levels normalize. After 1–5 years your risk of heart attack is halved. You can also try hypnosis, which has proved successful in helping some smokers to quit. If you're finding it hard to quit just yet, take a good multivitamin and mineral supplement daily to help counteract the depletion of nutrients.**

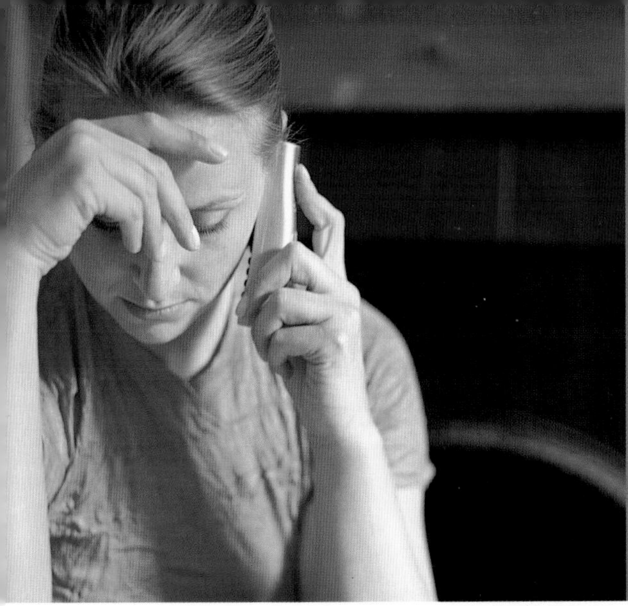

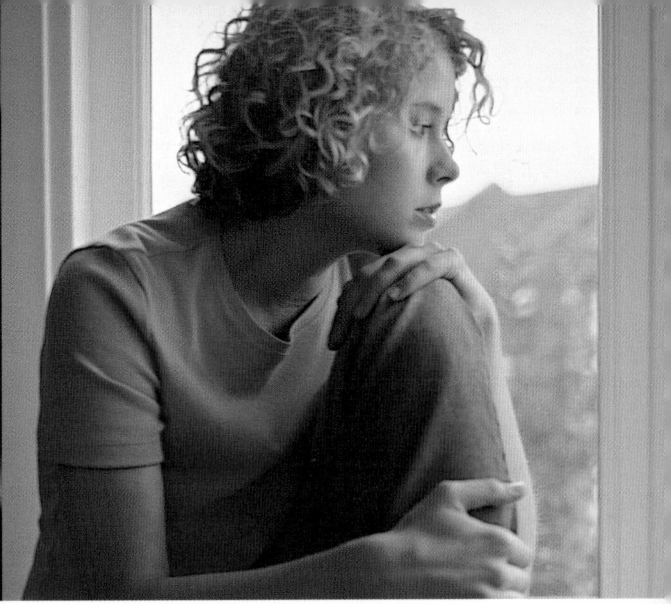

Constantly dealing with family problems or suffering relationship difficulties can sap your emotions.

emotional ENERGY DRAINS

Apart from demands on your physical energy, you may also experience emotional drains that can come in many guises. Partners and family can wear you down with constant claims on your time. You may have certain demanding friends who zap your energy with selfish requests. At work, colleagues or bosses who undermine your position can lower your self-esteem. While in the home, entertaining the kids can sometimes make you feel isolated.

A loving relationship

The relationship you have with a partner can give you the most incredible energy highs and lows, depending on how well it is going. If you have a selfish partner and you seem to be the one that makes the compromises to keep the relationship going, there is an energy imbalance and you may feel unhappy and resentful. And if you constantly argue with a partner, your emotional energy will be at a low ebb.

Take action **Talk through your feelings with your partner and suggest changes to bring the relationship back on an equal footing. And try to see if you can both work out why you constantly disagree. If a serious rift has occurred, joint counselling may well help to save the relationship.**

Children and ageing relatives

Both young and old can upset your emotional energy as they make demands on your time. Children can be easily upset by problems at school and young ones may have tantrums or upsets to get your attention. You may also find that older relatives, especially ones that are bedridden, think all your spare time should be spent with them.

Take action Conserve your energy by making a special time each day for your children to talk through their day with you; perhaps turn it into a story time for younger ones. Also, be realistic with needy relatives. It is a good idea to see them on a regular evening or weekend, so that they can look forward to the visit.

Friends

Most of us have at least one friend who we would describe as self-obsessed or unreliable, or both. These 'energy vampires' will 'drink' you dry. You know the type. They phone you late at night with their current problems or crisis and never want to hear your news. Or they call you just as you are leaving to meet them to cancel with the weakest of excuses.

Take action Save your energy for yourself by limiting the amount of time on the phone to 'draining' friends. Reappraise your friendships. If one is over, explain why and move on. As you get older, your energy levels change and so will your friends.

Colleagues or bosses

People at work can sometimes be unsupportive, which can take its toll on your emotional energy and undermine your self-esteem.

Take action With an unappreciative boss, discuss a way to resolve your problems. Talk to unhelpful colleagues and see how you can work better together.

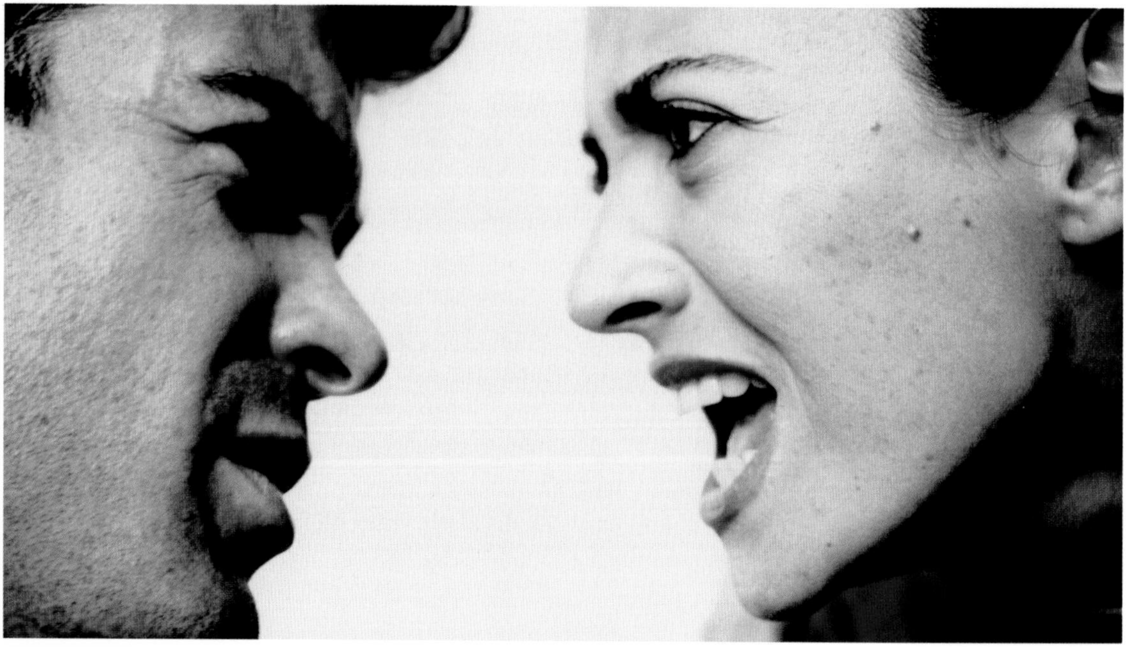

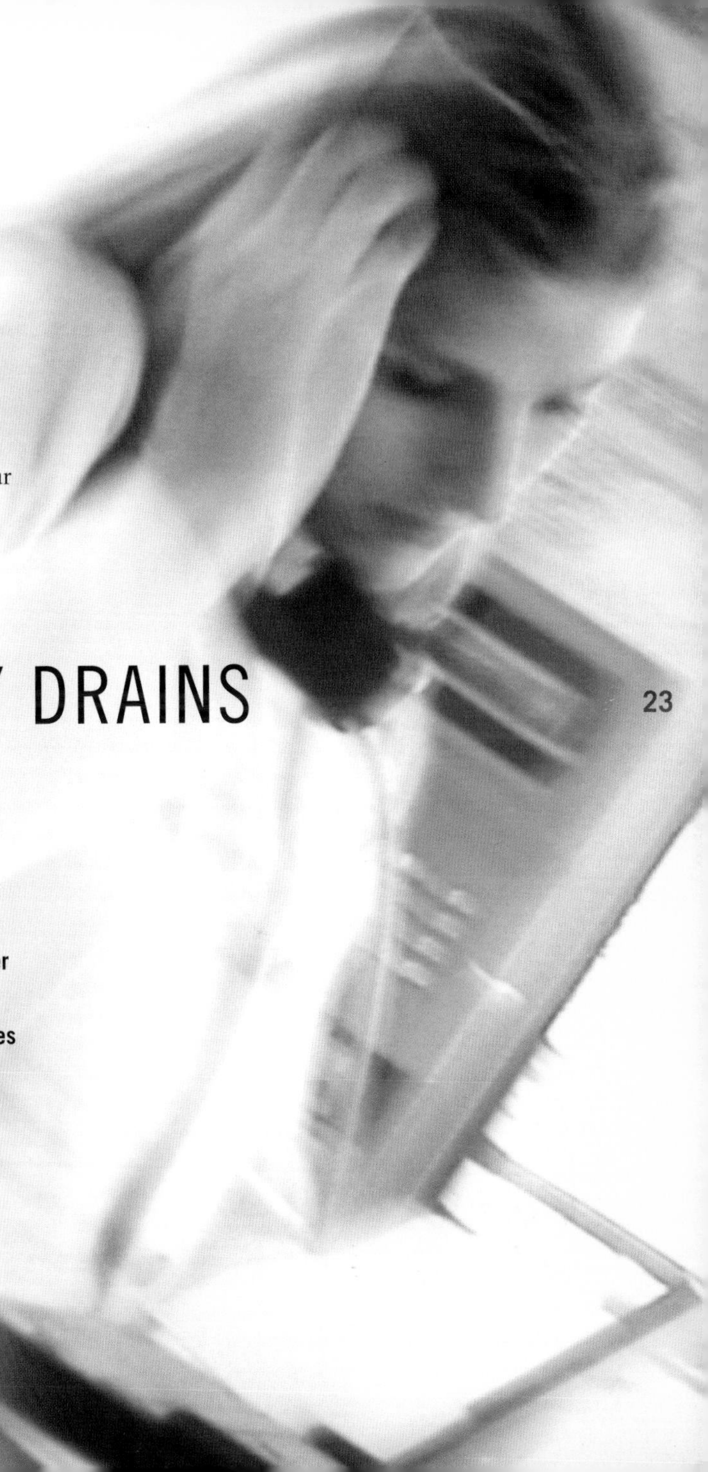

Our spiritual needs are often low on the agenda. But if these are neglected, we will never achieve the perfect inner and outer harmony that we seek. Think about your life as it is today and study any areas where you are not happy that may be draining your spiritual energy. Watch your attitude, if you are constantly negative, your life will continue on that path. You may have a desire to paint or play an instrument but are not making the time to do it. Or, maybe your dream is to buy a property abroad, but you can't get round to doing the research on your chosen area. Perhaps you are in a mundane job that pays well, but you really desire to be a photographer or social worker.

spiritual ENERGY DRAINS

Take action **Make some regular time to connect to your inner self, as it harbours all your dreams and desires. Be positive and work to achieve your aims. Practise writing things down (journalling, see pages 128–129); you may be surprised at what you discover about yourself. Meditate (see pages 41 and 133) regularly in a quiet room to hear those inner messages that will keep you on the right path and let you fulfil your true desires.**

Be more selfish in the future and give yourself more attention if you want to feel really balanced again.

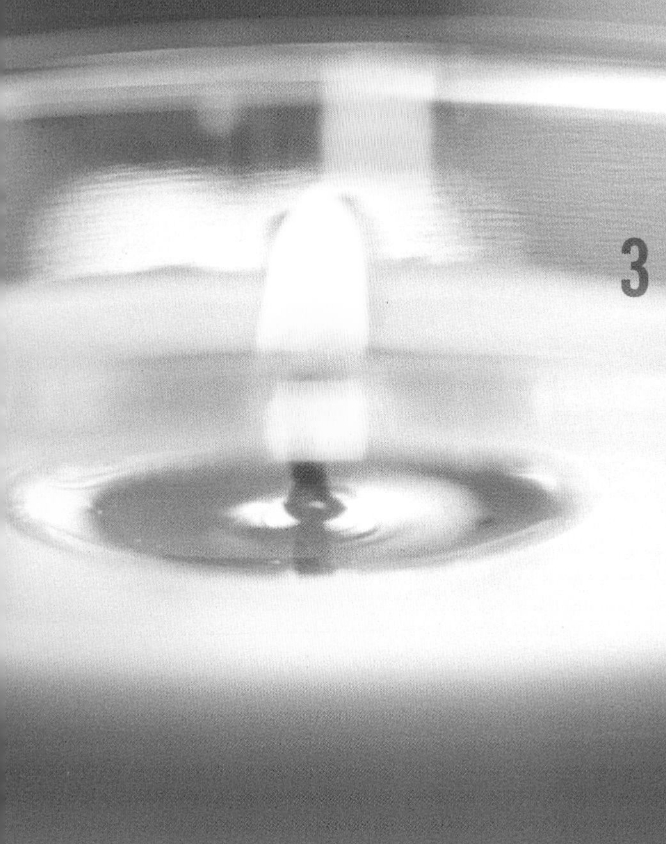

3 First steps

One of the first steps is to recognize that your energy levels are being drained on a daily basis. The next step is to accept that you need to be more selfish in the future and give yourself some attention if you want to feel really balanced once again. Your family or friends may feel a little resentful initially when you decide to do this as your focus is taken from them to you. But this is the only way you are going to feel really good and have the energy you need to enjoy your life to the full.

Discover what your energy drains are by completing the questionnaire opposite so that you can deal with them. You may well find that there are more emotional or spiritual causes than physical ones.

What are your daily energy drains?

Complete the questionnaire below to find out how your energy is being zapped from your mind, body and spirit on a daily basis.

		Yes	No	Sometimes
1	Do you smoke more than 20 cigarettes a day?			
2	Do you have a boss who never appreciates your work?			
3	Are your constantly arguing with your partner?			
4	Do you get anxious or worry about minor problems?			
5	Are your drinking more than six cups of coffee daily?			
6	Do you regularly not get enough sleep or sleep badly?			
7	Are you stuck in a relationship that you don't know how to end?			
8	Do you constantly feel that your life is going in the wrong direction?			
9	Have you got achievable dreams that you are not putting into practice?			
10	Are you always running yourself down?			
11	Do you consistently work late?			
12	Does your lunch often consist of a hurried snack such as chocolate or crisps?			
13	Do you feel you give everything to your family but get little in return?			
14	Is your computer, work space or home office full of clutter?			
15	Do you get regular messages from your inner self, but choose to ignore them?			
16	Are you longing to live in the country but stay in town?			
17	Do you regularly get calls from friends who just offload their problems?			
18	Are you often drinking more than 14 units (women) or 21 units (men) of alcohol a week?			
19	Do you know that you are not in the right job, but are staying because of the money?			
20	Are you often wasting your energy in senseless disagreements?			
21	Is your normal attitude quite negative, do you view your life as 'half empty' rather than 'half full' in the glass analogy?			
22	Are you always talking about making changes in your life, but then don't put them into practice?			
23	Do you feel you have no time to take some spiritual space to meditate or do a yoga class?			
24	Do you fail to make regular exercise a priority in your life?			
25	Does your life seem empty right now, and you don't quite know why?			

Now, add up your score. Give yourself 2 points for a 'Yes', 1 for a 'Sometimes' and 0 for a 'No'. Total score =

Score of 35–50

Your energy levels are pretty depleted right now, so decide to make yourself your number one priority to refresh and restore them. Address any inadequacies or overindulgences in your diet and then look at improving your sleeping patterns. Next, take some time to analyse how you deal with family problems or unsupportive friends. Try to do some of the Instant energizers (pages 36–141) regularly to re-energize your life.

Score of 20–34

You are working hard but haven't totally neglected your overall energy levels. Still, they are lower than they should be, so look at any particular areas that need improvement. Make sure you have a nutritious lunch each day and that your alcohol intake is moderate. Work on any emotional drains in your life, such as a bad relationship. Follow your dreams and do a selection of the Instant energizers (pages 36–141) to give you the boost you need.

Score of 19 and under

Life is fairly under control for you; you have reasonable energy levels, but don't get complacent. You only need a difficult project at work or a crisis at home for them to start dropping. Look after yourself healthwise, and don't burn the candle at both ends. Keep physical, emotional and spiritual energy topped up by doing some of the Instant energizers (pages 36–141) so that you stay happy and in balance.

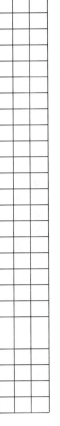

pinpointing YOUR LOWS

Now you have completed the questionnaire on page 25, you will be more aware of which factors are responsible for your energy dips or lows. Note down any regular stimulants you use (see pages 19–20) and make a pact with yourself either to cut down on them or to give them up right now! Make a list of your current emotional drains and write down how you plan to deal with them.

Energy slumps

Recognize which part of the day is worst for you. If you are a morning person, schedule important meetings or activities with children for the morning when you are at your most energetic. Note down the time when you start to feel tired and eat a high-energy snack (see page 10) half an hour before that time to even out your blood-sugar levels. If you are regularly exhausted and irritable by late afternoon, use a mid-afternoon boosting reflexology or breathing exercise (pages 86–105) to give you an energy boost. On the other hand, if you're a night owl who finds it difficult to wind down and get to sleep, cleanse your aura or do a clearing meditation before bed.

Long-term lows

Spiritual lows can take longer to deal with as they often involve making life changes that take you out of your comfort zone. It may be that you want a more creative job or crave some 'you time' and a lie-in at the weekend, when your partner can deal with the kids. Whatever your goal, ensure you set time limits to achieving them. In the meantime, use mantras, self-affirmations and visualization exercises (see pages 36–141) to turn your goals into reality.

Write down a key affirmation that you can repeat aloud (at least ten times) to give you a boost when you are feeling low or insecure, or when you feel that life is not going your way. Choose your words carefully and make them positive. Try something like: 'I am a wonderful person and I am successful at everything I attempt'; 'I happily accept everything this new day brings me' or 'I have great health, love and happiness in my life'.

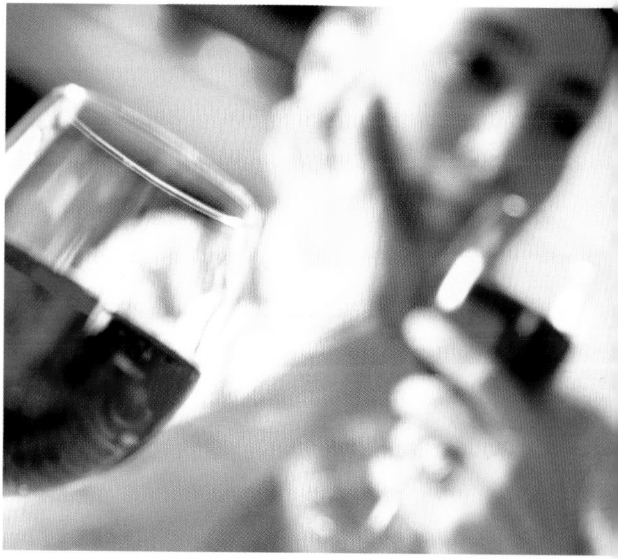

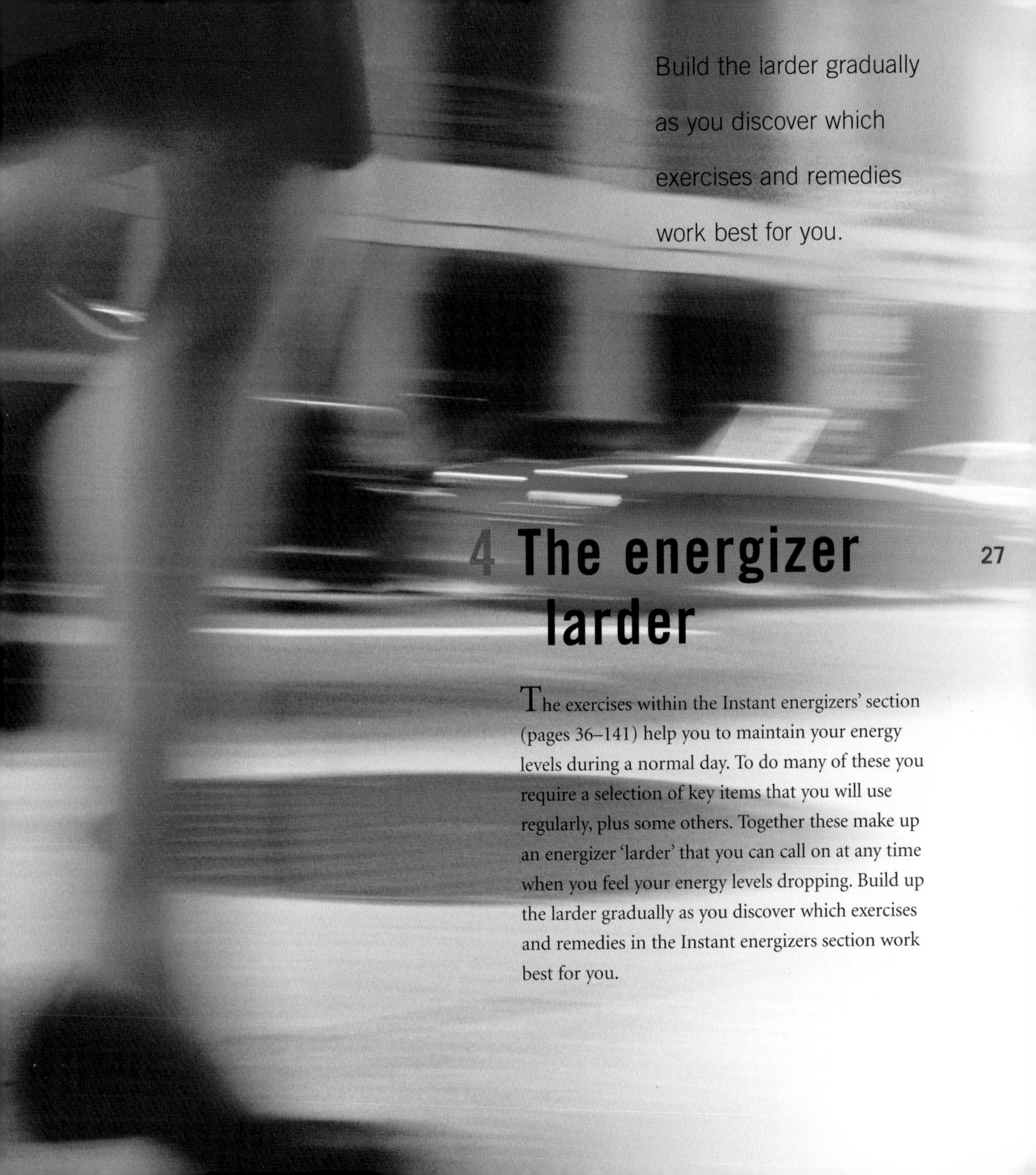

Build the larder gradually as you discover which exercises and remedies work best for you.

4 The energizer larder

The exercises within the Instant energizers' section (pages 36–141) help you to maintain your energy levels during a normal day. To do many of these you require a selection of key items that you will use regularly, plus some others. Together these make up an energizer 'larder' that you can call on at any time when you feel your energy levels dropping. Build up the larder gradually as you discover which exercises and remedies in the Instant energizers section work best for you.

You may decide to buy several Bach or Bush flower remedies to even out your emotional lows. Rescue remedy, for example, can help panic attacks. Or if you are a tea drinker, you may want to buy fresh herbs and spices, such as warming ginger, to make various healing teas. The versatile and aromatic essential oils, which have the innate power to calm or revive the senses, will become an essential part of your larder. Start with the cure-all lavender oil and add others as and when you need them. You may also want to keep some incense and smudge sticks at home to cleanse negative and dull energy and bring a 'zing' back into the atmosphere. Finally, let the healing vibrations of crystals restore diminishing energy levels. Why not carry a nurturing stone, such as amethyst, with you – in your pocket or bag – to protect you. You will soon find the ingredients in your larder to be an indispensable part of your energy-balancing programme.

Flower remedies

These natural liquid essences heal the mind, body and spirit. They harmonize any negative feelings stored in the subconscious mind. The essences are obtained when the healing vibrational quality or 'imprint' is extracted from certain flowers. This is normally done by the sun method: where the flowers are left in a bowl of water in strong sunlight, the resulting essence is poured into bottles half filled with brandy.

CHOOSING **remedies**

Bach flower remedy	Emotional cure
Elm page 59	Restores confidence in those who are overwhelmed with pressure from work or family commitments.
Hornbeam page 63	Gives emotional strength to face the new day for those who are mentally exhausted at the thought of too much work or too much to do.
Olive page 63	Replaces lost energy for those who are exhausted because of overwork or overexertion.
Rescue remedy (combination) page 63	Helps in emergencies or stressful events, such as taking a driving test, exam nerves or speaking in public, when there is emotional panic, loss of control and mental pain.
Willow page 63	Lifts the gloom and self-pity from an irritable and introspective pessimist who likes to wallow in misfortune.

Bush flower essence	Emotional cure
Alpine mintbush page 63	Gives joy and renewal to those suffering from mental and emotional exhaustion or from the weight of responsibility.
Calm and clear (combination) page 82	Encourages a person to relax and unwind when they feel overcommitted with no time for themselves.
Crowea page 63	Balances and centres the individual who is worrying and feeling 'out of sorts'.
Dog rose of the wild forces page 67	Provides emotional balance for the person who fears loss of control.
Emergency essence (combination) pages 100–101	Helps ease distress and panic in someone who has suffered a shock.
Five corners bush flower page 47	Gives love and acceptance of self to those suffering low self-esteem.
Space clearing spray (combination) page 97	Creates a safe and harmonious environment where there has been a build-up of negative mental and emotional energy.

Sometimes the boiling method is used: the flowers are simmered for 30 minutes in spring water and then decanted as before. The types used in this book are Bach flower remedies and Bush flower essences.

How to take flower remedies

With Bach flower remedies put 4 drops on your tongue or add them to a small glass of water 4 times a day. With Bush remedies, place 7 drops under the tongue, twice daily.

Smudge sticks and incense

Smudge sticks are made from special dried herbs that are tied in bundles. When lit, their purifying scent recharges the atmosphere. When smouldering, sweet-smelling incense can brighten the ambience in a room. Choose one of these scents to use in the exercises in the Instant energizers.

Smudge sticks see pages 122–123	Effects of scented smoke
Rosemary	Cleanses stagnant atmosphere.
Sage	Purifies atmosphere on a deep level.
Sweetgrass	Drives away negativity.

Incense see page 134	Effects of scented smoke
Cedarwood	Improves feelings of safety.
Cloves	Helps to boost concentration and lifts mood.
Jasmine	Relaxes the body for sleep and aids meditation.
Myrrh	Calms the emotions.
Sandalwood	Cleanses the atmosphere and enhances meditation.
Vanilla	Physically energizes but also calms the emotions.

Essential oils

These wonderful scented oils are aromatic essences that have been extracted from plants, flowers, trees, fruit, bark grasses and seeds. They have therapeutic psychological and physiological effects through their smell and through the skin. They can boost or relax our moods and promote healing in our bodies.

Essential oils have therapeutic effects through their smell and through the skin.

About 150 essences exist, each with a unique scent and healing property. All have antiseptic properties but some also have pain-relieving, relaxing, stimulating and antidepressant qualities. It's a good idea to buy the multi-use lavender and tea tree oils first, then experiment with others (see table opposite) until you find ones that suit you.

How to use essential oils

Some essential oils can be used neat while others have to be diluted or mixed with a base oil. See pages 56, 63 and 108 for some examples of how to get the best from essential oils.

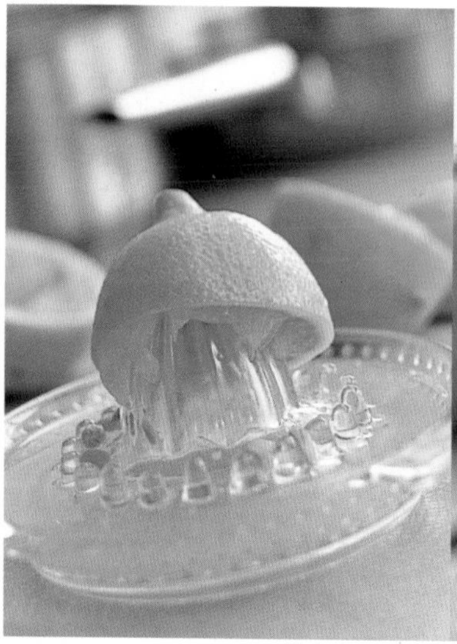

Lemon

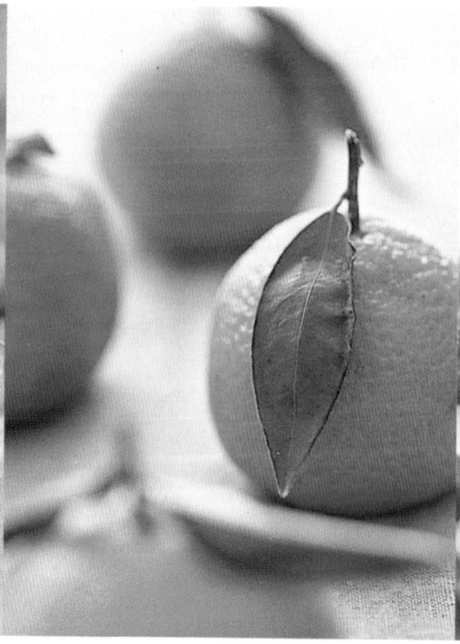

Orange

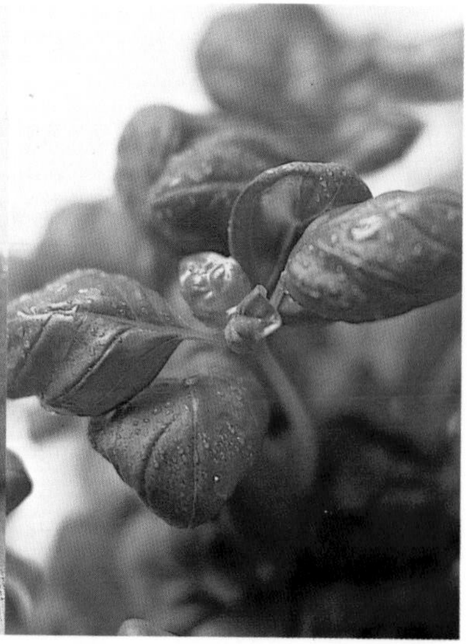

Basil

Essential oil	Properties
Basil page 108 (avoid during pregnancy)	Uplifting, harmonizing oil that increases concentration and clarifies thought processes.
Bergamot pages 43, 63 (use with caution in sunny weather)	Gentle, stimulating oil that is an effective antidepressant.
Camomile page 117	Relaxant that is antispasmodic, relieving tension headaches or an upset stomach.
Clary sage pages 43, 117 (avoid during pregnancy)	Antidepressant and relaxant that gives a euphoric feeling.
Eucalyptus page 97	Invigorating oil that cleanses the head and helps respiratory complaints.
Frankincense pages 56, 117	Calming, spiritually uplifting oil that soothes nervous conditions.
Geranium pages 108, 110, 117, 136	Refreshing antidepressant that is good for nervous tension and exhaustion.
Ginger page 43	Stimulates energy production.
Grapefruit page 117	Tangy oil that gives an energy boost and alleviates nervous exhaustion.
Jasmine pages 108, 136	Great fragrance that both relaxes and lifts anxiety, depression and lethargy.
Juniper page 131 (avoid during pregnancy)	Relaxing, purifying oil that can also refresh, particularly when run down.
Lavender pages 57, 108, 110, 117, 131, 136	Versatile, relaxing oil that eases stress symptoms. It mixes with other oils and can soothe tension headaches, nervous digestive upsets and aid restful sleep.
Lemon pages 43, 117	Cleansing, antiseptic oil that refreshes and boosts the immune system.
Lemongrass pages 56, 97	Stimulating oil that cleanses and tones the mind and body.
Lime pages 108, 117	Invigorating oil that can coax sluggish body organs into action.
Mandarin page 117	Refreshing and cleansing oil that aids digestion and soothes heartburn.
Marjoram page 84 (avoid during pregnancy)	Calming and warming oil that releases tight muscles and reduces anxiety and headaches.
Neroli page 63	Calming oil that lowers stress levels.
Orange page 43	Revitalizing oil that is a tonic and raises the spirits.
Patchouli page 136	Sensuous, relaxing oil that inspires the mind and lessens depression.
Pine pages 43, 117	Cleansing oil that helps to lighten fatigue and tired muscles.
Rose page 133	Fragrant, sensual oil that both soothes the emotions and eases muscular and nervous tension.
Rosemary pages 93, 97, 131	Stimulating, cleansing oil that eases nervous exhaustion and mental fatigue.
Sandalwood pages 56, 136	Heavy scented oil that is a relaxant and an antidepressant.
Tea tree page 43	Useful cleansing, antiseptic oil that is very stimulating.
Ylang ylang pages 108, 136	Soothing and sensual oil that is also good for stress, panic attacks, anxiety and depression.

Herbs and spices

Herbal remedies have been used since ancient times to heal, and they still play an important part in healthcare in our lives today. Herbs (and spices) contain vitamins, minerals, trace elements and healing agents, such as tannins, butters and glycosides, that are beneficial to the body. Full of healthy nutrients, they can act as tonics or stimulants but can also impart a more calming influence. The antispasmodic and antiseptic qualities of some herbs calm the digestive system and boost immune function.

How to use herbs and spices

Fresh herbs are best to use when making the teas in the Instant energizers' section so that you extract all the curative ingredients. See page 46 for the general principle of making herbal teas.

Full of healthy nutrients, herbs and spices can act as tonics or stimulants but can also impart a more calming influence.

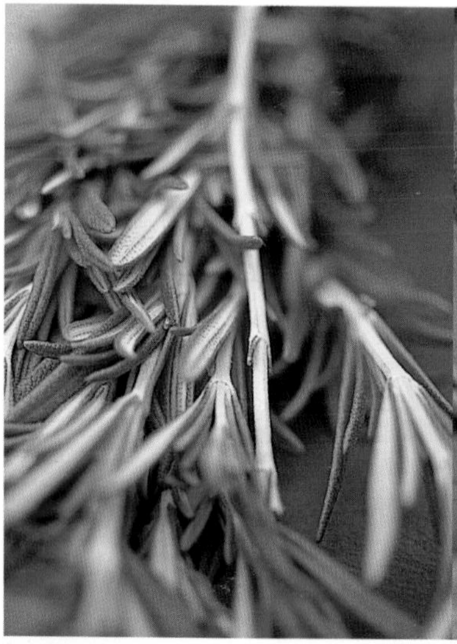

Rosemary

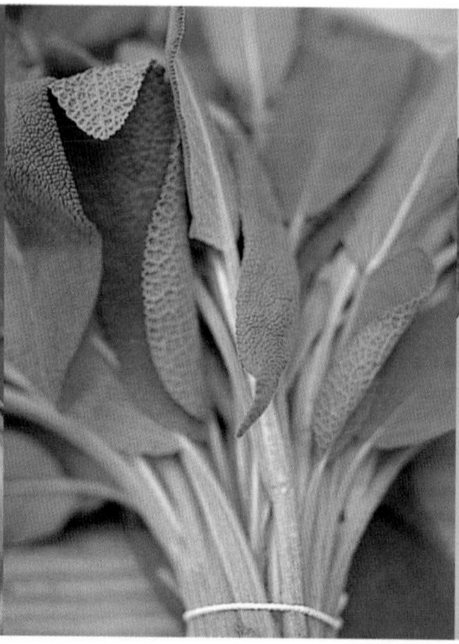

Sage

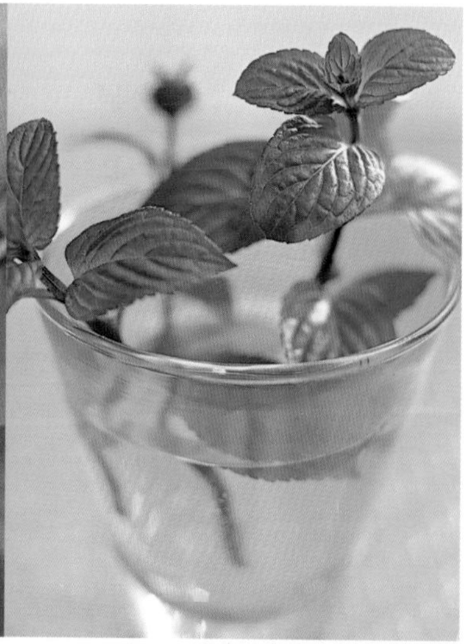

Mint

Herb or Spice	Uses	Properties
Ginger page 46	Warming and pungent spice that is best used fresh in tea.	Ginger aids fat breakdown and lowers blood cholesterol levels, speeding up digestion. It prevents nausea and is a good tonic encouraging blood flow, particularly in cold weather. It strengthens and heals the respiratory system.
Gingko biloba page 58	Ancient medicinal herb that can be drunk in tea to improve arterial circulation and increase memory.	It improves the use of glucose in the brain. It also increases mental alertness by stimulating the production of the brain's alpha waves.
Korean ginseng page 90	Root that is usually available as ginseng powder.	This stimulant increases energy levels, strengthens the immune system and decreases fatigue, thereby improving overall physical and mental efficiency.
Lemon balm page 58	Sweet-scented herb that has a pleasant flavour in tea.	Its antispasmodic qualities relieve muscle tension, alleviate nervous anxiety and help digestion.
Peppermint page 58	Herb containing menthol, which works as a carminative to reduce stomach tension or upset and feelings of nausea.	It has a fresh taste in tea, can aid concentration and can give you a 'lift' if you are suffering from exhaustion.
Rosemary page 46	Fragrant, aromatic herb that makes an all-purpose tonic as a tea.	Rosemary reduces the pain of a headache, can alleviate dizziness and strengthens the nervous system.
Sage page 46 (avoid if diabetic or pregnant)	Herb with a slightly bitter taste; add honey in tea to counter this bitterness.	Sage is a tonic that can also aid a griping stomach. It is also a relaxant that calms the nerves or overexcitement.
Green tea page 90	Eastern tea containing high levels of polyphenols and flavenoids that boost the immune system.	It has a strong antioxidant action that destroys free radicals that can increase the risk of cancer.

Crystals

When hot gases and mineral solutions bubbled to the surface from the Earth's molten layer millions of years ago, the first crystals were formed. As the gases and liquids cooled, their atoms formed three-dimensional lattices, becoming the crystals we know today. Their crystalline structure enables them to absorb, strengthen and then transmit electromagnetic energy. This energy is used in crystal healing to balance the vibratory level of the aura, *chakras* and body cells. In healing, crystals can remove stress and negativity, dissolve blockages and bring harmony into your life. Initially, buy the stones for the main exercises in Instant energizers and add in other suggested ones as and when you need them.

How to select crystals

Allow plenty of time in a crystal shop as the crystals you want will choose you. You will feel drawn intuitively to a particular stone, or when you pick one up you will feel an energetic connection or be comforted by it.

Cleansing crystals

When you buy crystals they will have taken on the energetic imprint of the shop they have been in, so cleanse them thoroughly to re-energize them.
If you use your crystals often to get rid of negative emotions, cleanse them regularly.

Water cleansing Hold a crystal under running tap water to cleanse it. Focus on transmuting any negative energies into positive ones as the water is running over the stone. Leave it to dry in the sun.

Sunlight cleansing Wash briefly under water and then leave on a sunny windowsill for 24 hours to renew its energy (avoid for amethyst and rose quartz as they are light sensitive).

Setting your intention

You can utilize the energizing properties of crystals for many different forms of healing, but before you do this you need to make the crystal your own by setting an intention for its use, to 'switch' it on or 'tune' it in.

- **Hold the crystal in your hand, placing your other hand on top, and promise you will only use it for the highest good.**
- **Become attuned to the crystal's energy; if you prefer, see a ray of white light connecting you.**
- **Focus on the purpose for your crystal, whether it be for healing, meditation or cleansing, then dedicate it by saying out loud: 'I intend this crystal to help with ... (add your intention)'. Repeat it several times.**
- **Keep a special crystal with you, in your car or by your bed at night.**

Crystals	Uses	Qualities
Agate page 63	Grounding stone that boosts self-esteem.	Promotes inner peace and improves perceptive skills.
Amber pages 76–77	Golden stone that heals the nervous system.	Promotes patience and brings wisdom and balance.
Amethyst page 130	Crystal that reduces physical and emotional pain.	Helps develop spiritual awareness and clear the aura.
Aquamarine page 83	Calming stone that reduces stress.	Makes the mind sharper and cleanses the Throat chakra.
Aventurine pages 60–61	All-round healing stone that promotes physical, mental and emotional wellbeing.	Enhances creativity and brings prosperity.
Beryl page 63	Crystal that encourages positive thoughts.	Alleviates stress and quietens the mind.
Bloodstone page 63	Stone that helps decision making.	Purifies the blood and grounds the body by cleansing the lower *chakras*.
Cat's eye page 63	Grounding stone that stimulates confidence and happiness.	Clears negativity from the aura and protects it.
Green tourmaline page 61	Powerful healing stone that opens up the heart chakra and promotes compassion.	Transforms negative energy into positive energy.
Jasper page 42	Nurturing and protective stone.	Promotes clear thought patterns and helps to balance the *chakras*.
Natural quartz page 91	Versatile crystal, which aids meditation, and amplifies the energy and the power of other crystals.	Reduces irrational fears and increases psychic abilities.
Rose quartz page 96	Wonderful healing stone that opens the heart.	Takes away negativity, heightens self-esteem and aids self-affirmations.

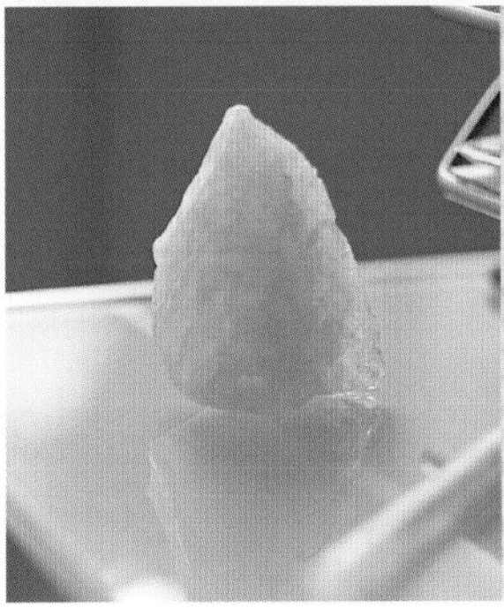

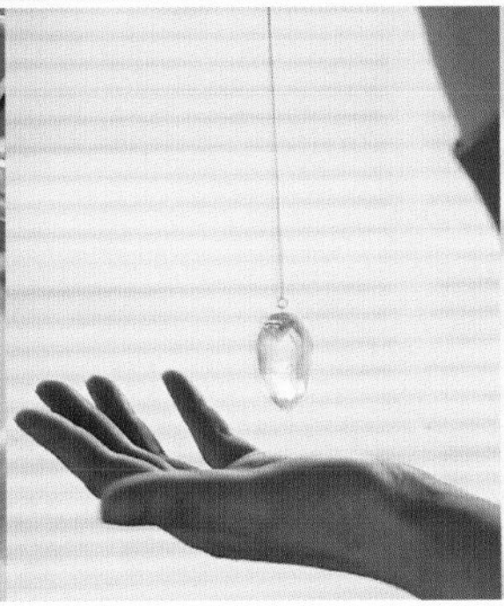

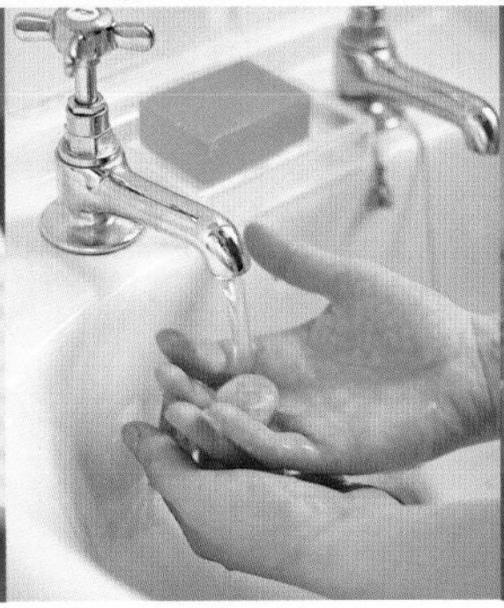

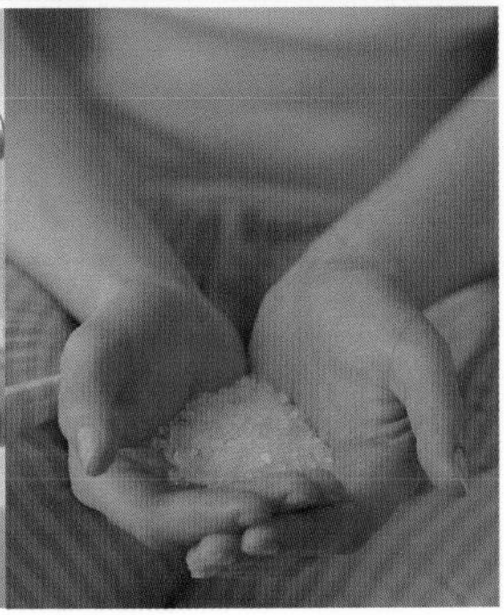

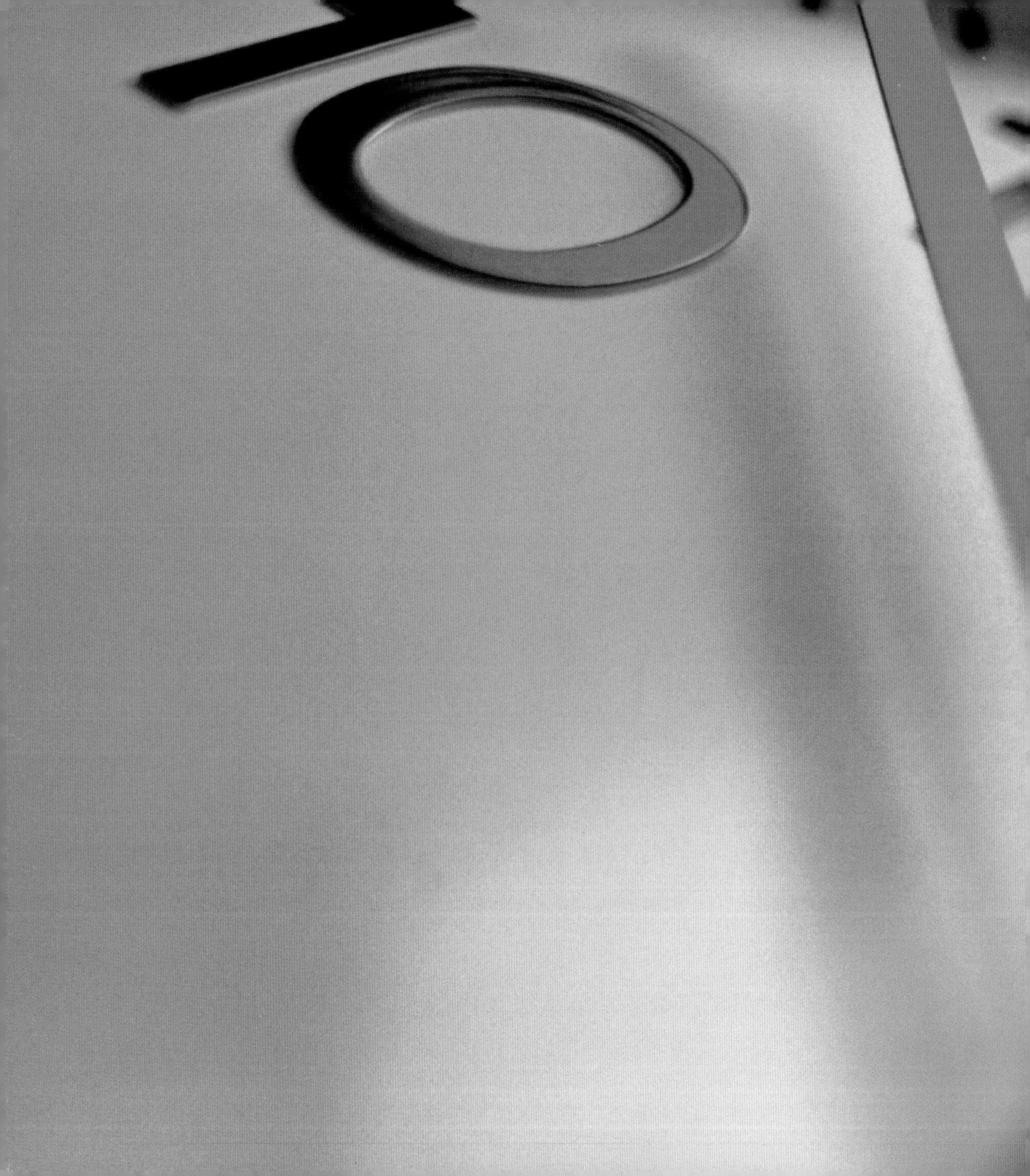

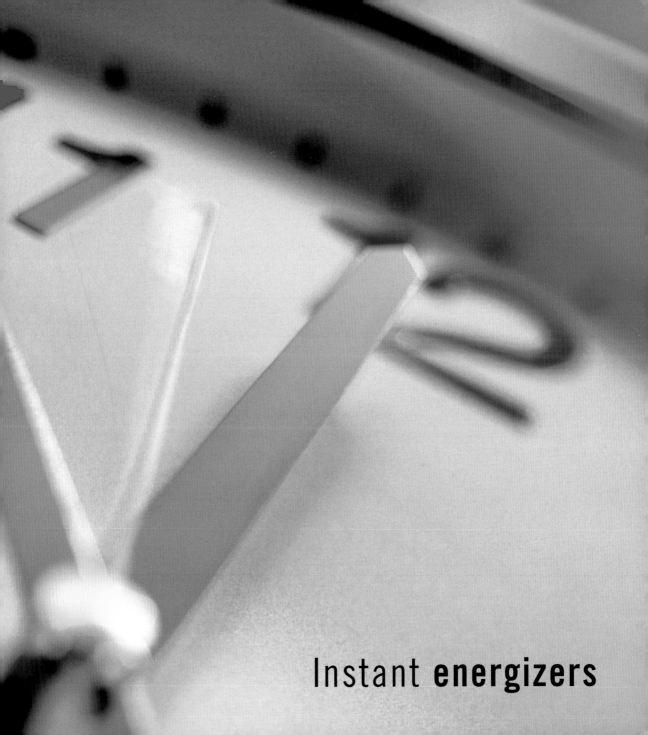

Instant **energizers**

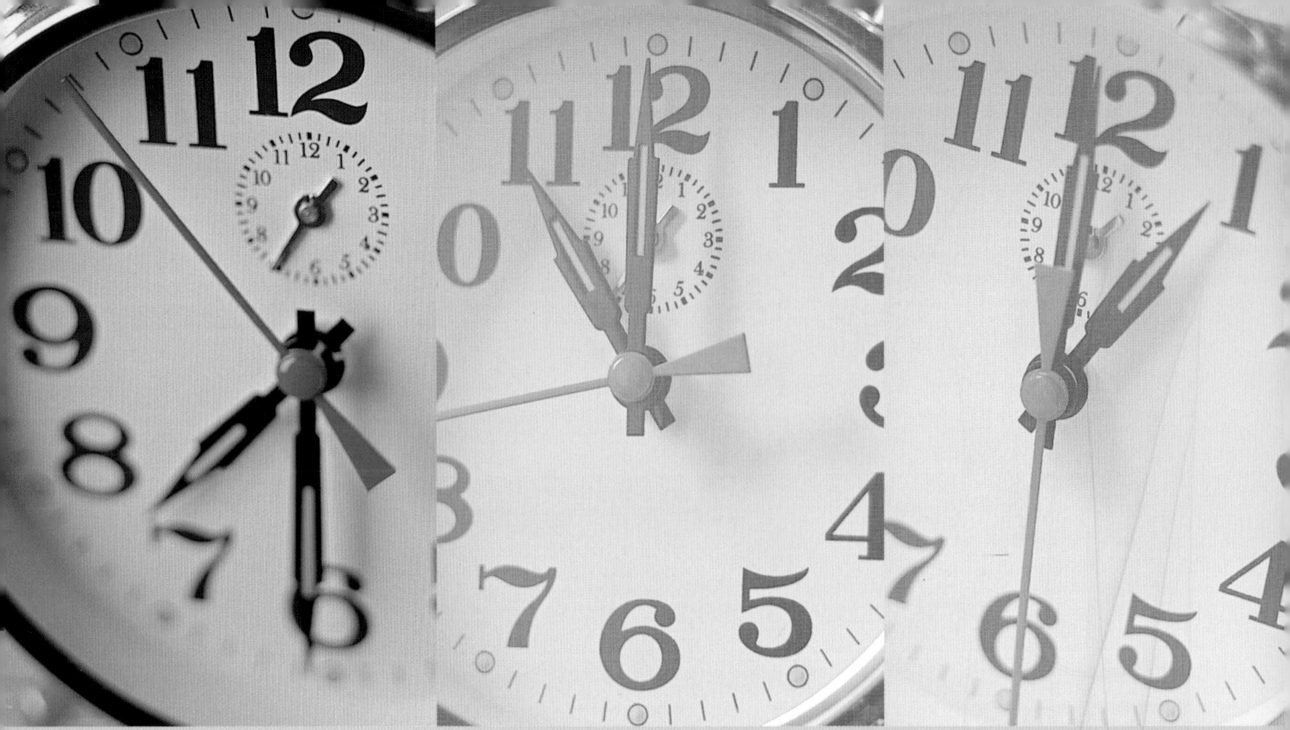

5 Wake up fresh

These early morning holistic energizing exercises aim to give you the initial energy boost you need – physically, mentally and spiritually.

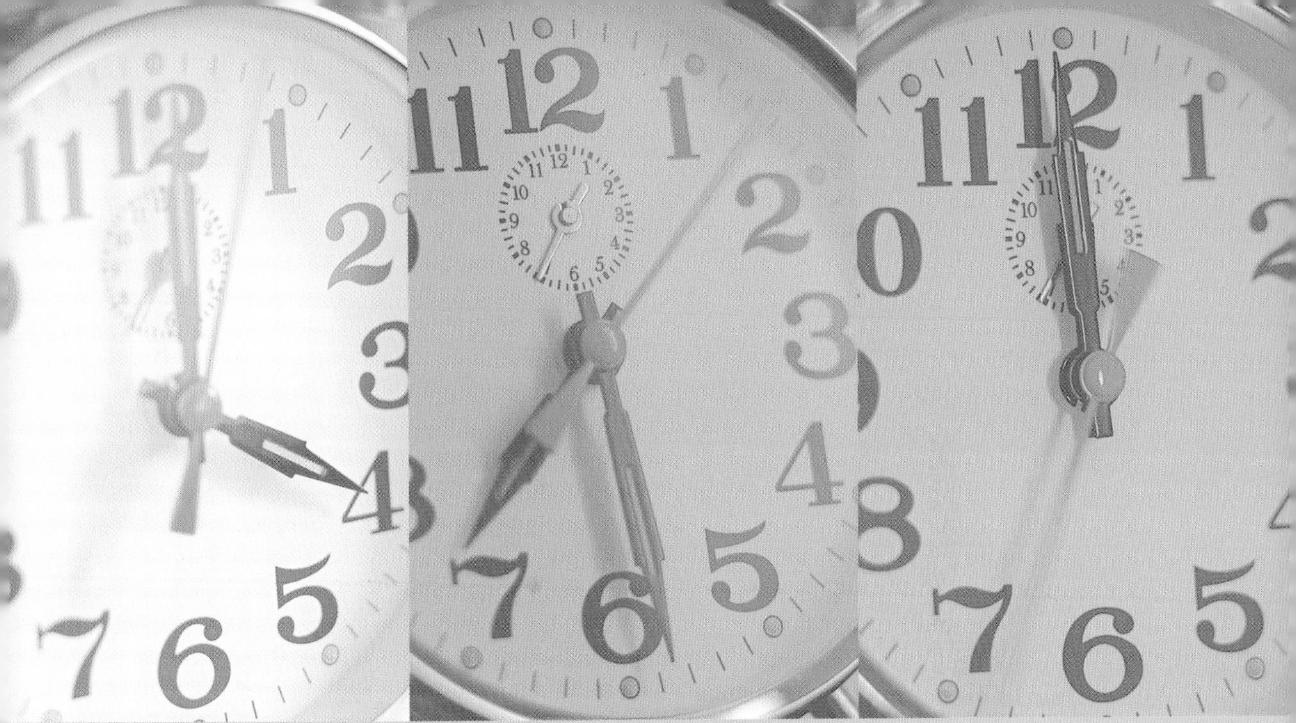

When you wake up in the morning your energy levels can be at a low ebb and you can feel sluggish and reluctant to begin the day. Your bodily systems will have slowed down for the long night's sleep and can need some encouragement to start working at full power again. Your mind may still want to linger in your pleasant dream world and not have the focus needed for the busy day ahead.

These early morning holistic energizing exercises aim to give you the initial energy boost you need – physically, mentally and spiritually. Clear and concentrate your mind with one of the meditative techniques, set your daily intent with an affirmation or work on both your body and your mind with some pre-breakfast yoga postures. The choice is yours; use one or two that seem appropriate. By practising these energizers regularly you will feel capable of handling all the challenges of the day ahead.

As your alarm sounds in the morning, it can be hard to rouse yourself to get up from your warm, cosy bed – and when you do get up you can feel lethargic and find it hard to get going. Doing a morning breathing exercise can give your body the stimulating uplift it needs.

The importance of proper breathing is often underestimated. As babies we instinctively breathe deeply from our diaphragms, but as we get older we become lazy and take shallower breaths from the chest. When we inhale, oxygen from the air is absorbed into our blood and is circulated to all body cells and organs; when we exhale all the waste carbon dioxide collected from the body is breathed out. The more oxygen our blood receives the healthier we are.

BREATHING **for energy**

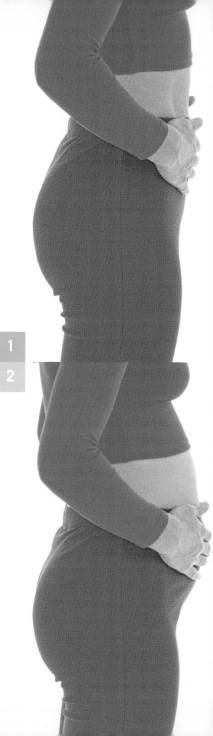

1

2

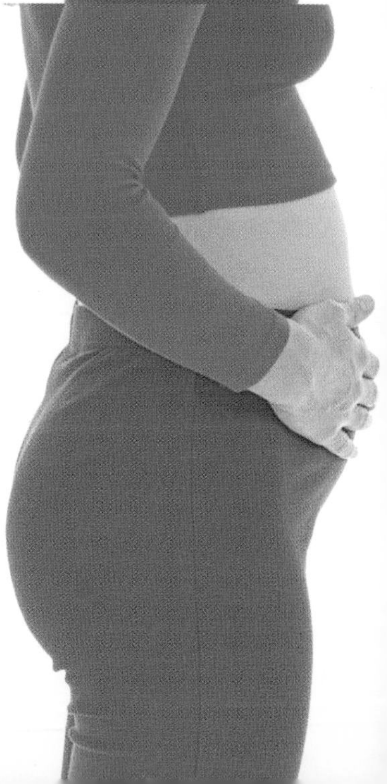

BREATHING DEEPLY

Take some deep breaths from your diaphragm to expand your lung capacity and boost oxygen levels in your bloodstream, to clear out toxins and to purify your internal organs before starting your working day.

1 Stand upright with a straight spine or sit cross-legged on a mat on the floor. Breathe in deeply, through your nose, from your diaphragm, drawing air into your lower lungs.

2 As you expand your ribcage feel the air working up through your lungs until it reaches the top. Hold for a few seconds.

3 Slowly breathe out, through your nose, releasing the air first from the top of your lungs and then downwards. Repeat this deep breathing technique for about 5–10 minutes every morning.

Meditation is a wonderful technique to quieten your mind and bring inner peace; what is more, it is simple to learn. It helps you to leave behind all your fears, slows down your busy thought processes and separates you from your ego so that you can communicate with your subconscious mind that influences everything you do. Meditating for a short time each morning can reduce your stress levels and improve your overall wellbeing.

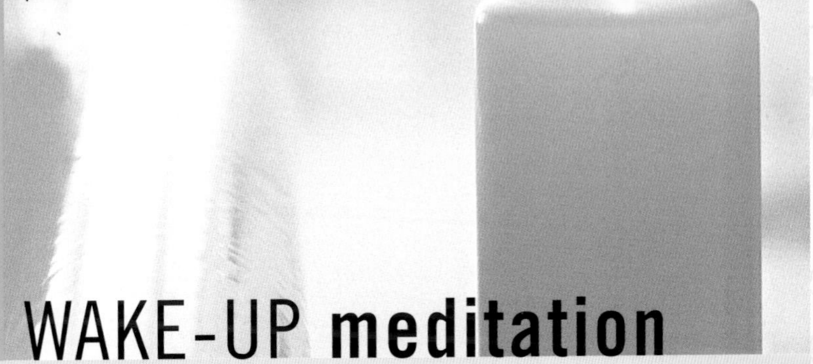

WAKE-UP **meditation**

Use a mandala

Another technique to try is to meditate with a Tibetan or Buddhist *mandala* (a magic circle representing eternity). Take a colour copy from a reference book and place it in front of you. Focus on the central point of the circle as you start to meditate.

MEDITATE TO ENERGIZE

Practise this meditation for about 5–10 minutes every day. It won't take long to see its benefits: much more energy for the day and you will feel better able to cope with stress and life's hassles.

1 Place a lit candle in front of a yoga mat (or similar) on the floor, then sit cross-legged with a straight spine and with your heels together to help maintain your concentration and slow your mind.

2 Consciously relax all your body muscles, working through from the top of your head to your toes. Slow your breathing down, inhaling and exhaling deeply from the diaphragm.

3 Now gaze at the candle's flame. After about 60 seconds close your eyes, but hold the flame's image in your mind for as long as you can to quieten your mind. Now start to meditate, focusing on just one thought. As other thoughts intrude, just let them drift by.

4 Towards the end of your meditation, start thinking positive thoughts about the day ahead. See yourself enjoying yourself and being successful at everything you attempt. Slowly open your eyes; you are now ready to face any challenge.

If you have a demanding day ahead, you may need some spiritual protection to help you cope. Everyone's bodies have a subtle spiritual energy field that surrounds them called the aura (see page 14). It has several layers and is filled with constantly changing colours that come from the light our bodies absorb. The aura also contains the seven main energy centres, known as the *chakras* (see page 15), that are situated from the groin area (the Root chakra) up to the top of the head (the Crown chakra). The aura reflects our emotional, mental and spiritual wellbeing, and its vibrational energies interact with our physical body, so they need refreshing regularly to stay healthy.

Energy tip

Hold a nurturing crystal, such as jasper, while you are doing this exercise.

The aura's vibrational energies need refreshing regularly to stay healthy.

REFRESH **your aura**

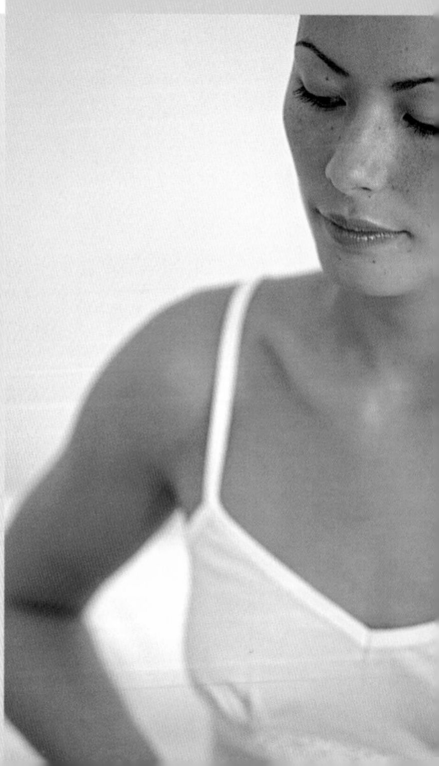

PROTECTING YOUR AURA

In addition to violet, white is another colour that links to the Crown chakra, our spiritual centre. Use it in this visualization exercise to fill your aura and protect it from daily negativity.

1. Sit cross-legged on a mat on the floor with a straight spine. Close your eyes and breathe deeply from your diaphragm.
2. Visualize a white light entering your Crown chakra on the top of your head; see it moving slowly through your body filling your organs and chakras until it reaches your feet. Sit for a few minutes and feel the warmth of this healing energy.
3. Now, see the white light expanding and forming a protective band around you. Feel its special power, then focus for a few minutes on your day ahead and slowly open your eyes. Repeat regularly to reinforce its powers.

Once out of bed in the morning, your body can feel it requires a kick-start to get its circulation moving and to galvanize the body organs into action. Essential oils (see pages 30–31) are absorbed through the nose; their scents stimulating or calming the senses. They can also be taken in through the skin's pores, from where they are carried into the bloodstream, and quickly affect how you are feeling. Using a fresh, tangy essential oil, such as lemon, in your morning shower will give you a welcome uplift: cleansing your body, clearing your sleepy mind and elevating your spirit.

Stimulating oils

- Citrus oils such as lemon, orange and bergamot are great tonics in the morning and are good skin cleansers to boot.
- Clary sage oil (avoid if you are pregnant) encourages creativity.
- Coriander oil brings inspiration.
- Spicy ginger oil boosts mental clarity.
- Pungent pine oil improves concentration.
- Tea tree oil both cleanses and energizes.

aroma CLEANSING

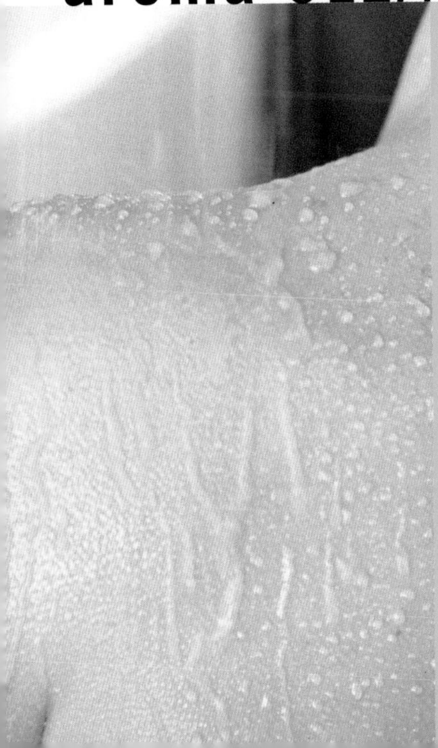

CREATING AN AROMATIC SHOWER

1 Mix 30–50 drops of your chosen oil in a 200–250 ml bottle of unscented shower gel; shake well. (Alternatively, mix 10 drops of your chosen oil in 15 ml of odourless vegetable oil. Dilute it half and half with water as you use it.

2 Run the shower until hot and steamy, step in and apply the gel direct to your body or pour some on a bath sponge and wash yourself.

3 Shower for about 5–10 minutes, allowing the aromatic scent of the oil to clear your head and inspire you for the day.

Shower power

Choose a stimulating essential oil from the list above to make your morning shower an especially invigorating experience.

Bringing fresh air into the home by opening windows in the early morning (and evening) is a wonderfully simple energizer to revitalize a home's atmosphere and release any stale energies from the previous evening. As the air pushes through, it takes with it moist kitchen or bathroom air, helping to avoid dampness and any fungal growth. If your air quality is low, it affects how you feel and can deplete your auric field (see page 14). So flush air through your home daily for instant purification and cleansing.

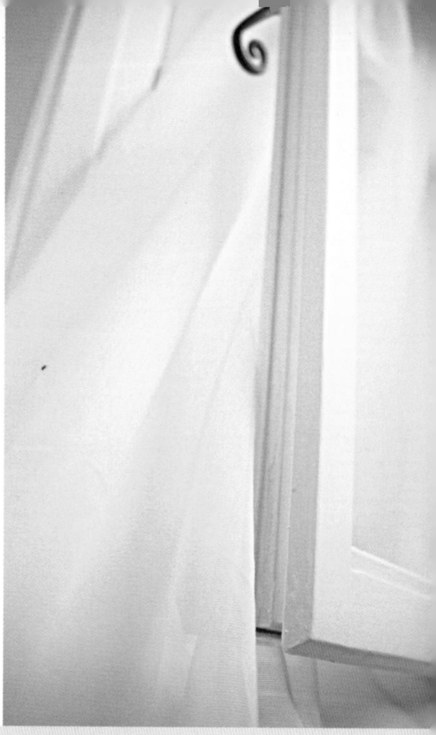

GREETING **the day**

Ionize your home

Improve the quality of the air in your home with an ionizer, particularly in rooms where there are televisions or computers. An ionizer removes detrimental airborne pollutants containing positive ions and creates a negative-ion-rich environment in which we thrive. The ionizer brings an air quality similar to that by the sea or in a forest.

LET IN THE FRESH AIR

Opening windows to allow air into your home can transform the atmosphere from stale and stagnant to fresh and inspiring in a matter of minutes.

1. Your home needs to breathe. So each morning open one window at the front and one at the back for 10 minutes to allow a through passage of air.
2. Stand by the open window in the front and feel it brushing over your skin. Breathe in the air, feeling how it wakes you up and invigorates your lungs. Silently connect with the 'Spirit of the Air' and thank it for entering your home and removing any negative vibrations.

Bringing fresh air into the home is a wonderfully simple energizer to revitalize its atmosphere.

Starting the day with a visualization exercise can reduce negative thinking and instil a new confidence in your capabilities. To make the most of the visualization first relax your body, which slows down your body organs and focuses your mind inwards, away from outside distractions. The visualization technique encourages 'right brain', more intuitive activity and the images that you will conjure up cancel out any destructive thoughts that the 'left brain', the ego or rational side, will try to engender.

Visualization tip

If you are finding it hard to visualize, practise first by seeing yourself on your last enjoyable holiday; savour all the images, losing yourself in the happy scenes.

Visualization can reduce negative thinking and instil a new confidence in your capabilities.

new day BEGINNINGS

A BRIGHT NEW DAY

Practise this visualization technique to create the day you want and to achieve your planned objectives.

1 Sit cross-legged on a mat on the floor. Take several deep breaths from your diaphragm and then consciously relax your muscles, working from the top of your head down to your feet.

2 As your body relaxes, visualize your ideal day. Don't worry if initially you find this hard, keep concentrating and the imagery will come.

3 Start visualizing what you want. If, for example, you are giving a work presentation, see yourself smoothly coordinating the visuals with your talk. See how confidently you answer any questions. Feel and sense your power as your colleagues listen to your talk. Hear the praise as it ends successfully. Or perhaps you are a parent worrying about hosting your toddler's birthday party. See yourself happily organizing the food, controlling the party games and having fun.

4 Stay with these images for about 10 minutes, then slowly open your eyes; you are now ready for a successful day.

The natural healing ability of herbs is well known: they are an excellent source of vitamins, minerals and amino acids and can encourage healing in the body on a deep physical level (see page 32–33). Some herbs have properties that calm and sedate the organs after a strenuous day, while others are better for getting you going in the morning, invigorating the body and cleansing the blood. Making a herbal or spice tea (infusion) when you get up takes a little time but your body reaps the benefits of absorbing more of the healing herbal properties.

Invigorating alternatives

Sage and rosemary both make refreshing teas. Infuse about 3 teaspoons of the fresh herb, or 1 teaspoon of the dried, in a teapot with the 2 cups of boiling water, as below. Leave for 10 minutes, strain and serve, adding the honey if needed.

'get up and go' TEA

GINGER AND LEMON TEA

A cup of this invigorating and fresh herbal tea benefits you from the properties of the ginger and the lemon. Ginger makes a fragrant, warming tea that promotes good blood flow, strengthens the respiratory system and boosts digestion. Meanwhile, the lemon offers you some antioxidant protection and provides vitamin C to increase your body's resistance to infection.

Ingredients

- 2 teaspoons fresh grated or dried ginger root
- 2 cups of boiling water
- 2–3 teaspoons fresh lemon juice
- 1–2 teaspoons fresh honey (optional)

Making the tea

1. Place the ginger in a china or glass teapot and add the boiling water. (Always make the tea in a non-metal teapot as metal can adversely affect the flavour of the herbs.)
2. Steep for 10 minutes, strain into a cup and then add the lemon, and honey if preferred.

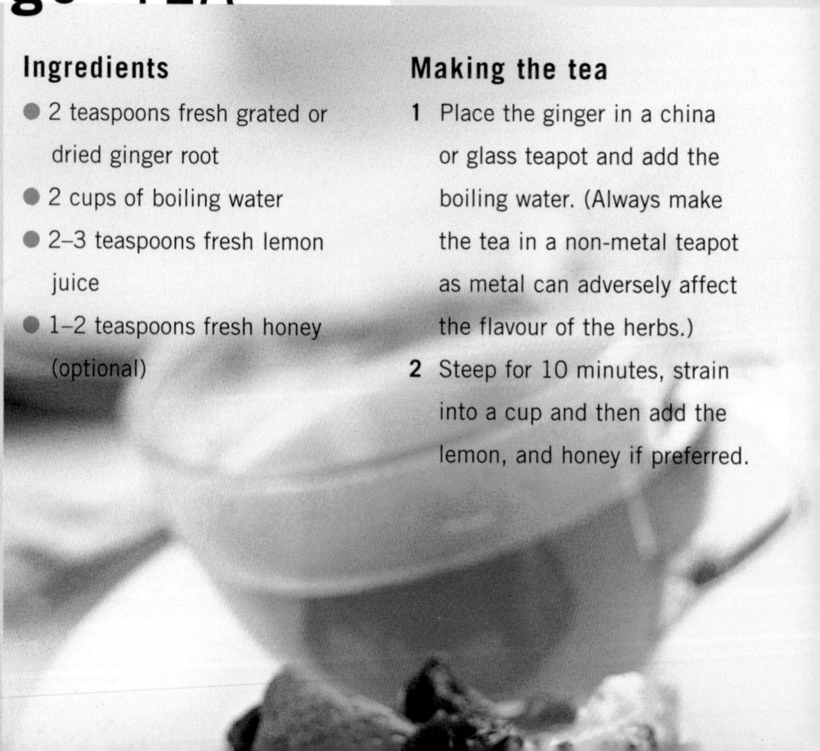

the power of POSITIVITY

Beginning your day with a positive affirmation to suit your forthcoming challenges will surround you with creative energies. You may want to boost your self-esteem, deal with a work situation or overcome a niggling problem at home. Compose your own affirmations with words that really mean something, as they reflect what your mind truly feels. By constantly repeating your affirmation in your head, you embed that thought deep within your subconscious so that eventually it becomes reality.

Choose your affirmation to suit your day.

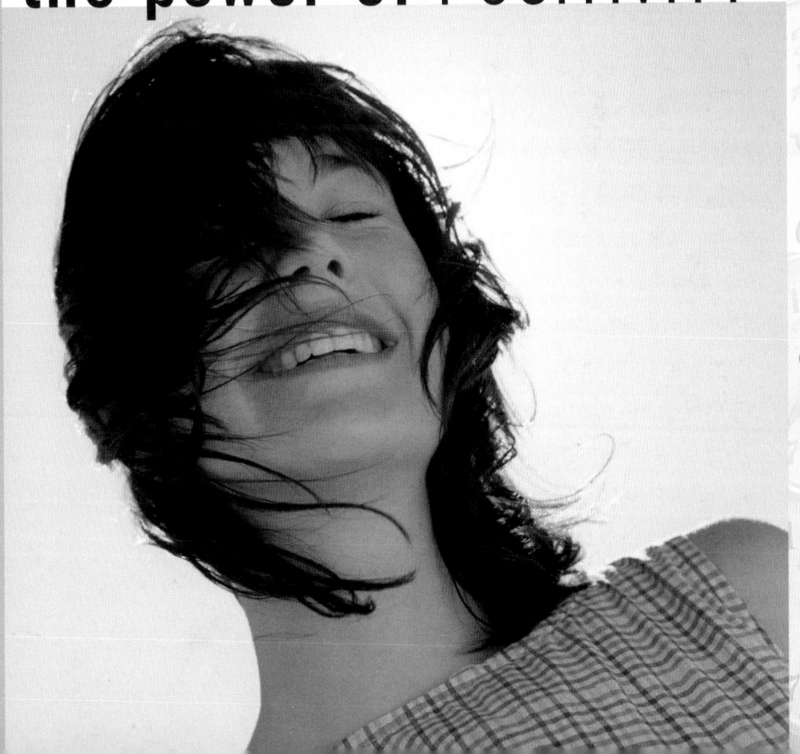

NEW DAY AFFIRMATION

Choose your affirmation to suit your day. Always use the present tense (or it won't work) and make sure your words support your aims. Write it down and say it aloud to enforce it.

1. Sit in a comfortable place or go for an early morning walk. Keep your affirmation short so that you can remember it.
2. Think of your affirmation, if it relates to self-esteem issues it may be something like: 'I love myself just as I am'; or maybe for a work situation: 'I am capable of communicating well with my colleagues'; or for a problem at home: 'I can resolve my conflict with the decorators'. Repeat your phrase 10–20 times to fix it in your subconscious.
3. Repeat the phrase throughout the morning as other negative emotions intrude.

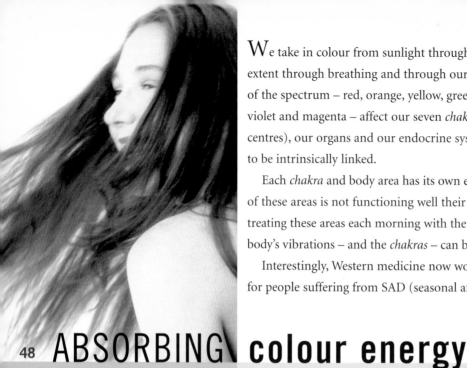

ABSORBING colour energy

We take in colour from sunlight through our eyes, and to a lesser extent through breathing and through our skin. The eight colours of the spectrum – red, orange, yellow, green, turquoise blue, indigo, violet and magenta – affect our seven *chakras* (our spiritual energy centres), our organs and our endocrine system, which are all believed to be intrinsically linked.

Each *chakra* and body area has its own energy vibration. When any of these areas is not functioning well their vibration weakens. By treating these areas each morning with the colours they respond to, the body's vibrations – and the *chakras* – can be brought back in balance.

Interestingly, Western medicine now works with light and colour for people suffering from SAD (seasonal affective disorder).

Other ways to take in colour

You can also absorb colour from food. For example, indigo food such as blueberries, damsons or olives can be eaten to aid sleep and soothe an over-stimulated brain. Yellow food such as bananas, grapefruit and melons can boost the digestive system and reduce stomach problems.

Absorbing colour

Colour therapy (or chromotherapy) was first researched in the 1930s by the American scientist Dinshah P. Ghadiali. He discovered that the various colour vibrations our bodies receive from sunlight boost the functioning of organs, glands and emotions.

Both the physical body and its spiritual energy field (the aura) are part of the process, receiving and 'selecting' colour for the body. Ghadiali found that specific colours could help heal sick body parts. Turquoise blue, for instance, when held near or placed on the skin, helps resolve problems of the throat and lungs, improves functioning of the thyroid glands and encourages clear self-expression.

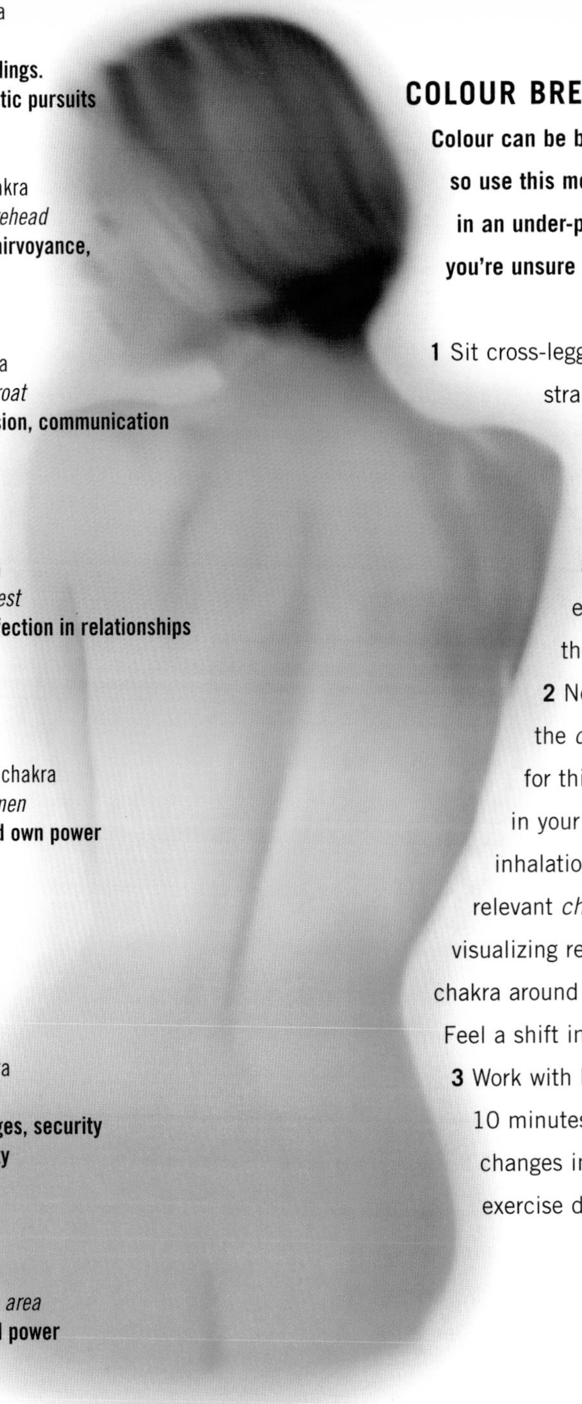

Crown chakra
Top of head
Spiritual feelings. Love of artistic pursuits

Third eye chakra
Middle of forehead
Intuition, clairvoyance, self respect

Throat chakra
Middle of throat
Self-expression, communication

Heart chakra
Centre of chest
Love and affection in relationships

Solar plexus chakra
Upper abdomen
Intellect and own power

Sacral chakra
Pelvic area
Creative urges, security and sexuality

Root chakra
Lower pelvic area
Survival and power

COLOUR BREATHING ENERGIZER

Colour can be breathed into the body through the air, so use this morning exercise to increase the energy in an under-performing *chakra*. Check the chart if you're unsure which colour you need.

1 Sit cross-legged on a mat on the floor with a straight spine, keeping your shoulders down and back and your chest open. Do about five practice breaths, drawing the air in through your nose and down to your diaphragm. Hold each breath for about two seconds and then exhale slowly to a count of four.

2 Now close your eyes and meditate on the *chakra* colour that your body needs for this morning. When you see the colour in your mind, breathe it in on your next inhalation, and as you exhale, see it filling the relevant *chakra* area. For example, if you are visualizing red, see it flooding through your Root chakra around the top of your legs and pelvic area. Feel a shift in your energy as the blockage clears.

3 Work with breathing in this colour for around 10 minutes, and then sit quietly feeling any changes in your emotions or feelings. Do this exercise daily to correct *chakra* imbalances.

Yoga is a wonderful movement discipline that originated in India. In Sanskrit the word 'yoga' means the union of mind and body. Hatha yoga is one of the physical forms and consists of a series of postures or *asanas* that help purify the body and mind. According to yoga teachings all bodily functions are controlled by an energy called *prana* (see page 11) that flows through channels called *nadis*. When you practise hatha yoga, prana moves positively through the body, clearing away toxins and promoting wellbeing.

Try out these simple yoga postures for 5–10 minutes in the early morning to increase the functioning of your body's organs, glands and nervous system. The postures also tone your muscles, increase your vitality and discipline your mind.

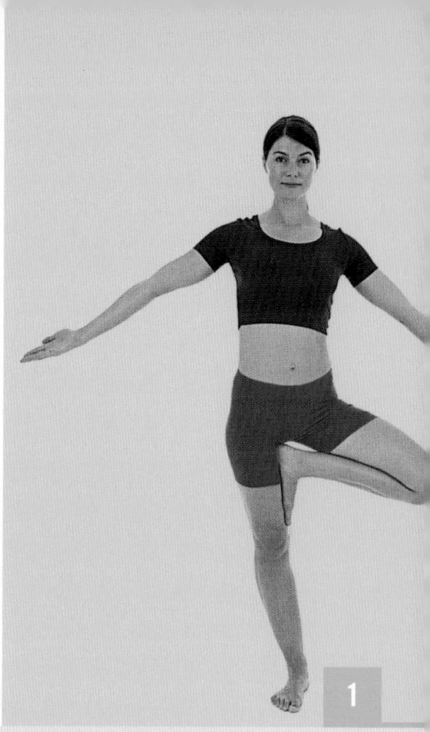
1

pre-breakfast YOGA

THE COBRA

This lying posture strengthens and tones the lower back, tightens the buttocks and boosts thyroid and adrenal gland function.

1. Breathe steadily while lying on your front on a mat on the floor, with your feet together. Place your palms under your shoulders next to your ribcage. Stretch your toes and point your chin towards the floor.
2. Inhale and lift your head off the floor, pushing up with your arms so that you look ahead. Keep your hip bones on the floor, breathe steadily and hold the position for about 10 seconds. As you exhale, lower yourself to the floor and return to Step 1. Repeat the movement.
3. Now, from Step 1, place your hands under your chest, this time with the palms facing inwards, and point your elbows outwards.
4. Inhale and pushing down lift your body off the floor. Look up, but keep your shoulders down and your hips just off the floor. Breathe steadily and hold for about 10 seconds. Exhale, then slowly lower yourself down. Perform 3–4 times.

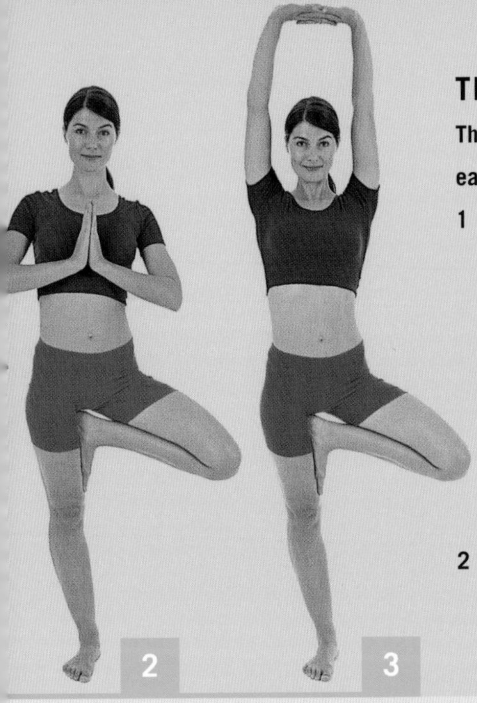
2
3

THE TREE

This standing posture teaches you to balance, focusing your mind in the early morning and connecting your physical and mental energies.

1 Stand up straight and take 10 deep breaths from your diaphragm. Breathing steadily, balance on your right leg, then place the sole of your left foot on your inner right thigh. Push your right hip out, keeping your hips square.

2 Look straight ahead, concentrating on the wall in front of you. Don't worry if you wobble, just grip firmly with your foot. When steady, put your palms together and hold.

3 Now stretch your arms above your head, clasping your fingers and hold for about 5 seconds. Feel the energy move from your feet up to your fingertips. Slide your right leg down, repeat on the other side. Perform twice on each side.

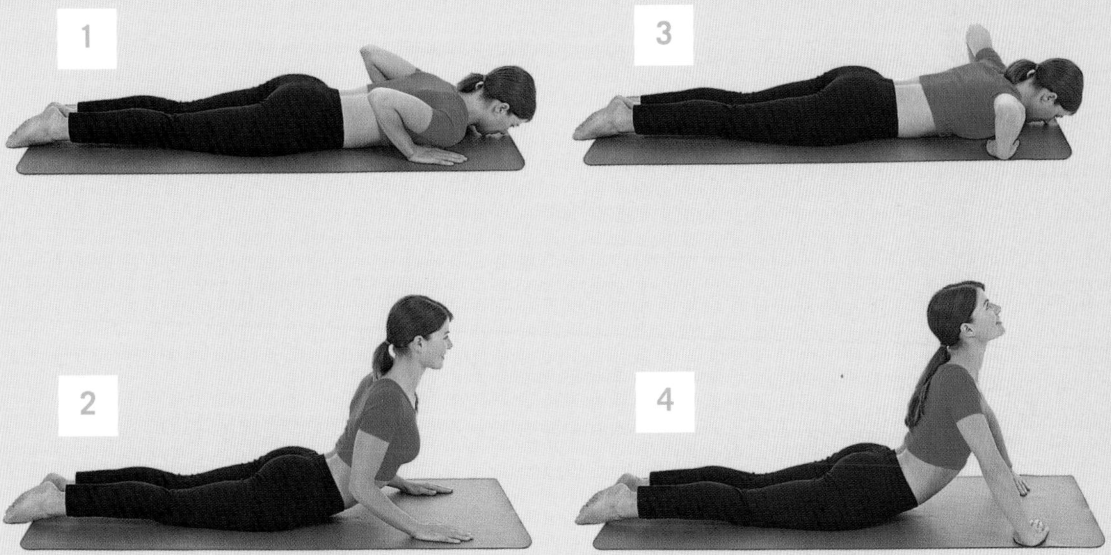
1
3
2
4

Saying a mantra out loud can energize your mind, body and spirit. In this meditative technique Sanskrit (ancient Indian) words are chanted repeatedly to focus the mind.

Chanting a mantra creates a sound vibration that harmonizes the body and mind. Saying the chosen phrase over and over removes outer distractions, connecting you with your inner wisdom. It also benefits your body, working your respiratory system and promoting increased blood circulation and waste removal.

Choosing mantras

Chant one of these mantras or find another that resonates with you.

- ***Om dum durgayei namaha*** – Greetings to the female energy that protects us from negativity.
- ***Om gum ganapatayei namaha*** – Greetings to the person who removes obstacles.
- ***Om namah shivaya*** – No direct translation, but means: Greetings to the person I am capable of becoming.

MORNING **mantra**

MANTRA FOR A POSITIVE OUTLOOK

Chant this morning mantra regularly and see the beneficial changes in your mind and body.

1 Sit in the meditation position and relax your muscles (see page 41). Set your intent for the day.

2 Choose your chant (see box above). You can start with a well-known one such as '*Om mani padme hum*' (hail the jewel in the lotus), often shortened to '*Om*'. You could use a word such as 'Peace', but chanting in another language is preferable as our words have many associations.

3 Close your eyes and chant your word establishing a rhythm as you do so and feeling a growing sense of peace. Chant for 5–10 minutes, then slowly open your eyes and become aware of where you are. You're now ready for anything.

Saying a mantra out loud can energize your mind, body and spirit.

Chanting a mantra creates a sound vibration that harmonizes the body and mind.

If you lack energy in the morning, use this simple acupressure routine to perk you up first thing. Acupressure is an ancient Chinese healing therapy that uses finger and thumb pressure on acupuncture points on the body to stimulate the flow of *chi* (energy) through 14 main channels or meridians. Working on the points removes blockages and encourages the flow of sluggish energy. It differs from reflexology (see pages 64–65), which follows the recent concept of zones, rather than meridians. Allied to shiatsu, the Japanese pressure therapy, acupressure is ideal for self-treating as it is easy to learn.

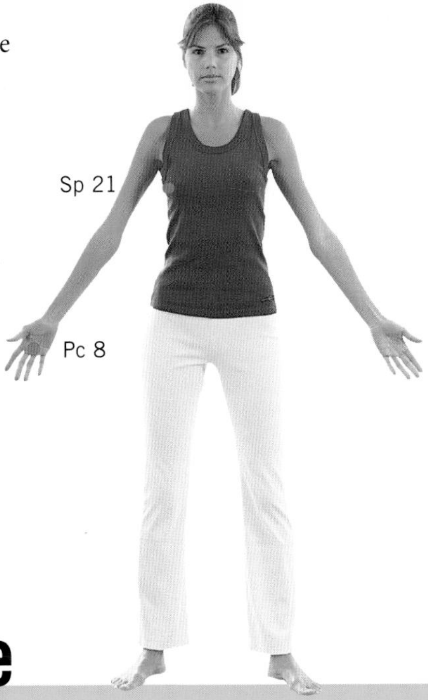
Sp 21
Pc 8

AWAKENING **acupressure**

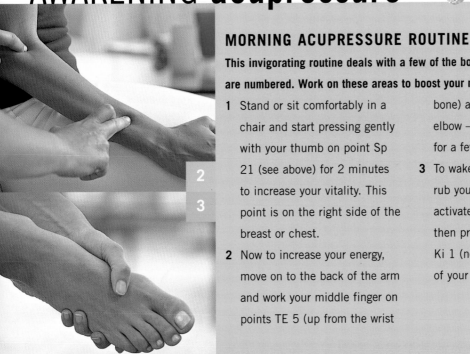
2

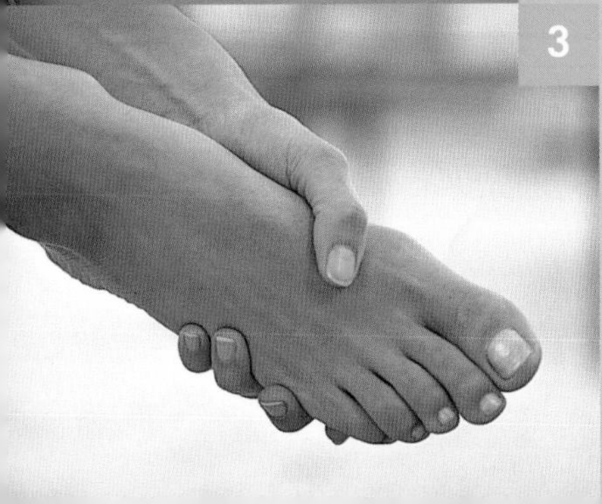
3

MORNING ACUPRESSURE ROUTINE

This invigorating routine deals with a few of the body points, all of which are numbered. Work on these areas to boost your morning energy levels.

1 Stand or sit comfortably in a chair and start pressing gently with your thumb on point Sp 21 (see above) for 2 minutes to increase your vitality. This point is on the right side of the breast or chest.

2 Now to increase your energy, move on to the back of the arm and work your middle finger on points TE 5 (up from the wrist bone) and LI 11 (middle of elbow – see also pages 12–13) for a few minutes.

3 To wake you up completely, rub your palms together to activate Pc 8 (see above) and then press them briefly on Ki 1 (not shown) on the soles of your bare feet.

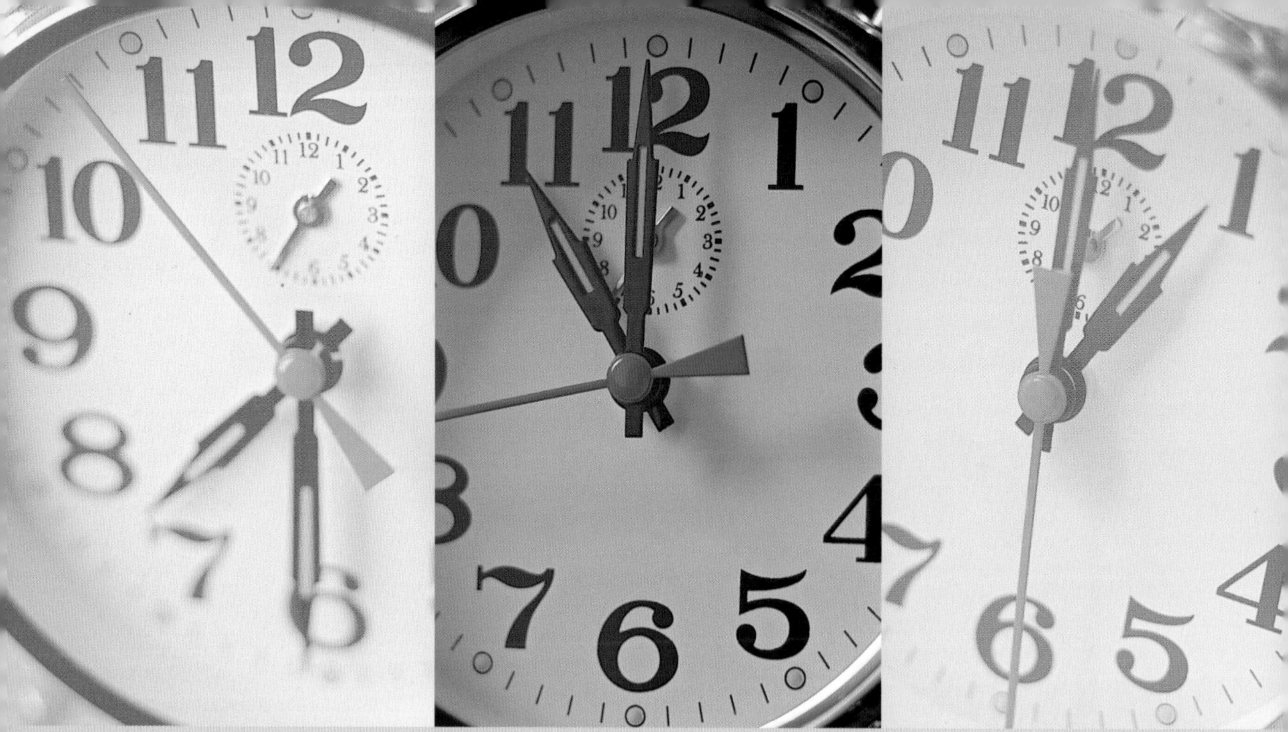

6 Mid-morning stress relief

Spend some time refreshing your body's energy levels and see how much more you are now capable of achieving by lunchtime.

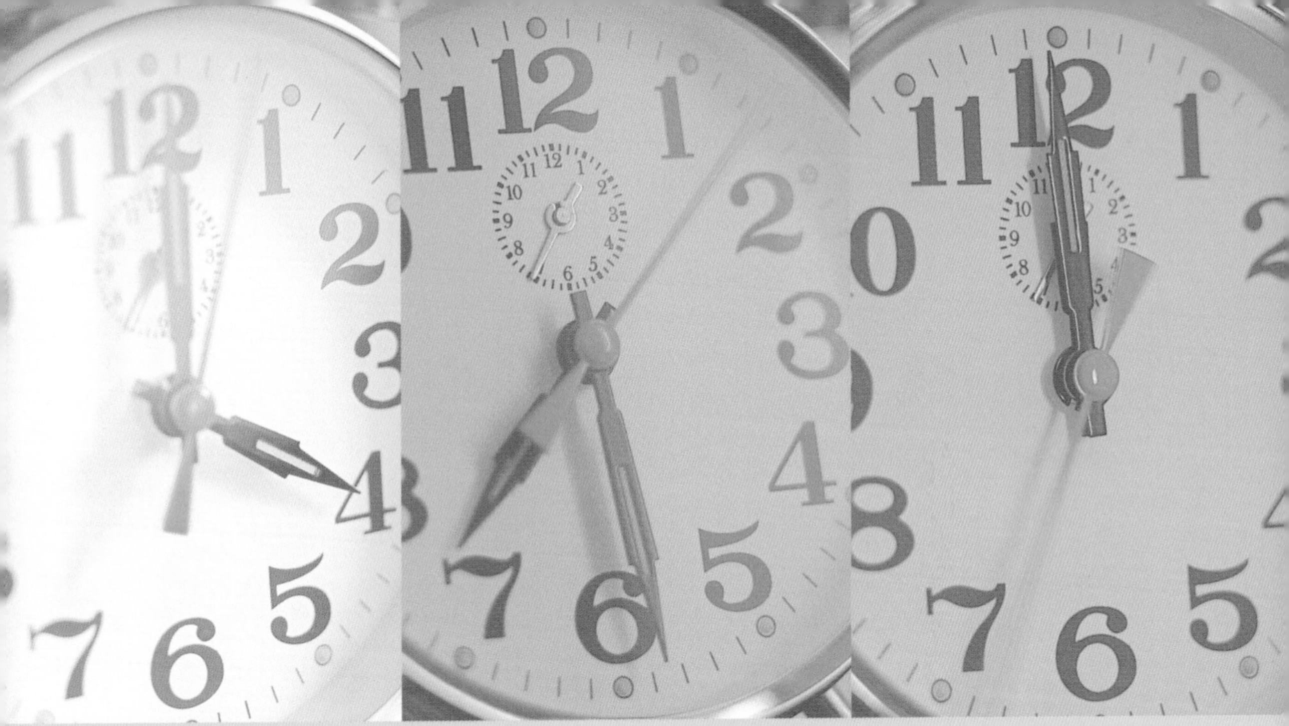

Mid-morning can bring a feeling of satisfaction for all the tasks you have already completed, but it can also bring some anxiety about what else you need to do for the rest of the day. Your physical energy levels may be dropping while your mind may still be 'buzzing' with your long 'to do' list.

This is an important time of day to stay in control and systematically plan the jobs to do next. Inevitably some stress is involved when you are busy, so aim to minimize it. The holistic energizers in this section can give you that physical and emotional boost. You can stimulate your senses with inspiring essential oils, drink a soothing herbal tea to balance your nerves, massage your temples and neck to ease tense and aching muscles or use a visualization technique to remove an energy block that is holding you back.

These energizers can be completed in a short break or a lull between tasks. Spend some time refreshing your body's energy levels and see how much more you are now capable of achieving by lunchtime.

If you are having a busy morning, you may be feeling the pressure and in need of a quick energy boost. Rather than reaching for a cup of coffee, try this aromatherapy boost. Essential oils (see page 30–31) enter our bodies via our nose and sense of smell, so they can have an immediate and beneficial effect on our emotions. Keep some invigorating oils to hand so that you have an easy stress-relief remedy that will increase your concentration mid-morning, leaving you to carry on with renewed enthusiasm.

Rather than reaching for a cup of coffee, try this aromatherapy boost.

Aromatherapy tip

If you plan to use essential oils regularly, it is a good idea to buy a plug-in electric burner that can be cleaned after use.

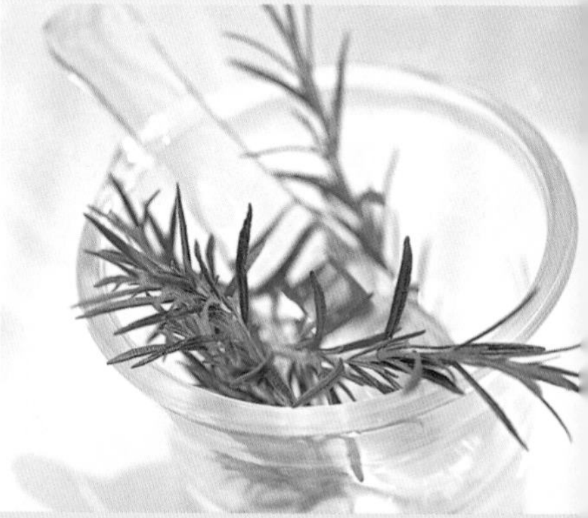

stimulating THE SENSES

AROMATIC UPLIFT

Try out the different oils listed below to see which aromas appeal to your senses, increasing your energy and giving you mental clarity.

Reviving oils

Tangy citrus oils, such as lemon, orange and bergamot, are refreshing and clarify your thoughts.

- Rosemary is revitalizing and balances the emotions.
- Lemongrass oil acts as a refreshing tonic.
- Frankincense soothes the nervous system and is spiritually uplifting.
- Sandalwood calms and reduces stress.

1. Put 4–5 drops of oil on a paper tissue or handkerchief. Hold the tissue to your nose and breathe in deeply for about a couple of minutes; feel the oil's instant effects.
2. Leave the tissue on your desk or kitchen table so that you can continue to inhale its aromas. Renew the oil hourly or as needed.
3. Alternatively, put the oil in a bowl of hot water and inhale deeply.

Lavender oil is a cure-all essential oil that can bring instant relief when applied to tense areas.

Aromatherapy tip

As an alternative to lavender, mix 2 drops of peppermint oil in 2 teaspoons of sweet almond base oil before applying.

When you are under pressure and working hard trying to keep everything running smoothly, tension from tight blood vessels in your head can build up, causing a throbbing headache in your temples. This can occur, for example, when you are looking after noisy children, or if you work in bad lighting conditions or spend too long in front of a computer. Lavender oil is a cure-all essential oil that can bring instant relief when applied to these tense areas. It induces calm and rebalances your emotions and energy, increasing *chi* flow to your Crown chakra – the spiritual energy centre (see page 15).

TENSION **relief**

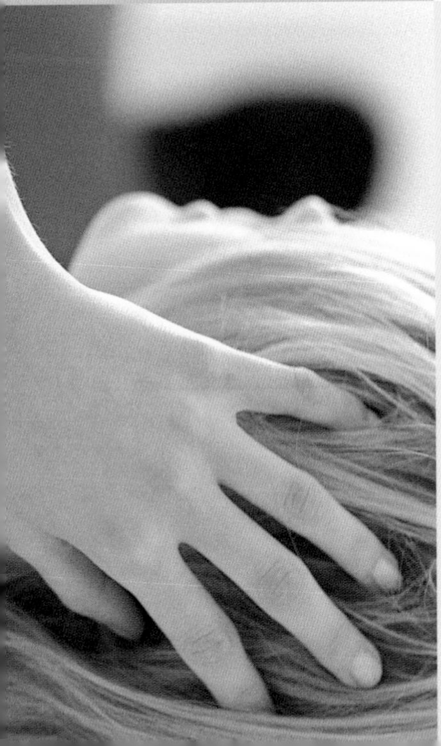

HEADACHE EASER

Take a few minutes away from your busy day to do this soothing routine. Use lavender essential oil and work it well in to your temples to relieve pain or any energy blocks in the temples.

1 Sit comfortably in a chair and put a few drops of lavender oil on your fingertips; lavender is one of the few oils that can be applied to the skin undiluted.

2 Rub the oil in a circular movement around your temples and along your forehead for a few minutes until the pain or tension eases.

Sipping a calming cup of herbal tea mid-morning can help you cope with a crisis, relieve your jagged nerves and balance your falling energy levels. Herbal teas are a healthier alternative to normal tea, which contains tannin and caffeine. The ingredients of some herbs (see pages 32–33 and 46) have the ability to act as a tonic and relieve irritability, nervous stomach cramps and anxiety. Making a tea from a fresh herb will give you the full benefit of its herbal properties, but if this is not possible use the dried herb or a herbal tea bag instead.

Calming alternatives

- Lemon balm helps to calm the nervous system. It has relaxant and antispasmodic properties and can help irritability and restlessness.
- Gingko biloba is a herbal stimulant and tonic that relieves headaches, improves blood and cerebral circulation, increasing short-term memory. Use it in tea bag form.

fortifying TEA

PEPPERMINT TEA

Peppermint makes a soothing tea that can boost your brain power, relieve headaches and clarify your thoughts. Its powerful menthol component can also help relax muscle tension or cramps in the stomach caused by stress. Drink this calming tea for added strength during the morning.

Ingredients

- 3 teaspoons of fresh peppermint or 1 teaspoon of dried peppermint
- 2 cups of boiling water

Making the tea

1. Place the peppermint in a china or glass teapot and add the boiling water.
2. Steep for 10 minutes, then strain and serve.

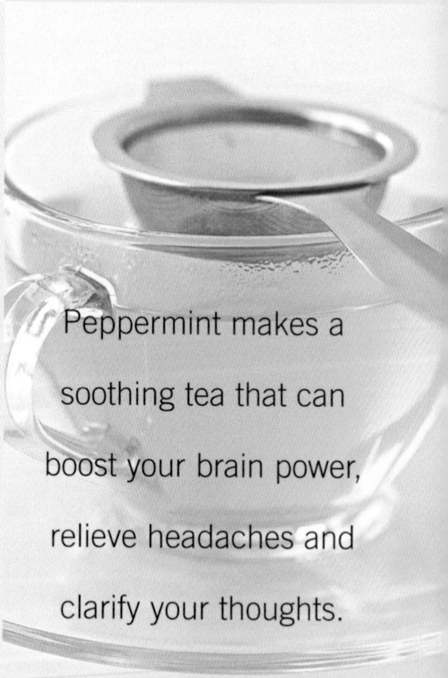
Peppermint makes a soothing tea that can boost your brain power, relieve headaches and clarify your thoughts.

MIRROR **power**

Energetically, mirrors are believed to have great powers; in fact, in ancient times it was only people such as pharaohs and kings who were allowed to use them. In feng shui terms they are believed to double the positive energy of the space in which they are placed. So to instil some positive vibrations in your psyche to enhance the morning's successes (perhaps completing a project) or over-ride any failures (possibly arguing with your partner), say a carefully chosen, upbeat phrase while looking straight in the mirror. You are supposed to see your spiritual self in a mirror, so get in touch with your subconscious as you speak and feel your personal power increasing.

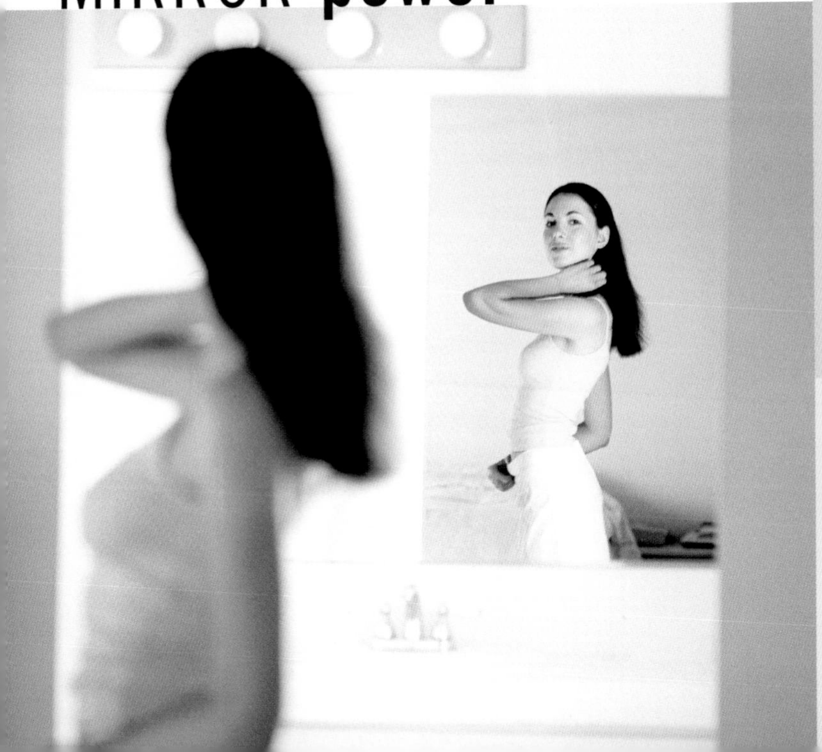

MIRROR WORK

Choose your phrase, then spend several minutes saying it in front of a mirror in the ladies' or men's room at work, in your work space or at home.

1 Take a few deep breaths to calm you, then look straight into your mirror and focus inwards. Connect with your spiritual image as you start saying your phrase out loud. It may be: 'My day continues well, I feel successful in everything I do', 'I am resolving this morning's problems' or 'I am a wonderful person, I can achieve anything'.

2 Repeat the phrase 10–20 times and feel a surge of spiritual vitality as you rebalance your energetic field.

Energy tip

Take 4 drops of Elm Bach flower remedy (see page 28) on your tongue or mix in water and drink for extra confidence as you say your phrase.

In times of stress a series of reactions is triggered in your body. As you panic the hypothalamus gland (your stress control centre) sets off a chemical chain reaction, triggering the release of the hormones adrenaline and noradrenaline, then cortisol into your bloodstream, activating all organs and cells. Your breathing becomes shallower, your heart races and your blood pressure rises, increasing blood circulation to the brain for quick thinking. You are now ready for action – to 'fight' or, conversely 'flee'. If this fight or flight response is followed by physical activity, this energy surge is used up and your body normalizes. But if you can't switch off, and still worry, you keep excess hormones in the body, putting pressure on your organs. By regulating your breathing you release pent-up tension and create inner harmony.

Stress-relieving tips

- Do some deep breathing for a few minutes to calm you down.
- If you are feeling a bit out of control, put 4 drops of Bach flower Rescue remedy on your tongue to relieve your anxiety.
- Spray Bush flower Emergency essence into the atmosphere to calm any panicky feelings you are experiencing.

BREATHING OUT **stress**

LETTING GO OF STRESS

When you know your body is under stress, take a few minutes to do this easy breathing exercise to ease your overworked organs.

1 Sit cross-legged on the floor with a straight spine and both feet flat on the floor. Keep your head in line with your neck and back. Focus on your abdomen and breathe in as you take your arms out to the side.

2 As you continue to breathe in and fill your lungs, lift your arms high above your head and look upwards.

3 Intertwine your fingers and continue stretching your arms. Breathe out forcefully, tilting your head back as you release all your stress and let your arms drop back down to your side. Repeat 5–10 times filling your lungs more deeply to clear all tension and re-energize your body.

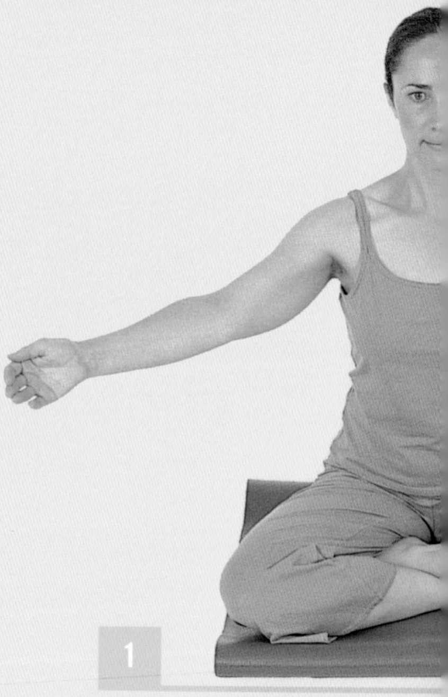

1

- Hold an aventurine crystal in your hands for about 10 minutes to balance your nervous system and blood pressure. Or use a tourmaline crystal to eliminate negative energy and strengthen your nervous system.

You can bring any morning stress symptoms under control with this simple breathing exercise.

By regulating your breathing you release pent-up tension and create inner harmony.

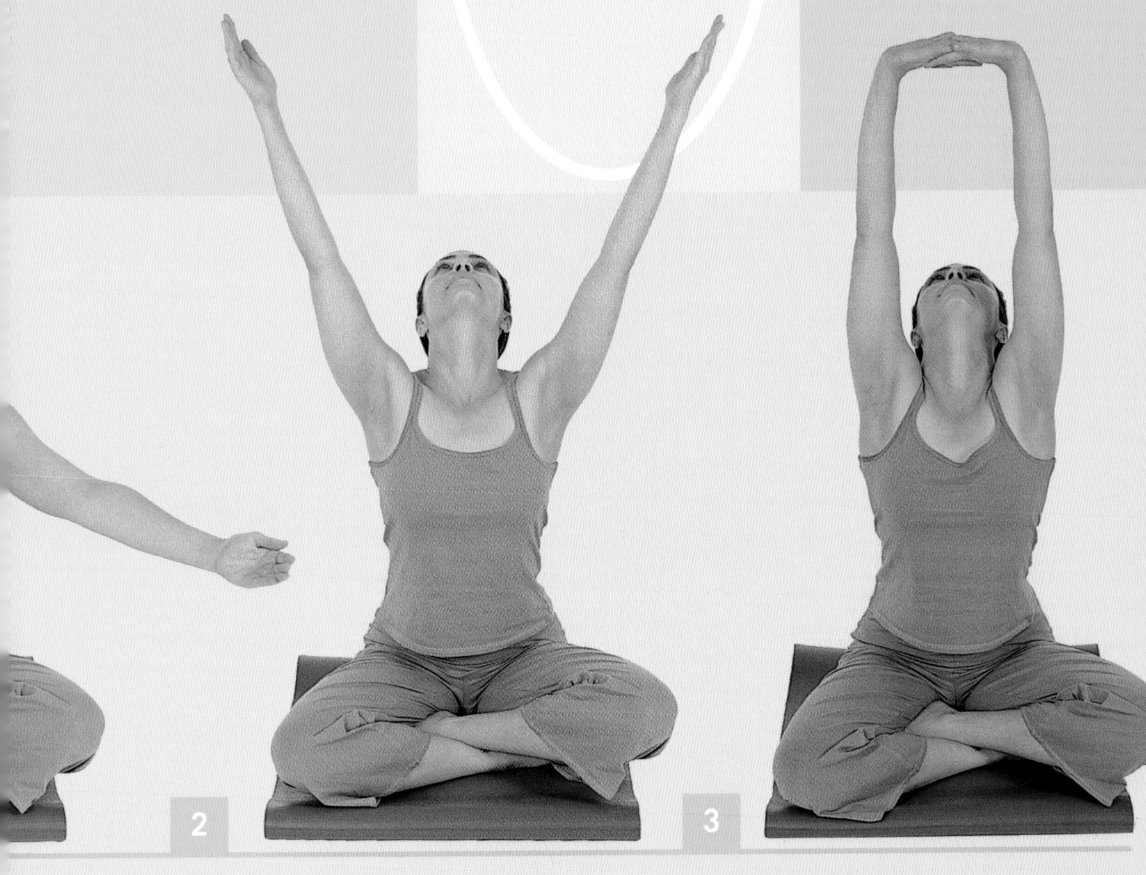
2
3

LETTING GO OF **anger**

If your morning is not going well and you are still seething or feeling very irritated after an argument with a colleague at work or because of an incident at home, take some time out to work on yourself. Anger is normal; it is a powerful agent of self-assertion and self-respect but it can become destructive if you are often having angry outbursts at the expense of other people. You may be projecting internal anger onto them because you are not handling your own stress well.

Suppressed anger is held as an energy blockage in the Solar plexus chakra (see page 15) in the abdomen. The blame and frustration here can be felt as a tight band in the stomach.

Working consistently on releasing this pent-up anger will bring balance to this chakra, letting you deal with any challenging occasions.

Working consistently on releasing this pent-up anger will bring balance to the solar plexus chakra.

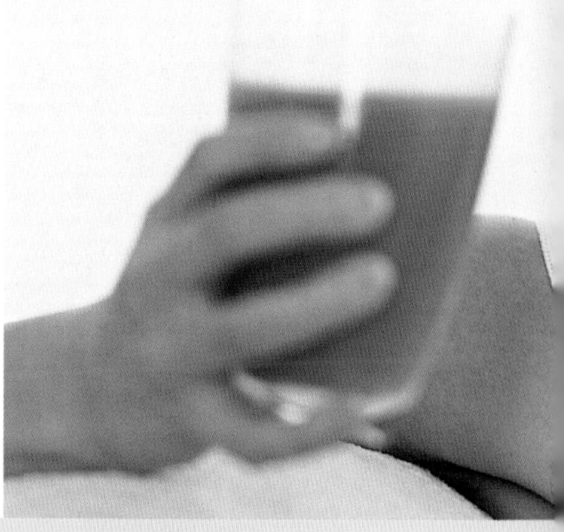

ANGER RELEASE

This exercise can be done during a brief break at work or sitting in a chair at home. Work for several minutes, ideally 5–10 minutes, on the Solar plexus chakra until you can feel less tension in your stomach.

1 Sit comfortably on a chair with a straight spine. Close your eyes, if you can, and take a few deep breaths from your diaphragm.

2 Take your mind to your Solar plexus chakra, just below your breastbone in your stomach. See your anger there as a large, tight ball. Feel the anger, recent and longer-term, the hurt or pain; don't resist the feelings, let them flood your body.

3 Now focus on the ball and see it becoming smaller, and sense your anger diminishing and your stomach relaxing. Instil some feelings of empowerment in the *chakra* as you slowly come to. Do this exercise whenever you are losing emotional control. To cleanse sustained anger, do this exercise often until the ball completely disappears.

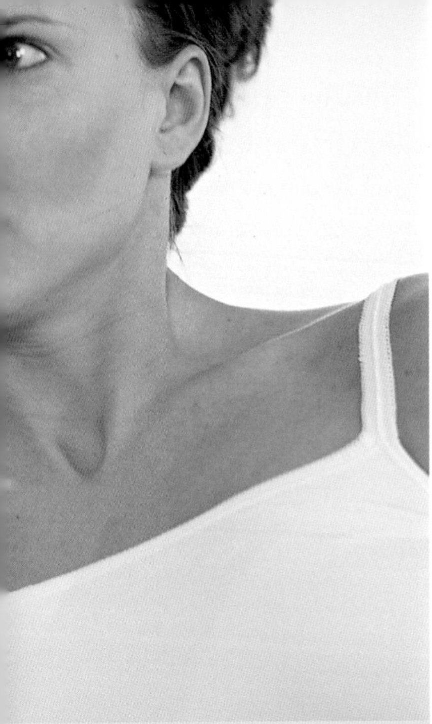

STRESS AND ANGER REMEDIES

Use the following Bach, Bush, essential oil and crystal remedies (see pages 28–35) for anger control, and to help lower your stress levels.

Remedy	Emotion	How to use
Bach flower		
Hornbeam	Mental exhaustion	See page 29
Olive	Exhaustion with little strength or energy	See page 29
Willow	Irritable and wallowing in self-pity	See page 29
Bush flower		
Alpine mint bush	Mentally and emotionally drained	See page 29
Crowea	Emotionally out of balance	See page 29
Essential oils		
Bergamot	Feeling stressed out	Put a few drops in an oil burner or use on a tissue
Neroli	Stressed and anxious	As above
Rosewood	Angry and irritable	As above
Crystals		
Agate	Bitterness and inner anger	Hold crystal in hands for 5 minutes and ask for cleansing
Beryl	Stressed and lacking courage	Place on Solar Plexus chakra and draw in healing energies for 5 minutes
Bloodstone	Feeling toxic and lacking energy	As Agate
Cat's eye	Feeling negative and lacking confidence	As Beryl

Energy tip

Put a few drops of Bach flower Rescue remedy in a small mister bottle (available from chemists) and spray around your work or home area after a disturbance to harmonize the atmosphere.

You may be projecting internal anger onto people because you are not handling your own stress.

reviving REFLEXOLOGY

Performing a short reflexology routine on your hands or feet in the middle of the morning can work wonders for flagging energy levels as well as alleviating any taut muscles in your shoulders and back.

This ancient therapy was first introduced into Britain in the late 1960s. Also known as zone therapy, reflexology is a treatment where pressure is applied to points and nerve endings on the feet and hands to encourage healing and good energy flow. As in acupuncture, the points are linked by ten 'reflex' zones to muscles and organs in the body, so that when stimulated the entire zone benefits. By massaging different points you can clear energy blockages and improve overall health. Ideally, take a break to do the reflexology, but if this is not possible you can work on a foot with one hand while still working.

INVIGORATING REFLEXOLOGY ROUTINE

Increase your energy flow and release the tension from your shoulders and back by spending a few minutes stimulating the points described below. Use both your hands and your feet to activate the relevant points.

A short reflexology routine can work wonders for flagging energy levels.

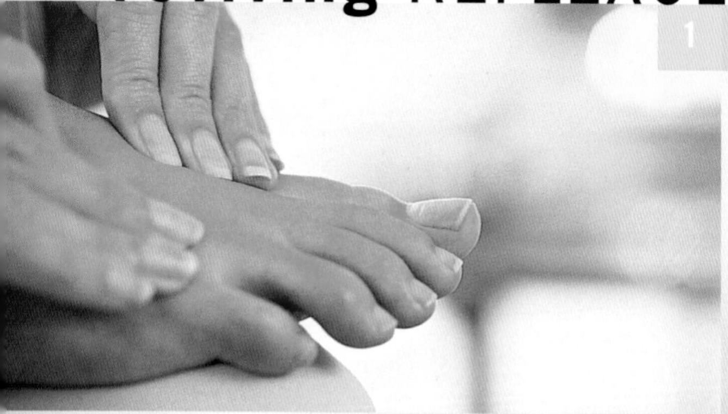
1

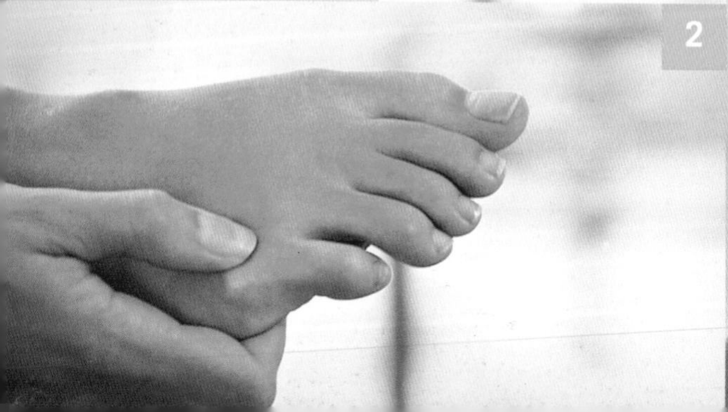
2

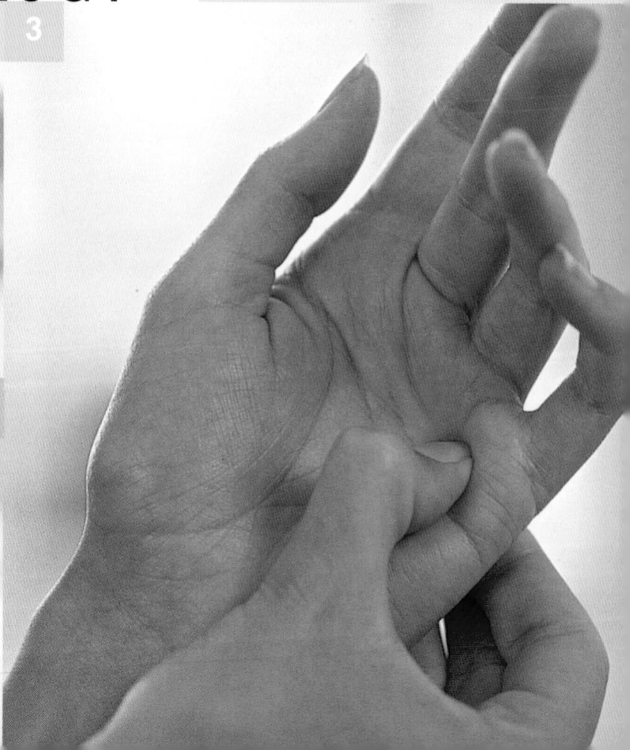
3

1 To release the stiffness in aching shoulders, press and knead the fingers of both hands across both the top and the sole of each foot, about 25 mm (1 in) from the toes.

2 Pinch, press and gently rotate your thumb to the count of five on the shoulder point, which is located between the base of the fourth and the fifth toes.

3 Alternatively, work your hand between the bases of the fourth and the fifth fingers.

4 To get the energy flowing, finger-walk your thumb or finger down the spine area, which is the bony ridge of your hand from the side of your thumb down to the wrist.

5 To ease aching back muscles use four fingers to knead or finger-walk horizontally along the bony ridge of your hand, pressing slightly harder on any sore areas. Finish with some soothing strokes down the hand over the spinal area.

Reflexology techniques

Most reflexology points are worked on with the fingertips and the edge of the thumb.

- **Thumb- and finger-walking** – Flex your thumb or finger as you slide it forwards in a similar movement to that of a caterpillar.
- **Rotating on a point** – Keep either your thumb or your index finger on one point and rotate it slightly to activate the point.

4

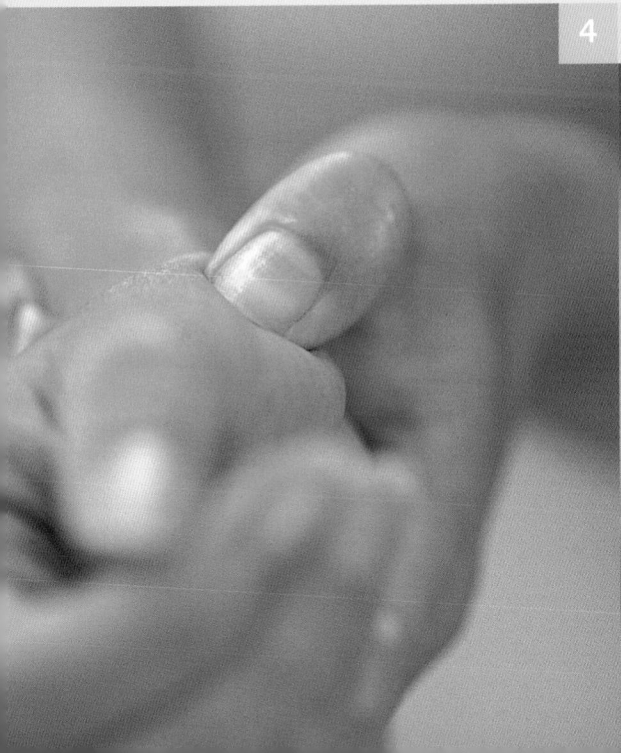

5

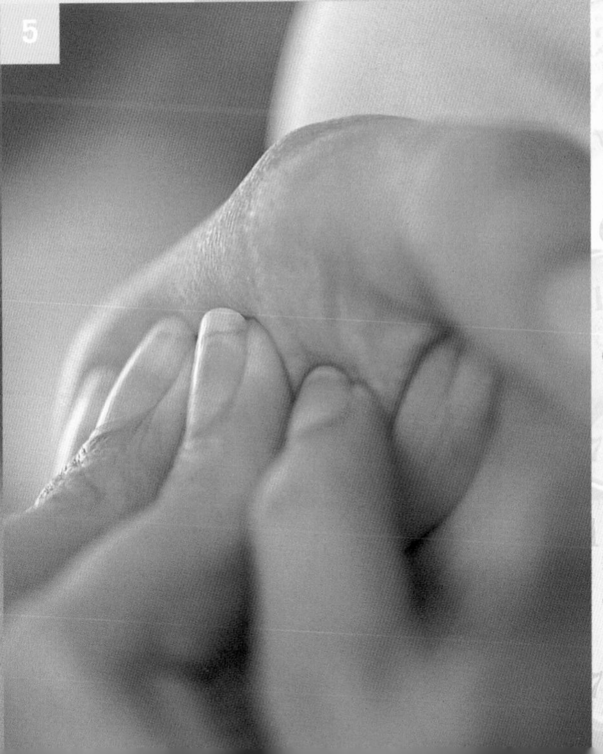

Mid-morning can seem quite late in the day if you have started work at a breakfast meeting or if you have been busy with children since the early hours. You may be feeling down and not quite right. You can sense that your energy is depleted and that a certain part of your body is causing the problem, but you don't know exactly where. You may even feel a bit shaky or queasy. These sensations are often an emotional imbalance causing an energy block in your body (see the *chakras* page 15).

Use the following exercise to discover the location of your blockage so that you can treat it with healing energy and continue your day with renewed vigour.

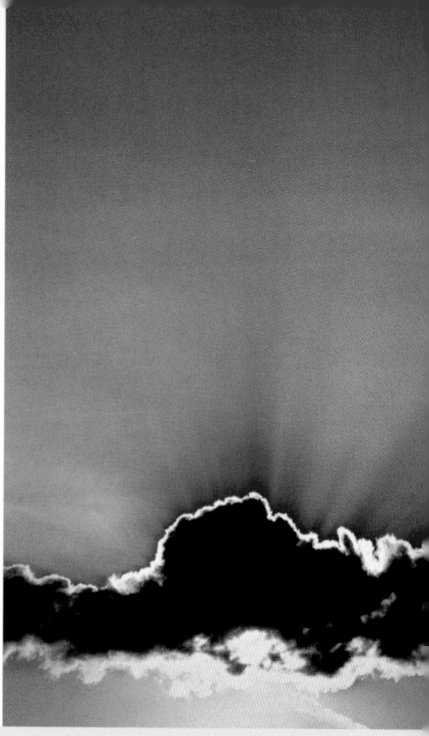

FREE-FLOWING **energy**

REMOVING ENERGY BLOCKS

After scanning your energy field (see opposite), try this visualization for about 5 minutes or so when you have a quiet moment at work or at home.

1 Sit comfortably in a chair with a straight spine. Close you eyes and breathe deeply from your diaphragm to calm you.

2 As your breathing slows, imagine yourself sitting in a field in mid-summer, the sky is completely blue but there is one dark cloud obscuring the sun. Now see this same imagery inside your body with the dark cloud being your blockage in your throat or stomach, for example.

3 Slowly see the dark cloud getting smaller and smaller as the sun starts to break through, feel its warmth as it breaks up the last pieces of the cloud, removing your blockage. Now let your whole body be filled with the healing yellow light. Sense your body relaxing as your energy starts flowing well again. Come to, energized and ready to tackle anything the rest of the day throws at you.

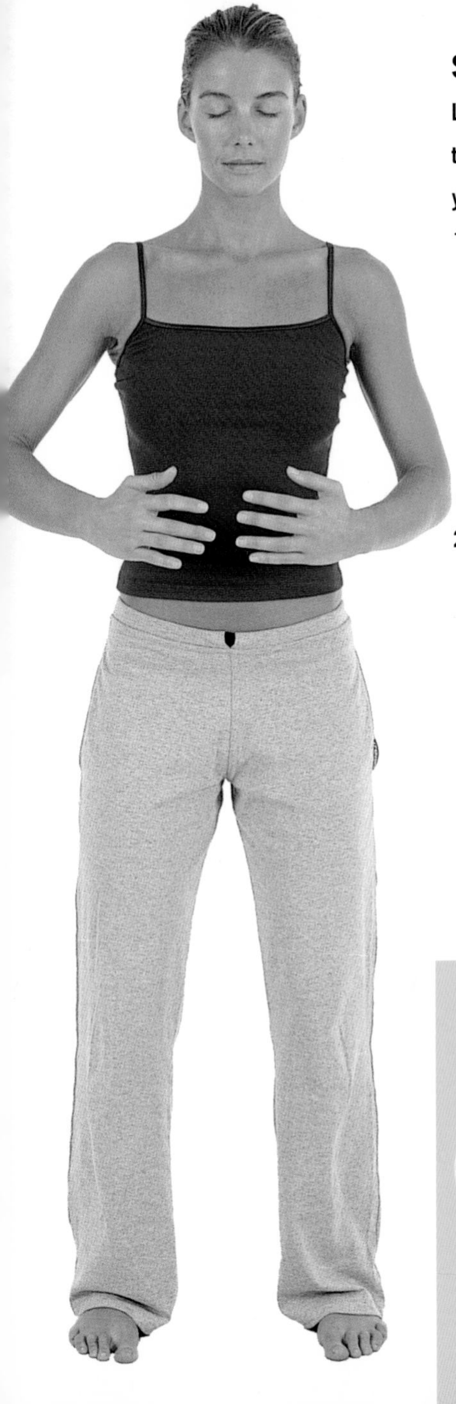

SCANNING YOUR ENERGY FIELD

Learning to scan your body to discover energy imbalances or blockages takes some practice, but you will soon get to know your body. Always scan your body before doing the visualization below.

1. Take off your watch and any rings or bracelets. Rub your hands together, then put your hands palms up and see if you can feel any 'tingles' – this is you own electromagnetic energy field.
2. Hold your palms facing each other, and then curve them slightly as if they were holding a soft ball, about the size of a football. Move this imaginary ball back and forth between your palms for a few minutes and sense the energy flow that exists between your hands.
3. Now your hands are sensitized, start to scan your body. Hold your hands out about 25 cm (10 in) in front of you, palms inwards and move them down your body from your head to your feet to find any blockages. Balanced areas usually feel warm; hot and tingly areas can indicate a painful or injured area, cold areas indicate an energy blockage. Note where your blockage is so that you can work on it (see opposite).

Energy tip

Put a few drops of Dog rose of the wild forces Bush flower essence in a small mister bottle (see page 63) and spray around you for emotional rebalancing.

This soothing acupressure routine can help to release any pent-up anxieties, release muscle pain, lower your stress levels and alleviate any mild depression that you are suffering.

As mentioned earlier (see page 53) finger or thumb pressure is used in acupressure on different acupuncture points to balance the body's energy flow. To reduce any symptoms of stress, it is necessary only to touch a few points to gain some relief and a calmer attitude that lets you cope with the rest of the day.

Soothing acupressure can help to release any pent-up anxieties and lower your stress levels.

HEALING **acupressure**

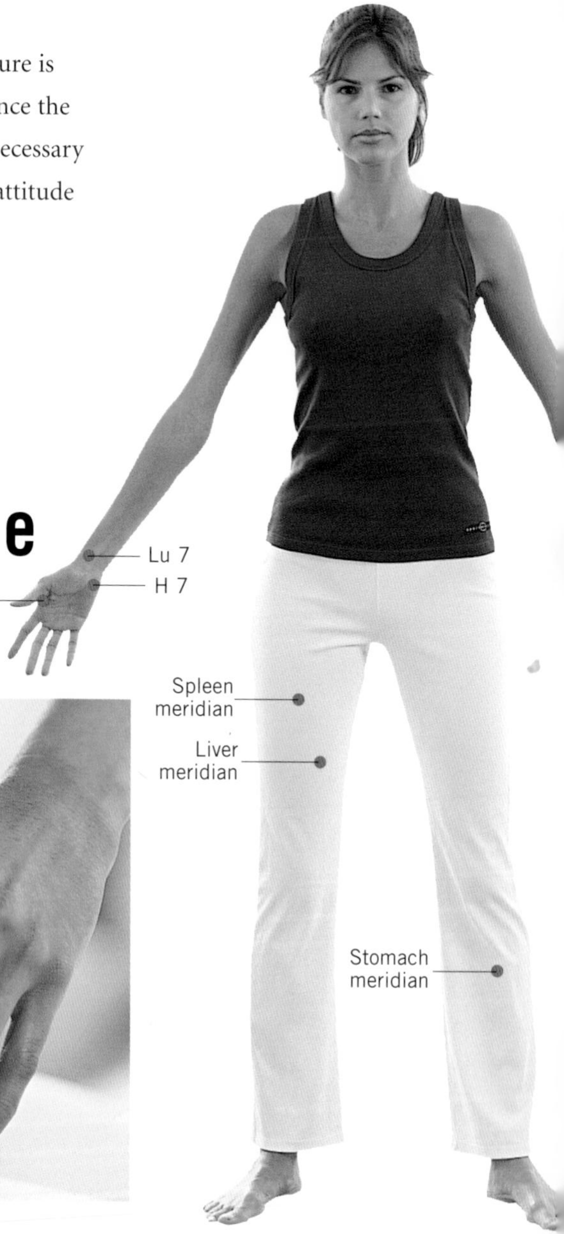
Lu 7
H 7
Lu 10
Spleen meridian
Liver meridian
Stomach meridian

Pressure principles

You can press into points with either your index finger or, for increased pressure, your thumb. Don't dig too hard so that it hurts, just massaging or stroking the area can be sufficient. With a tender area, massage with one finger in circles gently above and below it, before pushing the point itself very gently.

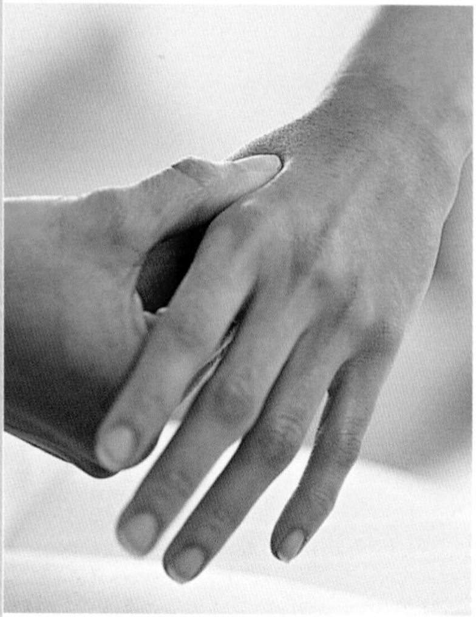

MID-MORNING ACUPRESSURE ROUTINE

In a quiet moment, work on the numbered points below for a few minutes, or until you feel your symptoms easing.

1 Sit comfortably in a chair, lift up your left lower leg and rub your fingers up and down the fleshy outer sides of the leg to stimulate the Spleen meridian and point St 40 on the Stomach meridian (see left). This can help to 'ground' you. Repeat on the other leg. Also work with thumb pressure on Lu 7 on your inner wrists and Lu 10 on the fleshy part of your thumbs (see left) to release stagnant energy that can make you feel down and free any blocked emotions.

2 To reduce tension and anxiety symptoms work with thumb pressure on Li 3 (between the second and big toes) on the Liver meridian (see picture), Li 4 – the great eliminator – (between the first finger and thumb in the fleshy part at the end of the thumb – see diagram on page 13), the Large intestine meridian (see diagram on page 13) and calming H7 (below the bony prominence of the wrist on the outer side of the little finger) on the Heart meridian (see left).

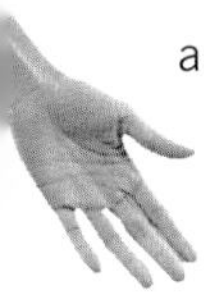

3 Stretch out your spine and breathe deeply from your diaphragm as you touch the 'sea of energy' CV6 on the Conception vessel, two finger-widths below the navel to bring energy down and alleviate muscle tension (see picture), or while you gently massage the heart point CV17 (see picture). When you are worried, rub your stomach with the base of your palm, clockwise and anticlockwise to relax the muscles.

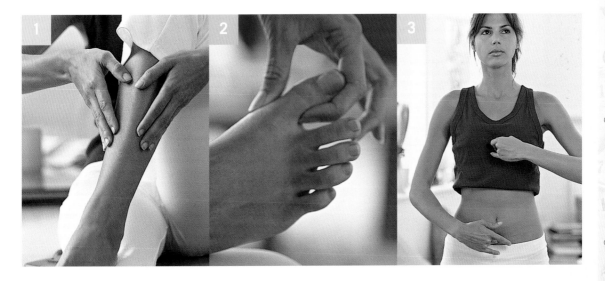

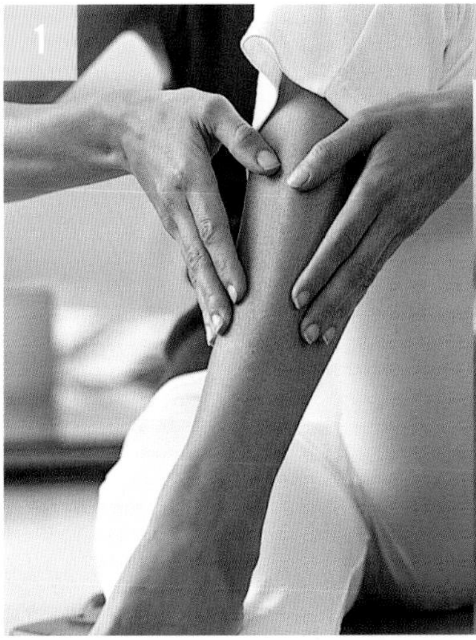
1

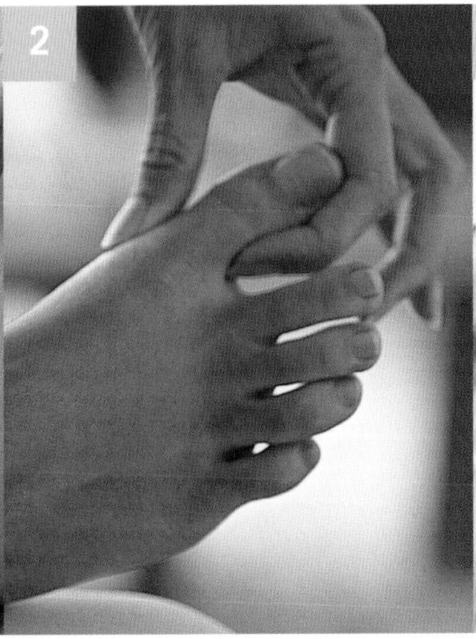
2

3

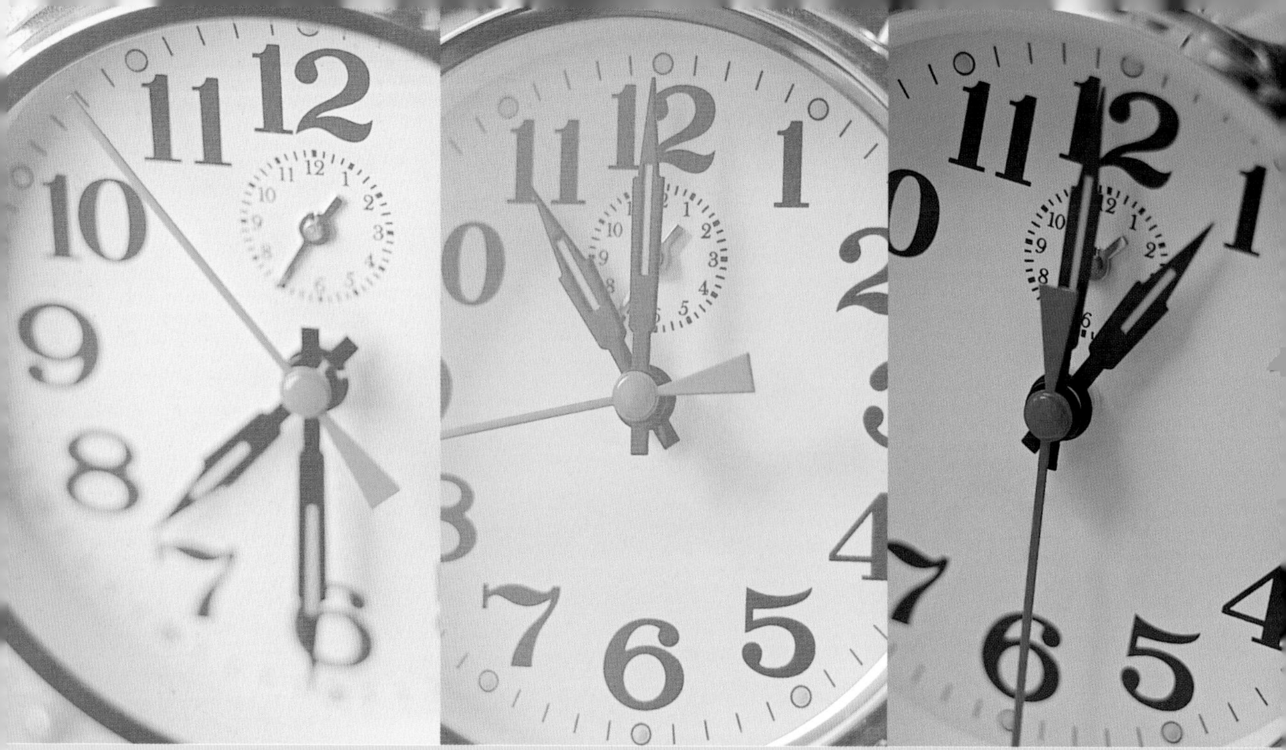

7 Lunchtime revivers

Just walking outside can help you reflect on what you have achieved in the morning.

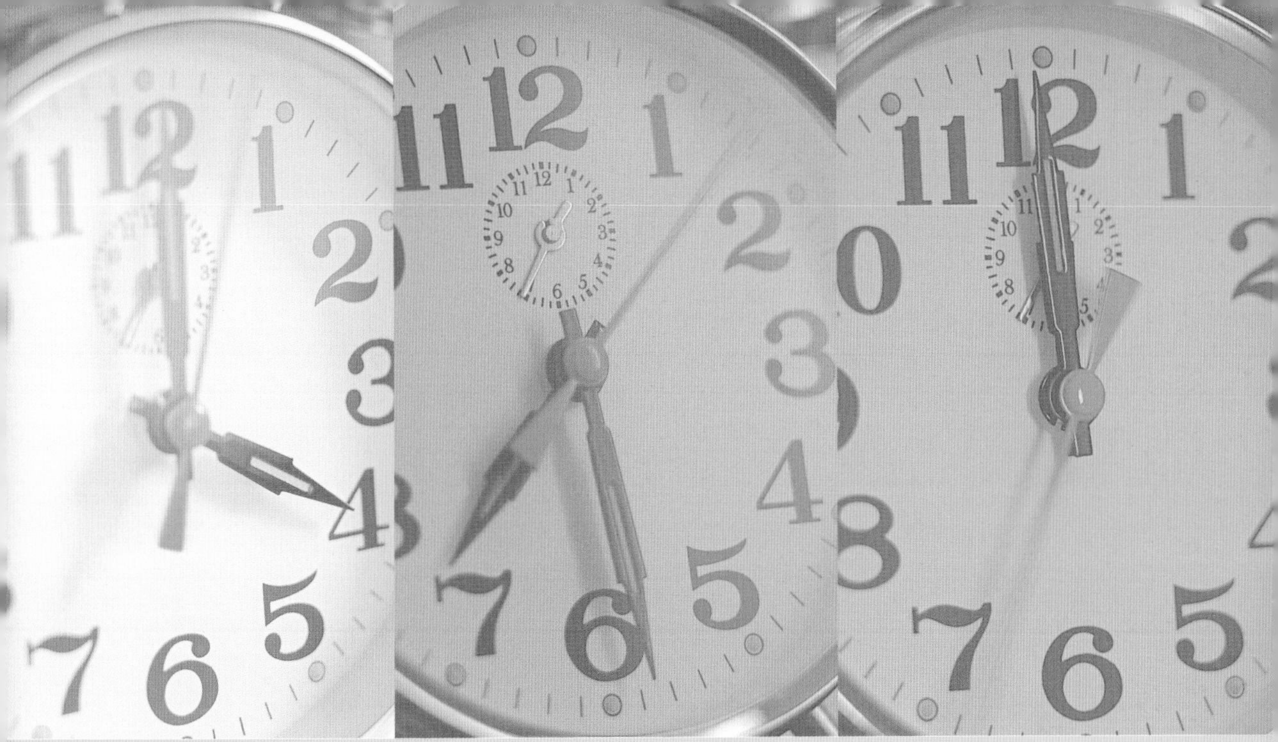

Taking some time for yourself over lunch gives you a chance to clear your head and lose the worries of the morning. Get away from a computer, phones or commitments, turn off your mobile and escape outside so that your body and soul can reconnect with the soothing rhythms of nature.

Doing these exercises outside replenishes your mind and emotions and inspires you to continue the afternoon with enthusiasm. Hug a tree to receive its wise and balancing energies or walk barefoot and sense the power of Mother Earth. But don't worry if you have to stay inside, you can still reduce the pressures of the morning by doing a mini Indian-type head massage to banish any irritations or the visualization exercise to dispel any tensions.

Find the energizer for you. If possible do two each day, and see how much more motivated you feel when you return to your afternoon tasks.

Leave behind the cares of the office or trials of home life to do this outside water meditation, which will cleanse your body of any worries.

Water is believed to have special purifying and sacred powers, and was often used in native healing ceremonies to soothe the spirit of an injured person. Today, water still retains the essence of a nurturing and healing energy. Looking into the hidden depths of water is supposed to be a source of wisdom, so sitting by a pond, lake or river can give you the chance to meditate and reflect on your life's purpose.

If you meditate by water regularly at lunchtime, you will soon see how its purifying influence helps you cope with your daily stresses. If there is no water nearby, sit in a green space and visualize a vast expanse of water in your mind first, before starting the meditation.

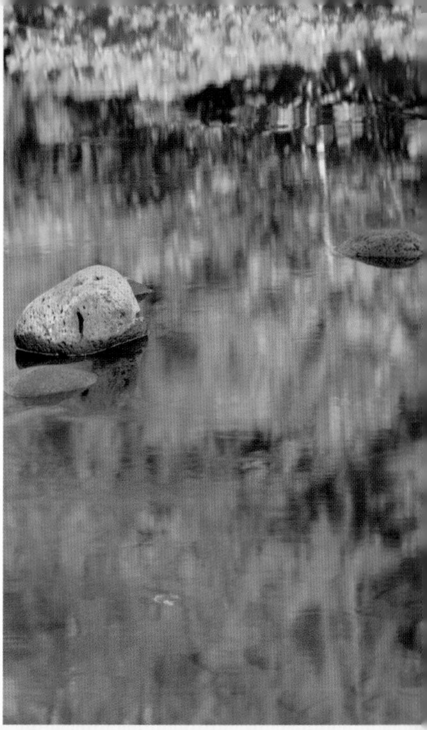

WATER **cleansing**

WATER MEDITATION

Practise this meditation for about 10 minutes, losing yourself in the nurturing influence of the water.

1 Sit comfortably on a bench in a park by a lake, on a riverbank or on the seashore on a calm day. Gaze into the water and start to slow your breathing, taking deep breaths from your diaphragm.

2 Feel the serenity and peace of the water and sense how it welcomes you. As you start to lose yourself in its infinite depths, let its cleansing presence wash through your mind, removing any anger, irritation or criticism that has occurred in the morning.

3 Let out any annoyances or emotional upsets and watch as they float away on the water. Feel positive thoughts about your capabilities entering your mind. See the challenges of the afternoon as a detailed list but only sense calm when you look at it. Slowly come to (or open your eyes) and return to face the afternoon with your energy levels recharged.

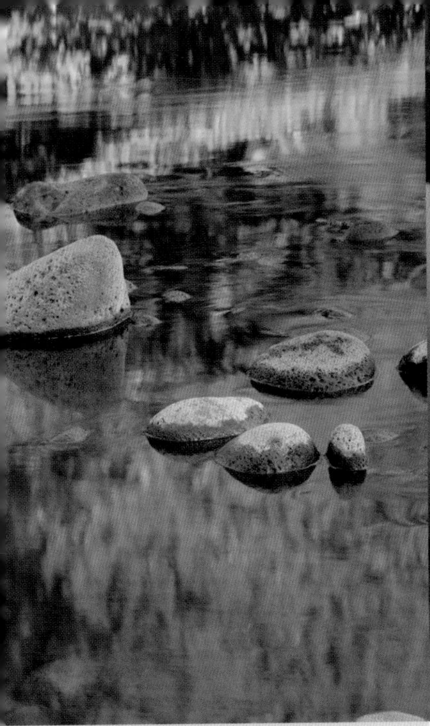

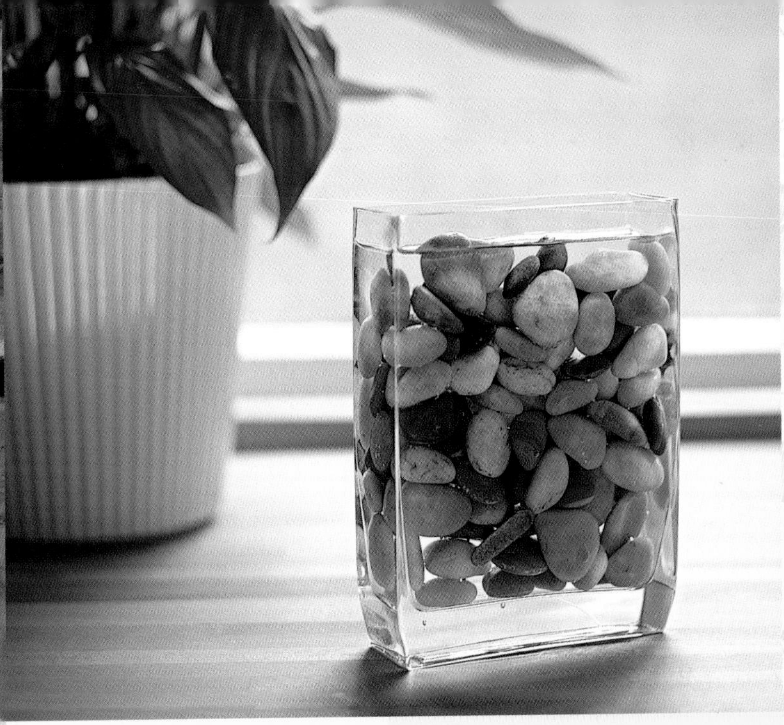

Energy tip

Water stimulates and encourages the flow of *chi*, so put a running water feature on the southeast corner (your wealth space in feng shui) of your desk or on a table in this area of your living room to encourage success.

Water feature

If getting outside is difficult and you want to try water meditation, place a water feature on your desk or on a table at home. Ideally, buy a small fountain with running water or one that runs over pebbles. Alternatively, place some chosen pebbles in the bottom of a square vase and fill with water. Gaze into the flowing or still water to inspire your meditation.

Water is believed to have special purifying and sacred powers.

Taking time out at lunchtime to go outside and walk barefoot on the ground, connects you with nature and inspires your soul.

In the Western world, most of modern life is spent indoors in artificially lit and centrally-heated buildings. We spend so much time indoors that we are rapidly losing our connection with the seasons and the natural energies of the planet.

Our bodies are familiar with the 'grounded' and strengthening electromagnetic fields that emanate from the earth, but by wearing shoes all the time we are losing our sensitivity to this powerful energy.

Walk barefoot outside during the summer months and whenever you can in the home to reinforce your connection to this ancient healing energy source.

Energy tip

Bring some earth energy inside. Keep a smooth pebble on your desk or on a windowsill at home. Buy one or preferably find one in a favourite place, perhaps by a river or the sea, so that you transfer the vibration of that beautiful place inside.

CONNECT with the earth

BAREFOOT WALK ON GRASS

Go barefoot walking in a local park or on your garden lawn for about 10 minutes to strengthen you in the middle of the day.

1. Take off your shoes and any socks or tights and stand upright on the grass for a few minutes to connect to the earth's energies. Deeply breathe in the fresh air and curl your toes a couple of times in the grass to feel its texture and freshness.
2. Now walk along the grass enjoying each step, let the sweet smell of the earth fill your nostrils and seep into your lungs. Feel the chatter of your mind quietening, and any tiredness or tension leaving you as you become at one with nature's grounding and creative source.
3. Walk for about 5–10 minutes and sense the profound intimacy of being in touch with Mother Earth. Put your shoes on and return inside feeling revitalized for the afternoon ahead.

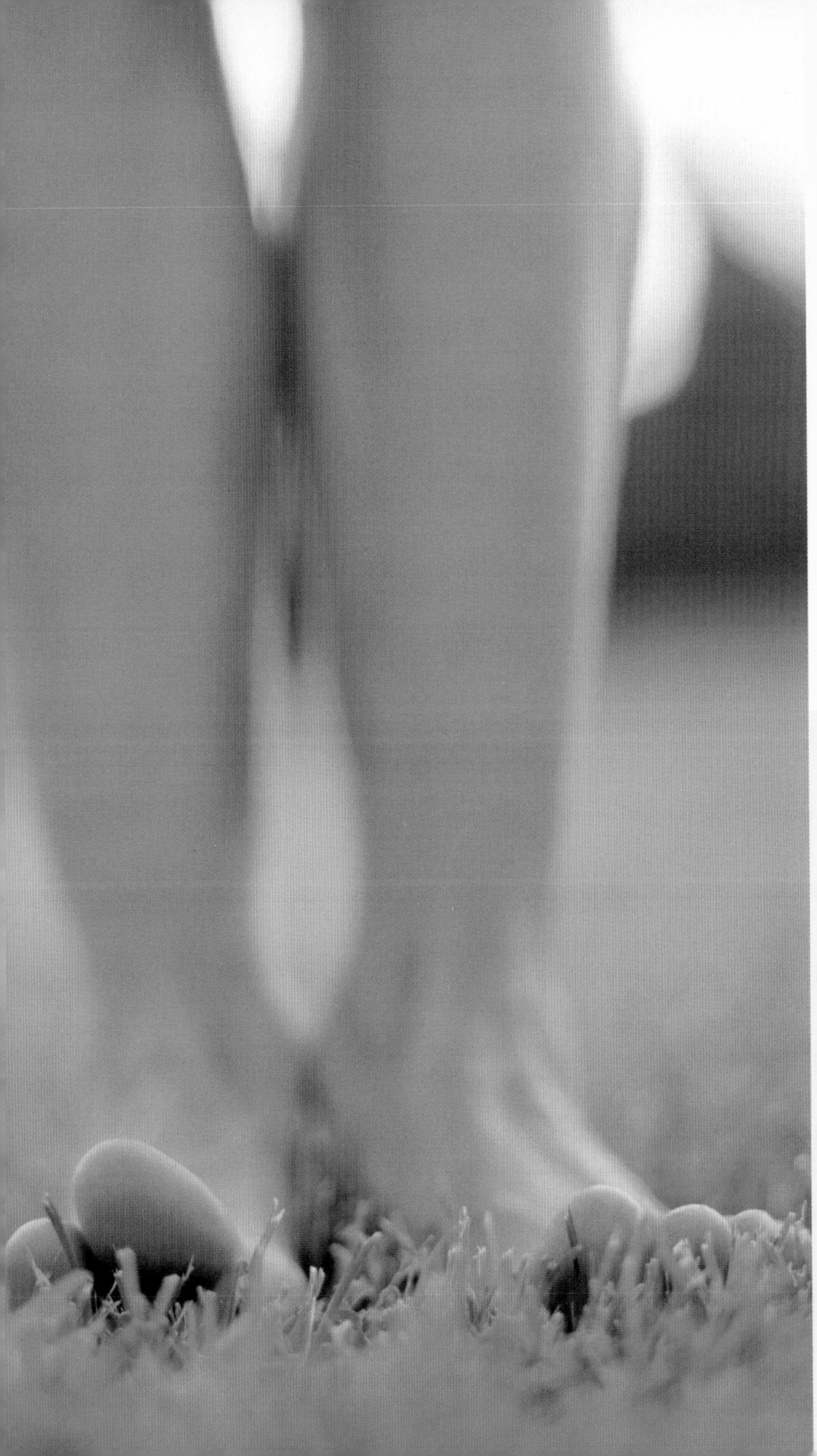

Walking barefoot on the ground connects you with nature and inspires your soul.

Mother Earth

Ancient civilizations that lived and worked on the earth, thought of Mother Earth as the fertile provider for all. There was a deep sense of partnership, of living with the earth. Pre-Christian peoples, such as the Druids, were so in tune with nature that they built sacred buildings in accordance with the elements, and where they felt strong earth energies. This connection is being revived today by people supporting the Gaia theory that what we do to the earth, we do to ourselves.

It may sound a bit wacky to escape outside at lunchtime to go and hug a tree, but the harmonizing and balancing energy they give out can calm and refresh you. The solid strength of an old tree is very protective and reassuring, and, once again, very 'grounding', especially if your morning has been challenging or chaotic.

The ancient Greeks worshipped trees as they thought they were oracles of the gods, while many Native American tribes consider them to be sacred and would never deliberately cut them down.

Trees put down deep roots into the ground; so spending some time with them can reassure you and literally 'bring you right back down to earth'.

EMBRACING tree energy

The solid strength of an old tree is protective and reassuring, and very 'grounding'.

Crystal tip

Put a piece of amber in your pocket as you hug your tree to facilitate the balancing of your energies and calming of your nervous system.

Shamanic healing

Shamans or healers of Native American tribes often used the roots of a tree or a tree stump as a pathway or gateway as they 'journeyed' (a deep visualization technique) from ordinary reality to the lower worlds in the spirit realm – the tree acted as the transition between the two worlds.

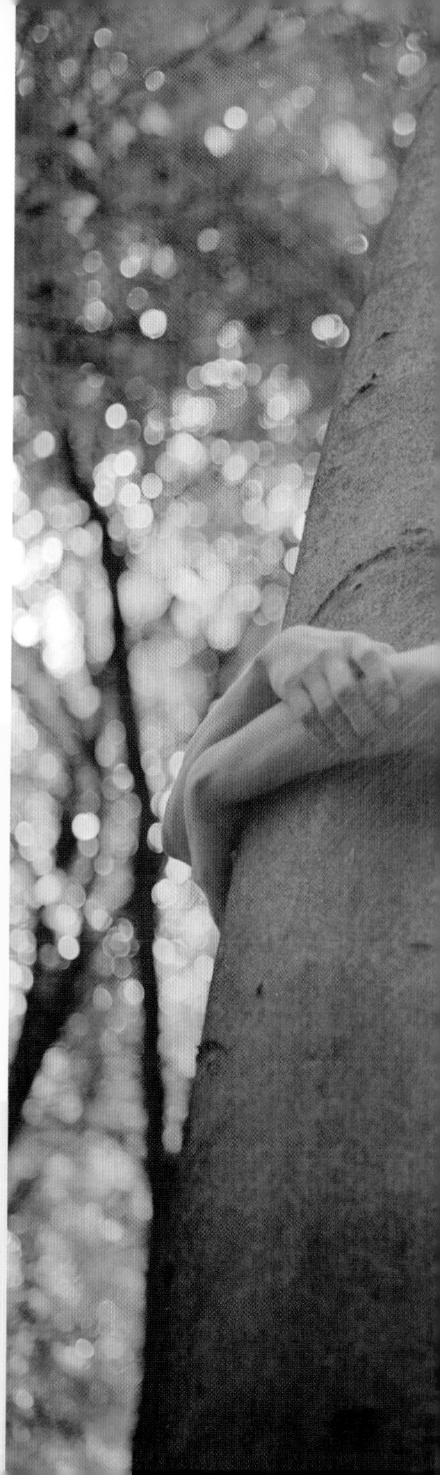

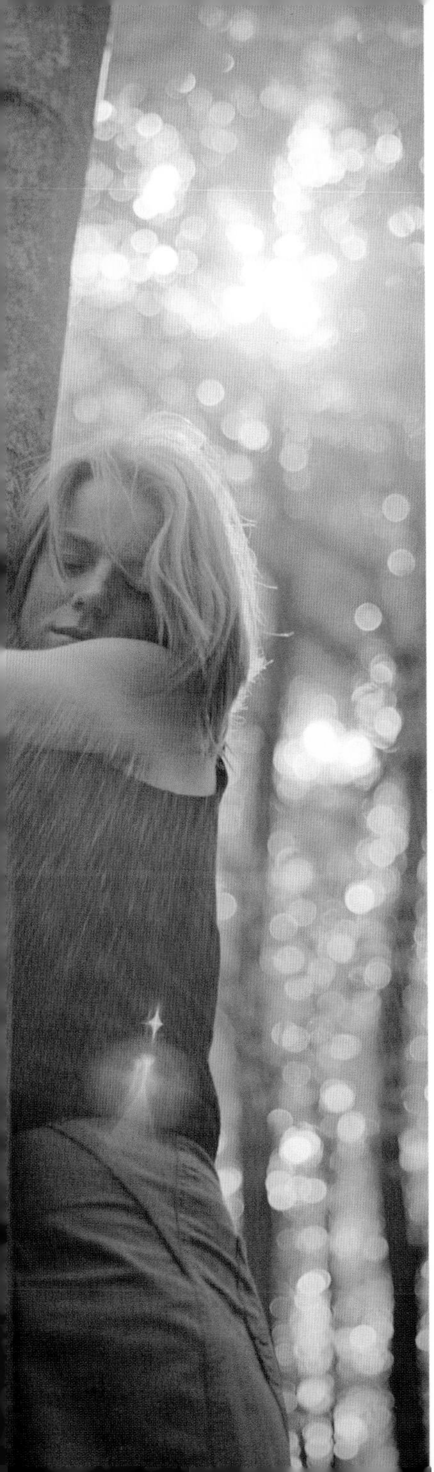

TREE HUGGING

Choose a quiet place and stand and hug your chosen tree or sit with your back next to a tall strong tree for at least 10 minutes; let its healing energies bring you mental clarity and emotional serenity.

1 Sit on the ground behind your tree and wrap your arms around it. Alternatively, sit with your back straight up against the tree.

2 Close your eyes and take some deep breaths from your diaphragm and relax your muscles. Remove your shoes, and put your feet flat on the ground so that you are 'rooting' yourself in the earth.

3 Now let go of any negative thoughts, anger or resentments that have been held for a while or that have built up during the morning. Visualize them being soaked up by the earth and dissipated by its healing energies.

4 When you have released all the negativity, imagine this healing energy coming up through the soles of your feet, working its way up through your legs, stomach, chest, through your arms, until it goes out through the top of your head. Sense this energy as a 'tingling' feeling.

5 As you absorb this earth energy, let some pure golden, protective universal light travel your body through the top of your head down to your feet. Keep breathing deeply as you feel the warmth of the two energies mixing. Slowly open your eyes, sensing how much more balanced and harmonized you feel. Let go of the tree, thanking it and Mother Earth for their loving, healing energies. If you want, leave a small token, such as a coin or a small crystal, as a thank you to your tree.

Chi kung or qigong literally means 'training the breath' or 'energy cultivation' (*chi* or *qi* means energy and *gong* means cultivation). It evolved in China many centuries ago and it is the exercise movement from which t'ai chi originates.

There are many forms of chi kung but the main aim of 'internal' chi kung is to manipulate the flow of *chi* inside the body to stimulate healing. The 'hard' martial art forms of this art are t'ai chi or kung fu, while a 'softer' form just works with moving *chi* internally. Aerobic conditioning, meditation and relaxation are all part of chi kung, as there is no extreme exertion it is suitable for all fitness levels.

Do this easy chi kung routine at lunchtime in the fresh air to remove any harmful *chi* from your aura.

LUNCHTIME **chi kung**

WARM-UP EXERCISES

Do a few of these warm-up exercises for several minutes before starting The shower of light routine.

1 Stand with your feet a shoulder-width apart. Start to bounce up and down on the balls of your feet.

2 Start to swing your arms back and forth energetically to get rid of stale air and toxins in the lungs. Inhale as you go up on your toes with your arms up and exhale as you go down and swing your arms behind you. Also swing from side to side to warm up the muscles.

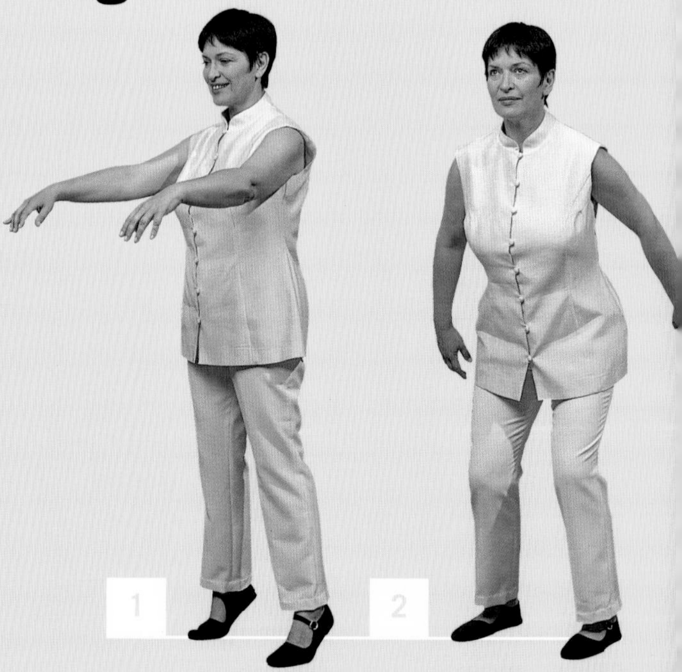
1
2

Chi kung tip

Practise the movements after a light snack but not after a heavy lunch.

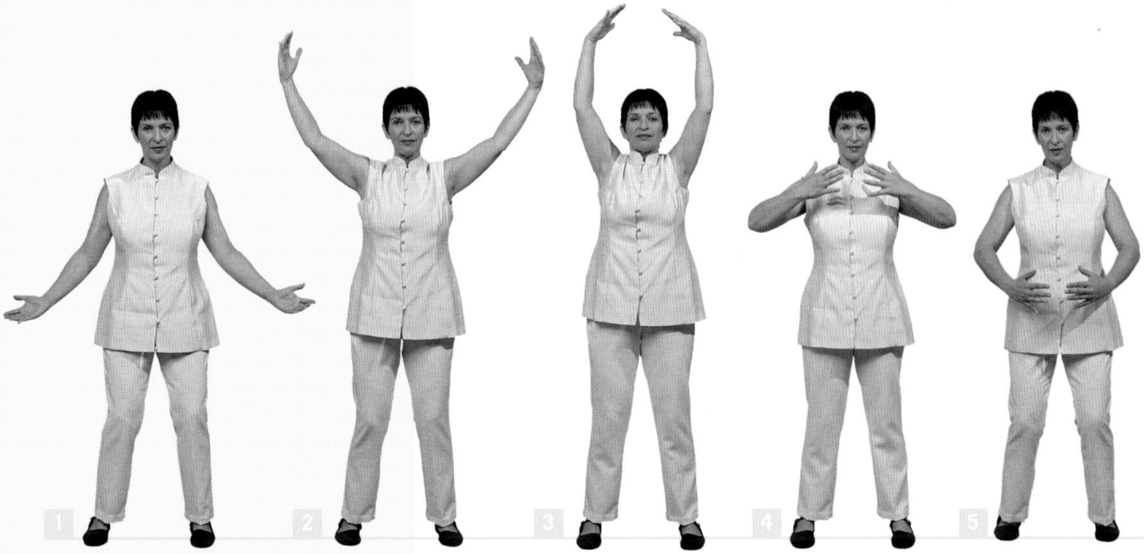
1
2
3
4
5

THE SHOWER OF LIGHT

Perform this routine for about 10 minutes to fill your body with new vibrant energy.

Chi kung or qigong literally means 'training the breath'.

1 Stand with your feet shoulder-width apart. Turn your palms outwards, breathe in and slowly raise up your arms in front of you.

2 Continue raising your arms up to your head height, keeping them slightly curved in shape.

3 When you arms are right over your head, imagine fresh *chi* filling your palms from the sky.

4 Breathe out, slowly bringing your arms down the front of your body, this time with your palms facing inwards.

5 Keep breathing evenly and continue to bring your arms down until they reach your navel. As you do this movement, visualize the fresh *chi* flowing down your front, your back and sides through the body's meridians (see page 12), flushing out any negative *chi*. Bring your hands back to your side, and repeat the sequence about 6 times.

Having a break at lunchtime often gives you a chance to go outside in the fresh air to revive you and lift any tiredness you are feeling.

As was discussed earlier (see page 40), breathing deeply and slowly improves your body functions and increases your general wellbeing. Check your breathing throughout the day; it is very easy to breathe shallowly if you are stressed. Stop to take a few deep breaths, and maybe yawn and stretch out your arms to get in touch with your body.

Cleansing breathing, preferably out in the open air, can release any anxieties or disperse any stagnant energy from the morning into the outside atmosphere.

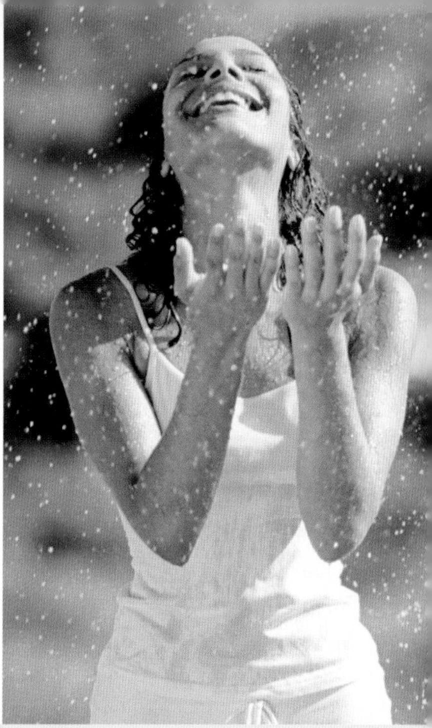

CLEANSING **breathing**

BREATHING OUT STALE ENERGIES

Perform these breathing exercises for 5–10 minutes and let the new energy you absorb revive your body and spirit.

1 Sit comfortably outside or in a quiet space inside. Take a deep cleansing breath through your nose, pulling the breath right up from your feet through your body. Breathe out forcefully through your mouth, blowing out any stagnancy or anxiety held inside. Repeat for several minutes.

2 Now, breathe in deeply and imagine a fountain in your lungs that rises up, getting taller and taller until it overflows through the top of your head as you exhale. Repeat for a few minutes until you feel energized.

Breathing tip

Bring yourself into the 'now' by breathing in future dreams and breathing out negative aspects of your past.

Breathing deeply and slowly improves your body functions and increases your general wellbeing.

After a busy morning where it feels like you haven't stopped since you got up, you may be feeling emotionally drained. If you can make time and find a quiet space outside, or inside, to sing you will ease any jaded emotions and bring some joy back into your soul.

When you sing you also improve the resonance and flexibility of your speaking voice. As you sing confidently, you naturally raise your spirits by breathing more deeply and releasing any anxieties that you are holding inside. You also benefit from the higher levels of oxygen being absorbed into the bloodstream. Our body cells and organs react to different sound vibrations, which can change when an area is under stress, so singing can help restore these vibrations to their normal level.

When you sing you also improve the resonance and flexibility of your speaking voice.

LUNCHTIME **singing**

UPLIFTING SINGING

Find a quiet space, outside if you can, where you won't be disturbed and sing your heart out for 5–10 minutes. If it's difficult to find a quiet space, why not sit in your car?

1. Choose a favourite song that you can remember well. Start to sing softly at first until you get into the natural rhythm of the song.
2. As you become more confident, you will breathe in deeply and sing more loudly; at the same time, you can sense how any tension in your chest or stomach simply dissolves. Feel the vibrations coursing through your body, giving you a feeling of joy and happiness.

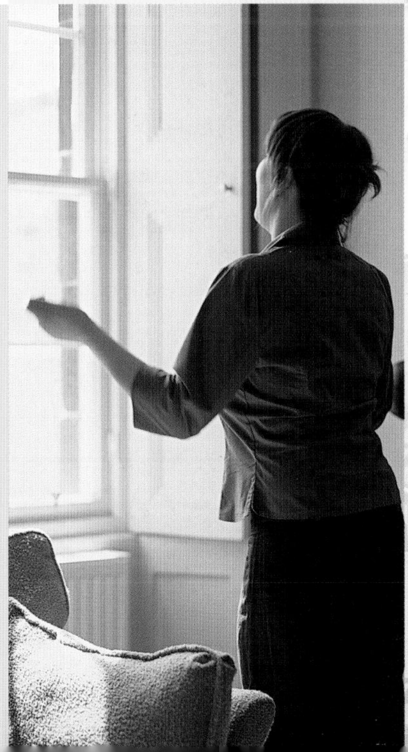

Even with only half an hour to spare at lunchtime, you can do this visualization exercise outside or inside to take you to a favourite place and leave behind the morning's upsets.

The visualization technique consciously uses your imagination to create attractive and positive imagery to heal negative thoughts or to make changes in your life. If you think of the stress symptoms you experience when you worry, the opposite effects are achieved with visualization. The strong positive images the brain receives brings serenity, over-riding any destructive thoughts. The body releases tension and positive physical effects take place.

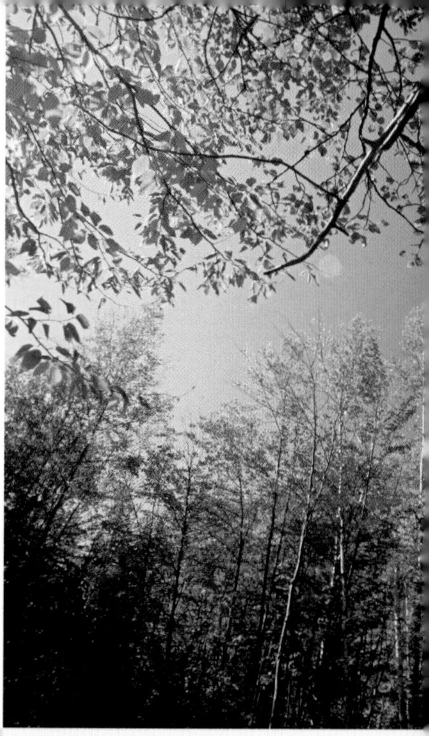

CREATING **bliss**

INDUCING CALM

Spend 10 minutes on this visualization technique to visit your special haven and find peace.

1 Sit comfortably and relax. Close your eyes and think of a favourite scene where you always feel at peace. It may be on a beach from a dream holiday, by a lake or river or even in your garden.

2 Now take yourself to this place and lose yourself in the environment. See the colours, hear the wildlife, smell the scents. Feel the tranquillity of the place rejuvenating your body and resolving any problems; see hassles just drifting off into the atmosphere.

3 Slowly open your eyes and come to, knowing you can return here at any time to feel this calm and to deal with any worries.

Energy tip

Spray some Calm and clear Bush flower combination essence into your aura (see page 29) before your visualization to help you wind down.

The strong positive images the brain receives brings serenity, over-riding any destructive thoughts.

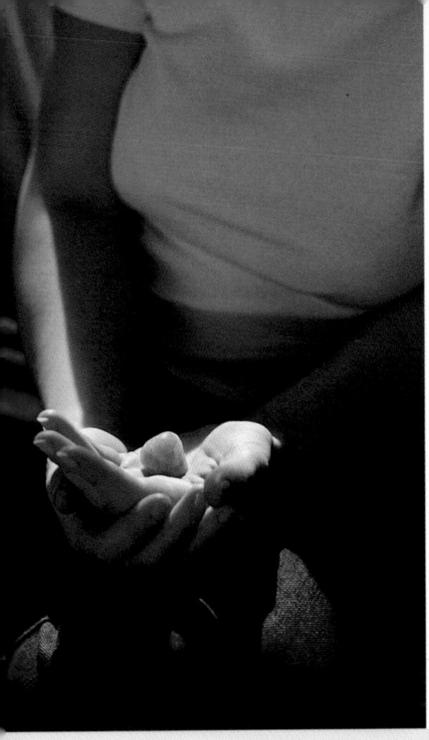

For thousands of years crystals have been used for healing and protection (see pages 34–35). Every *chakra* (see page 15), cell and organ in our body is believed to vibrate at its own frequency. If these become unbalanced or upset, illness can result. By setting a mental intent you can send healing energy (directed from the universal life force) into a crystal so that it emits the electromagnetic vibrations needed to restore the healthy functioning of a *chakra* or body part.

Working with an aquamarine crystal regularly at lunchtime will help you speak out and give your mind a therapeutic workout.

crystal CLEARING

CRYSTAL HEALING FOR MENTAL CLARITY

Work with a cleansed aquamarine crystal (see page 35) for 5–10 minutes to clear your mind and restore any blocked communication.

1 Sit comfortably in a chair, close your eyes and hold your crystal for several minutes. Tune into its energies, having already set its main intent (see page 34). Ask the crystal to clear your mind of any distractions and fears.

2 Now hold your crystal for a few minutes over your Throat chakra in the middle of your throat and ask for any communication problems to be removed. Open your eyes and thank your crystal for its healing energies.

Crystal tip

You can also cleanse your crystal by smudging. Light a herbal smudge stick (see page 122), hold over a flameproof dish and waft the purifying smoke over your crystal; you can cleanse several crystals together in this way.

If you don't have time or can't get outside at lunchtime, you can still boost your energy levels by using the power of your hands.

Your hands can be used for two different healing routines: by massaging your hands, you can relieve any aches and strains in your fingers; by working on your head with strong fingers, you can release tension that has built up during the day.

The hands are often neglected but they respond as well to massage as the rest of the body.

LUNCHTIME HAND MASSAGE

The hands respond as well to massage as the rest of the body. By massaging them you can get the blood flowing and shift any tension in the muscles and joints caused by rigid or repetitive movements. Try this relaxing massage with essential oils to ease aching fingers when you have been typing on a keyboard all morning or driving for a long time without a break.

healing HANDS

The massage routine

Work on your hands using these circling, kneading and stretching techniques for 5–10 minutes to reduce nagging aches and pains.

1 Mix 3 drops of marjoram essential oil to 3 teaspoons of your base oil in small plastic bottle.

2 Sit comfortably in a chair. Rub some massage oil into your right hand. Breathe in and out gently as you squeeze out tension between each finger on your left hand with your right thumb and fingers. Then press and rotate your right thumb into the back of your left hand, working over the whole area.

3 Turn your hand over and repeat the circles on your palm, kneading the hand with strong strokes to release contracted muscles.

4 Turn your hand back over and finish by pressing the side of each finger with your right thumb and finger from the top to the base, then gently pull each one. Repeat on the other hand.

2

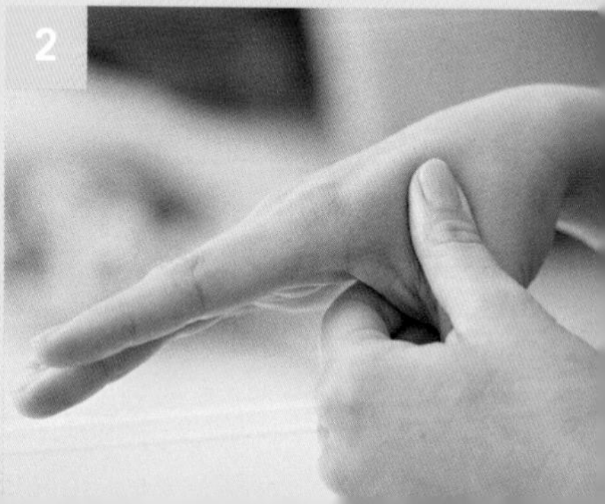

MINI INDIAN-TYPE HEAD MASSAGE

This invigorating head massage complements the temple and neck sequence on pages 100–101. Working on your scalp in this way at lunchtime releases any taut muscles, improves your concentration, induces a feeling of wellbeing and gets any sluggish energy moving again.

Our heads are our power centres, where our brain organizes our busy days. It is not surprising, then, that they suffer from anxiety, emotional tension or headaches. Finger massaging around the crown of the head is very therapeutic, it recharges your energy levels, activates the lymphatic system to clear out toxins and soothes your tired spirit.

Oils to use

- Marjoram essential oil.
- A proprietary base oil such as grapeseed, sunflower or safflower oil.

The massage routine

Massage your head (no oil is needed) for 5–10 minutes. Concentrate on easing any tight or knotted scalp areas.

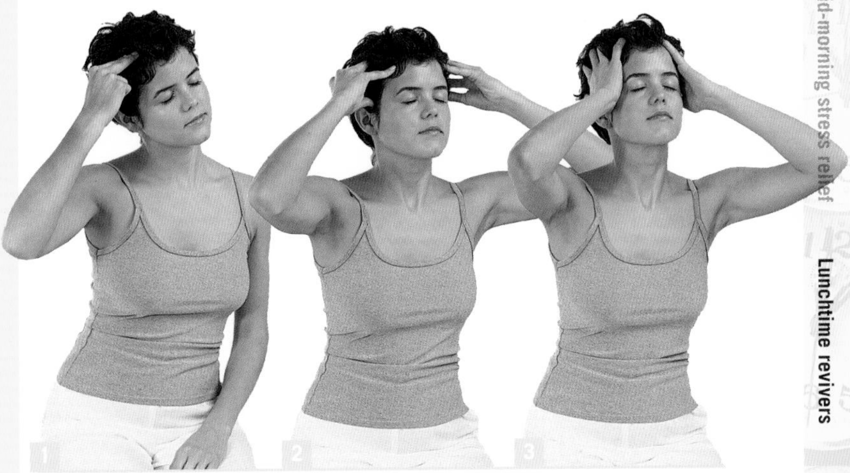
1
2
3

1 With your forefinger and middle finger of one hand massage your scalp in a circular movement, slightly lifting your hair as you do so. This invigorates your scalp and revives flagging energies.

2 Using both hands, make circular movements with your fingertips all around your scalp. Grasp small handfuls of hair and give them a tug for instant tension relief.

3 Run your fingers over your face and then push them through your hair savouring the immediate energy surge and mental release. Repeat the process from the nape of your neck up to your crown, reducing any neck stiffness from your morning's concentrated work.

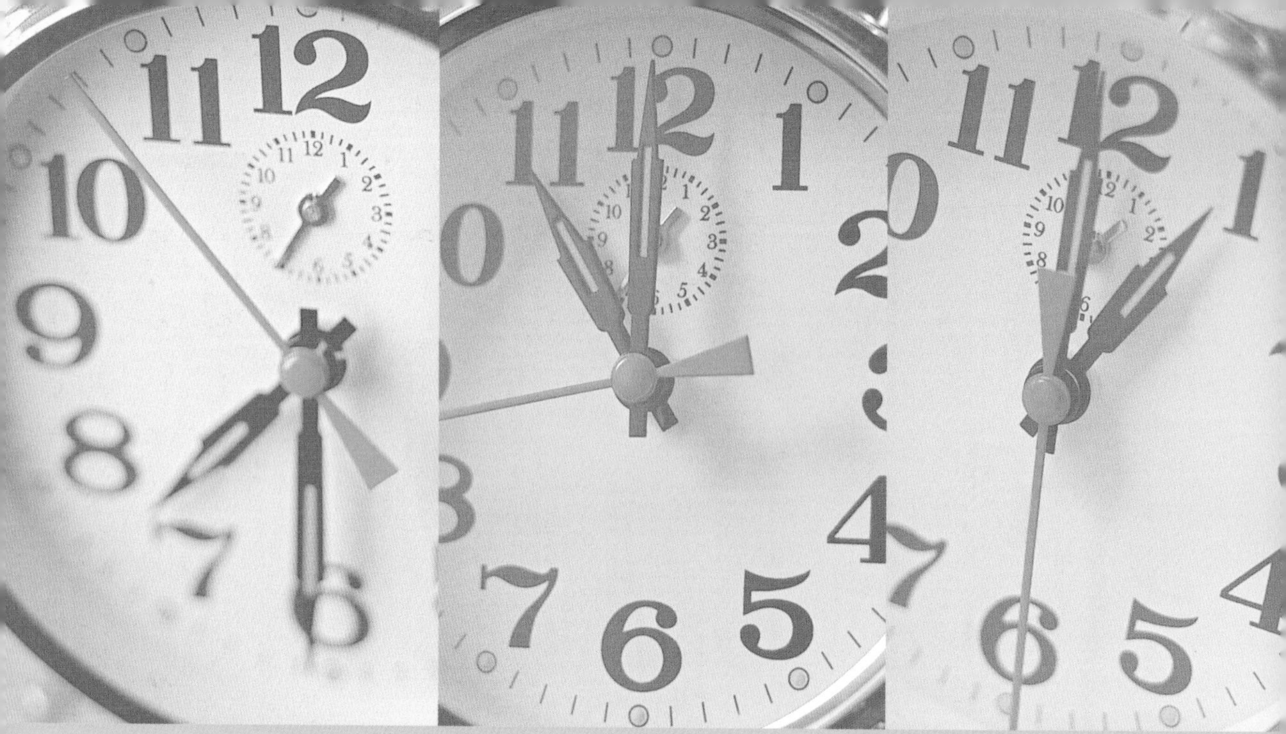

8 Mid-afternoon boosters

At this time of day your energy levels really start to flag and you need to re-energize to get through the remainder of the afternoon.

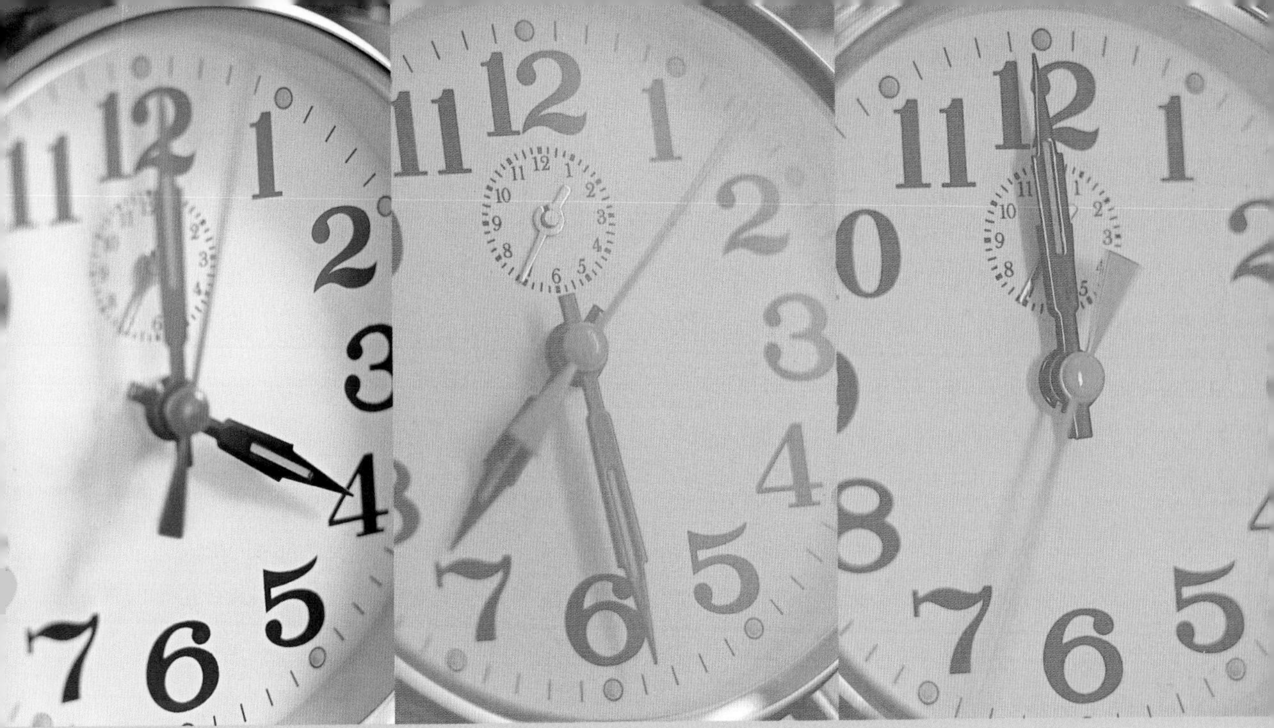

Mid-afternoon is when your energy levels can start to take a real dip, especially if the frustrations of the day are catching up with you. You may be feeling tense, have a slight headache or finding that some of your muscles are starting to ache. Try to stay upbeat, though, and let go of the day's anxieties. Don't dwell on any negative outcomes but focus on your successes.

Use the holistic energizers in this section to release the strains of the day and give you that last energy surge to keep you going for the rest of the afternoon.

Try to set aside a time to do the short energizer that recharges your physical state and emotional mood. By releasing any stress or rebalancing your inner energies, you can face the final responsibilities of the day with a lighter heart and renewed vigour.

As your working day continues you may find that your eyes become dry, tired and gritty from reading, driving or sitting in front of a computer for long periods. Bad lighting and air conditioning can also aggravate the problem making your eyes feel very dry and sore. Your neck muscles may also be starting to feel painful as they 'lock' and stiffen from constantly leaning forwards or staying too long in one position.

Taking time out briefly to ease the strain that has accumulated in your eye and neck muscles will give you that necessary energy surge to finish your day.

Exercise tip

Always make sure that your shoulders do not round or stoop during these exercises as this posture can pull rather than relax the neck muscles. Try shrugging your shoulders to relax them first: squeeze your shoulders up towards your ears and then push them down as far as you can into your body. Repeat this sequence a few times and you'll feel tension simply disappear.

PALMING

Covering your eyes so that they are in complete darkness can clear your head and refresh your eyes (see also pages 100–101).

1 Either sit with your elbows supported on a desk or table, or sit upright with your elbows on your chest, and cup your hands over your eyes. If you are at home, you can lie down to do this, but keep your knees bent.

2 Rub your palms together until they feel warm and then gently place your cupped hands over your closed eyes but do not touch them.

3 Breathe deeply as you enjoy the complete darkness, letting your mind empty as the warmth of your hands soothes your tired eyes. Breathe in stimulating energy into your eyes and breathe out any strain. Maintain your breathing rhythm for 5–10 minutes.

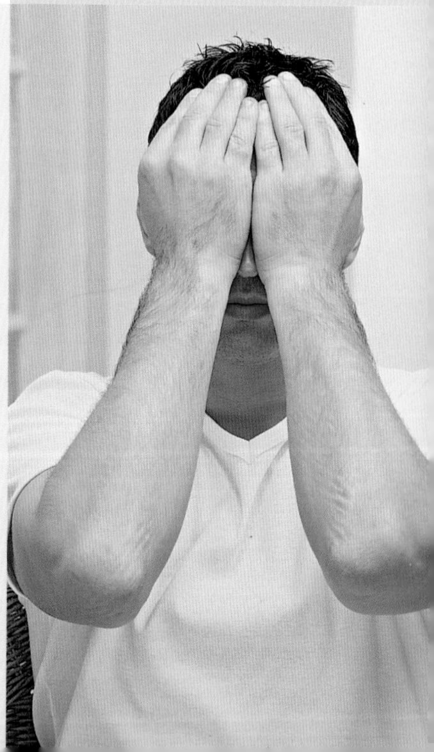

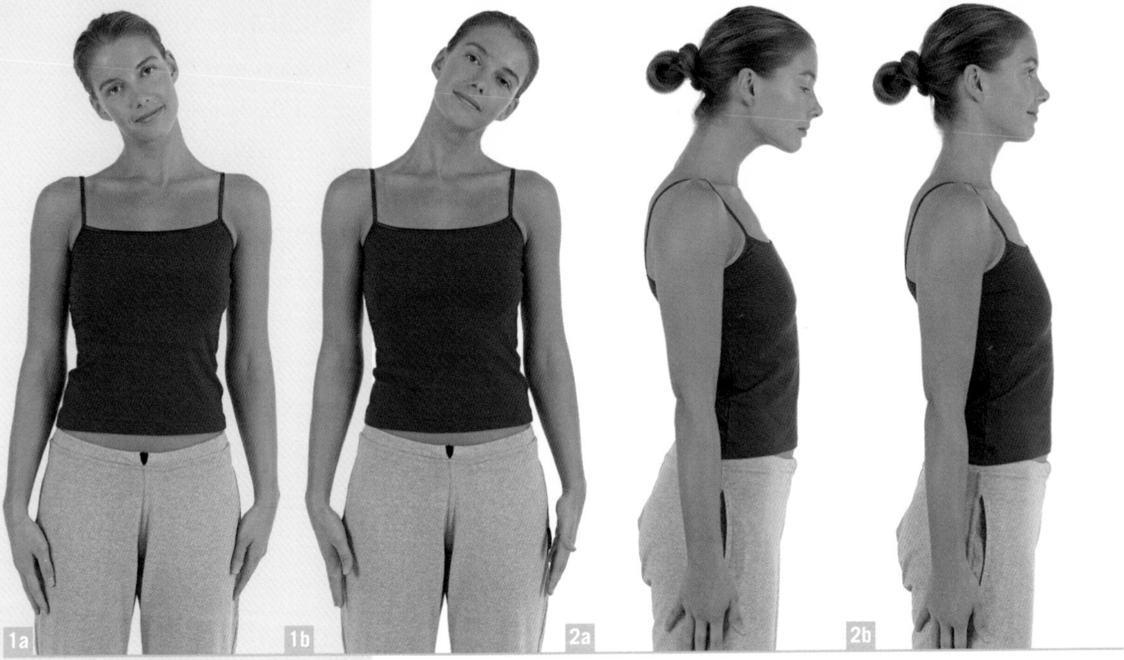
1a
1b
2a
2b

NECK ROLLS

Gently rub your tense neck muscles, then spend about 5 minutes doing these neck rolls to relax and loosen up any rigid muscles.

Exercise tips

- Blink constantly for about 15 seconds to moisten dry eyes.
- To perk up tired eyes, splash them alternately with hot and cold water for a few minutes.

1 Stand or sit upright in a chair keeping your spine straight. Keep your shoulders down as you lean your head towards the right (see picture 1a). Hold for 30 seconds, feeling the stretch in your neck and left shoulder. Relax your head, bring it back to the centre and repeat on the left side (see picture 1b). Repeat several times on each side.

2 Drop your chin slowly down towards your chest and feel the stretch in the back of your neck (see picture 2a); hold for 30 seconds then gently release (see picture 2b). Repeat several times.

3 Take your right hand and put it on the back of your head. Push forwards gently with your hand to get an increased stretch in your neck; hold for 30 seconds then release. Repeat several times.

The middle of the afternoon, particularly around 3–4p.m., is when energy levels slump and sometimes it can be hard to continue. Sipping a cup of herbal tea can act as a tonic (see also pages 32–33, 46 and 58), cleansing the blood and revitalizing the body organs. Some herbs, such as ginseng, are 'adaptogens' that fight or adapt to whatever problem the body is experiencing: if you are feeling tired, it will energize you; if you feel stressed it will calm you. If you are unable to buy ginseng powder, use a herbal tea bag instead. (Please note: you should avoid Korean ginseng if you are pregnant or have high blood pressure.)

Green tea

There are many health benefits of drinking green tea, which is readily available in tea bags. As well as boosting the immune system, it contains powerful antioxidants that slow ageing and destroy free radicals (harmful reactive molecules that can damage body cells), thereby reducing the risk of cancer and heart disease.

A TEA tonic

GINSENG AND HONEY TEA

Ginseng makes a potent revitalizing tea that reduces physical or emotional stress. It can normalize blood sugar levels and stimulates the functioning of the brain and nervous system, aiding mental clarity.

Ingredients

- 3 teaspoons Korean ginseng powder (available from health stores or herbal shops)
- 1 cup of boiling water
- 1–2 teaspoons honey (optional)

Making the tea

1. Dissolve the ginseng powder in the boiling water and leave it to stand for 10 minutes.
2. Ginseng has a pleasant flavour of its own but some people prefer to add honey.

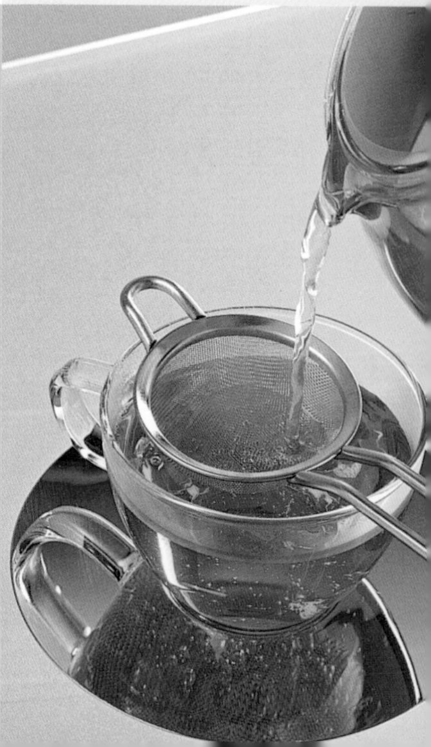

Feng shui tip

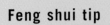

Place your crystal in the northeast corner of your desk or study to stimulate your education and knowledge – your learning space.

Crystals are wonderful aids to healing as discussed on pages 34–35 and page 83. The vibrational frequencies they emit can bring your body and spirit back into balance. Natural quartz is one of the most versatile crystals. In a practical capacity its silicon chips are adapted for use in everyday commercial life to receive, store, amplify and transmit data in computers and in credit and smart cards. In healing, the crystal's ability to amplify energy, can harmonize all the *chakras* (see page 15), particularly the Crown chakra – your spiritual centre.

Use this natural quartz crystal in the middle of the afternoon to restore depleted energy and aid your mental awareness.

crystal POWER

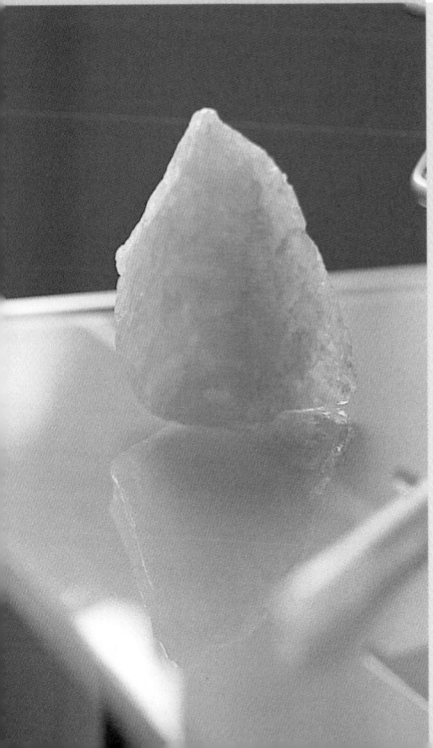

CRYSTAL HEALING FOR ENERGY REBALANCING

Hold a cleansed crystal (see page 34) for 5–10 minutes to boost your *chakras* and to give you spiritual inspiration.

1 Sit comfortably in a chair holding your crystal next to your Solar plexus chakra (just below the breastbone, see page 15). Close your eyes and tune in to the crystal's power, having already set its main intent (see page 34). Ask for increased energy flow through your *chakras*.

2 Now, place the crystal briefly on your Crown chakra on the top of your head and then your Third eye chakra in the middle of your forehead. Ask for spiritual and intuitive insight into current problems. Open your eyes and thank the crystal for its help.

The middle of the afternoon is a time when you can feel lethargic and a bit low, weighed down by the events and aggravations of the day. Spend a few minutes breathing out negative emotions that have accumulated inside to soothe you mind and spirit. This exercise can evoke a sense of calm as you realign your body's energies, smoothing out the flow of energy. Physically your heart and lungs will also benefit as they receive extra health-giving oxygen.

By the end of this exercise your whole mind and body will feel energized and ready to cope with any challenging events that confront you later on in the afternoon.

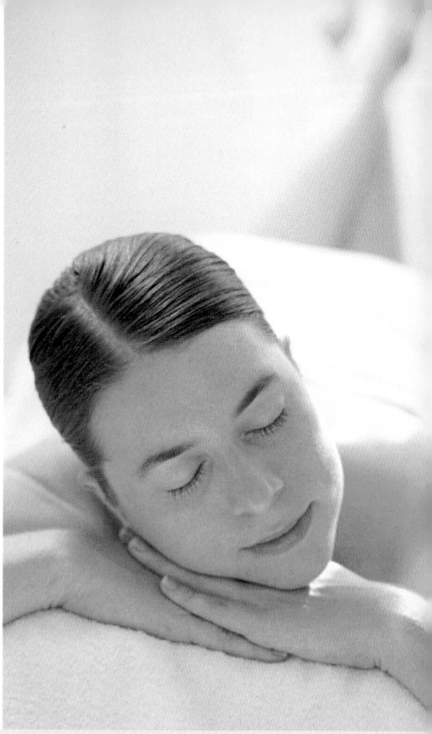

centering

BREATHING TO REBALANCE

Practise this breathing exercise for about 5–10 minutes until you feel all irritations leaving you.

1 Sit comfortably in a chair, close your eyes and start taking slow, deep breaths from your diaphragm. When you have a regular breathing rhythm start to imagine that you are going down a well into the centre of your being.

2 As you inhale, take in the warm healing energy that is at the bottom of the well. As you breathe out, let go of all the negative thoughts and emotions that have built up during the day.

3 As you go deeper inside yourself, appreciate the silence, peace and self-love – no arguments, criticisms, fears or doubts can reach you here. Experience the bliss of connecting with your inner spirit in every part of your body. Slowly return up the well and come to, refreshed and ready for the rest of the afternoon's challenges.

AFTERNOON AFFIRMATION

Choose your positive phrase carefully, and make it short and to the point. Write it on a Post-it and stick it somewhere you can see it.

1 Sit comfortably, or walk up and down, as you repeat your phrase (out loud, preferably). In connection with the examples right, it may be: 'I am getting the extra staff I need for my project' or 'The headteacher offers a helpful strategy to improve my child's school performance'.

2 Really feel and mean what you are saying. Repeat 10–20 times to fix it in your subconscious and say it regularly throughout the afternoon.

Energy tip

Smell some rosemary essential oil from a tissue (see page 56) as you do your affirmation to help increase your concentration.

Positive affirmations can help you achieve what you want, but you have got to believe they are going to happen. If you undertook the other affirmations earlier in the day (see pages 47 and 59) you will have benefited from the strength and confidence they have given you.

This afternoon affirmation can work on your goals later in the day or even the next morning. You may have an important meeting before you go home that is crucial to a current project so focus on a favourable outcome. Or you may have an appointment with your child's headteacher about his poor school-work performance, so use a phrase that shows the situation being mutually resolved.

achieving YOUR AIMS

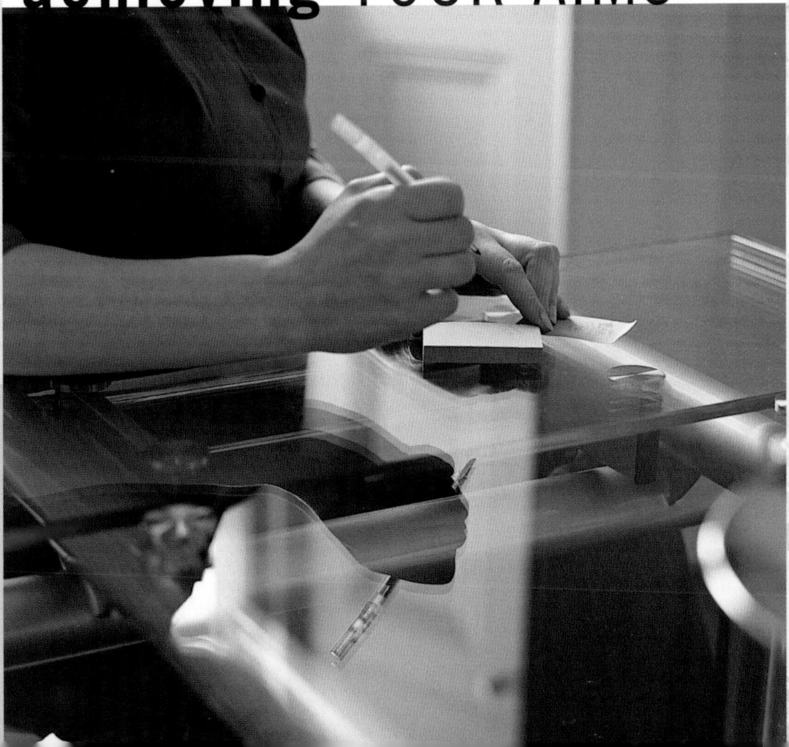

A work space, in an office, at home or any environment, needs to be well ordered, tidy and have good storage facilities for a good energy flow that encourages clear decision-making, creativity and business success. In feng shui, the art of furniture placement and energy flow, *chi* (energy) moves in spirals around a room. When this flow is obstructed by junk on the floor or surfaces, it becomes sluggish, slow and sticky affecting the atmosphere of your work area, so that you lack direction or enthusiasm for your projects.

Clearing out unwanted rubbish or clutter in mid-afternoon spurts over a week will create a substantial energy shift that allows space for new people or new projects to enter. Furthermore, it helps you to work with more confidence and drive.

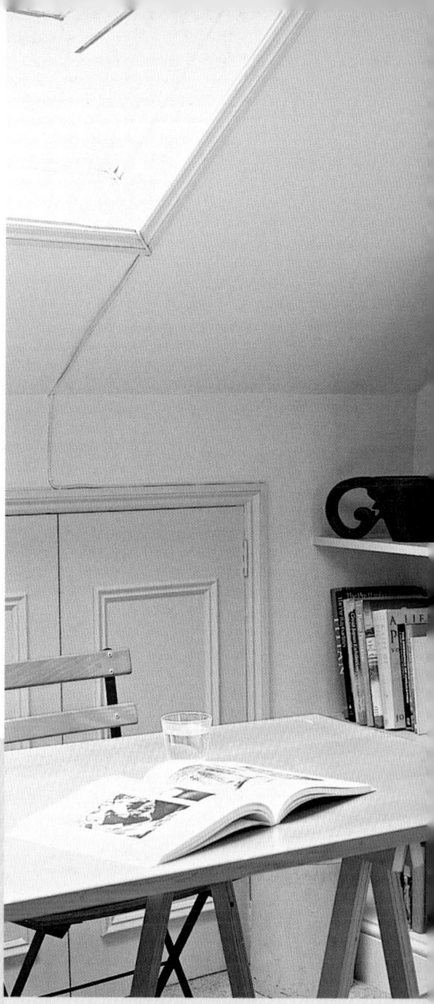

clearing OUT

Clever storage

If you have had a big clear-out but still have essential items that need to find 'homes', see where you could add new storage units; slim ones can fit in small spaces. Could you build more shelves above or below existing ones or fit more under sloping ceilings? Keep an eye out for clever storage items that can do more than one thing: space-saving shelves or tables that open up and store books or magazines hidden inside. Buy insert trays for slim metal cabinets that can sit under tables or desks to hold small pieces of stationery, home crafts, samples or other business items.

Any environment needs to be well ordered, tidy and have good storage facilities for good energy flow.

Clutter tip

The definition of work clutter is:

- Something no longer needed or wanted.
- A broken item or one that can't be fixed.
- Something disliked or outmoded.

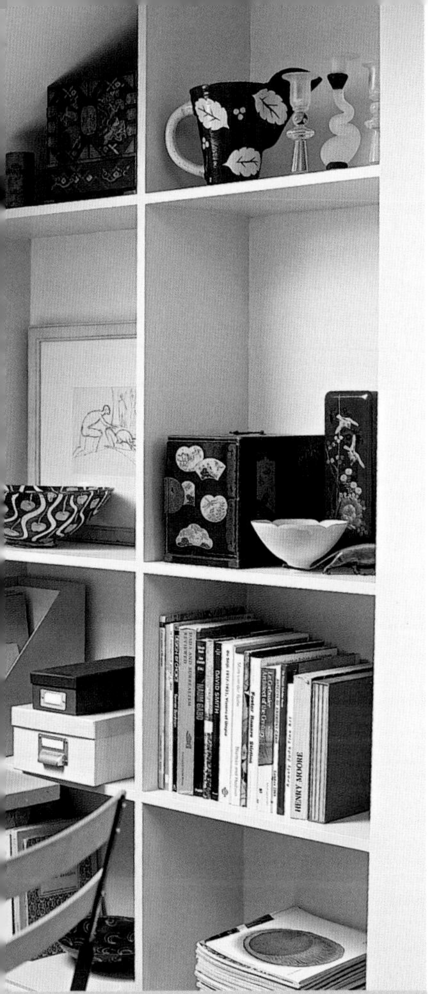

CLEARING YOUR WORK SPACE

Write a list of your worst clutter piles and start on them first.

Spend 10–15 minutes clearing every day until the piles are gone.

1. Make the floor area a priority. Recycle any unwanted papers, magazines (file any clippings of interest) or outdated stationery. Go through boxes of old materials and be ruthless, keeping only what you use. In terms of storage, try to set up files on shelves to keep the floor free. Clear box files and, again, arrange them on shelves. Store anything that's not current in a cabinet or cupboard.
2. Empty wastepaper bins daily – they are pools of stagnancy.
3. Go through filing cabinets and thin house or work files down; save what is current, remove anything that is redundant and recycle what's not needed.
4. Clear your desk space. Keep invoices or bills in a bring-forward file or a pending tray. Refer on files or reports or store them in a cabinet as soon as you have dealt with them. Remove old Post-its and business cards, transferring phone numbers or useful information to your personal organizer or notebook. Deal with correspondence immediately, then file. Throw out broken pens, pencils, rulers and other old stationery, store essentials in a holder on the desk. Aim to leave your desk completely clear at the end of the day.
5. Sort through your bookshelves. Give away any duplicate books and any books that are no longer used. Save only up-to-date reference books and arrange logically on shelves; ditch any old ones as they keep you stuck in the past.

Write a list of your worst clutter piles and start on them first.

CLEAR your computer

You're probably feeling renewed after clearing your work space (see pages 94–95), now it's time to sort out your computer. When both the hard disk and RAM are overloaded your computer becomes slow and inefficient. Conflicts between different software programs can also cause frustration, such as the computer 'freezing' or 'crashing'. When your computer is full and taking a long time to carry out simple commands, it can negatively affect you mentally and emotionally; the result is that you feel frustrated and out of control with your projects.

Try to spend 10 minutes or so each afternoon to clear out unwanted files, programs and correspondence. Have a plan of attack; how are you going to sort through all your various folders? Even after a day or two, you'll notice how your spirits rise as extraneous work disappears.

Computer tip

Put a rose quartz crystal next to your computer. This healing stone will protect you from any electromagnetic stress.

When your computer is full and taking a long time to carry out simple commands, it can negatively affect you.

MAKING COMPUTER SPACE

Spend 10–15 minutes daily freeing up space on your computer so that you reduce any confusion in finding what you want. After a while, you may find you become almost obsessive about any unfiled items and you'll be delighted to see how organized your hard disk has become.

1 Go through your email inbox and delete any old messages. Print out or file onto the hard disk the ones you have to keep for reference. Remember to delete any sent mail as well.

2 Look through your hard disk and delete or archive onto storage disks correspondence files or projects that are no longer current. Remove software programs that are out of date (or get some professional help if you are unsure) or redundant.

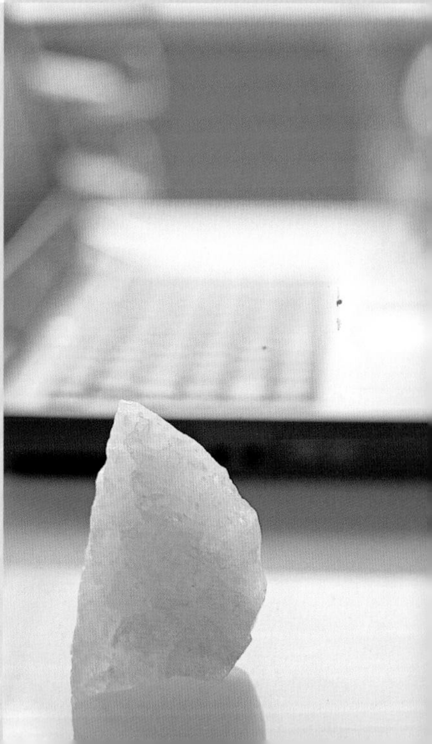

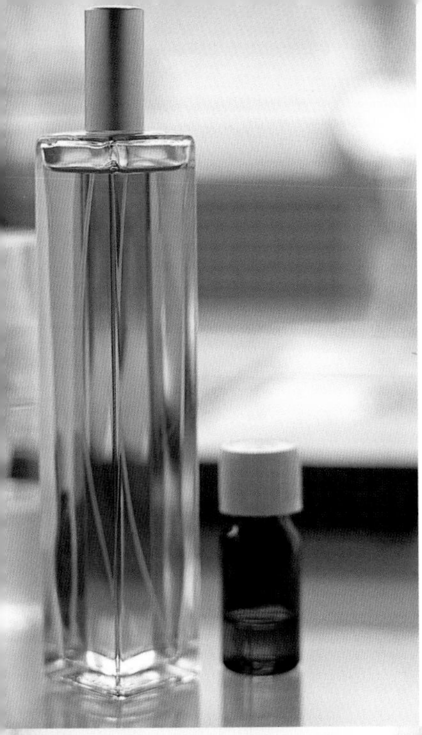

After your clear-out, you may be left with a slight, musty atmosphere as old dusty articles have been shifted from the floor and surfaces. Once you have cleaned everywhere thoroughly, spend a short time space clearing the room or desk to dispel any lingering stagnancy. The technique can cleanse the existing *chi*, leaving a new bright, vibrancy that will encourage a positive working attitude.

There are several methods of space clearing (see pages 116–123) but if you work in an open-plan space (where other people are involved), the simplest is misting essential oils.

PURIFYING **a work space**

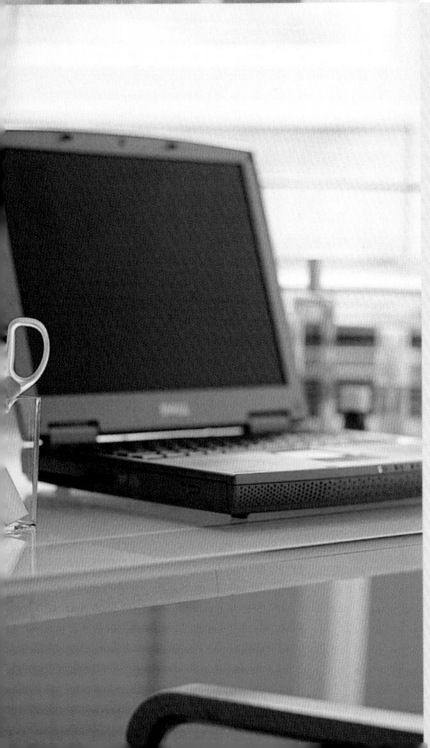

SPACE CLEARING YOUR WORK AREA

Spend a few minutes spraying aromatic essential oils around your work area to change the atmosphere and boost productivity.

Stimulating and cleansing oils

- Use eucalyptus, lemongrass or rosemary essential oils.

1. Put 4 drops of oil in a mister bottle and half fill with water; mix (see also page 117). Spray around you first to revitalize your aura (see also page 131).
2. If you have a contained work space, spray round it in a clockwise direction, misting high into the corners, asking for a more positive, successful and creative space. Also mist round and under your desk and over your computer and chair.

As your energy levels plummet mid-afternoon, try this colour exercise to boost your body organs and glands and your *chakras* (see page 15 and 49).

The healing colour vibrations that enter our bodies and *chakras* (see page 15) through sunlight are necessary for them to function well. Spending so much time indoors, working or doing chores at home, can mean we don't always get a natural 'top up' of this sunlight energy, which later in the day can leave us feeling a bit drained and lacking in motivation. Visualize the seven colours entering your body and flooding it with colour to rebalance your energy.

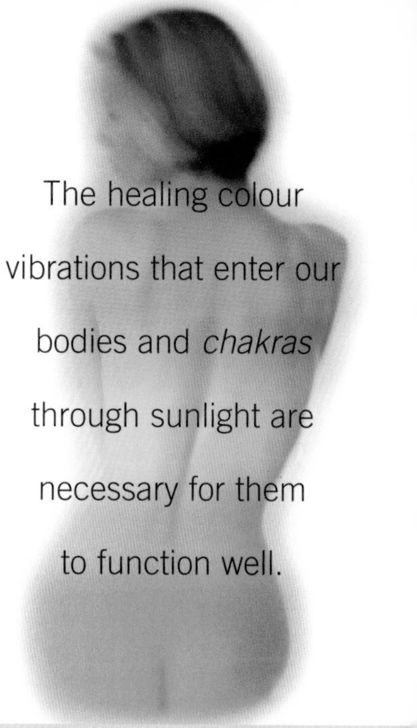

The healing colour vibrations that enter our bodies and *chakras* through sunlight are necessary for them to function well.

COLOUR VISUALIZATION

Spend 5–10 minutes regularly filling your body with the healing colours of the rainbow.

1. Sit comfortably and take some deep breaths from your diaphragm. Now visualize a bright red colour coming up your legs into your Root chakra (lower pelvis); feel it dispelling your fears.
2. Now, change the colour to a rich orange and see it filling your Sacral chakra (lower abdomen) and bringing joy. Next, see the colour as a bright yellow flooding your Solar plexus chakra (upper abdomen) and clearing your mind and emotions.
3. As the yellow fades, bring in a loving, purifying green colour to your Heart chakra (over the heart). Then visualize a turquoise in your Throat chakra (upper chest and throat) and sense how it helps your self-expression.
4. Let the blue fade to a deep indigo that washes over your Third eye chakra (middle of your forehead) and boosts your intuitive powers. Finally, see a soft violet colour entering your Crown chakra (top of your head), stimulating your spirit (your 'higher self'). As the colour disappears, come to, feeling revitalized and recharged.

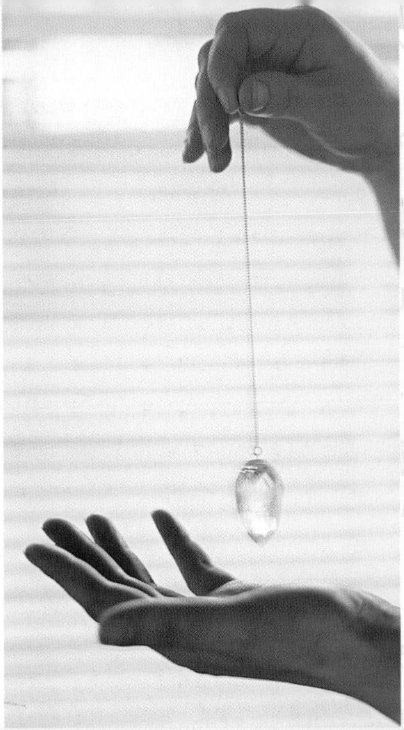

If you lack energy but don't quite know what *chakra* or which body area body is suffering, find out the colour you currently lack by using the dowsing technique.

Dowsing is an ancient technique that utilizes divining rods or pendulums to detect the presence of substances such as water and oil or unnatural earth energies. The technique works by asking questions of your subconscious mind (your inner self). Responses come through the electromagnetic energies emitted by your hands. This method also works on your body, so you can easily check which *chakra* is not balanced or underfunctioning.

DOWSING **for colour**

Essential equipment

- Buy a pendulum with a clear quartz crystal or make one by hanging a bead on a cord 15 cm (6 in) long.
- Make seven small cards of the *chakra* colours in red, orange, yellow, green, turquoise, indigo, violet.

THE DOWSING TECHNIQUE

Spend a few minutes daily dowsing to find out which colour (sometimes more than one) your body is lacking.

1 Hold your pendulum loosely in your hand and ask it which direction is 'yes'. It will spin either clockwise or anticlockwise. Ask it for 'no' and note these directions down. Finally ask for a 'don't know' response, which is normally swinging from side to side.

2 Now, hold the pendulum over each coloured card and ask in turn 'do I need this colour today'. Write down the responses. Keep the coloured card or cards you need in front of you, or with you, to look at regularly to absorb their healing vibrations.

Massaging your head mid-afternoon with simple hand movements is a wonderful release for any mental or emotional stress that has developed. It can also remove the strain from taut muscles and prevent the onset of a painful and debilitating headache (see page 57).

When your body is under stress, blood flow becomes restricted through the veins and arteries creating that 'tight' uncomfortable feeling, particularly in areas such as the head. As adrenaline is released from the adrenal glands to help you cope with a situation where quick reactions are needed, your heart beats faster and your muscles begin to ache as they tense or 'harden'. Working long hours hunched over a desk or driving for too long in a rigid position can also cause a stiff neck and eye strain.

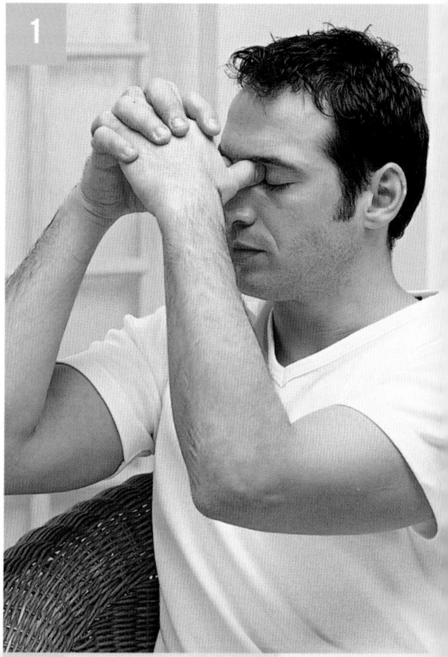
1

Mind and body release

Research by an Austrian psychoanalyst called Wilhelm Reich in the mid-twentieth century first reinforced massage as a holistic therapy. He expressed the belief that the mind and body were interconnected and that emotions such as anger or despair could be held in tense body areas and require release for good health and wellbeing.

Massaging your head is a wonderful release for any mental or emotional stress.

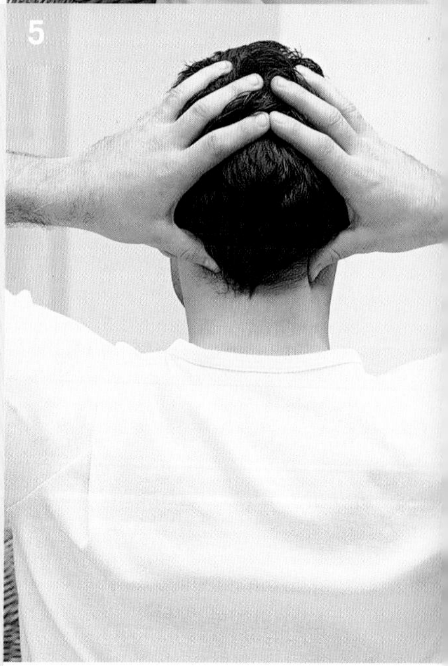
5

2

6

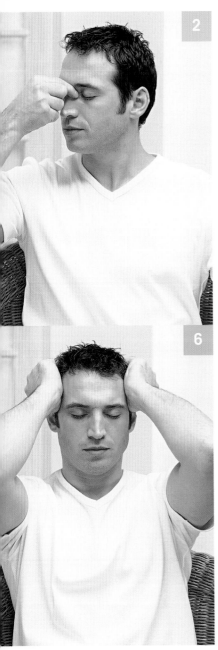

HEAD MASSAGE TECHNIQUE

This easy routine takes only 5–10 minutes and requires no oils. By applying pressure around your eyes and doing fingertip massage around your temples and the back of your neck, you can improve blood flow, release tension and encourage better oxygen flow to create a sense of wellbeing.

1. Close your eyes. Intertwine your fingers and press your thumbs into the corners of your eyes. Hold for about 3 seconds and then repeat 6 times to reduce eye strain.
2. With your right forefinger and thumb pinch your nose at the top; left-handers may prefer to use their left hand. Hold for about 3 seconds, release, then repeat 6 times to clear your vision and ease tiredness.
3. With you right forefinger, press on your Third eye chakra in the centre of your forehead. Hold for about 6 seconds, then release and repeat 4 times to shift any energy blockages.
4. With the first and second fingers of your right hand, push up from your eyebrows and over to the temple area to ease tension. Move across the face from right to left.
5. With your fingers apart, hold the back of your head and circle your thumbs around the fleshy area at the base of your skull to relieve neck muscle tension. Work around the area for a couple of minutes, stopping if it feels painful. Repeat once more.
6. Put your hands at the base of the back of your neck and move them up to your crown. Clutch a handful of hair each side and tug for a few seconds. Now slide your fingers to the temples at the side of your head, clutch your hair again and tug gently from side to side. Repeat both actions 2 or 3 times, then smooth your fingers through your hair and feel your mental frustrations lifting.

The afternoon is often the time when the pace of a busy day catches up with you. If you have been on the phone constantly or typing important emails, or spent hours in meetings or rushing about organizing children you may well feel pressured. These short reflexology routines can give you instant benefits and reduce unpleasant stress symptoms.

Reflexology (see pages 64–65) is a massage technique that works on pressure points on the hands and feet to increase energy flow in the ten 'reflex' zones and to remove any existing blockages in the muscles and organs that may be causing pain. The two routines here work mainly on the hands and help smooth out energy blocks to reduce the gripes of a stressed stomach and the twinges and soreness of early repetitive strain injury (RSI) symptoms in your fingers, hands, wrists and shoulders.

These short reflexology routines can give you instant benefits and reduce unpleasant stress symptoms.

SOOTHING **reflexology**

RELIEF FOR A STRESSED STOMACH

Work on the points for several minutes if your stomach is reacting badly to a stressful day.

1 Press with your left thumb on the liver point of your right hand, halfway down from your little finger. Also work on the gallbladder point, in and down from your second finger.

2 If you have cramping stomach pains, work on the thyroid point on the outside of your right hand in between your thumb and your forefinger.

3 Also work on the parathyroid reflexes (see step 2) between your thumb and your forefinger and the solar plexus point in the middle of your hand under the third finger. Stimulate the diaphragm point, too, which curves across the middle of the hand from under the little finger.

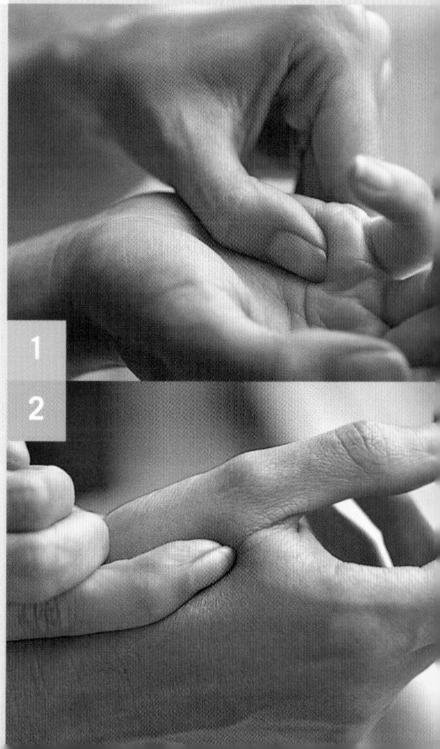
1
2

The afternoon is often the time when the pace of a busy day catches up with you.

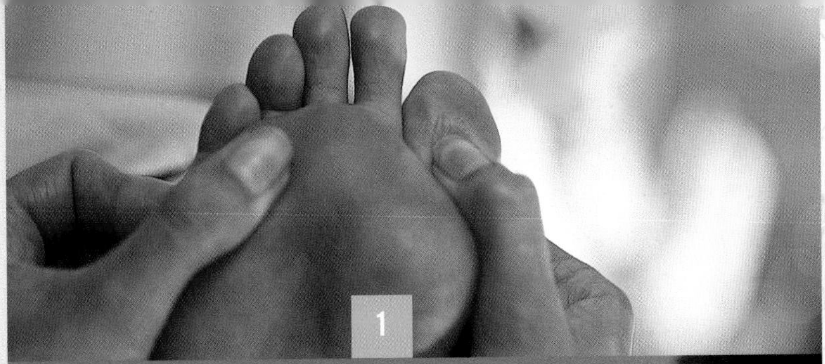
1

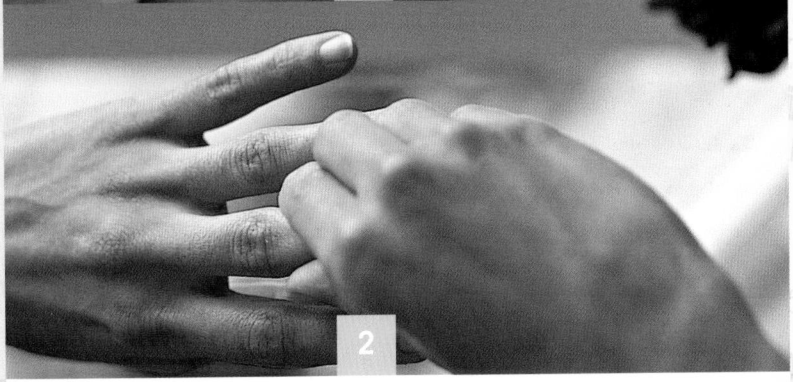
2

Reflexology tips

- Wash your hands before and also after a treatment as you are working with stagnant energy.
- Work gently on any sensitive areas with the tips of your middle finger and forefinger.

RELEASING RSI-TYPE SYMPTOMS

Press on these points for several minutes to ease strain in your hands, arms and shoulders.

1 Start working with your thumbs across the top of the sole of one foot, concentrating on the neck (under the big toe) and shoulder girdle (under the little toe, see picture). Do the same on the other foot. Then work on the arm and hand reflexes down the top half of your right foot from your little toe. Alternatively work on your hands.

2 Work on the hip and leg reflexes further down the side of the right foot to move energy down the body. Finally stretch and rotate each finger of both hands to break the stress-holding patterns (see picture).

As the evening draws near, you can become aware of many tense areas in your muscles from the rigours of the day. Recognizing where they are, and how they have become tense, is the first step towards loosening or relaxing them, and preventing it happening again. When you release muscle tension you can also relieve a headache or backache that has built up during the day. The process also benefits and helps clear your mind as it automatically quietens as you focus on letting go.

Once you know the muscle-releasing technique well, you will sense when your muscles are tightening and be easily able to relax them.

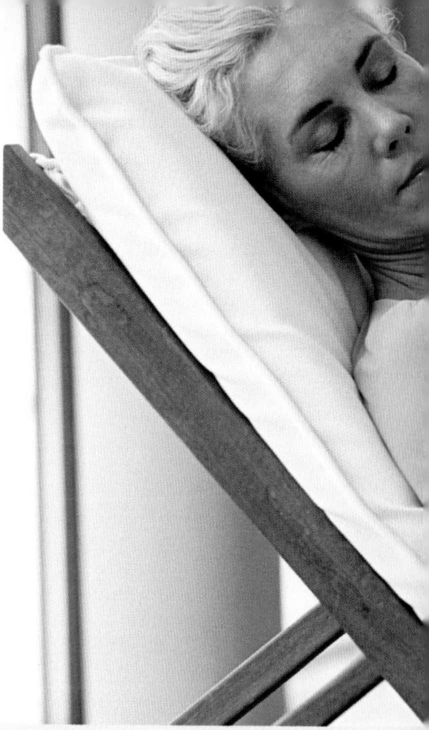

LETTING GO **of tension**

THE MUSCLE-RELEASING TECHNIQUE

Work with this technique for at least 10 minutes, maybe more, to loosen up your body and inspire your mind.

When you release muscle tension you can also relieve a headache or backache.

1 Sit comfortably or lie down. Close your eyes or focus on a fixed point ahead of you. Take 4 long, deep breaths from your diaphragm, and then breathe with a light, even rhythm.

2 Now take your attention to your toes, breathe in and tense them for about 5 seconds, then let go as you breathe out, feeling all the tightness flowing out. Notice what effect it has on your whole body. Repeat once or twice, then move on to your lower legs and repeat the movement there, again seeing how it feels in the rest of your body.

3 In the same way, work up your body tensing and releasing the major muscle groups in turn: your thighs, buttocks, lower back, stomach, chest, shoulders, arms, hands and neck, noticing any tense or tight areas loosening up.

4 When you get to your face, screw it up tightly, hold for

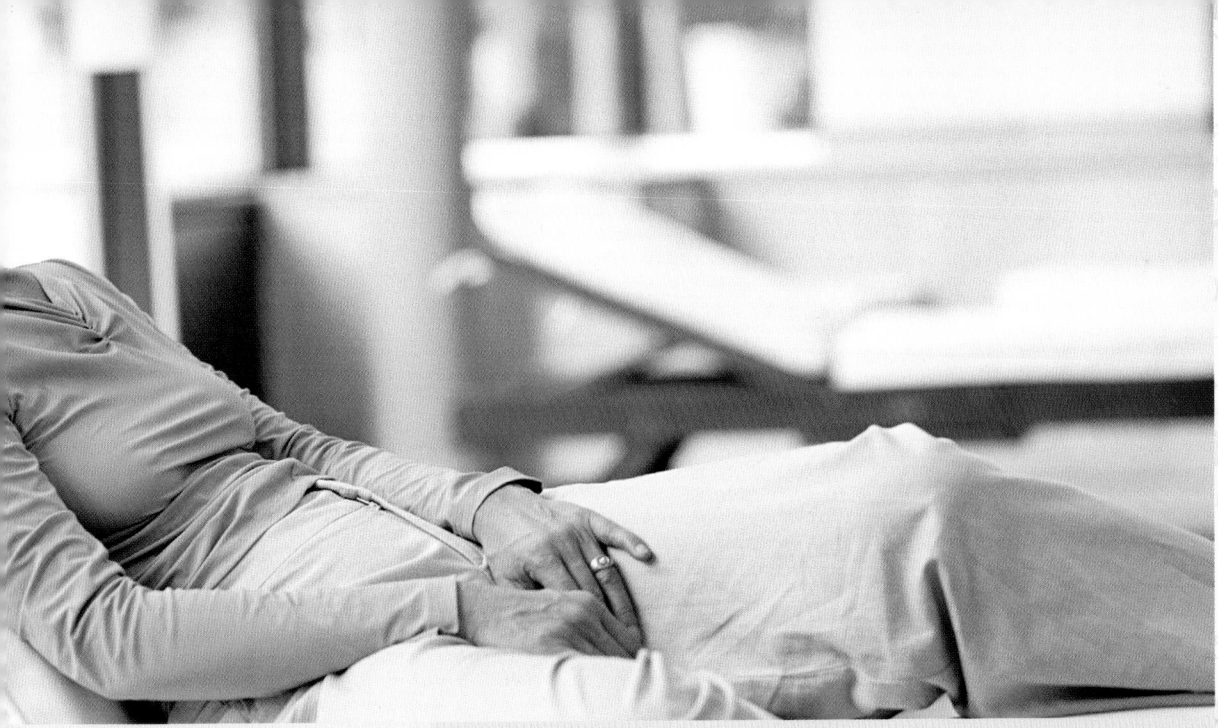

5 seconds and release. Then open your eyes and mouth wide, again holding for 5 seconds before releasing. Repeat twice.

5 Now tense your whole body from your toes to your head, hold for a few seconds and let go: see how heavy and loose your body feels when you let go. Relax for a few moments, and then open your eyes, feeling recharged and ready to continue your afternoon.

QUICK RELAXATION ROUTINE

If you have an important meeting or want to unwind before going out and your muscles feel very taut, carry out this 2–3-minute routine, to release any tension.

1 Concentrate on breathing slowly and choose a cue word such as 'Release' and repeat it in your mind as you start to relax.

2 Take a deep breath and at the same time clench a group of muscles in areas of your body where tension gathers, such as your face, neck, shoulders, chest and stomach.

3 As you breathe out, let go of your muscles, feeling all the tightness and tension simply slipping away.

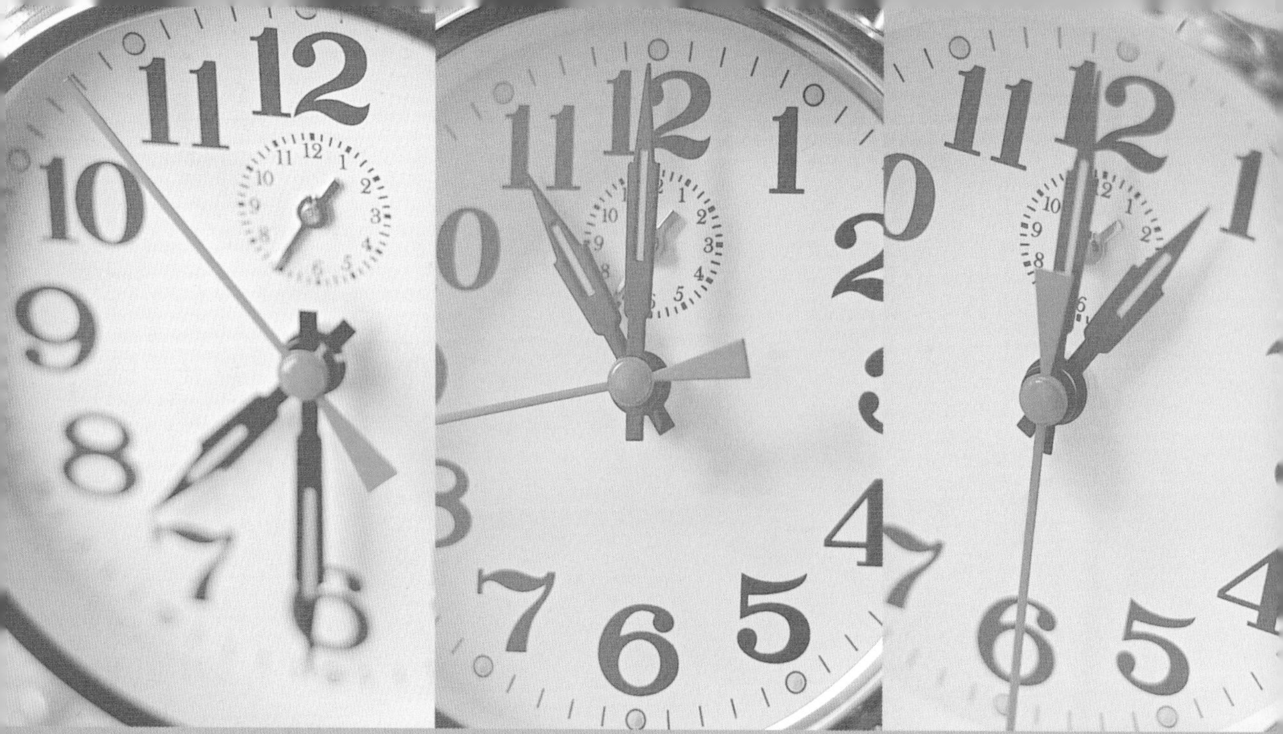

9 Evening refreshers

Sit down and reflect on your day; some are best forgotten, but for most days you can look back on your achievements with satisfaction.

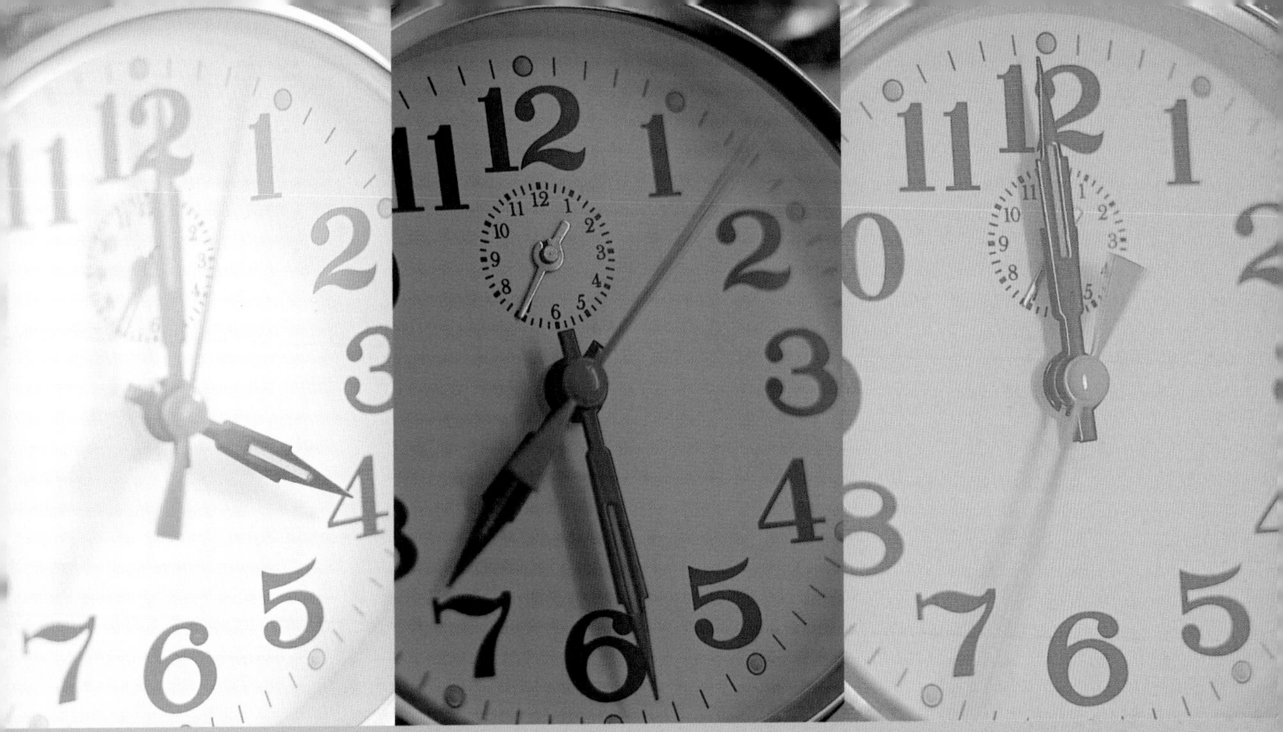

When you reach the end of a busy day, you can feel quite drained, mentally and emotionally. What is more, if you have a long journey home from work or need to put your children to bed before you can wind down, you can feel even more exhausted when you finally get some time to yourself. Sit down and reflect on your day; some are best forgotten, but for most days you can look back on your achievements with satisfaction. Give yourself some well-deserved praise for everything that you have done.

Now you have started to relax, choose an exercise from this section to harmonize your inner and outer *chi.* Lift your spirits with a wonderful scented bath, dismiss the cares of the day by dancing to some lively music, do some drumming to raise the energy levels in your living room or ease the aches of the day with a neck and shoulder massage with oils.

Select the evening energizer that you know will work best for how you feel and will give you optimism and verve for the hours ahead.

Letting go of the physical and mental tensions of a busy day coping with children, dealing with customers or spending hours in front of a computer is essential to your wellbeing. If you work outside the home, you also have the added aggravation of commuting. One of the best ways of freeing all the day's stresses, and restoring your energy for the evening ahead, is to spend some time on your own soaking in a perfumed bath.

Essential oils (see page 30–31 and 56–57) evoke the wonderful scents of the plants or flowers from which they are extracted. When they are added to a warm bath their therapeutic aromas are breathed in and are also absorbed by your skin, producing immediate psychological and physical benefits that will last all evening.

One of the best ways of freeing all the day's stresses is to spend some time on your own soaking in a perfumed bath.

CANDELIGHT **bathing**

FRAGRANT BATH WITH MAGICAL CANDLES

Choose from the essential oil blends below or experiment with mixing your own to find the one that calms your soul and lifts your spirits. (Safe note: always remember to extinguish all candles after finishing your bath.)

Healing oils

- Lavender and basil oil to calm emotions and clear the mind.
- Geranium and jasmine oil to ease nervous tension and lift the mood.
- Lime and ylang ylang oil to reduce any anxiety and stimulate sluggish organs.

1 Run a bath. When it is full put 3–4 drops each of your chosen oil blend in the water and agitate gently to mix them in.

2 Sink into the bath, close your eyes and let the oils do their work. Shut down your mind and feel all the aches of the day dissolving into the water. Stay in the bath for at least 15 minutes to absorb the curative qualities of the oils.

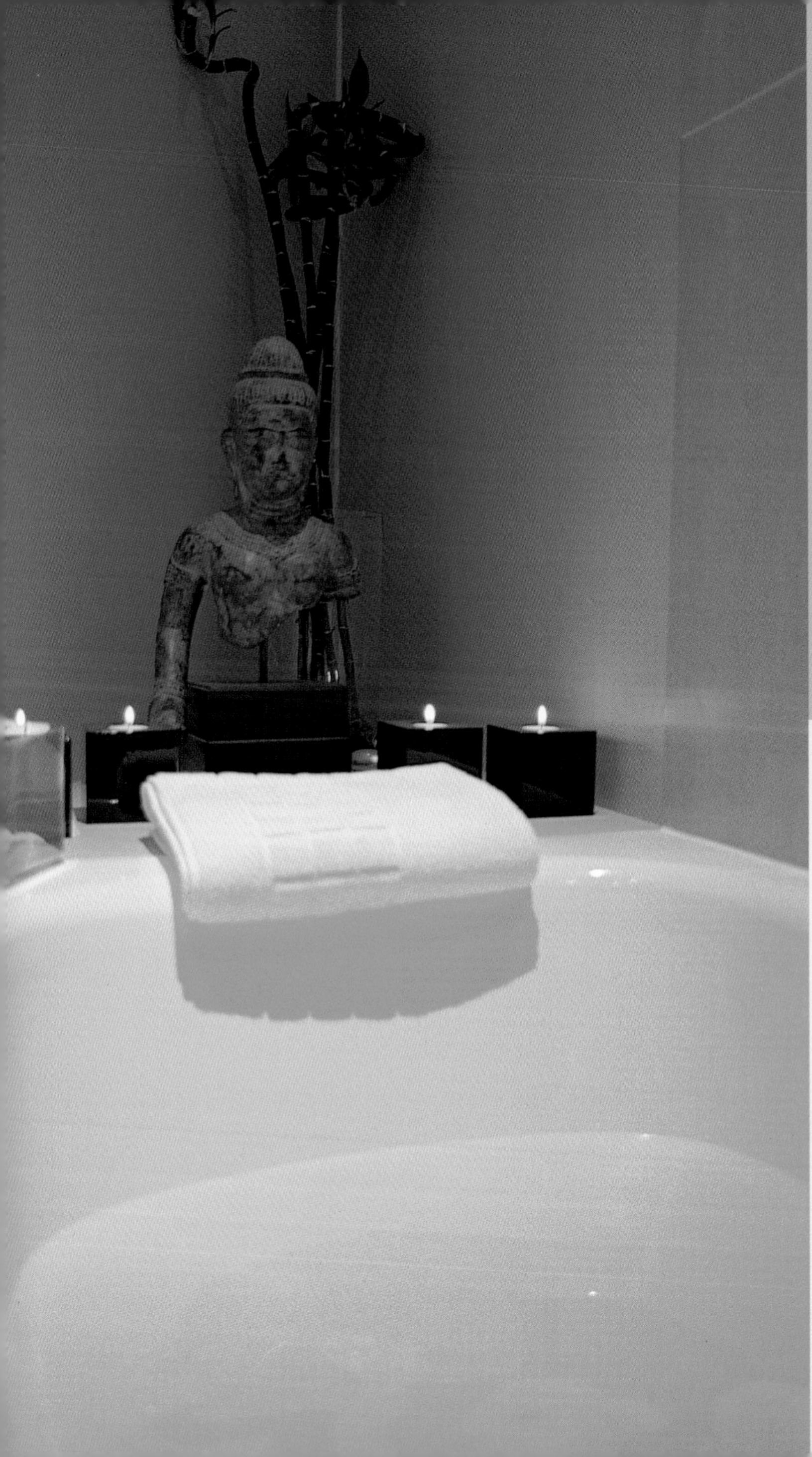

Inspiring candles

Soft, flickering candles around the bath or in wall sconces can create a soft, relaxing ambience when you are soaking the day away. They can also lift the energy flow in a bathroom, which is naturally sluggish and yin (passive). This is because candles link to the Fire element in feng shui and are considered yang (positive). You can also bring in some colour therapy by using green candles to harmonize your energy; white candles can bring protection.

Oil tip

Maximize your benefits by making a blend of oils for massaging into your skin. Mix 3 drops of each chosen oil into 20 ml/4 teaspoons of sweet almond or grapeseed base oil. After your bath, rub the oil well into your skin, starting at your feet and working upwards towards the heart.

Neck and shoulder tension often builds up over a working day. Being rigid in the same position for a long time is a common trigger. When muscles are tight they feel sore and uncomfortable, and the veins and arteries become restricted, resulting in poor blood flow. The lymphatic system can also become sluggish and does not pick up toxins so easily. Knotted muscles are also thought to restrict the flow of *chi* (see page 11) around the body and can affect your mental and emotional outlook.

Massaging taut muscles releases endorphins ('happy hormones') in to the body.

Energy tip

As you are stretching your upper body, repeat this relaxing mantra out loud 10 times: 'I am releasing all stress and tension from my neck and shoulders'.

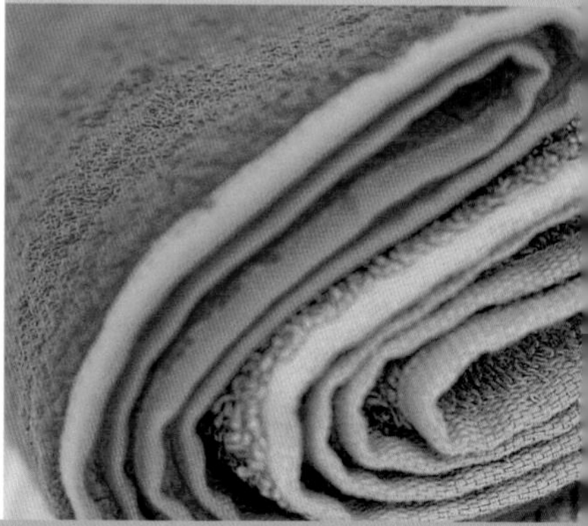

SOOTHE **and stretch**

NECK AND SHOULDER MASSAGE

Massaging taut muscles eases the tension, releases endorphins (the 'happy hormones') into the body, increases blood flow to the organs and slows your breathing. Knead a soothing oil mixture into your shoulder and neck muscles for about 5–10 minutes to remove daily strains.

A soothing oil mixture

- Mix 3 drops each of lavender and geranium essential oil into 20 ml/4 teaspoons sweet almond or grapeseed base oil.

1 Remove your top or slip it over your shoulders. Sit in a chair and rub oil into your hands. With your right hand, work on your left shoulder, kneading the muscles to loosen the tension. Move up and down the shoulder several times. Then, repeat on your right shoulder using your left hand.

2 With both hands, use your fingers to squeeze and release the neck muscles, working from the bottom of your neck up to the base of the skull and down again. Repeat several times. Finally, with your right hand only, knead or grip your neck muscles, several times until any tightness relaxes.

NECK AND SHOULDER STRETCHING

If you return home from work with a knotted neck and stiff shoulders but have insufficient time to do the neck and shoulder massage opposite, try this quick routine. It is a simple stretching exercise using a rolled bath towel that can alleviate the tension in your aching muscles in just a few minutes, leaving you rejuvenated for the evening ahead.

The stretching routine

You can get your blood circulation flowing more smoothly by stretching your neck and shoulders muscles with a bath towel in this simple routine.

1 Kneel on a mat on the floor in your bedroom or bathroom. Roll up a warm bath towel and put it round your neck, holding it with both hands. Lean back and arch your neck and hold for a few seconds, then release, feeling the tension lessening. Repeat 6 times.

2 Pull the ends of the towel down and wrap around your shoulders. Holding the towel tightly, push your fists into the small of your back, moving your elbows back to increase the pressure on your tight shoulders, and open your chest. Hold for a few seconds then release, feeling tension knots dissolving as you do so. Repeat 6 times.

1

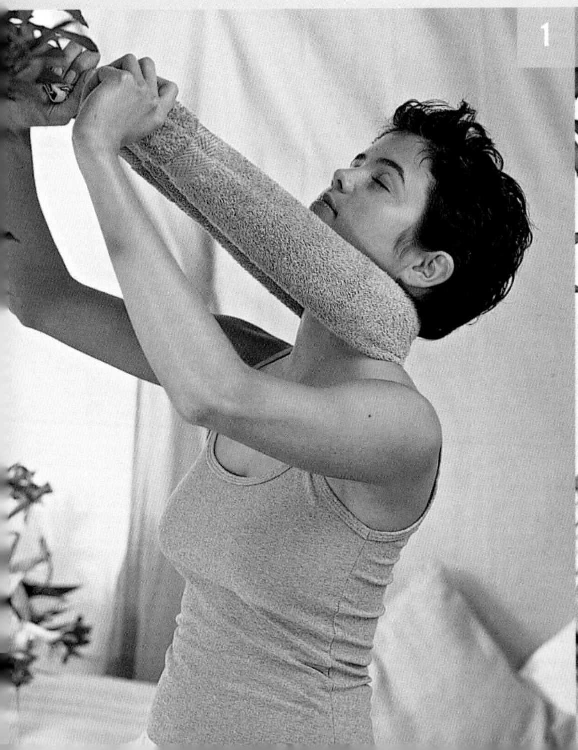

2

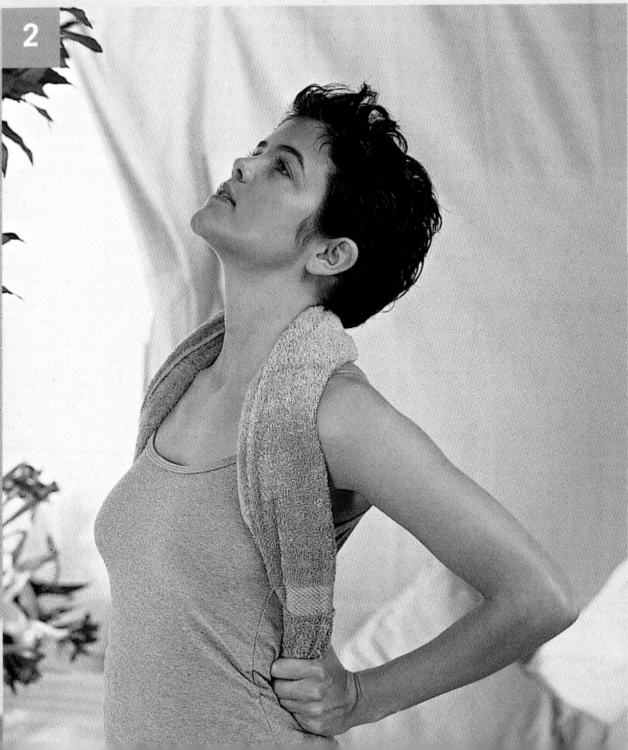

This type of breathing is a form of *pranayama* (breath control) that is used in yoga (see page 17). Practising this technique, where you breathe in through the left nostril and then the right, encourages the breath to flow smoothly through the seven main *chakras* in the body (see page 15) and remove any negative energy blockages that it encounters. It balances the body's masculine (the right nostril) and feminine (the left nostril) energies that need to be in harmony for complete wellbeing. This powerful breathing technique also helps to purify the nervous system, clear the mind and relax the body. It is often used before meditation.

Practise this in the early evening to clear the worries and anxieties of the day and leave you refreshed to enjoy the rest of the night.

POWERFUL **breathing**

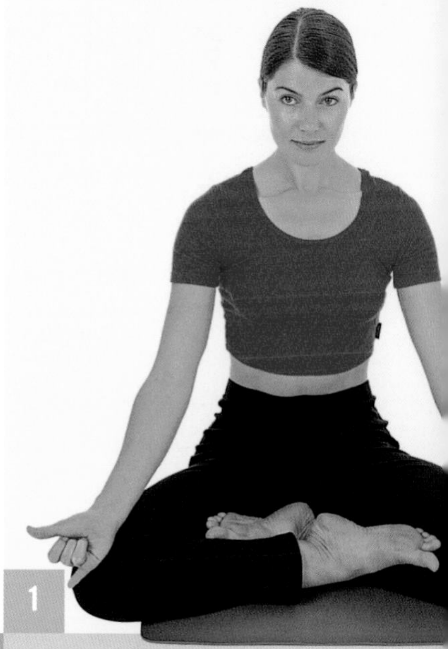

1

Mini meditation

Do this short meditation for about 5 minutes at the end of your working day to quieten a busy mind.

- Sit cross-legged on the floor and follow the meditation technique on page 41. As you focus on one thought try to let go of the day. As work thoughts or problems intrude let them float past you and visualize them flying out of a nearby window.
- As your mind stills and you start to relax, feel a sense of peace filling your body and mind. Just before you open your eyes, praise yourself for what you have achieved during the day, don't focus on any negatives, instead just send good energy towards the following day.

Practising this technique encourages the breath to flow smoothly through the seven main *chakras* in the body and remove any negative energy blockages that it encounters.

2
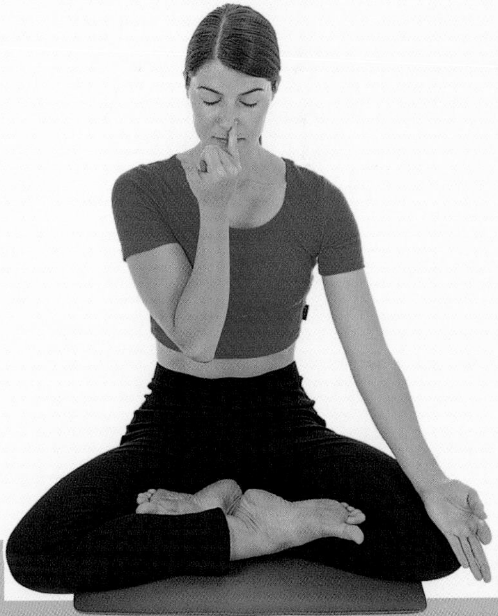

3
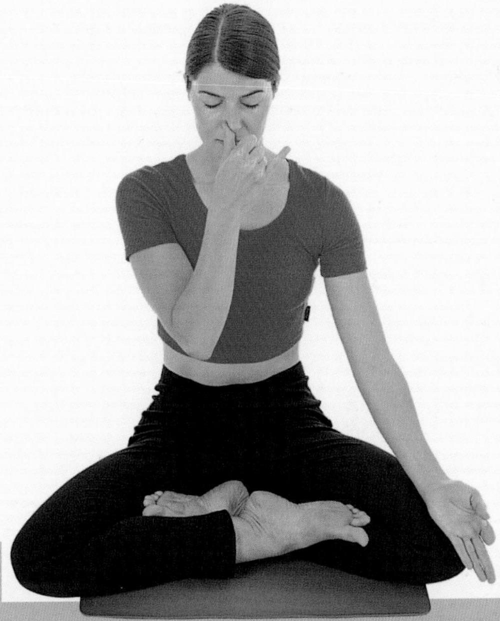

ALTERNATE NOSTRIL BREATHING

Use this method to breathe for a few minutes. You will notice that the breath is stronger and louder on the right.

1 Sit cross-legged on the floor or in the lotus or half-lotus position with your spine straight. Put your arms on your knees. Touch your first finger and thumb together of your left hand and fold in the middle three fingers of your right hand, keeping your thumb and little finger extended. These gestures are hand *mudras*, which are subtle movements that embody a spiritual meaning. Breathe deeply and evenly from the diaphragm.

2 Lift up your right hand and block your left nostril with your little finger. Breathe in and then out deeply through the right nostril letting all the air out of your lungs. Repeat this breathing process for 10 breaths.

3 Now block the right nostril with your right thumb and breathe in and out for about 10 seconds. Repeat the exercises 3–5 times on each side, and then finish by breathing deeply through both nostrils again as in the first step.

Dance movement is an arts therapy that shows how a person expresses any emotional disturbance through their body movements. Everyone has an individual way of moving; in a class a therapist analyses each person working out their strengths and sees where they may benefit from developing more self-awareness and group interaction.

In a simpler way you can use the dance technique at home in the early evening to release any emotional upset and angst from the day. Dancing can also increase your energy levels as you enthusiastically move all your limbs, shaking out all held tension. Music evokes powerful emotions in everyone: classical pieces can uplift our spirits, soothe our souls or even make us cry, while popular music can make us shout with joy as we sing along to a favourite number.

Regularly dancing to stimulating music with a strong beat, such as rock, jazz or Latin music, such as salsa, can give your body and mind a welcome release and some escapism after a busy, demanding or upsetting day.

expressive DANCING

DANCE AWAY FRUSTRATIONS

Create your own special space to dance away your daily frustrations for about 10 minutes each night. It can help remove energy blocks and give you the mental stimulation to enjoy the evening ahead.

1 Prepare the room in which you are going to dance. Make sure it is warm, dim the lights, close the curtains, turn off the phone so you are not disturbed. Wear some loose and comfortable clothing and choose a lively dance track.

2 Turn the volume up to a reasonable level and start to dance, building up from a slow rhythm to something faster and more energetic. If there are lyrics you love, express yourself further by singing along with them (see page 81).

3 It may feel strange to start with, but don't worry if you are not used to dancing by yourself – no one can see you. Get into the rhythm of the music, feel the beat moving through your legs, hips, shoulders and arms. Start to dance faster, doing more energetic movements and feel how your muscles become less stiff and move with more fluidity. Dance for about 10 minutes or more until you lose the worries of the day and feel new energy freely surging through your body.

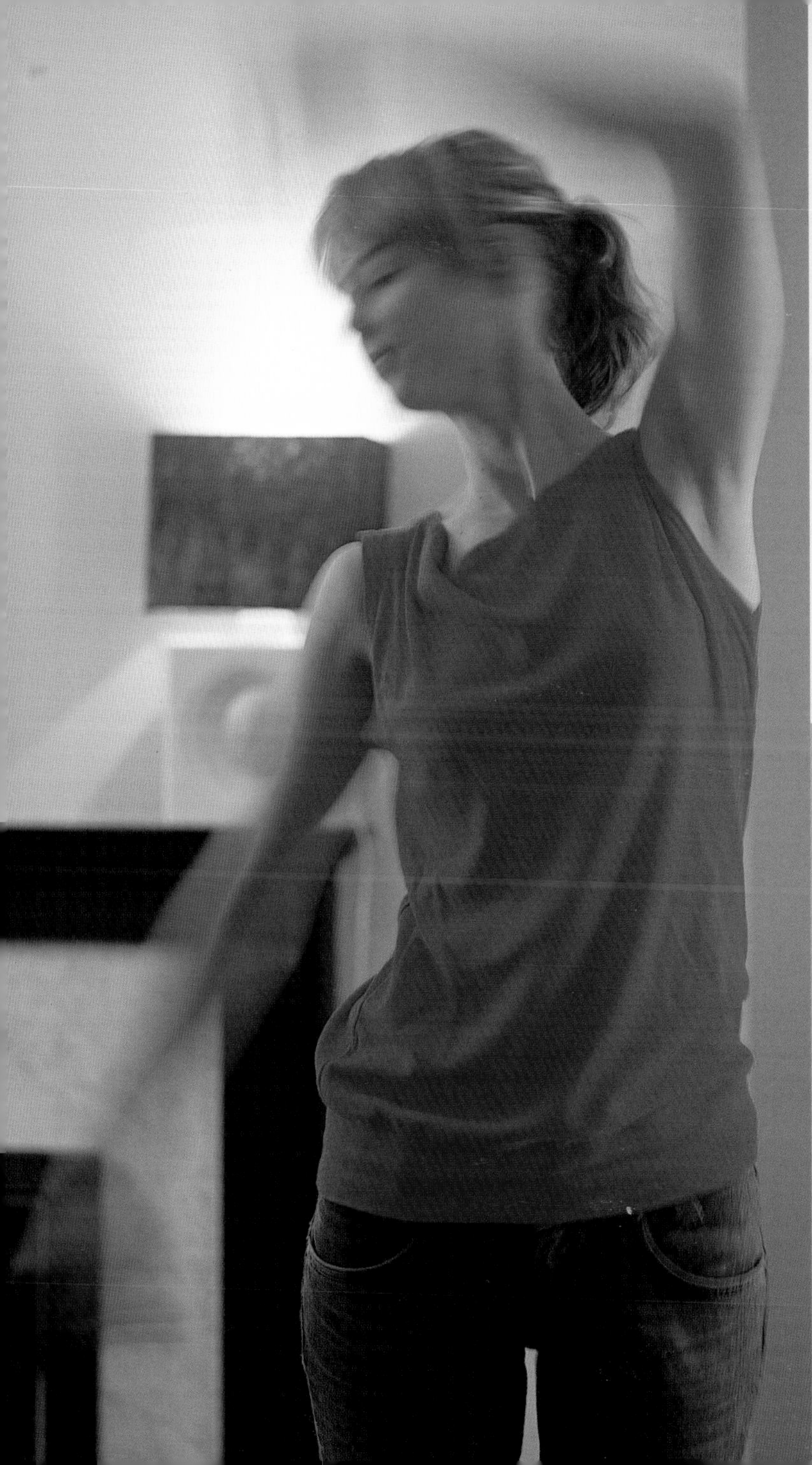

You can dance at home in the early evening to release any emotional upset and angst from the day.

Dance classes

If you really enjoy dancing, consider joining a weekly dance class locally, such as Ceroc or Le Roc (jiving techniques) or salsa. Classes are available in many areas and can be very sociable. They normally start with lessons in the early part of the evening with a 'freestyle' section later, where everyone has the opportunity to dance with each other.

Hoarding junk in your home can block its positive energy flow, while arguments, upsets, illness and other incidents all leave their energetic imprint on the building. By removing clutter and using a purifying technique you can raise the energy frequency, creating balance and harmony once more.

At the end of a long day the atmosphere in certain rooms of your home can often seem a bit sluggish or dull. If this is left unchanged, you can start to feel lethargic and uninspired about the evening ahead. Try these easy, refreshing techniques to lift the flagging energy levels and clear out negative energy. You'll feel instantly better, and able to look forward to a great night out or a creative evening at home.

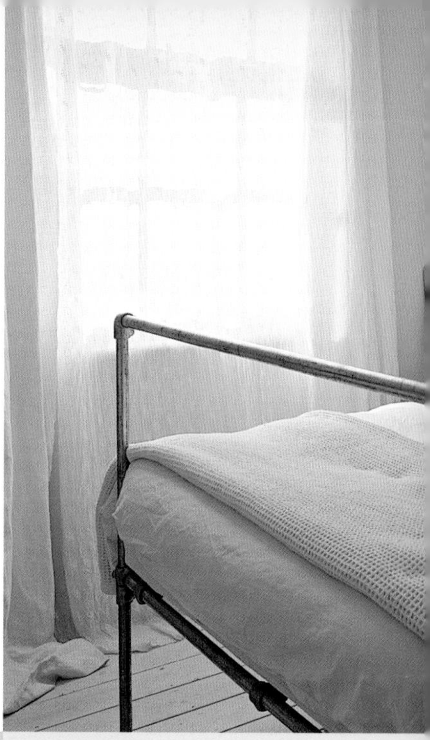

ROOM **purifying**

CLAPPING

Clapping is a wonderful, simple sound technique that gets rid of any stagnant or low energy areas in a room by loosening the energetic imprint. Clap for 5–10 minutes, first practising a few fast claps in a corner. If they sound muffled or very dull, the *chi* (energy) is very low and you will need to clap from floor to ceiling to disperse it.

1 Stand in the doorway of your room and focus on clearing dead energy as you clap clockwise round the room, doing small, fast claps in corners to see if the energy is depleted. Do louder, larger claps when the energy sounds muffled or dull and needs extra clearing.

2 When the dead energy has lifted, your claps will sound sharp and clear. Clap round each room that needs cleansing, until all the negativity has dispersed.

3 After about 10 minutes clapping, stand still in the room and sense the brighter, clearer energy. The changed and revived atmosphere feels similar to when you have opened all the windows to let in fresh air.

Clapping is a wonderful, simple sound technique.

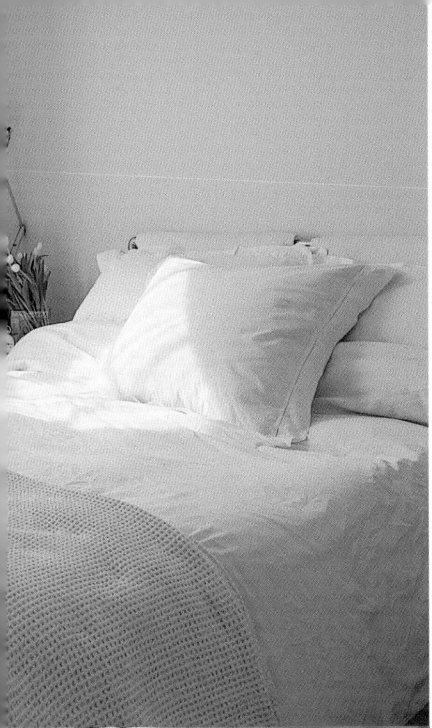

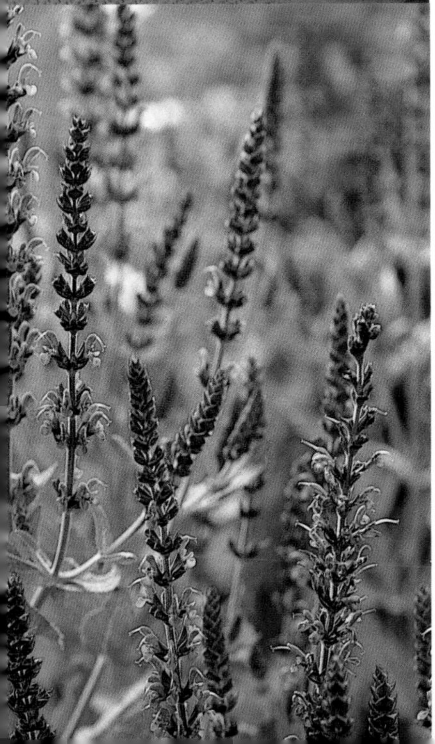

SPACE CLEARING WITH OILS

Essential oils stimulate the olfactory nerves in our nostrils, producing an immediate mood change. Many different oils are available (see page 31), and when heated in vaporizers or added to baths, they stimulate or calm the senses. By misting oils into a room's atmosphere you can immediately produce a vibrant and uplifting or calm and relaxed atmosphere, depending on the oil used. You are also left with a wonderful residual fragrance.

Useful oils

- For an invigorating, refreshing ambience try tangy oils such as mandarin, lime, grapefruit or lemon.
- To calm use lavender, geranium, camomile or frankincense.
- For a deep cleansing of stale energy juniper, clary sage or pine oils are best. (See also page 31 for oils and their effects.)

1 Fill a mister bottle (ideally made of glass, as it keeps better) with water and mix in about 5–6 drops of your chosen oil.

2 Starting at the door, spray your aura first (see page 131) and concentrate on your personal energy clearing. Then mist the scent into the atmosphere as you walk clockwise around the rooms that need purifying for about 10 minutes, spraying more of the oil mist into any dark, unused corners.

3 Stand back and sense how the energy in the room has changed for the better. For a serious uplift, repeat daily for a week.

Energy tip

If you don't have essential oils, spray rooms with spring water for a quick energy uplift and a healthy negative-ion rich environment (a feeling similar to being by the sea).

Drumming is another sound technique that can change the atmosphere in a room in your home for the better, especially if an upset has occurred there the previous evening. The drum's powerful rhythm and vibrations can immediately create a substantial energetic shift in a room, improving the flow of *chi* and the overall atmosphere.

Many Native American Indian tribes used drums, believing that the drumbeat represented the heart of Mother Earth and that drums carried the life spirit. Modern shamans still use the drum to get them in a trance-like state for 'journeying' (a technique similar to visualization) to seek advice from spirit guides. The hypnotic beat actually affects their brain waves putting them in a state of altered consciousness.

rhythmic DRUMMING

Drumming tips

If you do not want to buy your own drum, choose a shamanic drumming CD (available from alternative shops) and play it quite loud to clear your chosen room.

- Drumming is a very absorbing practice, if you drum in the early evening you may find you lose yourself in its hypnotic rhythm and forget all your cares and worries.
- Drumming is particularly effective in clearing emotional energy, when there have been tears or an angry outburst, for example.
- Drumming is the best technique to use if you feel the energy in a room is very congested and uninviting.

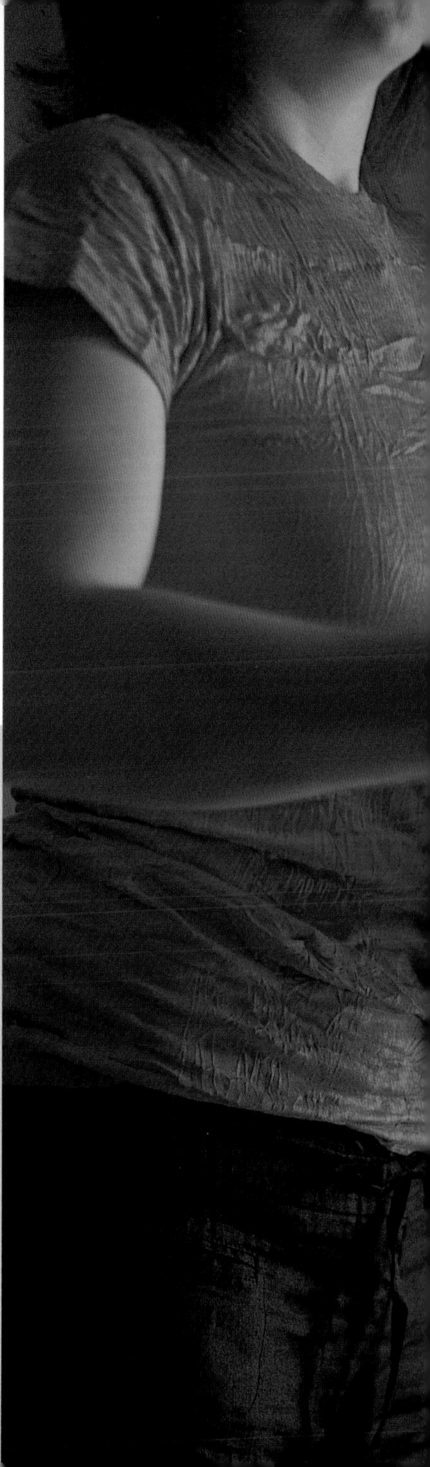

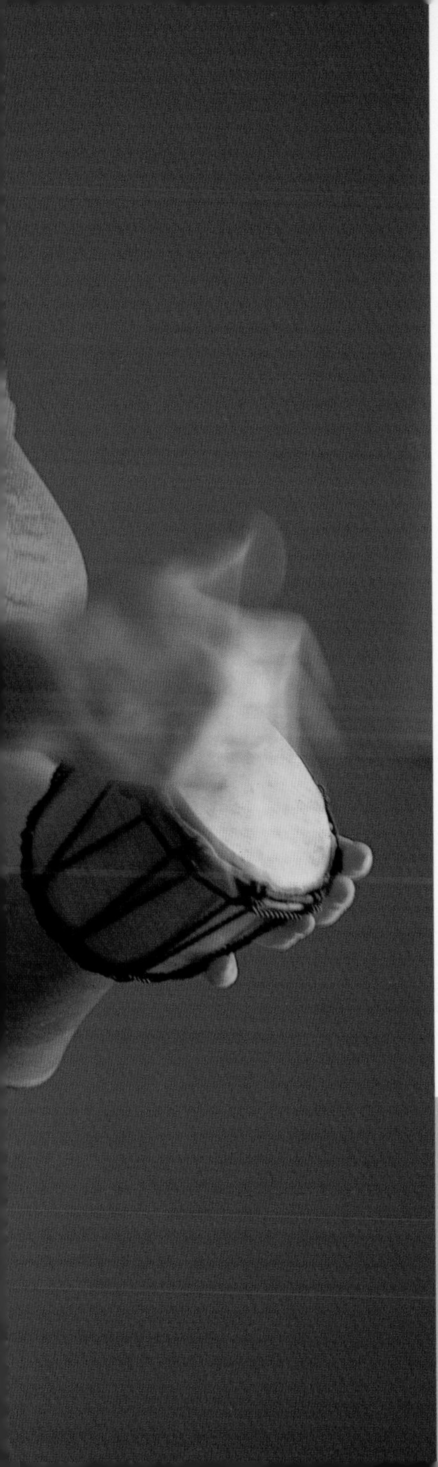

DRUMMING TO INCREASE POSITIVITY

Hand-held circular-frame drums made from animal skin are the most common types used for space clearing but any type can be used. Drum for about 10 minutes or until you feel the energy in the room has changed.

1 Many drums are held between the knees when you are drumming, so if you buy this type sit in the middle of the room to drum. But, if you use a hand-held drum, walk clockwise around the room from the doorway.

2 Hold the drum quietly in your hands for a few minutes to connect to it. Start drumming with a two-beat rhythm, keeping your wrists loose. This is the beat you first heard in the womb: the lubb-dupp of your mother's heartbeat. Let your body relax and your breathing deepen. As you develop the rhythm and strengthen your connection with your drum, instinctively quicken or slow the beat when it seems right. You will naturally start to drum faster when you encounter some stagnant energy.

3 If you are sitting to drum, towards the end of your 10 minutes, stand up and go to drum in each corner of the room to lift sluggish energy there. When you have finished, thank your drum for its help in space clearing the room and store it in a safe place.

The drum's powerful rhythm and vibrations can immediately create a substantial energetic shift in a room.

Toning is a simple purifying technique where you use the power of your own voice to change the energy flow. Anyone can use this technique; you just need to be able to hold one note for an extended time. If you arrive home and feel the atmosphere is flat in your living room, go round the room toning for a short time and notice how quickly you bring the 'buzz' back into the space.

Before your start toning a room, you need to find your own unique sounds. So, relax your body, particularly your face and jaw, and practise with a vowel tone such as 'ahhhh' or a musical scale such as 'doh'. Say it louder and louder and see how it grows from inside your body and reverberates around the room.

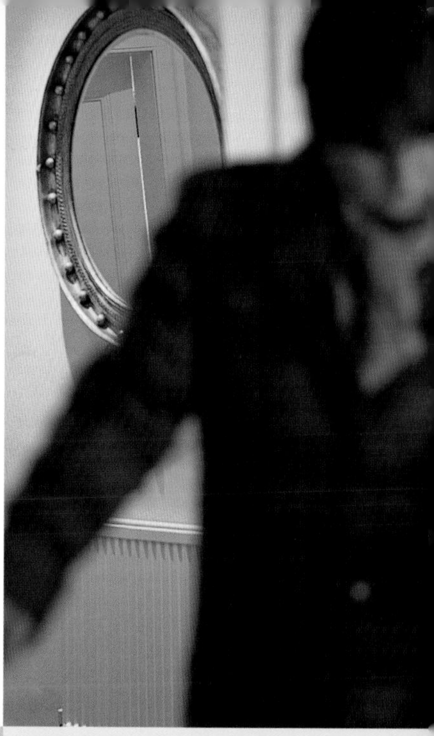

uplifting TONING

PURIFYING A ROOM WITH TONING

Practise with your chosen tone until it is strong and clear. 'Tone' round the room for about 10 minutes until you feel a new vibrancy in its energy.

1 Start toning at the room's doorway. Walk clockwise around the room, increasing the volume as you walk round. Feel the sound you are making and the 'sound' of the room becoming one.

2 Walk round and round in circles, stopping and toning louder in any stagnant areas where you hear the tone changing and becoming more muffled.

After toning for a short time you will notice how quickly you bring the 'buzz' back into the space.

Practise with a vowel tone such as 'ahhhh'.

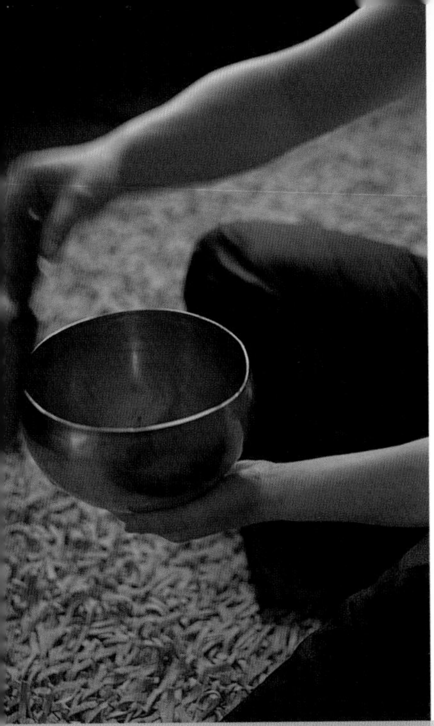

A singing bowl is another potent sound instrument that quickly lifts dull energy in living areas in the early evening. It can also literally 'clear the air' and harmonize the vibrations if you have had people staying, or workmen in.

Authentic singing bowls come from Tibet or Nepal and are made of seven metals, one of which must be gold, silver or platinum. The round bowl represents a vessel that can receive good luck but which can also capture bad energy and transform it into good energy. Stroking the bowl with a mallet produces a wonderful humming, energy field that spirals out from the bowl and back into its centre, dispelling any stagnancies while also pulling in positive vibrations.

USING **a singing bowl**

CHANGING ENERGY WITH A SINGING BOWL

Play your singing bowl for about 10 minutes to clear a room and see how vibrant the atmosphere becomes.

1 Sit in the middle of your room; your bowl needs to be stationary to reach full volume. Connect with your bowl, then place it on the flat palm of one hand and start stroking its outer or inner edge with its wooden mallet.

2 Move the mallet around your bowl firmly, feeling it start to 'sing'. Ask it to clear your inner energies as the beautiful sound whirls around you, purifying the room. Thank your bowl for its help and store wrapped in a silk scarf.

Singing bowl tips

Tap the side of the bowl at a medium pace to create a higher-pitched sound. Singing bowls are handmade and need to be stored carefully. Never allow the bowl to fall on a hard surface as this destroys its clearing power instantly.

One of the strongest ways of cleansing negativity from a room is smudging. It is well known for clearing predecessor energy when you move home and is particularly effective for cleansing a room after a bad argument or if someone has been ill. So use this purifier in the early evening if you feel a substantial change is needed in the energy levels of some of your rooms.

Smudging is an ancient Native American tradition that uses smoke from burning herbal sticks to purify a space. Smudge sticks, which are available from alternative health shops or via mail order, are commonly made from sage, sweetgrass and rosemary (see page 33) because of their strong purification powers, which have been known about since ancient times.

purifying SMUDGING

Feathers are traditionally used to waft the smoke around the room when you are smudging, as they are believed to connect you to the spirit world. If you buy or find a feather to use, always honour it and the bird it came from, and store it in a special place. Some countries restrict taking any part of a bird from the wild, so check your local regulations before taking a feather from outside.

Smudging tips

- When you light your smudge stick, let it burn for a few seconds before blowing out the flame so that it smoulders well, giving out a good smoke trail.
- Open all the windows in a room to let the smoke out after smudging.
- After smudging with a feather, shake it well to discharge its energy.

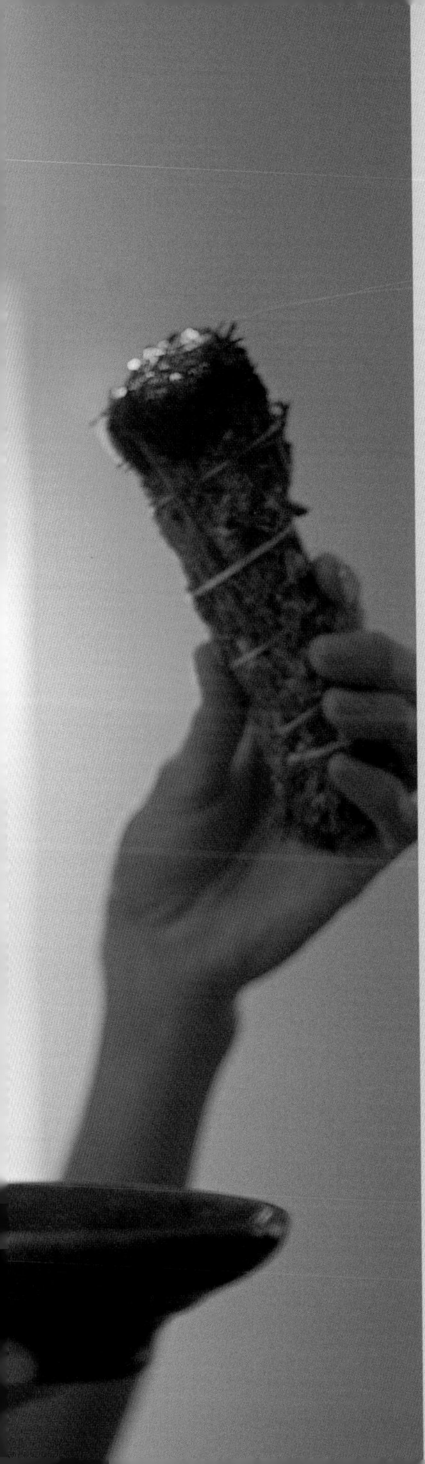

SMUDGING TO SHIFT NEGATIVITY

Smudge the healing smoke around the room for 5–10 minutes to remove any negative vibrations from the space. Use one sage smudge stick and a feather, if you have one, for this exercise.

1. Light your smudge stick and blow out the flame. Hold it over a flameproof dish to catch any embers. When it is smoking well, flick smoke with your hand or your feather all round your body to cleanse your aura (your body's spiritual energy field) of all the 'debris' you have picked up during the day.
2. Now, from the doorway of your room, walk round in a clockwise direction wafting the smoke with a flick of your wrist in front of you, make sure it reaches right into corners where energy tends to stagnate. Focus in your mind on cleansing the room of any specific problem.
3. If you feel any 'sticky' areas in the room where the energy seems different, spend a little longer there wafting the smoke around. When you have finished, put out your smudge stick in an ashtray or dowse it quickly with water under a running tap. Store in a cupboard for using again another time.

Use this purifier in the early evening if you feel a substantial change is needed in the energy levels of some of your rooms.

At the end of a long day your body and mind can be in need of some rejuvenation to enjoy the evening ahead. Yoga (see pages 50–51) is a wonderful exercise discipline that can relieve both mental and physical stress. The moves encourage suppleness and promote better inner energy flow, bringing harmony to the mind, body and spirit.

These easy poses take only 5–10 minutes and help to release accumulated tension in the spine, calm the mind and clear your thoughts and emotions. The Child's pose releases any spinal tension while the knee twists that follow tone and realign the spine. Always wear loose, comfortable clothing for your yoga session (see page 51).

EVENING yoga

KNEE TWISTS

These twists can release any stress still held in your muscles and spine. They also relieve backache and boost the blood supply to the spinal discs and nerves.

1 Lie flat on the floor on your mat with your knees bent and your arms stretched out to the side, palms facing downwards. Make sure your neck and head are in line with your spine.

2 Breathe in and as you breathe out, start to take your knees down to the floor on your right in one fluid movement, letting your stomach muscles facilitate the twist. As your knees reach the floor, turn your head to the left. Only move your pelvis, do not twist your shoulders and chest as this can put strain on your back.

3 Breathe in and bring your knees back to the centre and hold briefly.

4 Now take your legs down to the left and turn your head to the right. Perform the exercise for several minutes or until you feel all your body tension has gone.

CHILD'S POSE

This exercise takes a few minutes and relieves all the spinal tension of the day, soothes your mind and nervous system, and alleviates any stiffness in the neck and shoulders.

1 Kneel on all fours on a mat on the floor. Put your arms out in front of you and breathe in, keeping your head in line with the rest of your spine.

2 Breathe out, pushing your hips all the way back so that you sit

on your heels, your head looks at the floor, your arms go forward and your chest balances on your knees.

3 Move your arms behind you so that they hold your heels, as you breathe in and out deeply. Then move your hands further up your feet. Hold for a few minutes until you feel all your tension releasing. Repeat a few times if your back is very tense.

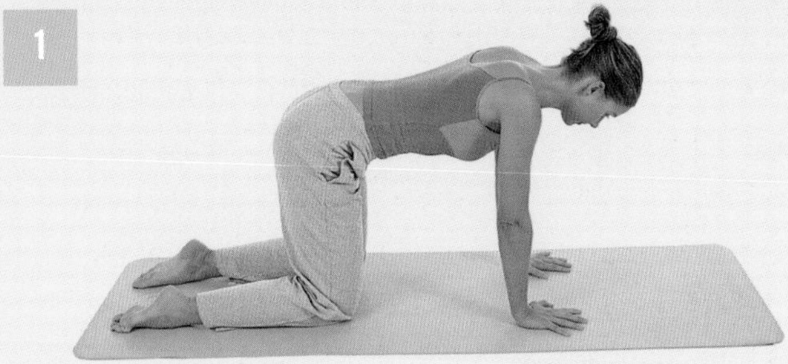
1

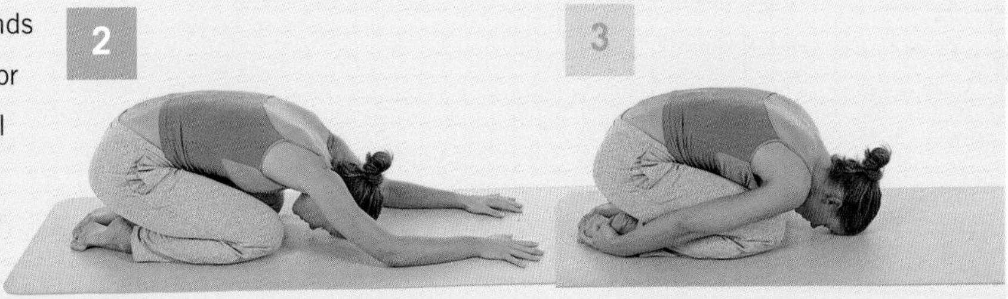
2
3

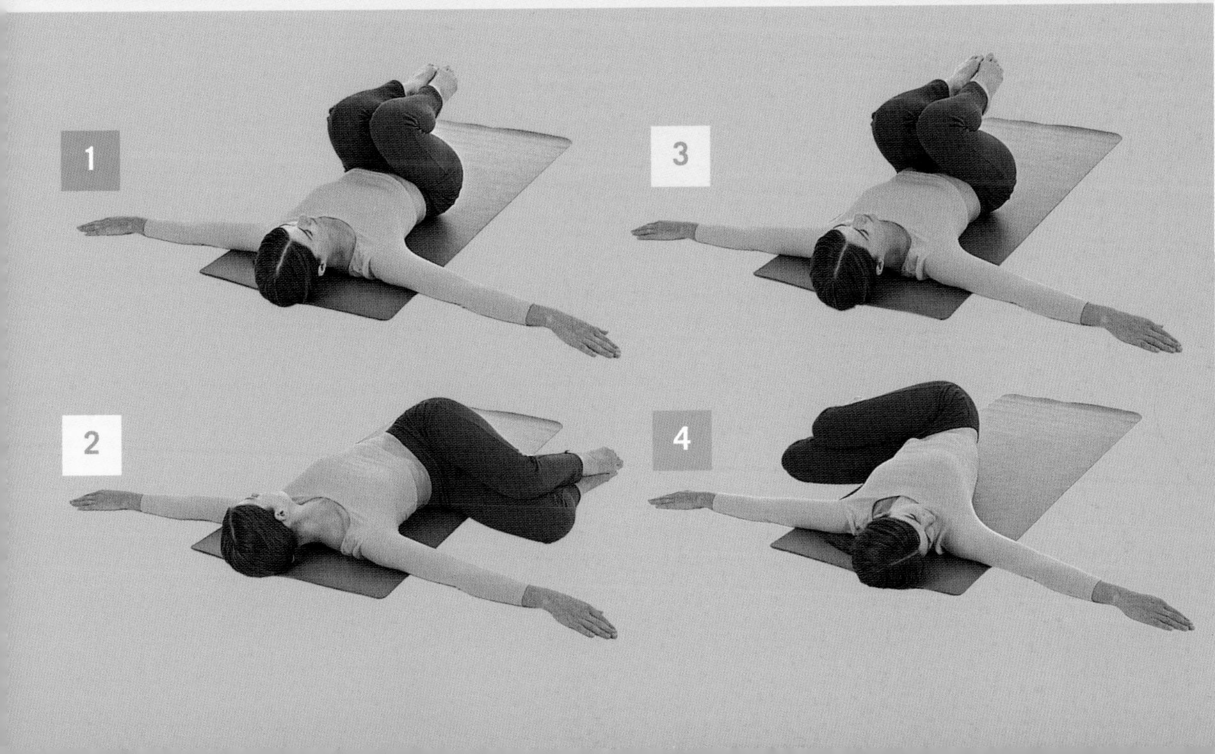
1
3
2
4

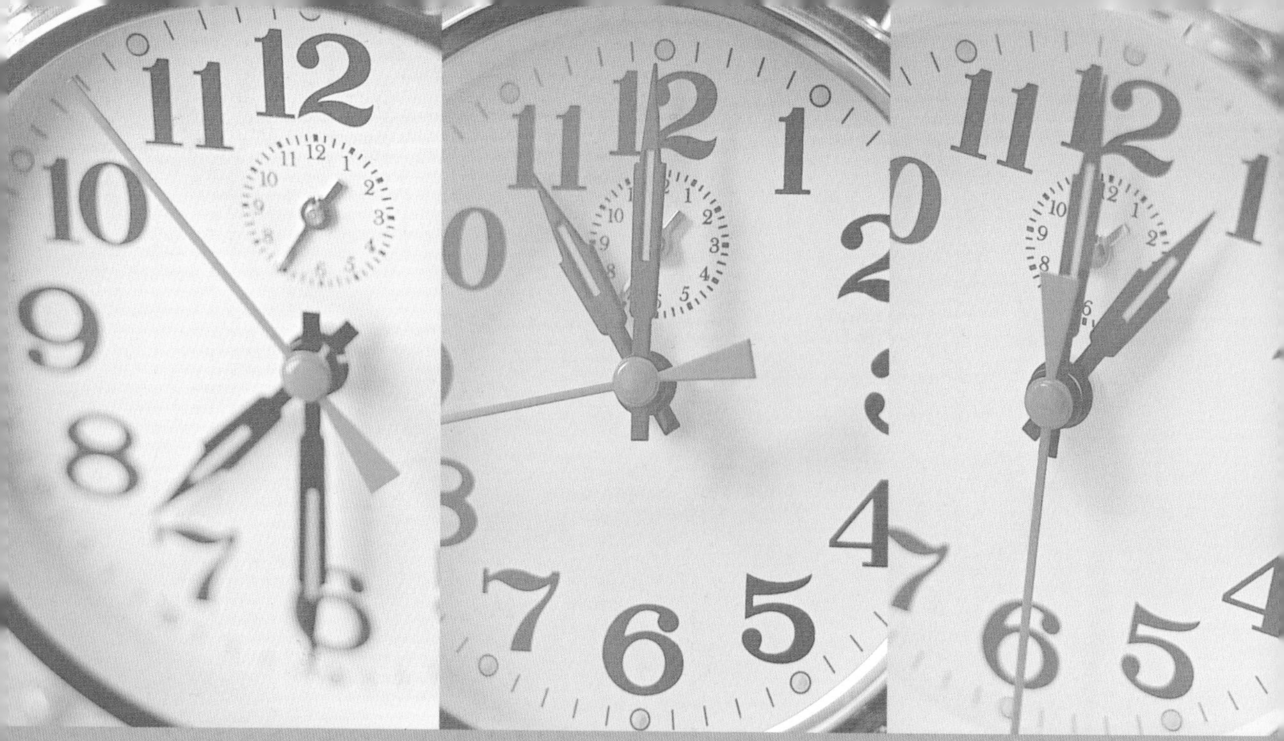

10 Late-night cleansers

Late evening is the time for a major cleanse of your mind, body and spirit so that you are revitalized for the next day.

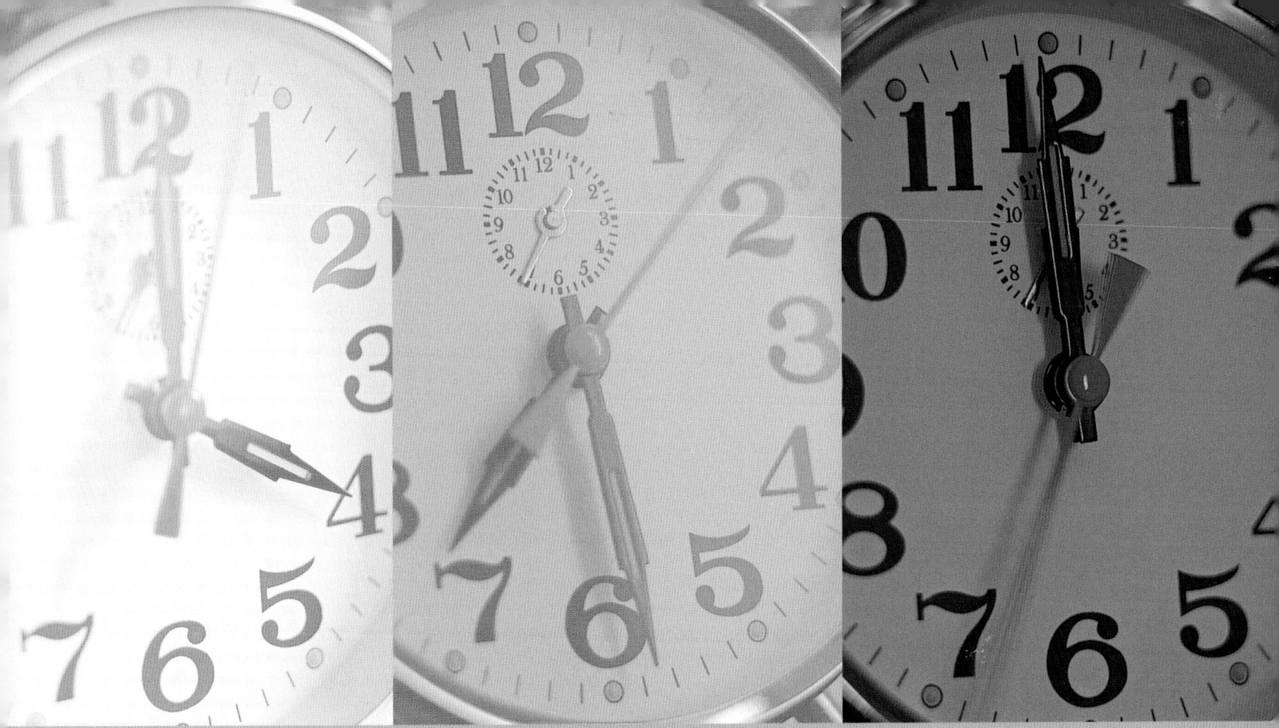

In the early evening you will have started to wind down from the day's activities and be feeling more relaxed. Late evening is the time to work on harmonizing your energy levels and making yourself feel good.

Let the exercises in this section clear your inner and outer realities – purify yourself and your home for true balance, as one is believed to reflect the other. Try releasing the emotions of the day by writing in a special journal, improve how you sleep with a purifying salt ceremony or ask for a solution to a problem by focusing on it just before you fall asleep and dream.

Perform one or more of the energizers that you know will help free you from your daily pressures, to leave you rested and relaxed for a blissful night's sleep.

If you feel upset and raw after a turbulent day, 'journalling' is a positive way of writing down your feelings and emotions about what has happened. You can write whatever you like. Perhaps you are angry with a colleague or you are upset because your childcarer has let you down at short notice. Just let all your thoughts come out.

Journalling is a technique often used by life coaches to get people to connect with their inner selves and find their true path. Too often we are so busy with our external lives, we do not listen to our inner 'voices' or messages. These are our internal thoughts that link us to our future.

If you do some journalling on a daily basis it can help support you emotionally and give you insight to old problems and the bright new future you want to create.

The inner child

Part of our subconscious mind contains our 'inner child' – the part of us that stood still at about four or five years old. This inner child holds our fears and worries and longs to be loved. It also hangs on to childhood beliefs: so if you were told as a child 'You'll never be a success' or 'Earning money is a struggle', your inner child will still believe this, until, that is, it receives different instructions. Journalling gives you a chance to update and rewrite these beliefs.

INSIGHTFUL **journalling**

JOURNALLING TO CLEAR THE DAY

Write down your daily 'ups and downs' in a special journal, or on your computer, to let go of any emotional upsets, and to seek guidance for any changes you need to make.

1 Sit comfortably at a table or at your computer. Close your eyes and take some deep breaths from your diaphragm. As your breathing slows stare ahead of you at a fixed point in the wall and quieten your busy mind.

2 When you are really relaxed, start writing in your journal or on your computer. Write what you are feeling inside, do not worry if it does not seem to make sense or you seem to be ranting. Don't let your ego question what you are doing, just let all your thoughts flow out; you will find a reason for them later.

3 If any old emotion or memory pops into your head as you are writing, put it down, everything comes out for a reason. After about 10 minutes or when you have covered three or four sides of your journal (if writing) stop writing. Sit still for a moment to recover from your emotional release and to disconnect from your subconscious mind before continuing your evening.

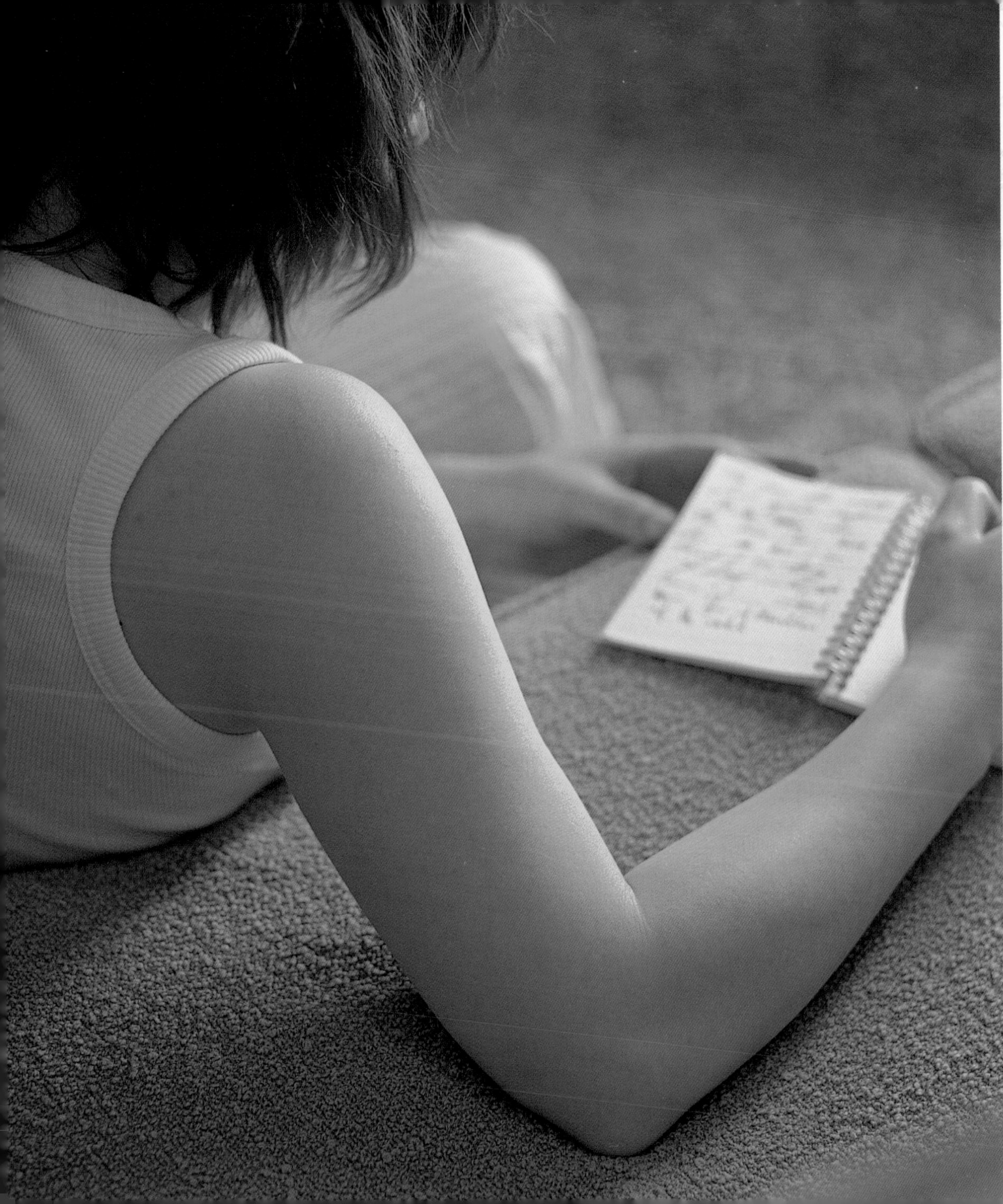

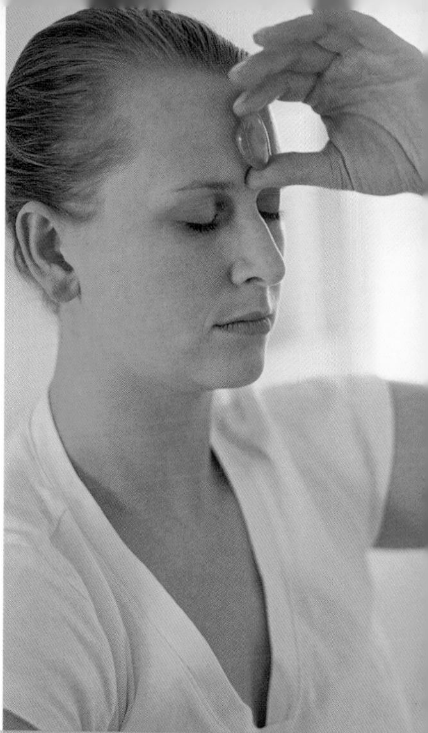

Crystals are powerful healers as they can harmonize any existing distortions in the rhythms of our bodies and *chakras* (see also pages 34–35, 83 and 91). Amethyst is one of the best healing stones to use as it has the ability to absorb the negativity of the day, and can also calm and purify the body and spirit. Furthermore, it can draw out any anger, fears or resentment that have built up in the body.

Use a piece of amethyst in the late evening to physically and psychically cleanse you, so that you are ready to enjoy a calm and peaceful night's sleep.

crystal HEALING

CRYSTAL CEREMONY FOR MIND AND BODY

Hold a cleansed amethyst crystal (see page 34) for about 10 minutes in your lap and then hold briefly to your Third eye chakra (the middle of your forehead) and your Crown chakra (the top of your head) as its powers are strongest there.

1 Sit in a comfortable chair with a straight spine or, if you prefer, sit cross-legged on a mat on the floor. Hold your piece of amethyst quietly in your hands and ask it to take away all the negative debris of the day that is clinging to you both physically and spiritually.

2 Sit quietly and let the crystal do its work for 10 minutes, then place it on your Third eye chakra to boost your intuitive powers. Finally, place it briefly on your Crown chakra to increase spiritual awareness.

Use a piece of amethyst in the late evening to physically and psychically cleanse you.

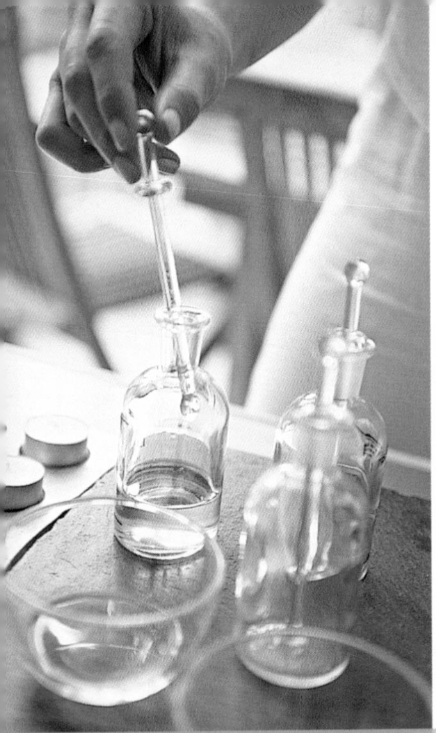

If you did the Protecting your aura with colour exercise on page 42, you will have gained some protection from the upsets of the day. But for a calm evening, mist your aura (your spiritual energy field) with oils to clear away the daily irritations. If you leave your aura with any 'damage', your energy field becomes depleted and you will feel washed out. If this damage is not corrected, you become more vulnerable to illness. You may have also encountered an 'energy vampire' (see pages 21–22) during the day, who has drained precious energy from you. Make this cleansing routine a nightly ritual for your health and wellbeing.

aura CLEANSING

CLEARING YOUR AURA

Spend a few minutes in a quiet space, such as your bedroom, to do this energetic cleansing.

Oils to use

- Juniper and rosemary are powerful and invigorating cleansers.
- Soothing lavender has the ability to bring your energy levels back to normal.

1 Fill a large mister bottle (ideally glass) with water and mix in 5–6 drops of your oil.
2 Hold the bottle for a moment and ask for help to remove any negative vibrations from your aura. Then, stand upright and mist all around your body. Start at the top of your head, spraying down your left side to your feet. Spray down your right side, then down your front and send some to your back.
3 Rest briefly; then breathe in the fragrance of the oil and let it do its work.

Aura tip

You can also cleanse your aura with a smouldering sage smudge stick (see pages 122–123).

Once you have mastered the art of visualization (see also page 82) you can use it in many ways to create positive thoughts or images in your psyche.

With this late-night exercise you can symbolically dispose of any worries from the day in a beautiful garden environment, so that your subconscious mind is convinced they are really gone. When you come to, you will have a lighter heart, a memory of an idyllic place and you'll be able to go to sleep soundly without a care in the world. You can also use this technique to release a past hurt.

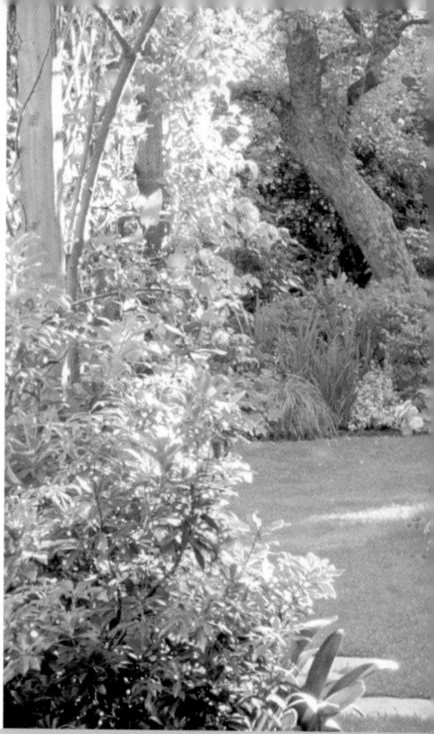

NIGHT visualization

RETREATING TO A SPECIAL PLACE

Spend about 5–10 minutes nightly going to this special place to offload your worries. Either hold or place in your pocket a rose quartz crystal that you offer symbolically at the end of your visit.

1 Sit comfortably in a chair in a warm place. Close your eyes and breathe deeply. Visualize a beautiful summer garden. See the lush green lawns, the neat flower borders full of roses, carnations, chrysanthemums and other blooms. Smell the scented air and watch the flitting butterflies.

2 As you look around, you notice an empty flower border. Dig a small hole here with a nearby trowel. Now, visualize all your worries as a small black box. Place this box in the hole, covering it with soil.

3 Ask Mother Earth to accept your worries and transform them into joy. Leave her a gift of your rose quartz crystal and walk away feeling completely free. Slowly come to and open your eyes.

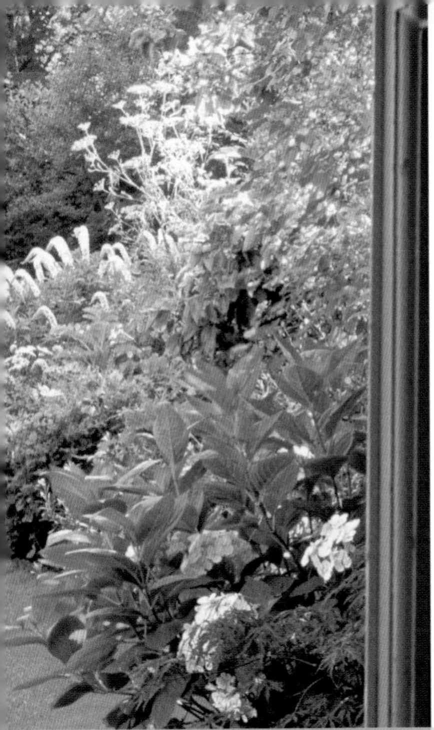

Meditating shortly before you go to bed can calm an overactive mind and allow the brain to shut down properly in preparation for restorative sleep.

When you meditate (see also page 41) your brain activity slows down to the alpha wave level, which induces relaxation and brings healing. It is also a very cleansing process as it allows the subconscious mind to bring to the surface any suppressed information or feelings. If negative thoughts appear, maybe filling you with anger or pain, allow them to pass through you while breathing deeply; don't resist them, let them release through you.

A CLEARING **meditation**

A NIGHT-TIME MEDITATION

Spend 5–10 minutes meditating each night to slow down your mind and to connect with your inner self.

Meditation tip

Burn some soothing rose essential oil (see page 31) in the room while you are meditating.

1. Sit comfortably on an upright chair or cross-legged on a mat on the floor in a warm, dimly lit room. Start breathing deeply from your diaphragm to calm you.
2. Follow the meditation technique on page 41 and feel your mind and body relaxing as all your stresses leave your body. As thoughts or current concerns come to mind just let them float by, knowing that you will resolve any problems.
3. Acknowledge any inner or past emotions that surface, even if you want to resist them, as these deep-rooted hurts need healing and processing so that you can move on. After about 10 minutes, slowly open your eyes, feeling ready for a good night's sleep.

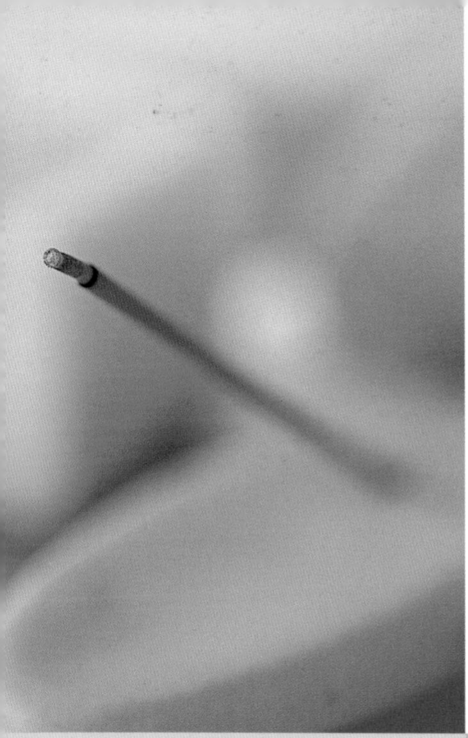

Burning scented incense in the late evening can relax you before going to bed. It can also enhance your mood, especially when combined with a night-time meditation (see page 133).

Incense has its roots with primitive humans, who found that certain burning woods released a pleasant aroma that affected the emotions (see also page 29). In the past, incense was used in many forms: as raw woods, crushed herbs, powders, pastes and even oils. The popular modern form, however, that will purify your living areas is incense sticks and cones; these are usually made from a mixture of fragrant plant oils, tree resins or gums, wood powders, herbs and spices.

purifying INCENSE

Types of incense

There are combustible and non-combustible forms of incense.

The combustible forms – sticks, cones or coils – are the ones mainly used in the home. They contain saltpetre (potassium nitrate), which keeps the incense alight once lit.

Non-combustible incense will not burn by itself so needs to be placed on a combustible source. Incense suppliers sell charcoal blocks containing saltpetre specifically for burning this incense.

BURNING FRAGRANT INCENSE

Incense is not a strong cleanser for heavy energies but it enlivens and balances the ambience of a room to improve your mood.

Incense to use

- Jasmine or myrrh calm and prepare the body for sleep.
- Cloves lift your emotions.
- Vanilla energizes your body but soothes moods.

1. Use a combustible incense fragrance (see right). Place your incense stick or cone firmly in or on its holder.
2. Light the tip. When it is burning well, blow out the flame so that the scented smoke wafts around the room. Sit nearby for a while and let the herbal aroma inspire your senses.

Performing a mantra in the late evening can help to clear your mind of the clutter and negative vibrations of the day and release any stress that you are still holding in your body. Chanting a chosen phrase continuously brings your body and mind into harmony (see page 52). The powerful vibration that the mantra creates corresponds to a specific spiritual energy and a state of consciousness. In time (this varies from person to person), the mantra absorbs and stills all other vibrations until your energy becomes totally in tune with the spiritual state represented by, and contained within, the mantra. Practising a mantra regularly can make you more in tune with yourself.

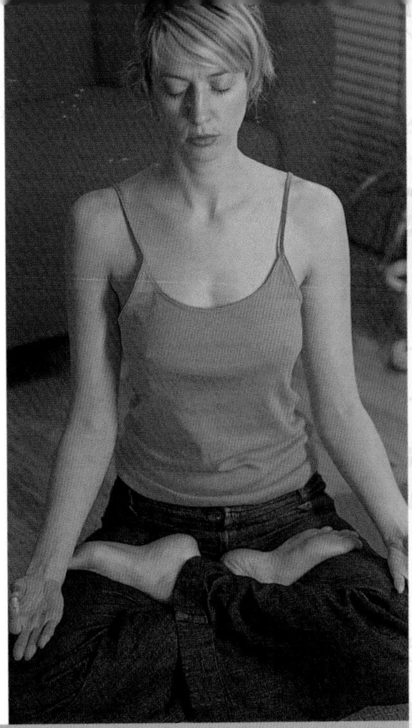

calming MANTRA

MANTRA FOR THE LATE EVENING

Chant this mantra regularly at night to get in touch with your spiritual self.

Chanting a chosen phrase continuously brings your body and mind into harmony.

1 Sit cross-legged with a straight spine and relax your muscles (see page 41). Set any intent to cleanse your worries of the day or to help a current aim in your life.
2 Use the chant '*Om shrim mahalakshmiyei swaha*' (approximate translation: salutations to that feminine energy which bestows all manner of wealth, and for which shrim is the seed). You can also abbreviate the chant to 'shrim', a word that basically means abundance (the more you say it the more abundance you will attract into your life).
3 Close your eyes and chant your phrase in a steady rhythm as you feel yourself relax. Chant for about 10 minutes, then slowly open your eyes and come to, feeling very at peace with yourself.

Your bedroom is a very important space. It is where you are very vulnerable as you rest your spirit for seven to eight hours a night, so the room's atmosphere needs to embrace you and make you feel very secure.

If the ambience is not right, you have been ill, had a disagreement with your partner in bed or if you have cleared out old clutter stored under the bed, the energy (*chi*) in your bedroom will be sticky and stagnant and may be affecting your sleep.

Burning a soothing essential oil combination (see page 31) in your bedroom before sleep will clear the negativity in the air and leave a sensuous scent to encourage a deep and sound sleep.

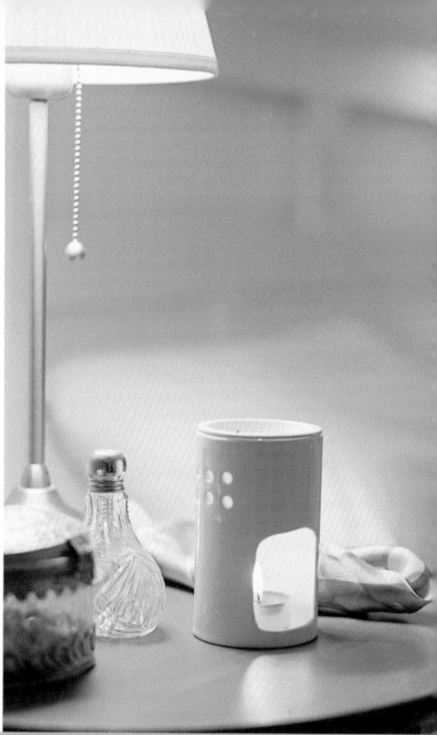

CLEARING **energies**

SPACE CLEARING THE BEDROOM

Burn your chosen essential oils for a short time in your bedroom before you sleep to calm your mind and spirit.

Oil combinations to use

- 4 drops lavender oil, 2 drops geranium oil, 2 drops patchouli oil to calm, balance and inspire.
- 4 drops jasmine oil, 2 drops sandalwood oil, 2 drops ylang ylang to reduce stress and to soothe.

1 Place your oil mix in the bowl of a vaporizer and fill with water; vaporizers are often ceramic and are heated by a lit tea candle underneath the bowl. Alternatively, use an electric burner (see page 56).

2 Leave the oils burning for 10–15 minutes before you go to bed. Breathe in the delicious fragrance as you turn off or blow out the vaporizer's candle and slip into bed.

CLEANSING **worries**

It is important to let go of any final niggling worries that are still circulating in your head before going to bed so that your mind slows down and clears, allowing rejuvenating sleep to come naturally.

Water is a wonderful cleanser and healer (see pages 72–73) that can be used in a waterfall visualization technique to purify and remove all the mental, psychic and physical disturbances that you still carry at the end of the day. The more you immerse yourself in the technique, seeing, feeling and tasting the water, the more effective it is.

Cleansing tip

For extra *chakra* cleansing, see the water changing to their seven colours as it flows down you (see page 49).

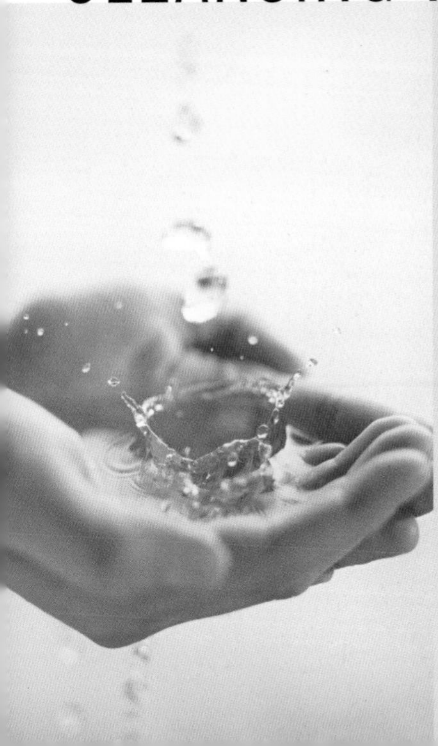

WATERFALL CLEANSER

Practise this technique for 5–10 minutes nightly to disperse any impurities that still cling to you.

1 Stand upright with a straight spine and relaxed shoulders. Close your eyes and see yourself standing beneath a running waterfall with crystal-clear water.

2 Feel the water raining down on your head; taste it as it passes your lips and then flows down your shoulders, over your stomach and down your legs. Sense any physical aches or pains disappearing with the flowing water.

3 Visualize your concerns and any energetic negativity being washed away with the healing water. See the water pooling at your feet and disappearing into the ground to be purified by Mother Earth. Slowly open your eyes and come to.

Salt has amazing purifying properties and since ancient times has been used in ceremonies to cleanse negativity. The large amount of salt used by the early Christians was thought to copy the Romans who liberally sprinkled it to repel evil demons or an unpleasant atmosphere. Its power lies partly in its antiseptic qualities and also in its crystalline structure, which is believed to realign the energy flowing through our bodies and our homes.

If you are experiencing bad dreams, having a difficult time at work or suffering emotional problems that are affecting your quality of sleep, you can use salt in the bedroom to offset these negative influences.

Keeping a bowl of salt by the bed or making a protective circle in the bedroom can make you secure and help you to sleep restfully.

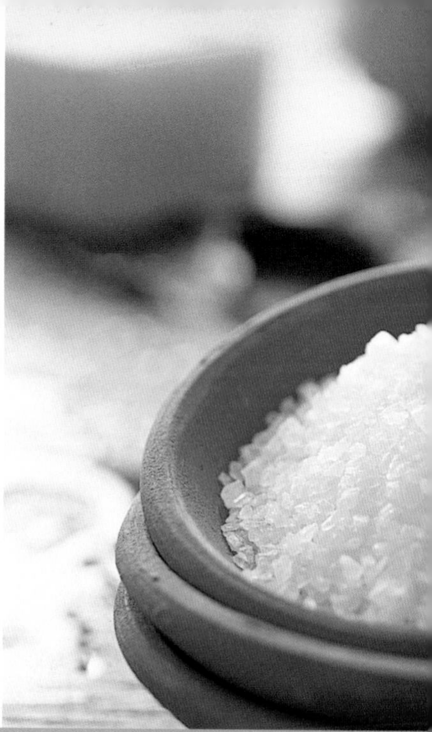

SALT **protection**

Salt has amazing purifying properties and since ancient times has been used in ceremonies to cleanse negativity.

PERFORM A SALT CEREMONY

Using salt in the bedroom can improve troubled sleep and dispel any lingering stagnant energies.

Types of salt to use

Unrefined sea salt (which evokes the power of the sea) and rock salt (which calls upon the power of the earth) are the best types to use for protection or purifying. Keep the salt in a sealed container until you want to use it, because as soon as it is exposed to the atmosphere it will start to absorb any impurities.

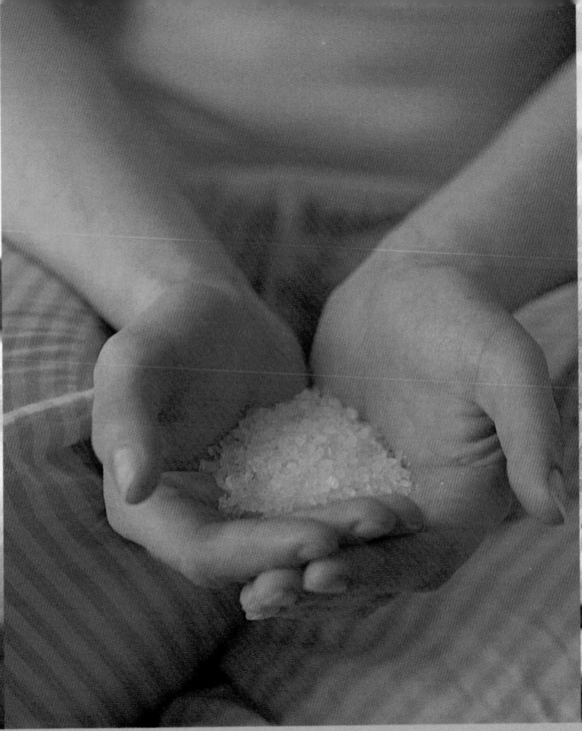

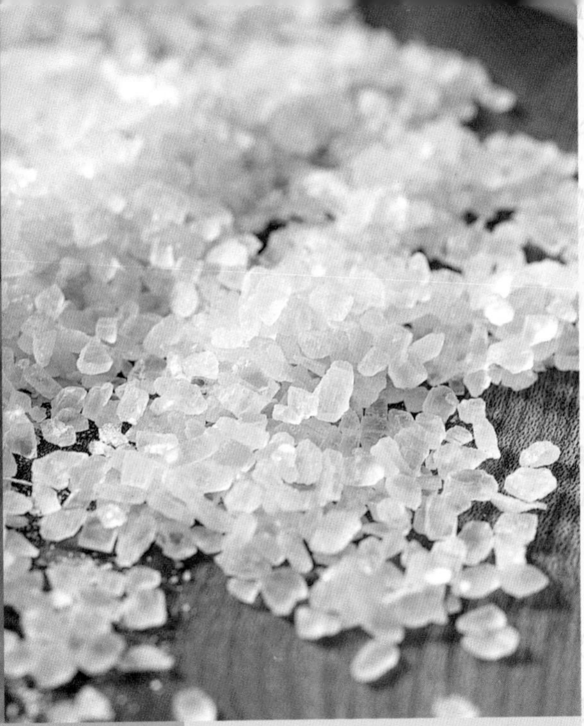

Protective salt circles

A salt circle is an effective protective barrier when you are sleeping; this is the time when you are at your most vulnerable and open to suggestion. The circle will keep out other people's thoughts and feelings. It will also allow your mind to clear out any upsets or irritations that have occurred, so that you can process the events of the day in a healing and balanced way, leaving you to wake refreshed and energized.

1. Take a handful of salt and hold it in your hand for a few seconds asking for help from the universe to improve how you sleep, resolve your troubles and protect you from any negativity.
2. Now, walk round your bed, sprinkling the salt in a large circle to enclose it. If you don't want to make a large circle, place some salt in a bowl next to your bed.
3. Throw away the salt every morning to remove all the impurities of the night and the previous day.

In the same way as you use visualization techniques (see pages 45 and 132) to embed positive thoughts in your subconscious mind or to produce a positive outcome to different dilemmas, you can use your dreams to find solutions to troublesome problems.

Our dreams are often very graphic, detailed and emotional in their content as they relay messages to us from our subconscious. However, dreams use metaphorical symbols that you need to interpret and apply to your current situation.

By holding your dilemma in your mind as you fall asleep, you leave your subconscious mind free to work on the problem and offer a solution in your dreams. In the morning, write down your dream and analyse its meaning.

You can use your dreams to find solutions to troublesome problems.

POSITIVE dreamwork

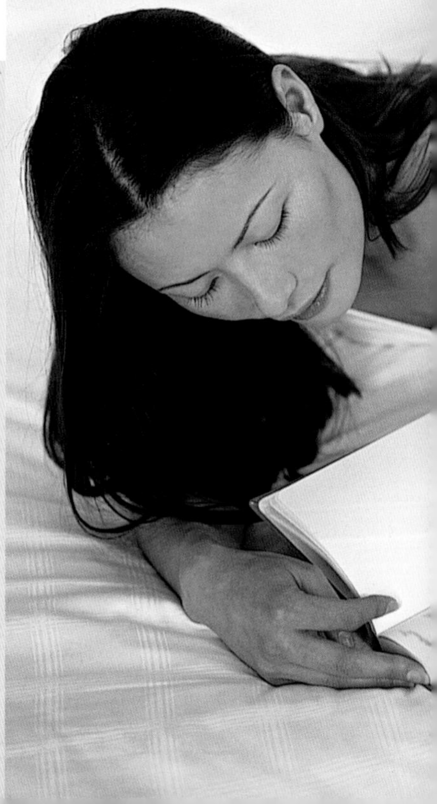

Dream symbols

If you receive symbols in a problem-solving dream that you do not understand, look them up in a dream book. Here are some common ones and their interpretation.

- Fire can signal new beginnings, or if out of control the need to control ambition.
- A hotel often signifies transition in a relationship.
- Funerals can represent the end, or the need to end a phase of life.
- A rainbow suggests good news or forgiveness.
- Snow represents transformation; melting snow shows fears and obstacles disappearing.
- Trains indicate you are receiving help on your journey.

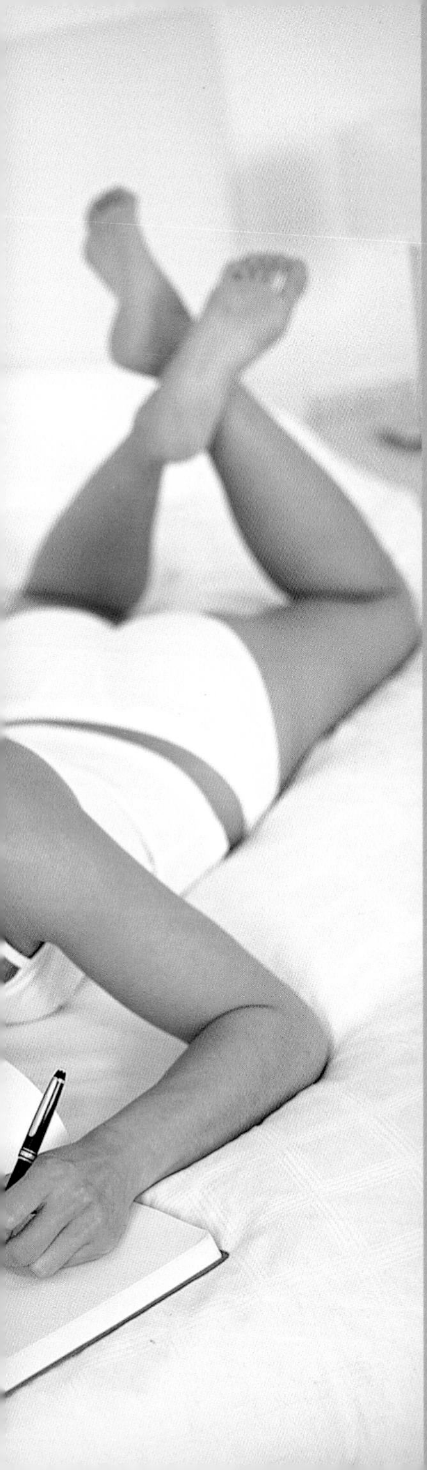

DREAMING TO SOLVE PROBLEMS

Focus on the problem you want answered in your dreams for some minutes before going to sleep. Keep a pen and pad by your bed to write down your dream when you wake.

1 Sit up in bed, breathe deeply for a few minutes to relax you, then start to focus on the problem you want resolved. If it is a problem with your work, picture your desk or work environment, or if it is a relationship problem with your partner, lock on to his or her image.

2 Say what your problem is and what is worrying you about it. Ask for a clear-cut answer to your situation. Keep the imagery in your head as you fall asleep.

3 In the morning, write down the details of your dream in the first few minutes when you wake up as your brain loses the content very quickly. The answer may come in clear images or in symbols for you to interpret. Repeat the exercise for several nights if nothing is forthcoming on the first night.

Dream tip

Sometimes a solution to a difficult problem will be in your mind when you wake up – your subconscious will have found the answer for you while you were sleeping.

INDEX

acupressure 12, 17
early morning 53
mid-morning 68–9
pressure points 68
acupuncture 16, 64
aerobic exercise 10
affirmations *see* self-affirmations
alcohol 19
alternate nostril breathing 112–13
amethyst crystals 34, 35, 130
anger, letting go of 62–3
aquamarine crystals 35, 83
aromatherapy *see* essential oils
aromatic showers 43
astra/emotional body 15
aura 14–15, 34
clearing 131
and colour therapy 48
protecting 42
spraying 117
aventurine crystals 61
Ayurvedic (Indian) medicine 11, 14

Bach flower remedies 28–9, 59
stress and anger 64
barefoot walk on grass 74–5
bathing, candlelight 108–9
bedrooms, space clearing 136
blood-sugar levels 6, 9, 26
books, sorting and storing 95
bosses, relationships with 22
breathing exercises 17, 26
alternate nostril breathing 112–13
breathing out stress 60–1
centering 92
cleansing breathing 80
colour breathing energizer 49
early morning 40
Bush flower remedies 28–9, 82
emotional rebalancing 67
stress and anger 64

caffeine 19–20
candlelight bathing 108–9
carbohydrates, and energy 9
centering 92
chakras 11, 14, 15, 34
and alternate nostril breathing 112
and anger 62
cleansing 137
and colour 15, 42, 48, 49, 98, 99
and crystals 34, 83, 91, 130
and head massage 101
chi 11, 53, 57, 116
and drumming 118
and water 73
chi kung/qigong 17, 78–9
child's pose 124–5
children 21–2
chromotherapy (colour therapy) 48
cigarette smoking 20
citrus oils 43
clapping 116
classes, dancing 115
cleansing breathing 80
clutter, clearing out 94–5
cobra posture 51
colleagues, relationships with 22
colour
auras 14, 42
chakras 15, 42, 48, 49, 98, 99
dowsing for 99
therapy 48–9, 98
computers, clearing 96
crystals 28, 34–5, 42
anger remedies 64
cleansing 34
and computers 96
dowsing for colour 99
healing 83, 91, 130
selecting 34
and stress relief 61, 64
and tree hugging 76
uses and qualities 35

dancing 114–15
desk space, clearing 95
diet, and energy levels 8, 9, 19
Dog rose flower essence 29, 67
dowsing for colour 99
'draining' friendships 22
dreaming 140–1
drinks
alcoholic 19
caffeine-free 20
drumming 118–19

early morning 38–53
absorbing colour energy 48–9
acupressure 53
aromatic showers 43
aura refreshment 42
breathing exercises 40
energy levels 39
fresh air 44
meditation 41
new day affirmation 47
tea 46
visualization 45
yoga 38, 50–1
earth energy 74–5
Eastern view of energy 6, 11–15
Elm Bach flower remedy 28, 59
emotional energy drains 21–2
energizer larder 27–25
crystals 28, 34–5
essential oils 28, 30–1
flower remedies 28–9
herbs and spices 32–3
incense 29
smudge sticks 29
energy blocks, removing 66
energy channels 7
energy levels 6, 8, 9
early morning 39
mid-morning 54
energy zappers 18–23
emotional 21–2
physical 18–19
questionnaire 25, 36
spiritual 23
energy-related therapies 16–17
essential oils 28, 30–1
aura cleansing 131
burners 56
candlelight bathing 108–9
hand massage 84
mid-morning stress relief 55, 56–7
neck and shoulder massage 110
room purifying with 97, 117, 136
stimulating 43
stress and anger remedies 64
etheric body 14–15
evening refreshers 106–25
breathing exercises 112–13
candlelight bathing 108–9
dancing 114–15
neck and shoulder massage 110
neck and shoulder stretching 111
room purifying 116, 116–23
yoga 124–5
exercises 10, 19
aerobic 10
chi kung/qigong 17, 78–9
instant energizers 27
muscle-releasing 140–5

stretching 10, 111
weight-bearing 10
see also breathing exercises; visualization
eyes 88–9

family–life balance 18
feathers, and smudging 122, 123
feet *see* reflexology
feng shui 16, 58, 73, 91, 94
flower remedies 28–9
food
absorbing colour from 48
and energy 8, 9
healthy snacks 10
right balance of 9
free-flowing energy 66–7
fresh air 44
friends 22

Gaia theory 75
Ghadiali, Dinshah P. 48
ginger and lemon tea 46
gingko biloba 58
ginseng and honey tea 90
grass, barefoot walk on 74–5
green tea 90

hand massage 84
see also reflexology
head massage 85, 100–1
headaches 85, 100
lavender oil for 57
healthy snacks 10
herbal smudge sticks 29, 83
herbal teas 46, 55, 58
herbs 32–3
hypnosis 20

incense 29, 134
Indian (Ayurvedic) medicine 11, 14
Indian-type head massage 85
inner child 128
ionizers 44

journalling 23, 128–9
jump-starting your energy flow 17

knee twists 124–5
kung fu 78

late-night cleansers 126–41
aura cleansing 131
calming mantra 135
crystal ceremony 130
dreaming 140–1
incense burning 134
journalling 128–9
meditation 133
salt protection 138–9
space clearing the bedroom 136
visualization 132
waterfall cleanser 137
lavender oil 28, 30, 31, 57, 108, 110
for headaches 57
lemon, ginger and lemon tea 46
lemon balm 58
lifestyle
and energy levels 6, 18
sedentary 19
loving relationships 21
lunchtime revivers 70–85
barefoot walk on grass 74–5
chi kung/qigong 17, 78–9
cleansing breathing 80
crystal clearing 83
embracing tree energy 76–7
hand massage 84
singing 81
visualization 82
water cleansing 72–3

mandala, using for meditation 41
mantras 26, 110
choosing a mantra 52
late evening 135
morning 52
marjoram oil 84
massage 17
hands 84
head 85, 100–1
neck and shoulders 110
meditation 17, 23
and chi kung 78
early morning 41, 52
mantras 26, 52
mini 112
night-time 133
using a *mandala* 41
water meditation 72–3
mental body 15
mental clarity, crystal healing for 83
meridians 11, 12–13, 16
and acupressure 69
mid-afternoon boosters 86–105
affirmation 93
centering 92
clearing out clutter 94–5
clearing your computer 96
colour healing 98–9
crystal power 91
head massage 100–1
muscle-releasing technique 104–5
neck rolls 89
palming 88
purifying a work space 87
reflexology 102–3
tea tonic 90
mid-morning stress relief 54–69
acupressure 68–9
breathing out stress 60–1
energy levels 55
essential oils 56–7
free-flowing energy 66–7
herbal teas 55, 58
letting go of anger 62–3
mirror work 59
reflexology 64–5
removing energy blocks 66
scanning your energy field 67
mini meditation 112
mirrors 58
morning people 26
Mother Earth 74, 75, 132, 137
muscle-releasing exercises 104–5

nadis 14, 50
neck
massage 110
rolls 89
stretching 111
new day affirmation 47
nicotine 20
night owls 26

older relatives 22
opening windows 44

palming 88
peppermint tea 58
positive affirmations *see* self-affirmations
prana 11, 14, 50
problem-solving by dreaming 141
protein, and energy 9

qigong/chi kung 17, 78–9
quartz crystals 91
questionnaire, daily energy drains 25

reflexology 16, 26, 102–3
and acupressure 53
mid-morning stress relief 64–5
releasing RSI-type symptoms 103
relief for stressed stomach 102
techniques 65
tips 102
Reich, Wilhelm 100
reiki 17
relationships, emotional energy
drains 21–2
relaxation
muscle-releasing technique 104–5
quick technique 105
room purifying 116–23
bedrooms 136
clapping 116
drumming 118–19
essential oils 117
salt protection 138–9
singing bowls 121
smudging 122–3
toning 120
work spaces 94–5
rose oil 31, 133
rose quartz crystals 34, 35, 96
rosemary oil 31, 56, 93, 97

rosemary tea 46
RSI (repetitive strain injury) 102, 103

SAD (seasonal affective disorder) 48
sage tea 46
salt protection 138–9
seasonal affective disorder (SAD) 48
sedentary lifestyles 19
self-affirmations 26
afternoon 91
new day 47
shamanic healing 76
shiatsu 16, 53
shoulders
massage 110
relaxing 88
shower of light 79
showers, aromatic 43
singing 81, 114
singing bowls 121
sleep 10
smudge sticks 29, 83, 122, 123, 131
smudging 122–3
snacks, healthy 10
space clearing *see* room purifying
spices 32–3
spiritual energy centres *see chakras*
spiritual energy drains 23, 26
stimulants 19–20, 26
stomach, relief for stressed 102
storage 94–5
stress 19, 60–1
see also mid-morning stress relief
stretching exercises 10
neck and shoulders 111

t'ai chi 78
tea
ginger and lemon 46
ginseng and honey 90
green 90
peppermint 58
rosemary 46
sage 46
tea tree oil 30, 31, 43
toning 120
tourmaline crystals 61
toxins 17, 19–20
traditional Chinese medicine 11, 17
tree posture 51
trees, embracing tree energy 76–7

visualization 17, 26, 55
a bright new day 45
colour visualization 98
creating bliss 82
mini meditation 112
night-time 132
removing energy blocks 66
scanning your energy field 67
waterfall cleanser 137

walking, barefoot walk on grass 74–5
warm-up exercises, chi kung 78
water features 73
water meditation 72–3
waterfall cleanser 137
weight-bearing exercise 10
Western concept of energy 6, 9–11
windows, opening 44
work
clearing out work space 94–5
relationships at 22
work–life balance 18
writing, journalling 23, 128–9

yin and yang meridians 12
yoga 17
child's pose 124–5
the cobra 50
early morning 38, 50–1
evening 124–5
knee twists 124–5
nadis 14, 50
the tree 51

zone therapy *see* reflexology

ABOUT THE AUTHOR
Mary Lambert is a feng shui consultant and reiki practitioner based in London and can be contacted for consultations or reiki healing on: maryliz.lambert@virgin.net

AUTHOR ACKNOWLEDGEMENTS
I would like to thank Sarah Tomley, Jessica Cowie and the editorial and design team at Hamlyn for their creative input and efficient organization in running this project. A big thanks to my sister Gill for as ever giving me support and encouragement, and also to my tennis crowd and friends Claire, Anna, Lynne, Liz, Steve, and Sarah who helped keep me smiling during the solitary writing process.

Executive Editor Sarah Tomley
Project Editor Jessica Cowie
Executive Art Editor Rozelle Bentheim
Designer Simon Wilder
Picture Research Jennifer Veall
Senior Production Controller Martin Croshaw

ACKNOWLEDGEMENTS

PICTURE CREDITS Special Photography: Unit Photographic
Corbis UK Ltd/SIE Productions 131 top left **Garden Picture Library**/Juliette Wade 132–133 top **Getty Images**/1/4 66 top right/Simon Battensby 36–37/Color Day Productions 23/Robert Daly 59 bottom/Kevin Fitzgerald 47 bottom/Larry Dale Gordon 8/Diana Healey 92 top right/Alberto Incrocci 26 bottom right/Frank Krahmer 82 top right/Ghislain & Marie David de Lossy 15 centre, 49 left, 98 top right/Jens Lucking 76–77 centre/Laurence Monneret 80 top right/Victoria Pearson 75 left/Andre Perlstein 22 bottom/Andreas Pollock 104–105 top/Farmhouse Productions 18/Trinette Reed 48 top left/David Seed Photography 137 bottom left/Steve Taylor 44 top right **Octopus Publishing Group Limited**/2–3 top/Colin Bowling 90 bottom right/Gus Filgate 32 right/Jerry Harpur 117 bottom left/William Lingwood 30 left, 46 bottom, 58 bottom right/David Loftus 32 left, 32 centre/Neil Mersh 30 right/Peter Pugh-Cook 21 right, 40 top, 40 bottom, 50, 51 top centre, 51 top left, 51 centre left, 51 centre right, 51 bottom right, 51 bottom left, 61 left, 61 right, 61 centre, 67 left, 89 left, 89 right, 89 centre left, 89 centre right, 112 right, 113 left, 113 right, 125 top, 125 bottom/ William Reavell 20 left, 20 right, 56 centre right, 139 top right/Russell Sadur 42 bottom right, 62–63 top, 140–141 centre/Gareth Sambidge 110/Ian Wallace 10 bottom right, 12 right, 13 left, 13 right, 17 top right, 24, 30 centre, 41 top, 43 bottom left, 53 centre left, 53 top right, 53 bottom left, 57 bottom left, 64 right, 64 centre left, 64 bottom left, 65 left, 65 right, 68 left, 68 right, 69 left, 69 right, 69 centre, 84 bottom right, 102 centre right, 102 bottom right, 103 top, 103 centre, 134 top right, 138 top right/Jacqui Wornell 78 bottom right, 78 bottom centre, 79 left, 79 right, 79 centre left, 79 centre, 79 centre right, 85 left, 85 right, 85 centre, 88, 100 top, 100 bottom, 101 top, 101 bottom, 111 left, 111 right/Polly Wreford 94–95 centre **The Interior Archive**/Edina van der Wyck/Designer: Atlanta Bartlett 116–117 top **Rubberball Productions**/27, 72–73 top **Science Photo Library**/Francoise Sauze 14 right